Evidence-based Dermatology

Evidence-based Dermatology

Edited by

Hywel Williams
Centre of Evidence-Based Dermatology, University of Nottingham, UK

Associate editors

Michael Bigby
Department of Dermatology, Harvard Medical School and Beth Israel Deaconess Medical Centre, Boston, USA

Thomas Diepgen
University Hospital, Heidelberg, Germany

Andrew Herxheimer
Cochrane Skin Group, UK

Luigi Naldi
Department of Dermatology, Ospedali Riuniti, Bergamo, Italy

Berthold Rzany
Centre for Evidence-based Medicine in Dermatology, Charité University Hospital, Humboldt University, Berlin, Germany

BMJ
Books

First published in 2003
by BMJ Books, BMA House, Tavistock Square,
London WC1H 9JR

www.bmjbooks.com

British Library Cataloguing in Publication Data

A catalogue record for this book is available from the British Library

ISBN 0 7279 14421

Typeset by SIVA Math Setters, Chennai, India
Printed and bound in Malaysia by Times Offset

Contents

Contributors

Damiano Abeni
Clinical Epidemiology Unit, Instituto Dermopatico dell'Immacolata (IDI–IRCCS), Rome, Italy

Fiona Bath
Centre for Evidenced-based Dermatology, Queen's Medical Centre, Nottingham, UK

Michael Bigby
Department of Dermatology, Harvard Medical School and Beth Israel Deaconess Medical Center, Boston, USA

Robyn Bluhm
Mediprobe Laboratories, London, Ontario, Canada

Ian F Burgess
Insect R&D Limited, Cambridge, UK

Jeffrey P Callen
Professor of Medicine (Dermatology) and Chief, Division of Dermatology, University of Louisville School of Medicine, Louisville, Kentucky, USA

Norma Cameli
San Gallicano Dermatological Institute, Rome, Italy

Robert JG Chalmers
Dermatology Centre, University of Manchester School of Medicine, Manchester, UK

Carolyn Charman
Specialist Registrar in Dermatology, Queen's Medical Centre NHS Trust, Nottingham, UK

Suephy C Chen
Emory University, Atlanta, USA

Olivier Chosidow
Pitié-Salpétrière Hospital, Paris, France

Pieter-Jan Coenraads
Dermatology Department, University Medical Center, Groningen, The Netherlands

A Marco van Coevorden
Dermatology Department, University Medical Center, Groningen, The Netherlands

Elizabeth A Cooper
Mediprobe Laboratories, London, Ontario, Canada

Fay Crawford
Dental Health Services Research Unit, Dundee University, Dundee, Scotland

Bernard Cribier
University Hospital Strasbourg, Strasbourg, France

Thomas Crosby
Velindre Hospital, Cardiff, Wales

Luis Gabriel Cuervo-Amore
BMJ Publishing Group, Clinical Evidence, BMA House, London, UK

Robert S Dawe
Photobiology Unit, Department of Dermatology, Ninewells Hospital and Medical School, Dundee, Scotland

Finola Delamere
Trials Search Coordinator, Cochrane Skin Group, Department of Dermatology, University Hospital, Queen's Medical Centre, Nottingham, UK

Thomas Diepgen
Department of Social Medicine, Occupational and Environmental Dermatology, University Hospital Heidelberg, Heidelberg, Germany

Ciara S Dodd
School of Bioscience, Cardiff University, Cardiff, Wales

Peter von den Driesch
University Hospital Eppendorf, Hamburg, Germany

Joseph C English III
University of Virginia, Department of Dermatology, USA

James Ferguson
Photobiology Unit, Department of Dermatology, Ninewells Hospital and Medical School, Dundee, Scotland

Sarah E Garner
Health Technology Analyst, National Institute for Clinical Excellence and Senior Research Fellow, Department of Public Health Sciences, St George's Hospital Medical School, London, UK

Pierre Dominique Ghislain
Department of Dermatology, Saint-Luc University Clinics, Brussels, Belgium

Sam Gibbs
Department of Dermatology, Ipswich Hospital NHS Trust, Ipswich, UK

Urbà González
Department of Dermatology, Clínica Plató, Barcelona, Spain

Aditya K Gupta
Division of Dermatology, Department of Medicine, Sunnybrook and Women's College Health Sciences Center (Sunnybrook site), University of Toronto and Mediprobe Laboratories, London, Ontario, Canada

Anne Hawk
Department of Dermatology, University of Virginia, USA

Roderick J Hay
Dean, Faculty of Medicine and Health Sciences, Queen's University, Belfast, Whitla Medical Building, Belfast, Northern Ireland, UK

Andrew Herxheimer
Cochrane Skin Group, London, UK

Susan Jessop
Division of Dermatology, Groote Schuur Hospital and University of Cape Town, Cape Town, South Africa

Jonathan Kantor
Department of Dermatology, University of Pennsylvania School of Medicine, Philadelphia, USA

Nonhlanhla Khumalo
Department of Dermatology, Groote Schuur Hospital, Cape Town, South Africa

Gudula Kirtschig
Department of Dermatology, Vrije Universiteit, Acadmisch Zickenhuis, Amsterdam, The Netherlands

Sander Koning
Department of General Practice, Erasmus MC-University Medical Center, Rotterdam, The Netherlands

Michael Kulig
Institute of Social Medicine, Epidemiology and Health Economics, Charité Hospital, Humboldt University of Berlin, Berlin, Germany

Laurence Le Cleach
Department of Dermatology, Sud Francilien Hospital, Corbeil, France

Tina Leonard
Review Group Coordinator, Cochrane Skin Group, Department of Dermatology, University Hospital, Queen's Medical Centre, Nottingham, UK

Nanette J Liégeois
Department of Dermatology, Lahey Clinic and Harvard Medical School, Burlington, USA

Imogen Locke
Meyerstein Institute of Oncology, Middlesex Hospital, London, UK

David J Margolis
Department of Dermatology and Department of Biostatistics and Epidemiology, University of Pennsylvania School of Medicine, Philadelphia, USA

Cinzia Masini
Clinical Epidemiology Unit, Instituto Dermopatico dell'Immaculata (IDI–IRCCS), Rome, Italy

Jacqueline Müller-Nordhorn
Institute of Social Medicine, Epidemiology and Health Economics, Charité Hospital, Humboldt University of Berlin, Berlin, Germany

Dédée Murrell
Consultant Dermatologist, St George's Hospital, Sydney, Australia

Luigi Naldi
Department of Dermatology, Ospedali Riuniti, Bergamo, Italy

Suzanne Olbricht
Department of Dermatology, Lahey Clinic and Harvard Medical School, Burlington, USA

William Perkins
Department of Dermatology, Queen's Medical Centre, Nottingham, UK

Mauro Picardo
San Gallicano Dermatological Institute, Rome, Italy

Peterson Pierre
Private practice, Agoura Hills, California, USA

Jane Ravenscroft
Specialist Registrar in Dermatology, Queen's Medical Centre NHS Trust, Nottingham, UK

Alfredo Rebora
Clinica Dermatologica, Universita di Genova, Italy

Mónica Rengifo-Pardo
London, UK

Dafydd Roberts
Consultant Dermatologist, Singleton Hospital, Swansea, Wales

Maria Roest
Department of Dermatology, The Churchill Hospital, Headington, Oxford, UK

J Claude Roujeau
Department of Dermatology, Henri Mondor Hospital, University Paris XII, Créteie, France

Jennifer Ryder
Mediprobe Laboratories, London, Ontario, Canada

Berthold Rzany
Centre for Evidence-based Medicine in Dermatology, Charité University Hospital, Humboldt University, Berlin, Germany

Asad Salim
Dermatology Department, North Staffordshire Hospital, Stoke on Trent, UK

Catherine E Scarff
University of Melbourne Department of Dermatology, St Vincent's Hospital, Fitzroy and Skin and Cancer Foundation of Victoria, Australia

Torsten Schäfer
Institute of Social Medicine, Medical University Lübeck, Germany

Rod Sinclair
University of Melbourne Department of Dermatology, St Vincent's Hospital, Fitzroy and Skin and Cancer Foundation of Victoria, Australia

Dominic Smethurst
Lecturer, Centre of Evidence-Based Medicine, University of Nottingham, Queen's Medical Centre NHS Trust, Nottingham, UK

Seaver L Soon
Department of Dermatology, Emory University, Atlanta, USA

Brian R Sperber
Resident, Department of Dermatology, University of Iowa, Iowa, USA

Daniel M Spinner
German Cochrane Centre, Affiliated medical member, University Hospital Freiburg, Institute of Medical Biometry and Medical Informatics, Freiburg, Germany

Margaret Spittle
Meyerstein Institute of Oncology, Middlesex Hospital, London, UK

Jacqueline E Swan
Mediprobe Laboratories, London, Ontario, Canada

Lisette WA van Suijlekom-Smit
Department of Pediatrics, Erasmus MC-University Medical Center, Rotterdam, The Netherlands

Kim Thomas
Clinical Trials Manager, Centre of Evidence-Based Dermatology, University of Nottingham, University Hospital, Queen's Medical Centre NHS Trust, Nottingham, UK

Vanessa Venning
Department of Dermatology, Churchill Hospital, Oxford, UK

Sam Vincent
BMA Publishing Group, Clinical Evidence, BMA House, London, UK

Victoria P Werth
Department of Dermatology, University of Pennsylvania, Philadelphia, USA

Ros Weston
Focus Freelance Writing and Research, Salisbury, UK

David Whitelaw

Sean Whittaker
St John's Institute of Dermatology, St Thomas's Hospital, London, UK

Maxine Whitton
Consumer contributor, Cochrane Skin Group, London, UK

Hywel Williams
Centre of Evidence-Based Dermatology, University Hospital, Queen's Medical Centre, Nottingham, UK

Fenella Wojnaworska
Department of Dermatology, The Churchill Hospital, Headington, Oxford, UK

Hans Wolff
Department of Dermatology and Allergology, Ludwig-Maximilians-University, Munich, Germany

Johannes C van der Wouden
Department of General Practice, Erasmus MC-University Medical Center, Rotterdam, The Netherlands

Preface

Evidence-based dermatology is no longer a swear word in dermatology. Most dermatologists are practising good evidence-based dermatology to different degrees. The challenge is to improve those skills. This book may help you.

This book has a been labour of love for me, my associate editors and chapter contributors and I wish to thank them all for their efforts.

It is a *different* sort of book to the usual textbok. Different in that we have introduced the whole rationale for evidence-based dermatology in a section at the start of the book. Different in that we then provide you, the reader, with a detailed "toolbox" to help you understand some of the basic concepts in *practising* evidence-based dermatology. But the biggest difference is in the way we have encouraged our chapter contributors to follow a common structure when summarising the evidence base for different skin diseases – the "meat" of the book.

We have taken care, where possible, to separate the evidence found in studies from our opinions about that evidence, and we have tried to help the reader by providing summaries of key points at the end of each chapter. This has not been easy – I for one certainly find writing such highly structured chapters much harder work than the traditional "expert" book chapter.

The book is also different from other books in that it is accompanied by a website (http://www. evidbasedderm.com) that will include additional chapters and updates which will grow between this and the next edition. Complete coverage of the 2000 or so dermatology diseases is going to be a tough challenge, but we aspire to get there in successive editions and on our website.

We have strived to keep the book grounded in reality by making it as patient-based as possible by discussing the evidence around commonly encountered real patient scenarios. At the end of the day, it is patients who are at the heart of evidence-based dermatology.

Hywel Williams

Foreword

Fifteen years ago, when drafting an introductory chapter for a book on the effects of care during pregnancy and childbirth,[1] I decided to use contrasting quotations from a distinguished statistician and a distinguished dermatologist. In 1952, Austin Bradford Hill had Written:

> In my indictment of the statistician, I would argue that he may tend to be a trifle too scornful of the clinical judgement, the clinical impression. Such judgements are, I believe, in essence, statistical. The clinician is attempting to make a comparison between the situation that faces him at the moment and a mentally recorded but otherwise untabulated past experience.[2]

Twenty years later, Sam Shuster cointed the memorable pharse:

> Lies, damned lies and clinical impression[3]

My draft went on to discuss the fundamental importance and great dangers of clinical impressions: in obstetric practice they have led both to important therapeutic discoveries and to iatrogenic disasters. I doubt that people treating skin disease have the capacity to do unintended harm on the scale achieved by obstetricians and neonatologists, but I also doubt there is any justification for complacency in matters of dermatological therapy.

The variability that exists in the management of common chronic skin diseases is clear evidence of collective uncertainty about the effects of alternative management strategies, even if a majority of individual clinicians are certain that they are doing the right thing. For example, I gather that fumaric acid esters have been used widely to treat psoriasis for nearly 40 years in Germany, but that they have hardly been used anywhere else, although their use is supported by very strong evidence.[4] Some patients with warts are being put to the inconvenience (and expense) of attending hospital for cryotherapy; yet there is no strong evidence to suggest that they would be worse off treating their warts at home with salicylic acid paints.[5] As professionals concerned to do more good than harm to their patients, all who treat skin disease have a duty to reduce uncertainty about the relative merits of alternative treatments by paying attention to the results of well designed research.

To do right by their patients, people treating skin disease need to know what they know and what they don't know. This book tries to help them. Unlike traditional textbooks, it describes the methods that have been used to review the evidence upon which conclusions about the effects of treatment have been based, and gives references to more detailed reports of the systematic reviews on which the text has drawn.

There is no consensus about the materials and methods that should be used to assemble evidence to support treatment recommendations published in textbooks and review articles, nor even about the principles of systematic reviews. One senior dermatologist, for example, has written:

> The idea of a systematic review is a nonsense, and the sooner those advocates of it are tried at the International Court of Human Rights at the Hague (or worse still, sent for counselling), the better.[6]

Unfortunately, those who express reservations about applying systematic approaches to the synthesis of research evidence tend not to outline the alternative strategies that they deem preferable. This is a serious matter because it has been shown that reviews using explicit methods reach conclusions that differ from traditional reviews, with implications that can be matters of life of death.[7] In dermatology, too, the conclusions of reviews in which efforts have been made to reduce biases and the effects of chance can differ from those reached in traditional reviews of biases and the play of chance.[8] In the light of this evidence, I believe that continued acquiescence in reviews that have not attempted to minimise biases and, where possible and appropriate, the effects of chance, is not only scientifically unacceptable but also ethically highly questionable.[9]

The contributors to this book have tried to control biases, and – where they judged it appropriate – they have also reduced the play of chance by using statistical synthesis to analyse the results of similar but separate studies. As ways of improving the materials and methods used in such research synthesis are developed, researchers will apply them, taking advantage of the potential offered by electronic media to publish full and transparent accounts of their work, and to respond to new data and suggestions for improving their analyses.

In laying bare just how much cannot be known, the contributors to this book have also posed a very great challenge to everyone involved in treating skin disease. Can it be that a modest reduction in "doctor-assessed itch" is really the only demonstrable beneficial effect of the widespread use of evening primrose oil for people with eczema?[10] The book exposes the dearth of reliable studies addressing questions and outcomes that matter to patients, and it reveals the extent to which perverse incentives distort the dermatological research agenda. Those suffering from skin disease have every right to expect more from clinicians, researches, and those who fund research. This book should help to provoke them to do better.

1. Chalmers I. Evaluating the effects of care during pregnancy and childbirth. In: Chalmers I, Enkin M, Keirse MJNC, eds. *Effective care in pregnancy and childbirth.* Oxford: Oxford University Press, 1989:3–38.

2. Bradford Hill A. The clinical trial. *N Engl J Med* 1952;**247**:113–19.

3. Shuster S. Primary cutaneous virilism or idiopathic hirsuties? *BMJ* 1972;**2**:285–6.

4. Griffiths CEM, Clark CM, Chalmers RJG, Li Wan Po A, Williams HC. A systematic review of treatments for severe psoriasis. *Health Technol Assess* 2000;**4**:40.

5. Gibbs S, Harvey I, Sterling JC, Stark R. Local treatments for cutaneous warts (Cochrane Review). In: *The Cochrane Library*, Issue 4. Oxford: Update Software, 2002.

6. Ress JL. Two cultures? *J Am Acad Dermatol* 2002;**46**:313–14.

7. Antman EM, Lau J, Kupelnick B, Mosteller F, Chalmers TC. A comparison of results of meta-analyses of randomized control trials and recommendations of clinical experts. *JAMA* 1992;**268**:240–8.

8. Ladhani S, Williams HC. The management of established postherpetic neuralgia: a comparison of the quality and content of traditonal *v* systematic reviews. *Br J Dermatol* 1998;**139**:66–72.

9. Chalmers I, Hedges LV, Cooper H. A brief history of research synthesis. *Evaluation and the Health Professions* 2002;**25**:12–37.

10. Hoare C, Li Wan Po A, Williams H. Systematic review of treatements for atopic eczema. *Health Technol Assess* 2000;**4**:37.

Iain Chalmers
James Lind Inititative

Dedication

We, the editors, would like to dedicate this book to our patients who have helped us to understand the meaning of skin disease and who have given us insights into how to design better research studies to deal with the enormous gaps in knowledge for the treatment of skin disease.

Evidence-based Dermatology CD Rom

Features

Evidence-based Dermatology *PDF eBook*
- Bookmarked and hyperlinked for instant access to all chapters and topics
- Fully searchable text

Evidence-based Dermatology *PDA edition – sample chapter*
- A free sample chapter from the forthcoming PDA edition. Works on all PDA devices – Palm/Pocket PC/Psion etc.
- Requires Mobipocket Reader, free download available from http://www.mobipocket.com

BMJ Books *catalogue*
- Instant access to BMJ Books full catalogue, including an order form

Also included – instant access to the *Evidence-based Dermatology* update website

Instructions for use

The CD Rom should start automatically upon insertion, on all Windows systems. The menu screen will appear and you can then navigate by clicking on the headings. If the CD Rom does not start automatically upon insertion, please browse using "Windows Explorer" and double-click the file "BMJ_Books.exe".

Note: the *Evidence-based Dermatology* PDF eBook is for search and reference only and cannot be printed. A printable PDF version as well as the full PDA edition can be purchased from http://www.bmjbookshop.com

Troubleshooting

If any problems are experienced with use of the CD Rom, we can give you access to all content via the internet. Please send your CD Rom with proof of purchase to the following address, with a letter advising your email address and the problem you have encountered:

Evidence-based Dermatology eBook access
BMJ Bookshop
BMA House
Tavistock Square
London
WC1H 9JR

Part 1: The concept of evidence-based dermatology

Editor: Andrew Herxheimer

1
The field and its boundaries

Luigi Naldi

Evidence-based medicine represents the best way of linking and integrating clinical research with clinical practice.[1-6] The results of clinical research should inform clinical practice. Ideally, whenever a clinical question has no satisfactory answer it should be addressed by clinical research. Since clinical questions are innumerable and resources are limited, the process needs some control, and priorities should be set using explicit and verifiable criteria.[7-9] The public and purchasers have to be involved at this stage, and health needs and expectations in any given clinical area should be analysed and taken into account. In many instances, confirmatory studies are needed and systematic reviews can be used to summarise study results, or to explore results in specific subgroups with a view to further research. The results of clinical research should be applied back to individual patients in the light of their personal values and preferences. In the real world, forces other than those involved in such an ideal process often distort research priorities.[10,11] For example, strong industrial and economical interests partly justify the lack of data on rare disorders, or on common disorders if they occur mainly in less developed countries. This book may help to identify the more urgent questions that lack a satisfactory answer by summarising for physicians (and patients) the best evidence available for the management of a large number of skin disorders. It may thus be a starting point for rethinking the clinical research priorities in patient-oriented dermatology.

What is special about dermatology?

The skin is not a simple inert covering of the body but a sensitive dynamic boundary and is an important organ of social and sexual contact. Body image, which is deeply rooted within the culture of any given social group, is profoundly affected by the appearance of the skin and its associated structures.[12] The role that skin appearance plays in any given society is best understood from an anthropological perspective and using a narrative qualitative approach. This area is rather neglected in dermatological curricula.

Extensive disorders affecting the skin may disrupt its homeostatic functions, ultimately resulting in "skin failure", needing intensive care. This is rare but may happen, for example with extensive bullous disorders or exfoliative dermatitis. The most frequent health consequences of skin disorders are connected with the discomfort of symptoms such as itching and burning or pain, which frequently accompany skin lesions and interfere with everyday life and sleep, and the loss of confidence and disruption of social relations that visible lesions may cause. Feelings of stigmatisation, and major changes in lifestyle caused by chronic skin disorders such as psoriasis or leg ulcers have been repeatedly documented in population surveys.[13,14]

A vast array of clinical entities

Unlike most other organs, which usually count 50–100 diseases, the skin has a complement of

The chapter is based on: Naldi L, Minelli C. Dermatology. In: Day S, Green SB, Machin D, eds. *Textbook of Clinical Trials*. John Wiley & Sons, to be published in 2003.

1000–2000 conditions, and over 3000 dermatological categories can be found in the *International Classification for Disease* version 9 (ICD-9). Part of the reason is that the skin is a large and visible organ. In addition to disorders that primarily affect the skin, most of the major systemic diseases (for example disorders of vascular and connective tissues) have cutaneous manifestations. Currently, the widespread use of symptom-based or purely descriptive terms such as parapsoriasis and pityriasis rosea reflects our limited understanding of the causes and pathogenetic mechanisms of a large number of skin disorders. We still lack consensus on a detailed lexicon of dermatological terms used in research and everyday clinical practice.[15]

Extremely common disorders

Skin diseases are very common in the general population. Prevalence surveys have shown that skin disorders may affect 20–30% of the general population at any one time.[16] The most common diseases are also the most trivial ones. They include such conditions as mild eczematous lesions, mild to moderate acne, benign tumours and angiomatous lesions. More severe skin disorders which can cause physical disability or even death, are rare or very rare. They include, among others, bullous diseases such as pemphigus, severe pustular and erythrodermic psoriasis, and malignant tumours such as malignant melanoma and lymphoma. The disease frequency may vary according to age, sex and geographical area. In many cases, skin diseases are trivial health problems in comparison with more serious medical conditions. However, as already noted, because skin manifestations are visible they cause greater distress than more serious medical problems. The issue is complicated because many skin disorders are not a "yes or no" phenomenon but occur in a spectrum of severity. The public's perception of what constitutes a

"disease" requiring medical advice may vary according to cultural issues, the social context, resources and time. Minor changes in health policy may have a large impact on health and finance simply because a large number of people may be affected. For example, campaigns conducted to raise public awareness of skin cancer have led to a large increase in the number of people having benign skin conditions such as benign melanocytic naevi evaluated and excised.[17]

Large variations in terms of health care organisation

Countries differ greatly in the way in which their health services deal with skin disorders. These variations are roughly indicated by the number of dermatologists, ranging (in Europe) from about 1 per 20 000 patients in Italy and France to 1 per 150 000 patients in the UK.

In general, only a minority of people with skin diseases seek medical help while many opt for self-medication. Pharmacists have a key role in advising the public on the use of over-the-counter products. Primary care physicians seem to treat the majority of people among those seeking medical advice. Primary care of dermatological problems is not precisely defined and overlaps with specialist activity. Everywhere the dermatologist's workload is concentrated in the outpatient department. Despite the vast number of skin diseases, just a few categories account for about 70% of all dermatological consultations.

Generally speaking, dermatology requires a low technology clinical practice. Clinical expertise depends mainly on the ability to recognise a skin disorder quickly and reliably which, in turn, depends largely on awareness of a given clinical pattern based on previous experience, and on the practised eye of a visually literate physician.[18] The process of developing "visual skill" and a "clinical eye" is poorly understood and these skills are not formally taught.

Topical treatment is often possible

A peculiar aspect of dermatology is the option for topical treatment. This treatment modality is ideally suited to localised lesions, the main advantage being the restriction of the effect to the site of application and the limitation of systemic side-effects. A topical agent is usually described as a vehicle and an active substance, the vehicles being classified as powder, grease, liquid or combinations such as pastes and creams.

Much traditional topical therapy in dermatology has been developed empirically with so-called magistral formulations. Most of these products seem to rely on physical rather than chemical properties for their effects and it may be an arbitrary decision to consider one specific ingredient as the "active" one. Physical effects of topical agents may include cleansing, hydration and removal of keratotic scales. The border between pharmacological and cosmetic effects may be blurred and the term "cosmeceuticals" is sometimes used.[19] In addition to drug treatment, various non-drug treatment modalities exist, including phototherapy and photochemotherapy, and minor surgical procedures such as electrodesiccation and cryotherapy. Large variations in treatment modalities for the same condition mainly reflect local traditions and preferences.[20,21]

Limitations of clinical research

As in other disciplines, the past few decades have seen an impressive increase in clinical research in dermatology. However, the upsurge of clinical research has not been paralleled by methodological refinements and the quality of randomised controlled trials (RCTs) in dermatology seems to fall well below the usually accepted standards. Innovative thinking is needed in dermatology in order that clinical research addresses the important issues and does not simply ape the scientific design.

Disease rarity

There are at least a 1000 rare or very rare skin conditions for which no randomised trial has been conducted. These conditions are also those that carry a high burden of physical disability and mortality. Many of them have an annual incidence rate of below one case per 100 000 and frequently below one case per million. International collaboration and institutional support are clearly needed, but so far such efforts have been limited.

Patients' preferences

One alleged difficulty with conducting randomised clinical trials in dermatology is the visibility of skin lesions and the consideration that, much more so than in other areas, patients self-monitor their disease and may have preconceptions and preferences about specific treatment modalities.[22] The decision to treat is usually dictated by subjective issues and personal feelings. There is a need to educate physicians and the public about the value of randomised trials to assess interventions in dermatology. Motivations and expectations are likely to influence clinical outcomes of all treatments, but they may have a more crucial role in situations where "soft" endpoints matter, as in dermatology. Commonly, more than 20% of patients with psoriasis entering randomised clinical trials experience improvement on placebo independently of the initial disease extent. Motivations are equally important in pragmatic trials where different packages of management are evaluated, such as in the comparison of a self-administered topical product for psoriasis with hospital-based therapy like phototherapy. Traditionally, motivation is seen as a characteristic of the patient that is assumed not to change with the nature of the intervention. However, it has been argued that it is more realistic to view motivation in terms of the "fit" between the nature of the treatment and the patient's wishes and perceptions, especially with complex interventions that require the patient's active participation.[23] The public is inundated with uncontrolled and sometimes misleading or unrealistic messages on how to improve the body's appearance. All in all, there is a need to ensure that patient information and motivation are properly considered in the design and analysis of clinical trials on skin disorders.

The use of placebo in RCTs

Too many placebo-controlled randomised trials are conducted in dermatology even when alternative therapies exist. As a consequence, a large number of similar molecules used for the same clinical indication can be found in some areas, for example topical steroids. Many regulatory agencies still consider placebo controls as the "gold standard".[24] There is a need to establish criteria for the use of placebo in dermatology. The criteria should be developed with the active and informed participation of the public and should be considered by ethics committees and regulatory agencies. "Pragmatic" randomised trials conducted under conditions close to clinical practice and contrasting alternative therapeutic regimens are urgently needed to guide clinical decisions.

Long-term outcome of chronic disorders

Several major skin disorders are chronic conditions where no cure is currently available.[25,26] Whenever a definite cure is not reasonably attainable, it is common to distinguish between short, intermediate (usually measurable within months) and long-term outcomes. Long-term results are not simply predictable from short-term outcomes. Many skin disorders wax and wane

over time and it is not easy to define what represents a clinically significant long-term change in the disease status. This is an even more difficult task than defining outcome for other clinical conditions such as cancer or ischaemic heart disease, where death or major hard clinical endpoints (for example myocardial infarction) are of particular interest. In the long term, the way the disease is controlled and the treatment side-effects are vital, and simply and cheaply measured outcomes applicable in all patients seem to be preferable.[27] These may include the number of patients in remission, the number of hospital admissions or outpatient consultations and major disease flare-ups. Dropouts merit special attention because they may strongly reflect dissatisfaction with treatment.

Self-control design

Within-patient control studies (i.e. crossover and self-controlled studies) or simultaneous within-patient control studies are often used at a preliminary stage in drug development.[28] They are also used in dermatology, albeit improperly, at a more advanced stage. In a survey of more than 350 published RCTs of psoriasis (unpublished data), a self-controlled design accounted for one-third of all the studies examined and was relied on at some stage in drug development. The main advantage of a within-patient study over a parallel concurrent study is a statistical one. A within-patient study obtains the same statistical power with far fewer patients, and at the same time reduces variability between the populations being compared. Within-patient studies may be useful when studying conditions that are uncommon or show a high degree of patient-to-patient variability. On the other hand, within-patient studies impose restrictions and artificial conditions which may undermine validity and generalisability of results and may also raise some ethical concerns. The wash-out period of a crossover trial as well as the treatment schemes of a self-controlled design, which entails applying different treatments to various parts of the body, do not seem to be fully justifiable from an ethical point of view. Clearly, the impractical treatment modalities in self-controlled studies or the wash-out period in crossover studies may be difficult for the patient to accept.

Dropouts may have more pronounced effects in a within-patient study than in other study designs because each patient contributes a large proportion of the total information. The situation is compounded in self-controlled studies where dropping out from the study may be caused by observing a difference in treatment effect between the various regions of the body into which the patient has been "divided". In this case, given that dropouts are related to a difference in treatment effect between interventions, the effect of the interventions is likely to be underestimated.

The limitations of systematic reviews

The large number of clinical studies in dermatology and the lack of consensus on the management of many skin disorders point to systematic reviews as a way to improve the evidence and to guide clinical decisions. However, systematic reviews alone cannot be expected to overcome the methodological limitations in dermatological research we have noted. On the contrary, there are some indications that systematic reviews, if not properly guided by important clinical questions, might amplify the unimportant issues and may result in a rather misleading scale of evidence to guide clinical decisions. Since most randomised clinical trials are sponsored by pharmaceutical companies, it is quite plausible that data-driven systematic reviews will reflect the priorities as perceived by pharmaceutical companies and not necessarily by the public and clinicians. On the other hand, without a change in regulatory procedures, pharmaceutical companies will continue to pay

little attention to comparative RCTs and will continue to assess drugs for indications that are worth the financial investment, neglecting rare but clinically important disorders.

Systematic reviews alone cannot fill the gap and we urgently need fresh primary research and high-quality and relevant clinical trials.[29]

Evidence-based medicine: where do we go from here?

An evidence-based medicine approach should permeate medical education and inform academic medicine. Only if such a change is promoted can evidence-based medicine become central to clinical practice and not trivialised to "cookbook" medicine. If evidence-based medicine is successfully integrated into everyday practice, it may become easier to conduct primary clinical research based on clinical needs rather than on commercial interests.

More imaginative and effective research instruments are needed in primary research, and research strategies that take account of the peculiarities of dermatology should be developed. Qualitative research should not be neglected. It is the key to understanding intercultural variations in body image and of the ways health needs for skin diseases are expressed and perceived in different situations.[30–33]

References

1. McIntyre N, Popper K. The critical attitude in medicine: the need for a new ethics. *BMJ* 1983;**287**:1819–23.

2. Sackett DL, Rosenberg WMC, Gray JAM, Haynes RB, Richardson WS. Evidence based medicine: what it is and what it isn't. *BMJ* 1996;**312**:71–2.

3. Culpepper L, Gilbert TT. Evidence and ethics. *Lancet* 1999;**353**:829–31.

4. Vandenbroucke JP. Observational research and evidence-based medicine: what should we teach young physicians? *J Clin Epidemiol* 1998;**51**:467–72.

5. Vandenbroucke JP. Medical journals and the shaping of medical knowledge. *Lancet* 1998;**352**:2001–6.

6. Williams HC. Dowling Oration 2001. Evidence-based dermatology. A bridge too far? *Clin Exp Dermatol* 2001;**26**:714–24.

7. Klein R. Puzzling out priorities. Why we must acknowledge that rationing is a political process. *BMJ* 1998;**317**:959–60.

8. Kernick D, Stead J, Dixon M. Moving the research agenda to where it matters. *BMJ* 1999;**319**:206–7.

9. White KL. Fundamental research at primary level. *Lancet* 2000;**355**:1904–6.

10. Weatherall D. Academia and industry: increasingly uneasy bedfellows. *Lancet* 2000;**355**:1574.

11. Angell M. Is academia for sale? *N Engl J Med* 2000;**342**:1516–18.

12. Alam M, Dover JS. On Beauty. Evolution, psychosocial considerations, and surgical enhancement. *Arch Dermatol* 2001;**137**:795–807.

13. Ginsburg IH, Link BG. Feelings of stigmatization in patients with psoriasis. *J Am Acad Dermatol* 1989;**20**:53–63.

14. Phillips T, Stanton B, Provan A, Lew R. A study of the impact of leg ulcers on quality of life: financial, social, and psychological implications. *J Am Acad Dermatol* 1994;**31**:49–53.

15. Ackerman AB. Need for a complete dictionary of dermatology early in the 21st century. *Arch Dermatol* 2000;**136**:23.

16. Rea JN, Newhouse ML, Halil T. Skin disease in Lambeth: a community study of prevalence and use of medical care. *Br J Prev Soc Med* 1976;**30**:107–14.

17. Del Mar CB, Green AC, Battistutta D. Do public media campaigns designed to increase skin cancer awareness result in increased skin excision rates? *Aust NZ J Public Health* 1997;**21**:751–4.

18. Jackson R. The importance of being visually literate. Observations on the art and science of making a morphological diagnosis in dermatology. *Arch Dermatol* 1975;**111**:632–6.

19. Vermeer BJ, Gilchrest BA. Cosmeceuticals – a proposal for rational definition, evaluation, and regulation. *Arch Dermatol* 1996;**132**:337–40.

20. Peckham PE, Weinstein GD, McCullough JL. The treatment of severe psoriasis: A national survey. *Arch Dermatol* 1987;**123**:1303–7.

21. Farr PM, Diffey BL. PUVA treatment of psoriasis in the United Kingdom. *Br J Dermatol* 1991;**124**:365–7.

22. Van de Kerkhof PCM, De Hoop D, De Korte J, Cobelens SA, Kuipers MV. Patient compliance and disease management in the treatment of psoriasis in the Netherlands. *Dermatology* 2000;**200**:292–8.

23. Lambert MF, Wood J. Incorporating patient preferences into randomized trials. *J Clin Epidemiol* 2000;**53**:163–6.

24. Rothman KJ, Michels KB. The continuing unethical use of placebo controls. *N Engl J Med* 1994;**331**:394–8.

25. Al-Suwaidan SN, Feldman SR. Clearance is not a realistic expectation of psoriasis treatment. *J Am Acad Dermatol* 2000;**42**:796–802.

26. Krueger GG, Feldman SR, Camisa C *et al.* Two considerations for patients with psoriasis and their clinicians: what defines mild, moderate and severe psoriasis? What constitutes a clinically significant improvement when treating psoriasis? *J Am Acad Dermatol* 2000;**43**:281–3.

27. Wright JG. Evaluating the outcome of treatment: Shouldn't we be asking patients if they are better? *J Clin Epidemiol* 2000;**53**:549–53.

28. Louis TA, Lavori PW, Bailar JC III, Polansky M. Crossover and self-controlled designs in clinical research. *N Engl J Med* 1984;**310**:24–31.

29. Naldi L, Braun R, Saurat JH. Evidence-based dermatology: a need to reset the agenda. *Dermatology* 2002;**204**:1–3.

30. Greenhalgh T. Narrative based medicine in an evidence based world. *BMJ* 1999;**318**:323–5.

31. Elwyn G, Gwyn R. Stories we hear and stories we tell: analysing talk in clinical practice. *BMJ* 1999;**318**:186–8.

32. Herxheimer A, McPherson A, Miller R, Shepperd S, Yaphe J, Ziebland S. Database of patients' experience (DIPEx): a multi-media approach to sharing experience and information. *Lancet* 2000;**355**:1540–3.

33. Barbour RS. Checklists for improving rigour in qualitative research: a case of the tail wagging the dog? *BMJ* 2001;**322**:1115–17.

2

The rationale for evidence-based dermatology

Hywel Williams and Michael Bigby

What is evidence-based dermatology?
Definitions

Sackett, a clinical epidemiologist and one of the founders of modern evidence-based medicine (EBM), defined it as[1]:

> the conscientious, explicit and judicious use of current best evidence about the care of individual patients.

This definition reflects certain key concepts.

- "Conscientious" implies an *active* process which requires learning, doing and reflection.
- "Explicit" implies that we can describe the *process* that we use to practice EBM.
- "Current" implies being *up to date*.
- "Best" implies that we should seek the most *reliable* evidence source to inform practice.

As Chapter 12 elaborates, perhaps the most important and frequently forgotten phrase in this definition is "the care of individual patients". This is crucial – the place for EBM is not in trying to score intellectual points in the literature or in humiliating colleagues at journal clubs; it is at the bedside or in the outpatient consulting room. As chapter 12 emphasises, EBM is a way of thinking and working, with the improved health of our patients as its central aim.

Nowadays, the term evidence-based practice is often used instead of EBM. This reflects the *doing* rather than *talking* about EBM, and may be defined as integrating one's clinical expertise with the best external evidence from systematic research.[2] Evidence-based dermatology simply implies the application of EBM principles to people with skin problems.[3]

What evidence-based dermatology is not

Despite its clear definitions, the purpose of evidence-based dermatology (EBD) is often misunderstood in the literature.[4] Some of these misinterpretations are shown in Box 2.1. First, EBD does not tell dermatologists what to do.[1] Even the best external evidence has limitations in informing the care of individual patients. To use RE Clerk's metaphor, external evidence is just one leg of a three-legged stool, the other two being the clinician's expertise and the patient's values and preferences. Such clinical expertise and discussion of patient factors will always be at the heart of applying evidence during a dermatology consultation. EBM is not a cookbook of recipes to be followed slavishly, but an approach to medicine that is patient-driven from its outset. Patients are the best sources for generating the important clinical questions, answers to which then need to be applied back to such patients.[5]

Just as ordinary patients are at the heart of framing evidence-based questions, so too are ordinary clinical dermatologists at the heart of the practice of EBD. EBM is not something that only an exclusive club of academics with statistical expertise can understand and practise, but rather it is something that all dermatologists can practise with appropriate training. It is an essential skill that is as basic to being a doctor as the ability to examine and diagnose.

Contrary to popular belief, the prime purpose of EBM is not to cut costs. Like any information source, selective use of evidence can be twisted to support different economic arguments. Thus, the lack of randomised clinical trial (RCT) evidence for the efficacy of methotrexate in psoriasis should not imply that methotrexate should not be used/purchased for patients with severe disease when there is so much other evidence and long-term clinical experience to support its use. But this is not to say that a clinical trial comparing methotrexate and ciclosporin, acitretin or fumarates would not be desirable at some stage.[6]

EBM should not be viewed as a restriction on clinical freedom, if clinical freedom is defined as the opportunity to do the best for your patients, as opposed to making the same mistakes with increasing confidence. Searching for relevant information for your patients frequently opens up *more* rather than fewer treatment options.[7] The physician–patient partnership is free to choose or discard the various options in whatever way gives the most desirable outcome.

Guidelines are not the same as EBM, although the two are frequently confused.[8] Guidelines may or may not be evidence based, but guidelines are just that – guidelines. Many dermatology guidelines now incorporate a grading system that describes the quality of evidence used to make recommendations and their strength.[9]

Box 2.1 What evidence-based dermatology is not

- Something that ignores patients' values
- A promotion of a cookbook approach to medicine
- An ivory-tower concept that can only be understood and practised by an exclusive club of aficionados
- A tool designed solely to cut costs
- A reason for therapeutic nihilism in the absence of randomised controlled trials
- The same as guidelines
- A way of denigrating the value of clinical expertise
- A restriction on clinical freedom if this is defined as doing the best for one's patients

Problems with other sources of evidence
Working things out on the basis of mechanism and logic

Many physicians base clinical decisions on an understanding of the aetiology and patho-physiology of disease and logic.[10,11] This paradigm is problematic because the accepted hypothesis for the aetiology and pathogenesis of disease changes over time, and so the logically deduced treatments change too. For example, in the past 20 years, hypotheses about the aetiology of psoriasis have shifted from a disorder of keratinocyte proliferation and homeostasis, to abnormal signalling of cyclic AMP, to aberrant arachidonic acid metabolism, to aberrant vitamin D metabolism, to the current favourite: a T-cell-mediated autoimmune disease. Each of these hypotheses led to logically deduced treatments. The efficacy of many of these treatments has been substantiated by rigorous RCTs, whereas other treatments are used even in the absence of systematically collected observations. We thus have many options for treating patients with severe psoriasis (for example UVB, Goeckerman treatment, psoralen-UVA, methotrexate, ciclosporin and anti-interleukin-2 receptor antibodies) and mild-to-moderate psoriasis (for example dithranol, topical corticosteroids, calcipotriol and tazarotene). However, we do not know which is best, in what order they should be used, or in what combinations. We do not know how well methotrexate works (no well-designed clinical trials of methotrexate have been performed) or the optimal dose or dosing schedule for it.[6,10]

Treatments based on logical deduction from pathophysiology can have unexpected consequences. For example, the observation that antiarrhythmic drugs could prevent abnormal ventricular depolarisation after myocardial infarction logically led to their use to prevent sudden death after myocardial infarction. However, RCTs showed increased mortality in patients treated with antiarrhythmic drugs compared with placebo.[12,13] This highlights the dangers of using surrogate outcome measures, such as electrocardiograms, for more meaningful outcomes such as disability or death, simply because the surrogate measurements are easily made. The challenge with surrogate outcome measures is to ensure that they measure important things rather than trying to make measurable things important.

Some "designer" drugs such as topical tazarotene were promoted on the basis of their molecular mechanisms of action and may have appeared attractive at launch, but have been less exciting when tested in practice.[5] It might also be argued that the frequent narration of the superantigen story as a mechanism for antistaphylococcal treatments for atopic eczema is a smoke screen that obscures the real lack or uncertainty of evidence of clear benefit for such agents.[5]

Given these lessons, many dermatologists have become less interested in *how* treatments work and are now daring to ask questions such as: "*Does* it work?" and "How *well* does it work compared with existing, more established treatments?".

Personal experience

Although personal experience is an invaluable part of becoming a competent physician, the pitfalls of relying too heavily on personal experience have been widely documented.[14–16] These include:

- overemphasis on vivid, anecdotal occurrences and underemphasis on statistically significant strong evidence
- bias in recognising, remembering and recalling evidence that supports pre-existing knowledge structures (for example ideas about disease aetiology and pathogenesis) and parallel failure to recognise, remember and recall evidence that is more valid but does not fit pre-existing knowledge or beliefs
- failure to characterise population data accurately because of ignorance of statistical principles – including sample size, sample selection bias and regression to the mean
- inability to detect and distinguish statistical association and causality
- persistence of beliefs despite overwhelming contrary evidence.[17]

Nisbett and Ross[17] provide examples of these pitfalls from controlled clinical research, and simple clinical examples abound. Physicians may remember patients assuming that they who did not return for follow up improved, and conveniently forget the patients who did not improve. A patient treated with a given medication may develop a severe life-threatening reaction. On the basis of this single undesirable experience, the physician may avoid using that medication for many future patients, even though on average, it may be more efficacious and less toxic than the alternative treatments that the physician chooses. Few physicians keep adequate, easily retrievable records to codify results of treatments with a particular agent or of a particular disease; and even fewer actually carry out analyses. Few physicians make provisions for tracking those patients who are lost to follow up. Thus, statements made about a physician's "clinical experience" may be biased. Finally, for many conditions, a single physician sees far too few patients to draw reasonably firm conclusions about the response to treatments. For example, suppose a physician who treated 20 patients with lichen planus with tretinoin found that 12 (60%) had an excellent response. The confidence interval for this response rate (i.e. the true response rate for this treatment in the larger population from which this physician's sample was obtained) ranges from 36% to 81%. Thus, the true response rate might well be substantially less (or more) than the physician concludes from personal experience.[10,18]

Expert opinion

Expert opinion can be valuable, particularly for rare conditions in which the expert has the most experience or when other forms of evidence are not available. However, several studies have demonstrated that expert opinion often lags significantly behind conclusive evidence.[14] Experts suffer from relying on bench research, pathophysiology, and treatments based on logical deduction from pathophysiology, and from the same pitfalls noted for relying on personal experience.[18]

Textbooks can be valuable, particularly for rare conditions and for conditions for which the evidence does not change rapidly over time. However, textbooks have several well-documented shortcomings. They tend to reflect the biases and shortcomings of the experts who write them. By virtue of how they are written, produced and distributed, most are about 2 years out of date at the time of publication. Also, most textbook chapters are narrative reviews that do not consider the quality of the evidence reported.[14,18,19]

Uncontrolled data

Empirical, uncontrolled and non-systematically collected data form the basis of much of dermatology practice. This situation is justified by its advocates by two erroneous assumptions. The first is that it is acceptable to use such data because better evidence is not available – an assumption that is often not true. There is a surprisingly large body of high-quality evidence that is useful for the care of patients with skin disease. The second erroneous assumption is that the majority of dermatologists already base their practice on the best evidence that is already available. The base of knowledge for the practice of medicine is expanding exponentially. It is estimated that to keep up with the best evidence available, a general physician would have to examine 19 articles a day, 365 days a year.[2] Therefore, keeping up to date by reading the primary literature is now an impossible task for most practising physicians.[20] The burden for dermatologists is no less daunting.[5] The trick is to know how to find information efficiently, appraise it critically and use it well. Knowing the best sources and methods to search the literature allows a dermatologist to find the most current and most useful information in the most efficient manner, when it is needed. The techniques and skills needed to find, critically appraise and use the best evidence available for the care of individual patients have been developed over two centuries. These techniques and skills are currently best known as EBM.[10]

The process of evidence-based dermatology

Having discussed the definition and rationale of EBD, how does one actually do it? This process is best considered in five steps (see Box 2.2), although in real life they tend to merge and become iterative.[5] These steps are elaborated in subsequent chapters.

Box 2.2 The five steps of practising evidence-based dermatology

1. Asking an answerable structured question generated from a patient encounter
2. Searching for valid external evidence
3. Critically appraising that evidence for relevance and validity
4. Applying the results of that appraisal of evidence back to the patient
5. Recording the information for the future

Step 1: Asking an answerable structured question

Developing a structured question that can be answered requires practice. An example of a useless question would be, "Are diets any good in eczema?". A better question, generated from a real clinical encounter, would be, "In children with established moderate-to-severe atopic dermatitis, how effective is a dairy-free diet compared with standard treatment in inducing and maintaining a remission?". Such a question includes four key elements:

1. the patient population one wishes to generalise to
2. the intervention
3. its comparator
4. the outcomes that might make you change your practice.[21]

Unless one uses such a structure, it would be easy to waste time discussing and searching for data on the role of diets in preventing atopic disease, the effects of dietary supplements such as fish oil, studies that evaluate only short-term clinical signs, and those that deal with a "rag bag" of different types of eczema in adults and children. Rzany discusses further examples of framing answerable questions in more detail in Chapter 5.

Step 2: Searching for the best external information

Publication of biomedical information has now expanded so much that it is hard to contemplate searching for relevant information without some form of electronic bibliographic search, followed by reading the original key papers. Most of us (including the authors) are not experts at performing complex electronic searches, and need to learn such skills. These are dealt with in more detail by Bigby in Chapter 6. As pointed out earlier, traditional expert reviews are risky because often they have not been done systematically, and the links between the author's conclusions and the data are often unclear.[22] If one is searching for trials, then the Medline and Embase databases are also hazardous sources unless one is proficient, because simply searching by "clinical trials" type can miss up to half the relevant trials because of coding problems. The world's most comprehensive database of trials is now the Cochrane Central Register of Controlled Clinical Trials, containing over 340 000 records on 1 May 2002. Thankfully, it is also the easiest to search.

Step 3: Sifting information for relevance and quality

The usefulness of an article is a product of its clinical relevance times its validity divided by its accessibility.[23] Information sources need to be near the clinical area if they are to be used for patients. Getting distracted by irrelevant but interesting citations is also a real hazard when reading search results. Two filters need to be applied if one is to keep practising EBD: the first is to discard irrelevant information and the second is to spend more time looking at a few high-quality papers. Here it is timely to mention the concept of hierarchy of evidence,[24] which is discussed in more detail in Chapter 7. This means that if two RCTs deal with the question of interest (for example dietary exclusion in childhood atopic dermatitis), or better still, a systematic review deals with the same topic, one should critically appraise these sources rather than dilute what little time one has by reading lots of case series and case reports.

Step 4: Applying the evidence back to the patient

This is usually the most important step, but the least well developed in EBD. Key points to note here are:

- to consider how similar the patients in the studies are to the patient facing you now
- whether the outcome measures used in those studies (for example percentage reduction in erythema or induration score) mean something to you and the patient
- how large the treatment benefits were
- whether there were any serious side-effects of treatment
- how the evidence fits in with your patient's past experience and current preferences.

This difficult area is discussed in more detail in Chapter 12.

Step 5: Recording the information for the future

Having done so much work pursuing the above "evidence-based prescription" from question to patient, it might be useful to others and yourself to make a record of that information for future use as a critically appraised topic (CAT), although these have a limited lifespan if not updated.[2] The Cochrane Skin Group is now developing a site for storing and sharing dermatology CATs (http://www.nottingham.ac.uk~muzd). Such CATs could become the norm in dermatology journal clubs all over the country, replacing unstructured chats about articles selected for unclear reasons.

The key point to remember about the process of EBD is that it *starts and ends with patients*. A problem highlighted during an encounter with a patient is the best generator of an EBM problem.[25] Even if one then searches and critically appraises the best data in the world, the utility of this exercise would be zero if it is not applied back to that patient or other similar patients. Developing the skills to undertake evidence-based prescription requires practice.

Dermatologists will participate in the practice of EBD to different degrees depending on their enthusiasm, skills, time pressures and interest.[24] Some will be "doers", implying that they undertake at least steps 1–4 highlighted in Box 2.2. Others will be more inclined to adopt a "using mode", relying on searching for evidence-based summaries that others have constructed, thereby skipping step 3, at least to some degree. Finally, some will incorporate evidence into their practice in "replicating mode", following decisions of respected leaders (i.e. skipping steps 2 and 3). These categories bear some similarity to those of deduction, induction and seduction that Sackett used to describe the methods that physicians employ to make decisions about therapy.[14] Such categories are not mutually exclusive, since even the most enthusiastic EBM practitioners in "doing" mode will flit to "user" and "replicating" mode according to whether they are dealing with a common or rare clinical problem.

Conclusions

The objective of most physicians surely is to provide their patients with the best health care. To do so, a physician must be able to assess the patient's physical condition, know the best and most current information about diagnosis, prevention, therapy, prognosis and potential harm, and apply that knowledge to the specific patient. Medicine is advancing very rapidly, creating major changes in the way we treat our patients. We must keep up with such changes. We need to be up to date with such new external evidence. We frequently fail to do this if we rely on passive means or an occasional flick through the main journals, and our knowledge gradually deteriorates with time. Attempts to overcome this deficiency by attending clinical education programmes fails to improve our performance, whereas the practice of EBM has been shown to keep its practitioners up to date. EBM is a way of thinking that is intended to help accomplish these objectives. If we stick to thinking about patients' welfare when contemplating EBM, we are less likely to get things wrong.[5,10]

References

1. Sackett DL, Rosenberg WM, Gray JA, Haynes RB, Richardson WS. Evidence based medicine: what it is and what it isn't. *BMJ* 1996;**312**:71–2.

2. Sackett DL, Richardson WS, Rosenberg Q, Haynes RB. *Evidence-based Medicine. How to practise and teach EBM*. London: Churchill Livingstone, 1997.

3. Bigby M. Snake oil for the 21st century. *Arch Dermatol* 1998;**134**:1512–14.

4. Rees J. Evidence-based medicine: the epistemology that isn't. *J Am Acad Dermatol* 2000;**43**:727–9.

5. Williams HC. Evidence-based dermatology: a bridge too far? *Clin Exp Dermatol* 2001;**26**:714–24.

6. Griffiths CEM, Clark CM, Chalmers RJG, Li Wan Po A, Williams HC. A systematic review of treatments for severe psoriasis. *Health Technol Assess* 2000;**4**:1–125.

7 Hoare C, Li Wan Po A, Williams H. Systematic review of treatments for atopic eczema. *Health Technol Assess* 2000;**4**(37).

8. Seidman D. Compliance with guidelines is not the same as evidence-based medicine. *J Pediatr* 2001;**138**: 299–300.

9. Telfer NR, Colver GB, Bowers PW. Guidelines for the management of basal cell carcinoma. British Association of Dermatologists. *Br J Dermatol* 1999;**141**:415–23.

10. Bigby M. Paradigm lost. *Arch Dermatol* 2000;**136**:26–7.

11. Klovning A. Seminar 3: An introduction to evidence-based practice. http://www.shef.ac.uk/uni/projects/wrp/sem3.html.

12. Echt DS, Liebson PR, Mitchell LB *et al*. Mortality and morbidity in patients receiving encainide, flecanide, or placebo: the cardiac arrhythmia supression trial. *N Engl J Med* 1991;**324**:781–8.

13. The Cardia Arrhythmia Supression Trial II Investigators. Effects of the antiarrhythmic agent moricizine on survival after myocardial infarction. *N Engl J Med* 1992;**327**:227–33.

14. Sackett DL, Haynes RB, Guyatt GH, Tugwell P. *Clinical Epidemiology A Basic Science for Clinical Medicine*. Boston: Little, Brown and Company, 1991:441.

15. Bigby M, Gadenne A-S. Understanding and evaluating clinical trials. *J Am Acad Dermatol* 1996;**34**:555–90.

16. Hines DC, Goldheizer JW. Clinical investigation: a guide to its evaluation. *Am J Obstet Gynecol* 1969;**105**:450–87.

17. Nisbett R, Ross L. *Human Inference: Strategies and Shortcomings of Social Judgement*. Englewood Cliffs, NJ: Prentice-Hall Inc., 1980:330.

18. Bigby M, Szklo M. Evidence-based dermatology. In: Freedberg I, Eisen AZ, Katz SI *et al.*, eds. *Dermatology in General Medicine*. New York: McGraw Hill, 2002.

19. Greenhalgh T. *How to Read a Paper. The Basics of Evidence Based Medicine*. London: BMJ Books, 1997:196.

20. Guyatt GH, Sackett DL, Cook DJ. Users' guides to the medical literature II. How to use an article about therapy or prevention B. What were the results and will they help me in caring for my patients? *JAMA* 1994;**271**:59–63.

21. Straus SE, Sackett DL. Bringing evidence to the clinic. *Arch Dermatol* 1998;**134**:1519–20.

22. Ladhani S, Williams HC. The management of established postherpetic neuralgia: a comparison of the quality and content of traditional *v.* systematic reviews. *Br J Dermatol* 1998;**139**:66–72.

23. Shaughnessy AF, Slawson DC, Bennett JH. Becoming an information master: a guidebook to the medical information jungle. *J Fam Pract* 1994;**39**:489–99.

24. Bigby M. Evidence-based medicine in dermatology. *Dermatol Clin* 2000;**18**:261–76.

25. Shaughnessy AF, Slawson DC, Becker L. Clinical jazz: harmonizing clinical experience and evidence-based medicine. *J Fam Pract* 1998;**47**:425–8.

3

The role of the consumer in evidence-based dermatology

Andrew Herxheimer and Maxine Whitton

Bridging the communication gap

Dermatologists, like other doctors, now recognise the therapeutic value of an alliance with their patients (the "therapeutic alliance"), and the need to explain their advice and, as far as possible, to share management decisions with the patient. Different people may have very different values and preferences, and it is often wrong to assume agreement without explanation and discussion. Medical terms are often unfamiliar to patients. For example, to hear a rash or spot called an "eruption" or a "lesion" can be disconcerting. Using language the patient can understand, clinicians need to be able to explain the condition, its implications and treatment, as well as possible side-effects, and the consequences of not using the medication. If this can be achieved then patients are more likely to accept the requirements of the treatment and a true care partnership with the professional can be established. This could save time, and lead to quicker recovery and greater mutual trust. Unfortunately in most consultations there is not enough time to do this adequately, especially since some of the concepts that underlie diagnosis and treatment are unfamiliar to most patients and many patients lack necessary background knowledge. It is important to bridge this communication gap from both ends, by helping dermatologists and other professionals working with them to become more fluent and understanding of the patient's perspective, and by developing training and education for their current and future patients – or "consumers".

What are "consumers"?

It should be noted that "professional", "patient", "consumer", "health service user" and "citizen" are not different categories of people, but describe different roles, which often overlap. It is normal for a person to have different roles at different times, or even at the same time, and role conflict is not uncommon among health professionals. An obvious example is the doctor or nurse who is or becomes a patient, or a parent with a chronically ill child who becomes a patient advocate. The term "user of health services" is a neutral catch-all term for all those who use or have used any health service, public or private, and is easily extended to include potential users too – that is everybody. However, some people do not use this term because it may carry overtones of drug use or misuse. Also, the term tends to denote client groups who are disadvantaged in some way (for instance wheelchair users) and who use social services rather than the health service. The word *citizen* also covers everybody, but encompasses all spheres of activity, not only health and illness, and hints at civic responsibility, as in *citizens' jury*.

Taken at face value, the term "consumer" means the same as "user", but its connotations differ. This is evident from the two meanings given in

Collins' *English Dictionary* (1982): "1. a person who purchases goods and services for his own needs; 2. A person or thing that consumes". The commercial overtones of the first meaning displease some people. The word also evokes *consumerism*, defined as "the protection of the interests of consumers". This gives it a slightly assertive, even militant edge, suggesting that consumers of health services are more likely to insist on their rights than mere patients or users. The word is therefore particularly apt in connection with research ethics committees, health authorities, funding bodies and the like, where consumer voices are increasingly given parity with those of the professionals. It does, however, have the same universality as *user*: we are all consumers – whoever and whatever else we may be. It is clear that there is no perfect label for the many potential roles that patients and their carers may take in health that is free of certain connotations, but for simplicity, we will use the term "consumer".

The many roles of a consumer

The consumer has a number of potential roles in health care:

- to play an active part in self-care as far as his or her capacity allows;
- to work together with professionals in his/her own care and in the care of others in the family, the workplace and the locality;
- to communicate to health professionals and the healthy community the points of view, needs and wishes of people affected by a disease;
- to take part with professionals in the development and governance of health institutions (for example hospitals and nursing homes) and organisations, such as providers of primary care;
- to contribute to research policy and practice by helping to decide research priorities and funding, and helping to improve the design of research;

- to help recruit participants for worthwhile research;
- to contribute their own experiences of illness for the information and education of other patients and of professionals.

The visible nature of skin disease

All the above roles are relevant to dermatology, but not special to it. What distinguishes skin disease from other kinds of illnesses is that it is much more visible to the world. This means that its social effects are often far greater than for other illnesses of comparable seriousness, and that the patient's self-image is often harmed. Healthy people, including many health professionals, do not sufficiently understand these aspects, and do not cope adequately with them. Consumers and patients can help them understand and learn what matters to people with various skin conditions. In the case of vitiligo, for example, doctors sometimes base treatment decisions on how they perceive the degree of distress. Many think that white patients suffer less than those with darker skins, but studies as well as anecdotal experience have shown that this may not be true.[1] Nor is the extent of the disease always the most important factor in the patient's suffering. Self-esteem, self-image, the site of the lesions, the degree to which the patient feels disabled by the disease, and the support networks available to the patient all need to be considered. A study of psoriasis has found that the patient's opinion of disease severity can differ from the physician's and that the degree of distress depends on how far the disease affects everyday life.[2] These findings underline that the assessment of psoriasis (whether by doctor or patient) influences the choice of treatment. Patients may well prefer treatments that will address the disfiguring social effects of the disease to those that reduce the size of the lesions.

Although lip service is sometimes paid to the psychosocial aspects of skin disease, very little is done to address them. Treatment should include the option to refer patients for appropriate professional psychological help and this should be an integral part of treatment guidelines. It could be argued that some patient support groups (PSGs) perform this function. Although they can provide opportunities for members to share experiences and give practical advice, they are not equipped to give either medical advice or indepth psychological help. Commenting on a small study of cognitive behavioural therapy (CBT) used for vitiligo patients,[3] Picardi and Abeni[4] state that this approach might help patients with vitiligo, and possibly other skin diseases and suggest: "If the efficacy of CBT were confirmed, a new weapon could be added to the therapeutic arsenal of the dermatologist. This would be a substantial step ahead in the management of a disease for which no known cure can ensure complete clearance...".

Dermatology differs notably from other branches of medicine in the way it shades off into borderlands of cosmetics and cosmetic surgery, and in the often blurred boundaries between treatment, prevention and aggravation of skin problems. Even something as innocuous as washing can be a form of prevention (for example washing a chemical off one's hand), treatment (for example ridding the skin of an accumulation of excess scale) or aggravation (causing irritant contact dermatitis through frequent hand-washing with soap). The dual function of the skin as both a large and important organ and a superficial covering of the body that is important in social "display" can lead to trivialisation. Some skin conditions, like acne and vitiligo, are often considered purely cosmetic problems, particularly by some general practitioners.

Education and information for self-care

Before anyone with skin disease can hope to manage his or her own treatment, he or she has to learn about the condition and about the principles that underlie its treatment and how to apply them in everyday life. When this is achieved, the patient has much greater control and is more confident and self-reliant, although of course some advice and help from professionals will still be needed at times.

Many self-help groups or PSGs are founded by people who have been given no information about their condition, or whose questions have not been answered adequately. Often a PSG can resolve the practical everyday problems that health professionals are not aware of or avoid dealing with, through either embarrassment or a lack of understanding. Patients may have difficulty asking the questions that most concern them. They may be too embarrassed, or feel that the subject is too trivial and a waste of the doctor's time.

PSGs have a clear role to play in providing just such information, through fact sheets, leaflets, newsletters, in confidence on the telephone, CDs, videos or, increasingly, through their websites, so reaching wider international audiences. Most of this information is of course not yet rigorously evidence based, but as consumers acquire the skills of critical appraisal and an understanding of levels of evidence by working within organisations such as the Cochrane Consumer Network, information should become better and more reliable.

The UK Vitiligo Society is unique in publishing a book,[5] about to be revised and updated, on all aspects of vitiligo, its management and current research. Most self-help organisations have developed a raft of fact sheets, written in good lay language but with professional input where necessary to ensure accuracy. These help not only patients, but also professionals. Leaflets and fact sheets can be tailored to different groups, such as children, parents, teachers, health and other professionals, as well as to the general public.

Information produced by PSGs can cover a wide range of topics, including diet, clothing, complementary therapies and useful tips on various aspects of managing the disease. Some of the information provided may not be easily available from any other source. Here are some examples.

- The UK Raynaud's and Scleroderma Association gives information on heating aids and tips on how to keep warm, including the use of electrically heated gloves and socks provided by the UK NHS. Few patients are aware of this.
- The UK Psoriasis Association publishes handy hints gleaned from their members in their newsletter. They also give information on "Dead Sea therapy".
- The UK National Eczema Society publishes booklets on PUVA, itching and scratching, and wet wraps, as well as the psychological aspects of eczema, and fact sheets on diet, topical steroids, sun protection and the use of Chinese herbs for eczema.

PSGs are careful to state that they do not recommend alternative treatments but they give sound advice on things to look out for to minimise trouble, for example checking that alternative practitioners have appropriate qualifications.

Self-help groups can also make valuable contributions by helping to collect patients' own personal experiences of illness – which often raise concerns that medical accounts do not consider. These narratives can be systematically analysed and made accessible to patients, professionals and students, so that everyone can be much better informed. The Database of Individual Patients' Experiences of illness (DIPEx) is an ambitious project that is establishing such collections for a wide range of diseases.[6] So far it does not include experiences of any skin disease; that is planned for the future. The DIPEx website is at http://www.dipex.org.

The importance of all this work to the patient cannot be overstated. An understanding of the disease enhances the patient's ability to cope. An informed patient is empowered to take responsibility for his/her disease, and can learn to manage it more confidently. It is not uncommon for some patients to be better informed than their family doctor about their disease and its treatment. This can lead to problems in the doctor–patient relationship if it is not handled properly, but it can also contribute to much better collaboration between the patient and the doctor.

Consumers and research

Consumer involvement in clinical research is rare in dermatology. Most PSGs have the support and encouragement of research as one of their objectives. Many strive towards finding a "cure" for their particular condition, however unrealistic this may seem to health professionals. In general, however, PSGs tend to give financial support to projects that researchers have already chosen (i.e. the research agenda is mainly driven by university-based academics). Whilst not disputing their ability to carry out high-quality research, the "basic science" discoveries from such research rarely find their way back to the patient. The priority given to research over support and education varies between organisations.

PSGs do fund research, but the sums available from this source are modest compared with other disease areas. Among the UK skin groups. the biggest funder of research is the Psoriasis Association. Like many other PSGs, the association has a Medical and Research Committee to vet projects for research funding. The lay members on this committee help to ensure that the patient's perspective is included in their discussions. Projects are always referred to the National Council for a final decision and at this stage are sometimes passed back to the

Medical and Research Committee for review, often for a more patient-based approach.

Pharmaceutical companies fund the highest proportion of dermatological research projects, and they have been reluctant to involve consumers in such research in any meaningful way. Companies can establish strong relationships with groups, and sometimes work with them to devise quality-of-life questionnaires. Although these studies are mainly for marketing purposes, the results may also influence the choice of research topics and the design of clinical studies. For the most part, pharmaceutical companies tend to approach PSGs mainly for help with recruiting patients for trials, and most PSGs have contributed in this way. Because pharmaceutical companies often regard some of the data contained in their protocol to be commercially sensitive, PSGs rarely get much information to give to those wishing to take part in trials, apart from the exclusion criteria. Often participants are not given adequate information, are not thanked for their involvement and are not informed of the outcome of the trial. However, PSGs, because of the cumulative and combined experience of their members, have good insights into what research is needed. Skin diseases are by and large chronic illnesses with much higher morbidity than mortality. Patients who have been managing and living with their disease for many years have in some ways become experts at coping. However, they are also unaware that they can contribute to clinical research in other ways, not just as passive "subjects". Although their research concerns may differ from those of professionals, patients are well placed to pose relevant research questions and to contribute to the design of studies.

Some organisations, like the Raynaud's and Scleroderma Association, are beginning to suggest areas of research, based on their members' experience. For example, the association decided to offer funding for a project on calcinosis – a big problem for many people with the disease. This is not a particularly attractive topic and can be difficult to tackle. After several months waiting for a worthwhile proposal, a project was started in 2002. The association is also keen to fund a project to investigate the causes of childhood scleroderma. It is also worth noting that the UK National Eczema Society supported and funded the double-blind controlled study conducted at Liverpool University of the effect of housedust mites in adults and children with eczema.[7] Other organisations, such as the National Eczema Association for Science and Education based in the USA, have set up and supported international research meetings.

PSGs can play an important role in educating patients about ways in which they can become involved in clinical research. The National Eczema Society recognised this and encouraged its members and other dermatology patient groups to volunteer to join the Cochrane Skin Group (see Chapter 4) as consumer representatives. Under the auspices of an umbrella organisation of UK skin support groups called the Skin Care Campaign (formerly a project of the National Eczema Society), a meeting was held to inform consumers about the Cochrane Collaboration and how they as consumers could contribute to its work. Some consumers subsequently contributed by hand-searching journals, commenting on protocols and reviews, translating reviews and co-authoring a review (on vitiligo). From this meeting, a focus group was set up to help identify suitable questions for eczema research.

Examples of organisations that are committed to encouraging more consumer involvement in research should also be mentioned. Consumers in NHS Research was set up in 1996 to advise the NHS on how best to involve consumers in research and development (R&D). Members are drawn from the voluntary sector, research organisations, health information providers and health and social services management. The group aims "to ensure that consumer involvement in R&D in the NHS improves the way that research is prioritised, commissioned, undertaken and disseminated". This includes persuading researchers of the importance and value of consumer involvement by indicating ways in which consumers can be part of the research process, and offering information, advice and support to consumers, researchers and NHS employees through the Support Unit. Useful publications, available free on their website, include "Research; What's in it for Consumers?" (1998), "Involvement Works" (1999), and conference and workshop reports.

CERES (Consumers in Ethics and RESearch), was set up in the late 1980s to promote the idea that consumers can contribute to the design and conduct of medical research. CERES is an independent forum for those who believe that health service users should be involved at every stage of research affecting them and provides users with the means of publicising their views on new treatments and research. It is also for members of ethics research committees, health authorities and voluntary organisations. CERES is an independent charity run entirely by volunteers, with no office or paid staff, but it does have a website. CERES holds open meetings and publishes newsletters and reports, as well as leaflets to help patients taking part in research to understand the process and make informed decisions.

The Cochrane Consumer Network is a part of the Cochrane Collaboration. Its members include individual consumers as well as community organisations around the world. The network gives much needed support and training to consumers, encouraging them to take part in the work of the collaboration by helping to identify questions for review from the viewpoint of the person with the health problem, searching for the

trials, commenting on drafts of reviews and protocols and helping to disseminate the reviews. It works to keep consumers informed, develops training materials, helps to demystify scientific jargon to make reviews more accessible to the general public, and publishes a digest of new additions to the *Cochrane Library*, including full consumer summaries of reviews. Its website provides a means of commenting on issues and reviews and has links with other sources of evidence-based health care on the internet.

Consumer involvement in the process of evidence-based dermatology

Given the important and diverse roles that a consumer may play in the therapeutic alliance with his/her dermatologist, how do these roles become translated into the practice of evidence-based dermatology? This can be best answered by considering the four steps of evidence-based practice: i) asking an answerable question; ii) searching for relevant information; iii) appraising the validity of that information and then iv) applying it back to the patient.

1. **Asking an answerable question.** By definition, the question generated within an "evidence-based prescription" is derived from a patient encounter. For example, a woman aged 32 years with facial acne may want to know whether it is safe to take a combined anti-androgen/oestrogen pill, as opposed to continuing on prolonged oral antibiotics. Further discussion may reveal that she is mainly concerned about deep vein thrombosis as she has a family history of this. The structured evidence-based question emanating from this discussion would then be, "What is the increased risk for a woman in her thirties to suffer a deep vein thrombosis when taking the combined anti-androgen/oestrogen pill for her acne when compared with taking an oral antibiotic?". This will, of course, depend on other factors

such as whether she is a smoker, her weight, exercise profile etc. but it nevertheless illustrates how an evidence-based question needs to be tailored in a structured way around a particular individual.

2. **Searching for relevant information.** This may at first seem to be the domain of the dermatologist, yet the advent of the internet and many high-quality skin information websites has transformed this. Many patients now come to their first dermatology consultation armed with pages printed out from the internet. They may sometimes correctly self-diagnose conditions such as "cold urticaria" when even their family doctor was unsure. Whilst it is true that much of the information on the internet is of dubious value as a result of various vested interests and the lack of explicit criteria used to develop it, the internet can be a useful source of information for many rare and common skin diseases. In this sense, the "consumer" can play a useful role by helping their dermatologist to search for information that may be relevant to the evidence-based question.

3. **Appraising the quality of the data.** Again, although it might seem that only the dermatologist can appraise the validity of the data by checking for things such as adequacy of concealment of the randomisation schedule, and issues of blinding and intention-to-treat analysis, such an assessment is of little value if the dermatologist examines reported outcomes in a trial that means little to the patient. Consumers are ideally placed to help inform dermatologists about which aspect of the disease is important to them. For example, in patients with atopic eczema, is it short-term control of itching, duration or frequency of remissions, healing painful cracks in the fingers, coping skills, or ability to take part in sport and social activities?

4. **Applying the information back to the patient.** An "evidence-based prescription" is useless if that information is not then presented back to the patient who generated it. Patients are the only people who can ultimately decide if the treatment options they are offered fit in with their expectation for improvement, willingness to be inconvenienced by side-effects and frequent visits, and so on.

Thus it can be seen that the consumer has a central role in driving and informing the process of evidence-based dermatology in that the important questions begin and end with the patient. The dermatologist is seen as the patient's advocate, guiding and interpreting the evidence and applying it to the patient's unique circumstances through a caring and trusting partnership.

Conclusions

Given that many skin diseases are chronic, many patients and their carers want to know as much as possible about the causes and prognosis of their skin disease, and of the costs and benefits of the many treatments available to them. In many circumstances, the psychological effects of skin disease have been trivialised by doctors, and the involvement of consumers in skin research to date has been minimal.

Yet there is a huge opportunity for health professionals to work more closely and in partnership with consumers, particularly in the field of skin disease. Consumers are often in the best position to guide clinicians and researchers on what matters most to them in terms of therapeutic benefit, and they can provide psychological support and useful written information to fellow patients in ways that doctors cannot. Consumers are also well placed to help prioritise relevant research in dermatology by framing the research questions that are most important to them, by helping researchers choose meaningful outcome measures, and by recruiting patients through their networks.

Consumer groups are also ideally placed to disseminate research findings, and many are increasingly funding their own research.

Further information

Details of the PSGs and other organisations mentioned in this chapter are listed below. For a more comprehensive list of UK-based PSGs contact the Skin Care Campaign. There may be similar organisations in other countries but the authors do not have reliable information on PSGs in other parts of the world. The website http://www.patientsupportgroups.org may be helpful.

National Eczema Association for Science and Education

1220 SW Morrison, Suite 433, Portland, OR 97205, USA. Tel: +503 228 4430 or +800 818 7546; fax: +503 224 3363; website: http://www.eczema-assn.org

National Eczema Society

Hill House, Highgate Hill, London N19 5NA, UK. Tel: +44 (0)20 7281 3553; fax: +44 (0)20 7281 6395; website: http://www.eczema.org

Psoriasis Association

Milton House, 7 Milton Street, Northampton NN2 7JG, UK. Tel: +44 (0)1604 711 129; fax: +44 (0)1604 792894; website being developed

Raynaud's and Scleroderma Association

112 Crewe Road, Alsager, Cheshire ST7 2JA, UK. Tel: +44 (0)1270 872 776; fax: +44 (0)1270 883 556; website: http://www.raynauds.demon.co.uk

Skin Care Campaign

Address as National Eczema Society; website: http://www.skincarecampaign.org

Vitiligo Society

125 Kennington Road, London SE11 6SF, UK. Tel: 0800 018 2631; fax: +44 (0)20 7840 0866; website: http://www.vitiligosociety.org.uk

Consumers in NHS Research Support Unit

Wessex House, Upper Market St, Eastleigh, Hampshire SO50 9FD UK. Tel: +44 (0)2380 651 088; email: admin@conres.co.uk; website: http://www.conres.co.uk

Consumers in Ethics and Research (CERES)

PO Box 1365, London N16 0BW, UK. Email:info@ceres.org.uk; website: http://www.ceres.org.uk

Cochrane Consumer Network

PO Box 96, Burwood, Victoria 3125 Australia. Tel: +61 (0)3 9885 5588; email: info@cochraneconsumer.com; website: http://www.cochraneconsumer.com

References

1. Porter JR, Beuf AH. Racial variation in reaction to physical stigma: a study of degree of disturbance by vitiligo among black and white patients. *J Health Soc Behav* 1991;**32**:192–204.

2. Root S, Kent G, Al'Abadie MSK. The relationship between disease severity, disability and psychological distress in patients undergoing PUVA treatment for psoriasis. *Dermatology* 1994;**189**:234–7.

3. Papadopoulos L, Bor R, Legg C. Coping with the disfiguring effects of vitiligo: a preliminary investigation into the effects of cognitive-behavioural therapy. *Br J Med Psychol* 1999;**72**:385–96.

4. Picardi A, Abeni D. Can cognitive behavioral therapy help patients with vitiligo? *Arch Dermatol* 2001;**137**:786–8.

5. Lesage M. *Vitiligo: understanding the loss of skin colour.* London: The Vitiligo Society, 2002.

6. Herxheimer A, McPherson A, Miller R, Shepperd S, Yaphe J, Ziebland S. A database of patients' experiences (DIPEx): a multi-media approach to sharing experiences and information. *Lancet* 2000;**355**:1540–3.

7. Tan BB, Weald D, Strickland I, Friedmann PS. Double-blind controlled trial of the effect of housedust-mite allergen avoidance on atopic dermatitis. *Lancet* 1996;**347**:15–18.

4

The Cochrane Skin Group

Tina Leonard, Finola Delamere and Dédée Murrell

Background

The Cochrane Skin Group (CSG) is one of about 50 Collaborative Review Groups that together make up the Cochrane Collaboration. This international organisation has developed in response to a challenge issued by Archie Cochrane, a British epidemiologist, who, in his book published in 1972, pointed out the deficiencies of reviews of the medical literature and the lack of access to up-to-date information about health care.[1] In 1979 he wrote[2]:

> It is surely a great criticism of our profession that we have not organised a critical summary, by specialty or subspecialty, adapted periodically, of all relevant randomized controlled trials.

Archie Cochrane recognised that there was a great collective ignorance about the effects of health care. The amount of information available to both health professionals and the general public is overwhelming but much of it is not evidence based and some is contradictory. There was a great need for a systematic approach to organising and evaluating the information available from clinical trials. In 1987 (the year before he died), Cochrane referred to a systematic review of randomised controlled trials (RCTs) of care during pregnancy and childbirth as "a real milestone in the history of randomized trials and in the evaluation of care", and suggested that other specialties should copy the methods used.[3] This suggestion was taken up by the UK's Research and Development Programme, which had been set up to support the National Health Service (NHS). Funds were provided to establish a "Cochrane Centre" which would collaborate with people, both in the UK and elsewhere, to facilitate the production of systematic reviews of RCTs across all areas of health care.[4,5] The first "Cochrane Centre" was opened in Oxford in October 1992, and 6 months later the New York Academy of Sciences organised a meeting to discuss the possibility of an international collaboration.[6] Then, in October 1993, 77 people from 11 countries met to set up "The Cochrane Collaboration". This meeting was the first in what became a series of annual Cochrane Colloquia.

The principles of the Cochrane Collaboration

The Collaboration is based on ten principles:

1. Collaboration
2. Building on the enthusiasm of individuals
3. Avoiding duplication
4. Minimising bias
5. Keeping up to date
6. Ensuring relevance
7. Ensuring access
8. Continually improving the quality of its work
9. Continuity
10. Enabling wide participation

Structure of the Cochrane Collaboration

The Cochrane Collaboration has a number of elements, summarised in Figure 4.1.

Cochrane Collaboration

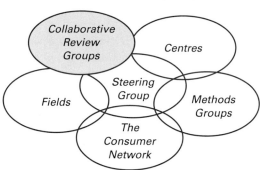

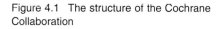

Figure 4.1 The structure of the Cochrane Collaboration

Collaborative Review Groups

The Collaboration has grown rapidly, and at the end of 2002 there were 49 review groups, between them covering all of the important areas of health care. Their main outputs are:

- systematic reviews, which are published electronically in the *Cochrane Library* and updated regularly
- a specialised register of clinical trials in their subject area.

Cochrane Methods Groups

Reviewers are supported by the work of various methods groups, for example statistical methods, health economics, non-randomised studies and health-related quality of life.

Cochrane Fields/Networks

These are groupings that represent a population, group, or type of care that overlaps multiple review group areas, for example: primary health care, child health, complementary medicine, vaccines, cancer.

The Consumer Network

Consumer participation is essential to the Collaboration, and the Consumer Network aims to:

- provide information and a forum for networking among consumers
- support the involvement of consumers throughout the Collaboration's activities
- liaise with consumer groups around the world
- encourage more consumers to become involved in the Collaboration, and to use its products.

Steering Group

This is the policy-making body of the Cochrane Collaboration.

The *Cochrane Library*

This is the main output of the Collaboration. It is the single best source of reliable evidence about the effects of healthcare interventions. It is updated quarterly and is distributed on an annual subscription basis on CD-ROM and via the internet. It includes several databases.

- **The Cochrane Database of Systematic Reviews** (CDSR) contains protocols and reviews prepared and maintained by Collaborative Review Groups. It includes a comments and criticisms system to enable users to improve the quality of Cochrane reviews.
- **The Database of Abstracts of Reviews of Effectiveness** (DARE) is assembled and maintained by the NHS Centre for Reviews and Dissemination in York, England. It contains critical assessments and structured abstracts of other systematic reviews, conforming to explicit quality criteria.
- **The Cochrane Central Register of Controlled Trials** (CENTRAL) contains bibliographic information on tens of thousands of controlled trials, including reports published in conference proceedings and many other sources not currently listed in other bibliographic databases.
- **The Cochrane Database of Methodology Reviews** (CDMR) summarises the empirical

basis for decisions about methods for systematic reviews and evaluations of health care.

- **The NHS Economic Evaluation Database** is a register of published economic evaluations of healthcare interventions.
- **The Cochrane Methodology Register** contains references to articles and books on the science of reviewing research.
- **The Health Technology Assessment Database** contains information on healthcare technology assessments.

The Cochrane Library also contains a handbook on how to conduct a systematic review, and a glossary of terms.

The Cochrane Skin Group

The CSG aims to provide the best evidence about the effects (beneficial and harmful) of interventions for skin diseases so that health professionals and consumers can make well-informed decisions about treatment.

History and structure

The CSG was established in 1997, after a workshop on dermato-epidemiology held at the World Congress of Dermatology. However, interest in forming the group had begun in 1992 and several exploratory meetings were held over the next 4 years.[7] The founder of the group and its Coordinating Editor is Professor Hywel Williams, of the Department of Dermatology, Queen's Medical Centre, Nottingham, UK, which is where the editorial team is based. The other members of the team are Dr Tina Leonard, the Review Group Coordinator, and Dr Finola Delamere, the Trials Search Coordinator.

An international board of editors consists of Dr Michael Bigby (Boston, USA), Dr Thomas Diepgen (Erlangen, Germany), Dr Sarah Garner (London, UK), Dr Sam Gibbs (Ipswich, UK), Sally Hollis (Lancaster, UK), Dr Sue Jessop (Cape Town,

South Africa), Philippa Middleton (Melbourne, Australia), Dr Dédée Murrell (Sydney, Australia), and Professor Luigi Naldi (Bergamo, Italy). The group's comments and criticism editor is Dr Urbà González (Spain). One of the CSG's particular strengths has been the involvement of consumers, who help it in many diverse ways. The Group currently supports about 280 reviewers worldwide and receives infrastructure support from the NHS Research and Development Programme.

Scope

A huge number of skin conditions need to be elucidated with clinically relevant questions about therapy. A full list of over 1000 of these skin conditions can be viewed on the CSG's website at http://www.nottingham.ac.uk/~muzd. The CSG's scope also includes cosmetic skincare products and the effectiveness of different models for delivery of health care for skin diseases. It does not include sexually transmitted diseases, which is now a separate medical specialty, and there is some overlap with other review groups such as the Musculoskeletal group for conditions such as lupus, which has important systemic aspects, and the Wounds group, which deals principally with venous ulcers.

Topics for review are chosen by potential reviewers with support and encouragement from the editorial base. All reviewers are volunteers. The Coordinating Editor and other editors also identify priority areas based on questions generated by colleagues. Public authorities in some countries provide grant support for specific topics. The CSG has no financial links with any pharmaceutical companies.

How does dermatology benefit from systematic reviews?

Dermatology can benefit from systematic reviews in three main ways.

- They provide a much more comprehensive literature search than a standard review. For example, when issues of *Clinical and Experimental Dermatology* from 1976 to 1997 were hand searched, 96 clinical trials were identified whereas Medline listed only 47.[8]

- People with skin problems are helped by clinical recommendations. For example, the CSG's review on "local treatments for cutaneous warts" found that simple topical treatments containing salicylic acid appear to be both effective and safe. There was no clear evidence that any other treatments have a particular advantage in terms of higher cure rates and/or fewer adverse effects.[9]
- Cochrane reviews have been criticised for not always providing evidence on which to base clinical decisions but a recent review examined all 26 systematic reviews relevant to dermatology in the CDSR and found sufficient evidence to make therapeutic recommendations in at least half of these reviews.[10] Even when no evidence is available, Cochrane reviews identify gaps in knowledge and frame the future research agenda. For example, the CSG's review on "Drugs for discoid lupus erythematosus" highlighted the need for RCTs looking at the use of potent topical steroid versus chloroquine/hydroxychloroquine.[11]

Editorial process

Each review is prepared in a defined manner to ensure consistency and high quality. First, before a review is attempted, the reviewers submit a protocol which includes an abstract, background, proposed method of searching the literature and who will check it, how articles will be selected for inclusion, and the type of data to be extracted consistently from these articles. This protocol is assigned to a "lead editor" who is responsible for guiding the authors through this preliminary stage. Support is also available from the Review Group Coordinator, usually via email. The reviewer also familiarises him/herself with the software that must be used for writing

the protocol and review. When the lead editor is satisfied, the protocol is sent out for peer review by the editors, an external content expert, a statistician and a consumer. The necessary revisions must be made and accepted by the Coordinating Editor before the protocol can be published in the *Cochrane Library*.

The review itself can take many months to complete. First, the required papers and other information have to be gathered. Then two independent co-reviewers decide on whether the papers qualify as suitably controlled and randomised trials that meet the inclusion criteria. The quality of these papers, based on the methods and analysis used, is also assessed. The data are extracted and analysed, a meta-analysis is done if appropriate and conclusions are drawn. The completed review is then resubmitted to the lead editor and if s/he is satisfied, it is again sent for peer review and revision before publication in the *Cochrane Library*.

After publication, comments and criticism about reviews can be made online directly from the *Cochrane Library*. There is also an obligation for all reviews to be updated every 2 years.

The role of consumers

Consumer involvement has been a strong feature of the CSG from the very beginning. This is because skin disease greatly affects the quality of life of the individual and because much of the trial work in skin disease has been dominated by answering questions that are important to the pharmaceutical industry. Consumers help us to redress that imbalance. At present (Autumn 2002) the skin group has 55 groups working on topics, both common and rare, such as acne, alopecia, bullous pemphigoid, eczema, excessive sweating, psoriasis, skin cancer and vitiligo. About 30 active consumers are involved at many levels. Initially they were recruited mainly through the National Eczema Society and the Vitiligo Society, but since we decided to always include a relevant consumer in the peer-review process, more consumers have become involved in this way. Increasingly consumers also take part in writing the review; two of the reviews in preparation have a consumer as lead author.

Our experience of consumer involvement is both positive and challenging. Consumers have little or no access to the support systems and infrastructure that professionals take for granted (for example information technology, administration, photocopying etc.). They have to meet many expenses themselves, from travel to telephone bills, and funding is often a major problem for them. However, their enthusiasm is boundless and infectious. Our consumers are highly motivated, and two of them even won stipends to attend the annual Cochrane Colloquium in Cape Town. Many of them also attend the UK-based meetings of the Collaboration and the CSG, and some are involved with the Collaboration at national level.

In particular consumers help us to ensure that our reviews are:

- relevant to patients and carers (i.e. outcomes are patient focused)
- written in language that is accessible to intelligent lay people.

Trials Register

An important part of the work of the Cochrane Skin Group is the development of a comprehensive international register containing reports of controlled clinical trials in dermatology. This register is a valuable resource for those preparing systematic reviews on dermatology topics.

Electronic search strategies have been developed by the Cochrane Collaboration to find reports of clinical trials covering all medical disciplines. These are regularly applied to Medline, Embase and other databases and are the main means by which the Cochrane Collaboration has built up the CENTRAL database of trials, which in May 2002 contained over 340 000 records.

Each review group develops its own search strategy related to its medical scope to find reports of trials that are relevant to its discipline. The CSG applies its "skin search strategy" to each new issue of the *Cochrane Library*. The records that result from this search are placed in a "pending" database and gradually transferred to the Specialised Skin Register once the paper copy of the reference has been checked. This "clean" electronic database contains only reports of RCTs and controlled clinical trials (CCTs) on subjects covered by the scope of the CSG. The database is sent to the *Cochrane Library* every quarter, where it becomes incorporated into the CENTRAL. Eventually this will build up within the *Cochrane Library* so that every record relevant to dermatology will have been checked for trial status and labelled, or will have been removed when it has been determined on closer inspection that the article is not a trial after all.

Hand searching

Electronic searches miss many reports of trials.[12] This may be because the articles were not written with a clear indication in the title or abstract that the contents describe a clinical trial, or because the journal has not been entered in a database. As there are well over 200 international dermatology publications, many of which are not on databases, electronic searching alone cannot identify trials that may have been published in these journals. The aim of the Collaboration is to identify reports of trials back to 1948. Much of this work can be done only by searching for trials by hand – "hand searching".

Hand searching refers to the task of physically turning each page of a journal looking for indications that an article reports a clinical trial. This huge task is being undertaken by the Collaboration as a "one-off" exercise to trawl systematically the medical literature worldwide for reports of trials. Each review group is responsible for searching for trials in journals relevant to their scope. This exercise includes searching journals that are listed on databases such as Medline. The advantage of hand searching is that as each article is examined page by page, references are found to trials that are mentioned only in the "Methods" section of a paper or in the correspondence pages. An example within our own review group shows the benefit of hand searching. When all the issues of *Archives of Dermatology* between 1976 and 1998 were searched, 270 trials were found. Of these 103 had not been identified by Medline because they had been classed as "journal article" or "letter", with no indication they were trial reports. In addition, there were 16 articles that were categorised as "randomised controlled trial", "controlled clinical trial" or "clinical trial" when in fact on closer inspection they were not trials at all. The Cochrane Collaboration and the National Library of Medicine are working together on the "Medline Re-Tagging" project to rectify these errors.

To prevent duplication of the considerable effort involved in hand searching, the Collaboration holds a Master List of the journals that are being searched. The Trials Search Coordinator of each review group is responsible for registering journals and for training the hand searchers.

A number of criteria must be met for an article to be a report of a clinical trial.

- A trial must be planned in advance and be a comparison of two or more interventions (where one may be a placebo).

- A trial must involve a single original population of human beings, or groups of human beings or parts of their body.
- If the allocation of the interventions to the single population is randomised and explicitly stated to be so this is classified as an RCT.

However, in many reports the method of allocation of interventions is not stated very clearly. These reports are classified as CCTs. There is much variation in the quality of the random allocation even among RCTs, so inevitably many of the CCTs turn out to be unreliable sources of evidence for the systematic reviewer. However, the hand searcher's task is to find reports of trials, not to make value judgements about the trials identified.

The future

The need for hand searching will diminish over the years as searching of older journals is completed. Also, journal editors are adopting the CONSORT guidelines (Consolidated Standards of Reporting Trials[13]), which aim to improve the standard of reporting of trials in publications. This will make it much easier to find trials electronically with simple search terms.

Other sources also need to be examined for valuable information about trials that have been performed. These are known by the term "grey literature" and include PhD and MD theses, pharmaceutical company records, conference proceedings etc. As it is known that trials with statistically significant results tend to be published more rapidly than those with less clear results,[14] it follows that a systematic reviewer needs to examine unpublished data that may contain valuable negative information about an intervention.

In the past it has been difficult to find out what research is already being done. There are now web-based clinical trial registers where trials can be registered, which should make it much easier in the future and help to prevent duplication of effort. The Current Controlled Trials Meta-Register[15] is an international searchable database of more than 125 000 ongoing RCTs and the National Research Register[16] is a register of research within the UK NHS. Within the CSG we have an Ongoing Trials web page[17] in which we invite dermatology trialists to lodge the (minimal) details of their clinical trial with their proposed outcome measures. This then provides a source of trial information for a systematic reviewer to refer to if the trial relates to their review topic. It also means that when the trial report is published the author will have proof that they have adhered to their original plans, particularly in relation to outcome measures.

The Specialised Skin Register is currently a database of reports of trials. However, many trials are carried out over several years and are multicentre studies, which often results in many publications relating to the same clinical trial. We therefore aim to gather these reports together to make the Register study based rather than report based. That should help the reviewer.

There is a unique obligation on Cochrane reviewers that they revisit their review periodically to update it in the light of new and newly unearthed evidence. This means that new reports of trials found by hand searching will be assessed. The Cochrane Collaboration is an international organisation but currently it is far too dominated by English-language publications, which may introduce their own bias.[18] As more studies are found in languages other than English and are incorporated into systematic reviews, we will all gain by having a more balanced and informed view about the usefulness of interventions.

Tasks undertaken by the Cochrane Skin Group

The work of the CSG encompasses:

- searching for trials (by hand and electronically)
- development and maintenance of a comprehensive register of trials (Specialised Skin Register)
- preparation of protocols and reviews
- disseminating the conclusions from the reviews as widely as possible – to healthcare managers, consumers and researchers.

The many roles for people in the CSG include:

- hand searchers, who systematically search dermatological journals, by hand, to identify trials and record these
- translators, as it is important to include evidence from all the literature, not just reports in English
- lead reviewers, who take responsibility for the review team preparing the protocol and the review
- co-reviewers, who help the lead reviewer to prepare the review
- peer reviewers, who help to ensure that the quality of Cochrane reviews is as high as possible
- consumers, who can take any of these roles and also help to write synopses of the reviews in lay terms, which are then published in various places, including the *Cochrane Library* website.

Contacting the Cochrane Skin Group

If you would like to help the CSG in any of the roles described above, please contact Dr Tina Leonard, the Group's Coordinator, who will be happy to send you further information about the CSG and the Cochrane Collaboration. The contact details of the editorial base are:

Cochrane Skin Group
Dermato-Epidemiology Unit
Queen's Medical Centre

University Hospital
Nottingham
NG7 2UH
UK
Tel: +44 (0)115 919 4415
Fax: +44 (0)115 970 9003

Coordinating Editor: Professor Hywel Williams
Tel: +44 (0)115 924 9924 extension 44539
Email: hywel.williams@nottingham.ac.uk

Review Group Coordinator: Dr Tina Leonard
Tel: +44 (0)115 919 4415
Email: tina.leonard@nottingham.ac.uk

Trials Search Coordinator: Dr Finola Delamere
Email: finola.delamere@nottingham.ac.uk

Useful websites

Cochrane Skin Group: http://www.nottingham.ac.uk/~muzd
Cochrane Centres: http://www.update-software.com/ccweb
Cochrane Library: http://www.cochrane.co.uk
Reviewer's handbook: http://www.update-software.com/ccweb/cochrane/revman.htm

References

1. Cochrane AL. *Effectiveness and Efficiency. Random Reflections on Health Services.* London: Nuffield Provincial Hospitals Trust, 1972. (Reprinted in 1989 in association with the BMJ.)
2. Cochrane AL. 1931–1971: a critical review, with particular reference to the medical profession. In: *Medicines for the Year 2000*. London: Office of Health Economics, 1979: 1–11.
3. Cochrane AL. Foreword. In: Chalmers I, Enkin M, Keirse MJNC, eds. *Effective Care in Pregnancy and Childbirth*. Oxford: Oxford University Press, 1989.
4. Chalmers I, Dickersin K, Chalmers TC. Getting to grips with Archie Cochrane's agenda. *BMJ* 1992;**305**:786–8.
5. Editorial. Cochrane's legacy. *Lancet* 1992;**340**:1131–2.
6. Chalmers I. The Cochrane Collaboration: preparing, maintaining and disseminating systematic reviews of the effects of health care. In: Warren KS, Mosteller F, eds. *Doing more good than harm: the evaluation of health care interventions. Ann NY Acad Sci* 1993;**703**: 156–63.
7. Williams HC, Adetugbo K, Li Wan Po A, Naldi L, Diepgen T, Murrell D. The Cochrane Skin Group. Preparing, maintaining, and disseminating systematic reviews of clinical interventions in dermatology. *Arch Dermatol* 1998;**134**:1620–6.
8. Delamere FM, Williams HC. How can hand searching the dermatological literature help people with skin problems? *Arch Dermatol* 2001;**137**:332–5.
9. Gibbs S, Harvey I, Sterling JC, Stark R. Local treatments for cutaneous warts (Cochrane Review). In: Cochrane Collaboration. *Cochrane Library*. Issue 3. Oxford: Update Software, 2001.
10. Parker ER, Schilling LM, Williams HC, Diba V, Delavalle RP. What's the point of systematic reviews in dermatology if all they show is "insufficient evidence"? *J Am Acad Dermatol* in press.
11. Jessop S, Whitelaw D, Jordaan F. Drugs for discoid lupus erythematosus (Cochrane Review). In: Cochrane Collaboration. *Cochrane Library*. Issue 3. Oxford: Update Software, 2001.
12. Adetugbo K, Williams H. How well are randomized controlled trials reported in the dermatology literature? *Arch Dermatol* 2000;**136**:381–5.
13. Moher D, Schulz KF, Altman DG *et al*. The CONSORT Statement: revised recommendations for improving the quality of reports of parallel-group randomized trials. *Ann Intern Med* 2001;**134**:657–62.
14. Clarke M, Hopewell S. Time lag bias in publishing results of clinical trials: a systematic review. 3rd Symposium on Systematic Reviews: Beyond the Basics. Oxford: Centre for Statistics in Medicine, 2000.
15. Current Controlled Trials. http://controlled-trials.com
16. Department of Health. Research and Development, Current Research: The National Research Register. http://www.doh.gov.uk/research/nrr.htm

17. Delamare F, Cochrane Skin Group. http://www.nottingham. ac.uk/~muzd/

18. Sterne JAC, Bartlett C, Juni P, Egger M. Do we need comprehensive literature searches? A study of publication and language bias in meta-analyses of controlled trials. 3rd Symposium on Systematic Reviews: Beyond the Basics. Oxford, 2000.

Part 2: The critical appraisal toolbox

Editor: Michael Bigby

5

Formulating well-built clinical questions

Berthold Rzany

Practising evidence-based medicine (EBM) centres on trying to find answers to clinically relevant questions based on individual patients. To make answering the questions feasible and practice of EBM possible, questions need to be structured.

Structuring well-built clinical questions

According to Sackett *et al.*[1] a well-built clinical question should be composed of four components:

1. the patient or problem
2. the intervention
3. the comparative intervention(s) (if necessary)
4. the clinically relevant outcome measure(s).[1]
   Well-built clinical questions about individual patients can be grouped into several categories: aetiology, diagnosis, therapy, prevention, prognosis and harm.

The first component of a well-built clinical question is an accurate description of the patient or problem. The next two components are accurate descriptions of the intervention(s). Interventions can be aetiologic factors, diagnostic tests, treatments, prognostic factors or harmful exposures. Several interventions (for example many treatments for psoriasis) might be appropriate for inclusion in the question. When

the focus is on treatment, the comparative intervention is usually an established treatment (for example. topical therapy with dithranol for psoriasis) or a placebo. The final component of the well-built clinical question is a clinically relevant outcome measure that is important to the treating dermatologist and the patient.

For example, a 71-year-old man presents with a painful cluster of vesicles on an erythematous base on his cheek. You suspect he has herpes zoster although herpes simplex is in your differential diagnoses. Examples of well-built clinical questions about diagnosis, therapy and prognosis would be[2]:

1. In an elderly man presenting with a vesicular eruption, is a viral culture or direct fluorescence antibody slide test more useful in establishing a diagnosis of herpes zoster?
2. In an elderly man with acutely painful herpes zoster, would treatment with antivirals alone or in combination with corticosteroids lead to more rapid resolution of pain and signs of infection?
3. If an elderly man who presents with acutely painful herpes zoster is treated or is left untreated, how likely is he to develop post-herpetic neuralgia?

Examples of poorly structured questions about this same patient would be:

Table 5.1   The four components of a structured question according to Sackett *et al.*[1]

Component	Patient or problem	Intervention	Comparison intervention (if feasible)	Clinically relevant outcome(s)
Explanation	Description of the patient based on demographic factors, past history and clinical presentation	Definition of the intervention. This could be a focused question (i.e. on one intervention) or a broader question (i.e. on several interventions)	Definition of the comparison intervention. Is there a gold standard?	Definition of what should be accomplished: Should the patient be healed? Should the condition (i.e. quality of life) of the patient be improved?
Example 1 (diagnostic procedure)	In this 28-year-old man with arthritis of the knees and circumscribed erythematous plaques with silvery scales on the extensor surfaces of the knees …	… are radiographs …	… compared with clinical criteria …	… helpful in securing the diagnosis of psoriatic arthritis?
Example 2 (therapeutic intervention)	In this 45-year-old man with recurrent plaques psoriasis of 10 years' duration …	… would PUVA treatment in combination with etretinate …	… compared with etretinate alone …	… lead to a longer period of remission?
Example 3 (prognosis)	What is the likelihood that children aged 4 years and under …	… with atopic eczema are more likely than …	… similar children who do not have atopic eczema …	… to develop asthma by the age of 13 years?

4. How do you make a diagnosis of herpes zoster?

5. What is the best treatment for herpes zoster?

6. What is the prognosis of herpes zoster?

There is no such thing as the one and only right question. In nearly every clinical situation, several well-built clinical questions are possible (Table 5.1). It is up to the physician and the patient to determine what the most important questions are.

The advantages of well-built clinical questions

A well-formed clinical question has two strong advantages: it makes finding the evidence easier and forces the clinician to specify the patient populations to which the evidence can be generalised and the outcomes that are clinically important.[2,3] A question like Question 4, 5 or 6 above will certainly lead to answers. However, obtaining the answer would require a considerable amount of time in searching and validating a vast amount of literature. Structuring the question as in Questions 1, 2 and 3 above would lead to more specific answers in considerably less time.

For example, consider the difference between searching Medline for Questions 2 and 4 above. Searching Medline to answer Question 4 using the search string "Herpes zoster and treatment" yields 3749 references, many of which are narrative review articles, bench research and case reports. Even limiting the search to randomised controlled clinical trials yields 211 references, many of which are poor-quality evidence. In contrast, searching Medline to answer Question 2 using the search string "Herpes zoster and (corticosteroid* or pred*) and (aciclovir or valiciclovir or famciclovir)" yields one reference that is a randomised controlled trial of the treatment of acute herpes zoster with aciclovir alone for 7 or 21 days and aciclovir plus prednisone for 7 or 21 days.[4]

What criteria might be used best to specify a question at the dermatology consultation? The answer to this question might vary according to patient attributes such as age, sex, past therapy and allergies. A question can be as only as good as the initial evaluation of the patient, which includes a detailed history and examination in order to obtain an accurate diagnosis. An exploration of which factors are important to the patient in terms of expectation of treatment outcome, willingness to put up with inconvenience of frequent medication, and tolerance of potential side-effects is also crucial at such an initial consultation. Specifying an outcome that means something to the dermatologist and patient is also important. For example, consider a 28-year-old man with psoriasis who is desperate for a remission of the visible plaques on his body because he is planning a once-in-a-lifetime holiday to the coast, where he wants to expose his skin whilst swimming. Finding trials that mention only 20–50% reduction in PASI scores as their sole outcome measure would be of little value. Of more interest to this man would be trials that specify the percentage of patients achieving complete remission after a course of therapy. Although a 30% reduction in PASI could be useful to another patient, it is simply a matter of choosing an outcome that seems clinically relevant to the patient in question.

Asking a clinically relevant and structured question is not as easy as it might appear, but it saves time and it is more likely to provide a useful answer than a vague unstructured one. Following the structure described in this section takes practice but increases the likelihood of ending up with a question that is a good base for the next steps in practicing evidence-based dermatology.

References

1. Sackett DL, Richardson WS, Rosenberg Q, Haynes RB. *Evidence Based Medicine. How to Practise and Teach EBM.* London: Churchill Livingstone, 1997.
2. Bigby M. Evidence-based medicine in dermatology. *Dermatol Clin* 2000;**18**:261–76.
3. Richardson W, Wilson M, Nishikawa J, Hayward R. The well-built clinical question key to evidence-based decisions (editorial). *ACP Journal Club* 1995;**123**:A12–13.
4. Whitley R, Weiss H, Gnann J *et al.* Acyclovir with and without prednisone for the treatment of herpes zoster. *Ann Intern Med* 1996;**125**:376–83.

6

Finding the best evidence

Michael Bigby

The ability to find the best evidence to answer clinical questions is crucial for practising evidence-based medicine. Finding evidence requires access to electronic searching, searching skills and available resources. Methods for finding systematic reviews and evidence about diagnosis, therapy and harm have been well developed.[1]

Evidence about therapy is the easiest to find. The best sources for finding the best evidence about treatment include:

- The *Cochrane Library*
- Searching the Medline and Embase databases
- Secondary journals and books (for example *ACP Journal Club, Evidence-based Medicine* and *Clinical Evidence*)
- Primary journals
- The National Guideline Clearinghouse (http://www.jcaai.org)
- Bandolier (http://www.jr2.ox.ac.uk/Bandolier)[2]

The Cochrane Library

The *Cochrane Library* contains systematic reviews of the treatment of diseases, a database of abstracts of reviews of effectiveness (DARE), and the Cochrane Central Register of Controlled Trials (CENTRAL). Volunteers, according to strict guidelines developed by the Cochrane Collaboration, write the systematic reviews included in the *Cochrane Library*. The latest issue of the *Cochrane Library* (2002, issue 3, accessed 13 Oct 2002) contained over 2000 completed systematic reviews. The number of

reviews of dermatological topics is increasing steadily.[1,2]

The CENTRAL is a database of over 300 000 controlled clinical trials. The registry is compiled by searching the Medline and Embase databases, and hand searching many journals. Hand searching journals to identify controlled clinical trials and randomised controlled clinical trials was undertaken because members of the Cochrane Collaboration noticed that many trials were incorrectly classified in the Medline database. As an example, Dr Finola Delamere of the Cochrane Skin Group hand searched the *Archives of Dermatology* from 1990 through 1998 and identified 99 controlled clinical trials. Nineteen of the trials were not classified as controlled clinical trials in Medline and 11 trials that were not controlled clinical trials were misclassified as controlled clinical trials in Medline.[3]

DARE is a database of abstracts of systematic reviews published in the medical literature. It contains over 3000 abstracts and bibliographic details on over 800 other published systematic reviews.[1,2]

The *Cochrane Library* is the best source for evidence about treatment. It is searched easily using simple Boolean combinations of search terms and by more sophisticated search strategies. The *Cochrane Library of Systematic Reviews*, DARE and the CENTRAL can be searched simultaneously. The *Cochrane Library* is available on a subscription basis on CD, and via the internet from Update Software (http://www. cochrane.co.uk). Subscriptions to the *Cochrane Library* are updated quarterly. The *Cochrane Library* should be available at your medical library.[1,2]

Medline searches

The second-best method for finding evidence about treatment and the best source for finding most other types of best evidence in dermatology is by searching the Medline database on a computer.[2,4] Medline is the National Library of Medicine's (NLM) bibliographic database covering the fields of medicine, nursing, dentistry, veterinary medicine, the healthcare system and the preclinical sciences. The Medline file contains bibliographic citations and author abstracts from approximately 3900 current biomedical journals published in the US and 70 other countries. The file contains approximately 9 million records dating back to 1966.[1,2,5]

Medline searches have inherent limitations that make their reliability less than ideal.[2] For example, Spuls *et al.* conducted a systematic review of systemic treatments for psoriasis.[6] Treatments analysed included UVB, PUVA, methotrexate, ciclosporin A and retinoids. The authors used an exhaustive strategy to find relevant references, including Medline searches, contacting pharmaceutical companies, polling leading authorities, reviewing abstract books of symposia and congresses, and reviewing textbooks, reviews, editorials, guideline articles and the reference lists of all papers identified. Of 665 studies found, 356 (54%) were identified by the Medline search (range 30–70% for different treatment modalities). No references beyond those identified by Medline searching were provided by the 17 of 23 authorities who responded.[6]

More than 20 vendors of Medline on line and on CD are available. Haynes *et al.* compared

several vendors of Medline on line and on CD to determine which was best in terms of finding relevant articles and excluding irrelevant articles. Assessed on combined rankings for the highest number of relevant and the lowest number of irrelevant citations retrieved, SilverPlatter CD-ROM Medline clinical journal subset performed best for librarians searches, whereas PaperChase online system worked best for clinician searches. For cost per relevant citation, Dialog's Knowledge Index performed best for both librarian and clinician searches.[7]

Regardless of the platform used, the key to Medline searching is to find relevant articles and to exclude irrelevant citations. Several useful techniques can greatly aid your ability to accomplish this goal. Searches are generally done on the basis of boolean combinations of search terms. For example, our search for best evidence about drug treatment of onychomycosis might read [onychomycosis and (terbinafine or itraconazole or fluconazole) and not case reports].* This search would identify articles on onychomycosis using any of the listed drugs and excluding case reports.[1,2]

It is important to understand the difference between textword and MeSH searching and to be able to do both.[2] Many of the programs used to search the Medline database automatically do textword and MeSH searches. MeSH terms include all of the terms in the medical subject headings, a controlled vocabulary of keywords used to index Medline. Each Medline citation is given a group of MeSH terms that relate to the subject of the paper from which it is drawn. Frequently, MeSH terms will have an additional subheading which further defines how the MeSH term relates to the article with which it is

---

*The convention used throughout for search entries is that Boolean operations within parentheses are done first.

associated.[2] This subheading is appended to the MeSH term, for example "onychomycosis diagnosis".

Indexing articles is not an exact science. The MeSH headings assigned by the NLM may not coincide with the intent of the author or the majority of searchers for several reasons: authors may not clearly express their intent; indexers are usually not experts in the field of the article they are indexing; and the mistakes associated with doing repetitive tasks occur.[2] Relevant articles may be missed when they are not assigned the appropriate MeSH heading. Irrelevant articles may be included in a MeSH search if they are assigned to the wrong MeSH heading. For example, the Cochrane Collaboration identified major problems in the Medline indexing of randomised controlled trials.[2]

Textword searches allow one to search articles for words within the title and abstract that are important to, and coincide with, the intent of the author. However, textword searches are subject to several problems – authors may not describe their methods or objectives well, or may make errors in spelling, omission or commission.[2] The problem of misspelling can be illustrated by doing a textword search for "pruritis" (pruritus spelled incorrectly). This search yielded more than 40 references in which the word has been misspelled. Many of these references may not be detected in a search for pruritus (spelled correctly).[2]

Boolean topic searches will often contain too many or too few references. They may contain many irrelevant citations and miss many relevant citations. Several techniques will help make searches more sensitive (i.e. pick up relevant citations) and more specific (i.e. exclude irrelevant citations).[2] To increase the sensitivity of searches, searching both textword and MeSH headings, exploding MeSH headings and using truncation

may be helpful. MeSH term searches can be "exploded" to include all terms that are logical subsets of the term entered.[2] For example, exploding the MeSH term "onychomycosis" will retrieve all the articles that use that MeSH term, whether they have subheadings or not. Many of the programs used to search the Medline database automatically explode searches of MeSH terms or MeSH major topics.

Truncation refers to searching using the root of a word to allow variants of the word to be detected. For example, a search of "onychomycosis and controlled clinical trial" will detect fewer studies than a search for "onychomycosis and control*" (where "control*" contains a wild card that will allow detection of all words that begin with the root "control"). Truncation can be performed on textword and MeSH heading searches.

To increase the specificity of searches, selecting specific subheadings of MeSH terms and limiting the search may be helpful. MeSH heading terms can be limited to specific subheadings to help narrow search results to relevant articles. For example, onychomycosis has subheadings that restrict retrieved articles to ones dealing with diagnosis or drug treatment.[2] Searches can be limited in many ways, including publication type, language, human subjects and date of publication. Restricting the publication type to randomised controlled trial or case-control study is a useful way to limit retrieved articles to those of highest quality.

Performing a sensitive or specific search from scratch is often a time-consuming task, and arriving at an efficient search strategy to suit one's particular needs is sometimes a work of art. Once accomplished, it is important to be able to edit, save and retrieve the search strategy. The saved strategy can then be used in future searches of different subjects without having to rethink or retype the whole search procedure. The methods for performing these techniques (textword and MeSH searching, exploding, truncation, using subheadings, limiting and saving) vary according to the platform used. Mastering them will greatly improve searching efficiency.

Specific search strategies – "filters" – have been developed to help find relevant references and exclude irrelevant references for best evidence about diagnosis, therapy, prognosis, harm and prevention.[8] You can limit your results to systematic reviews using the following strategy:

1. subjects of interest (for example onychomycosis)
2. REVIEW-ACADEMIC (use LIMIT)
3. REVIEW-TUTORIAL (use LIMIT)
4. Systematic$ and (review$ or overview$) (textword)
5. (meta?analy* or meta analy*) (textword)
6. 1 and (2 or 3 or 4 or 5) (combine).

The strategy to search the Medline database for evidence about diagnosis is to combine the subject or subjects with a combination of terms as follows:[2]**

1. Subject (for example onychomycosis)

Terms to use for maximum sensitivity of the search:

2. sensitivity-and-specificity (MeSH) or
3. sensitivity (textword) or
4. diagnosis (subheading) or
5. diagnostic use (subheading) or
6. specificity (textword)

Terms to use for maximum specificity of the search:

_____

**The terms used in the examples were specifically designed for use with OVID to search the Medline database. They may have to be modified for use with other searching platforms. The use of OVID is not an endorsement. It is an available platform with which the author has competence.

7. explode sensitivity-and-specificity (MeSH) or
8. (predictive and value*) (textword)

If in a hurry, the best one-term strategy:

9. sensitivity (textword)

For example, using OVID to search the Medline database, a specific search for tests to establish a diagnosis of onychomycosis would be [1 and (7 or 8)], a sensitive search [1 and (2 or 3 or 4 or 5 or 6)], and a quick search (1 and 9).

The strategy to search the Medline database for evidence about therapy is to combine the subject or subjects with a combination of terms as follows[2]:

Subjects:

1. disorder (for example onychomycosis)
2. treatment (for example terbinafine)
3. alternative treatment (for example itraconazole)

For maximum sensitivity:

4. randomised controlled trial (publication type, limit) or
5. drug trial (subheading) or
6. therapeutic use (subheading) or
7. random* (textword)

For maximum specificity:

8. double and blind* (textword) or
9. placebo* (textword)

Best one-term strategy:

10. clinical-trial (publication type, limit)

For example, using OVID, a specific search for therapy of onychomycosis with terbinafine or itraconazole would be [1 and (2 or 3) and (8 or 9)], a sensitive search [1 and (2 or 3) and (4 or 5 or 6 or 7)], and a quick search [1 and (2 or 3) and 10].

The suggested strategy to search the Medline database for evidence about harm is to combine the subject or subjects with a combination of terms as follows[2]:

Subjects:

1. medication (for example terbinafine)
2. alternative medication (for example itraconazole)

For maximum sensitivity:

3. explode cohort-studies (MeSH) or
4. explode risk (MeSH) or
5. odds and ratio* (textword) or
6. relative and risk (textword) or
7. case and control* (textword)

For maximum specificity:

8. case-control-studies (MeSH) or
9. cohort-studies (MeSH)

Best one-term strategy:

10. risk (textword)

For example, using OVID, a specific search for adverse effects of terbinafine or itraconazole would be [(1 or 2) and (8 or 9)], a sensitive search [(1 or 2) and (3 or 4 or 5 or 6 or 7)], and a quick search [(1 or 2) and 10]. High-quality case-control or cohort studies are not frequently found in the dermatological literature. Sensitive search strategies and scanning the long lists of articles retrieved are likely to yield the best evidence most efficiently.

These filters have been incorporated into the PubMed Clinical Search engine of the NLM and are available at http://www.ncbi.nlm.nih.gov/PubMed/clinical.html.[8] PubMed Clinical Search

is the preferred method for searching the Medline database for best evidence. It can be freely used by anyone with internet access.[1,2]

Embase searches

Embase is Excerpta Medica's database covering drugs, pharmacology and biomedical specialties.[9] Embase has better coverage than Medline of European and non-English language sources and may be more up to date.[9] The overlap in journals covered by Medline and Embase is about 34% (range 10–75% depending on the subject).[9–11]

Secondary journals

Structured abstracts of articles are published in secondary journals (for example *Evidence-based Medicine and Evidence-based Dermatology*). The articles are selected strictly on the basis of methodological quality and are accompanied by commentary that puts the information into clinical perspective. *Evidence-based Medicine* is available on line at http://ebm.journals.com/.

Evidence-based Dermatology is published quarterly in the *Archives of Dermatology. Clinical Evidence* is a 6-monthly updated compendium of evidence on the effects of common clinical interventions and many skin related diseases are included[2]. It is available through the American College of Physicians and the British Medical Association.[1,2]

Primary journals

Full text versions of many primary journals are available via the internet. Journals in this category include the *British Medical Journal (BMJ), New England Journal of Medicine, Annals of Internal Medicine, Journal of the American Medical Association (JAMA), The Lancet* and the *Canadian Medical Association Journal*. The

Wisdom website provides a handy portal to these journals (http://www.uib.no/isf/people/atle/ebm.htm#BM4_secondary).

The National Guideline Clearinghouse

The National Guideline Clearinghouse maintains a database of guidelines for the treatment of diseases, written by panels of experts following strict guidelines of evidence. The database is accessible via the internet (http://www.guideline.gov/index.asp). However, the current coverage of dermatological topics is limited.

Bandolier

Bullet points of evidence-based medicine (reviews and articles related to evidence-based medicine) are published in Bandolier, available via the internet at http://www.jr2.ox.ac.uk/Bandolier/. Reviews of treatment of warts and of new oral antifungals have appeared in it.[1,2]

References

1. Bigby M, Szklo M. Evidence-based dermatology. In: Freedberg IM, Eisen AZ, Wolf K, Austen KF, Goldsmith LA, Katz SI, eds. Fitzpatrick's *Dermatology in General Medicine, 6 ed.* New York: McGraw Hill, in press.

2. Bigby M. Evidence-based medicine in a nutshell. A guide to finding and using the best evidence in caring for patients. *Arch Dermatol* 1998;**134**:1609–18.

3. Delamere FM, Williams HC. How can hand searching the dermatological literature benefit people with skin problems? *Arch Dermatol* 2001;**137**:332–5.

4. Oxman AD, Sackett DL, Guyatt GH. Users' guide to the medical literature I. How to get started. *JAMA* 1993;**270**: 2093–5.

5. PubMed Overview. http://www4.ncbi.nlm.nih.gov/PubMed/overview.html (accessed 12 Jan 1998).

6. Spuls PI, Witkamp L, Bossuyt PM, Bos JD. A systematic review of five systemic treatments for severe psoriasis. *Br J Dermatol* 1997;**137**:943–9.

7. Haynes RB, Walker S, McKibbon KA, Johnson ME, Willan AR. Performance of 27 Medline systems tested by searches with clinical questions. *J Am Med Inform Assoc* 1994;**1**:285–95.

8. Haynes B. PubMed Clinical Queries using research methodology filters. http://www.ncbi.nlm.nih.gov/PubMed/clinical.html (accessed 29 July 1999).

9. Greenhalgh T. *How to Read a Paper. The Basics of Evidence-based Medicine.* London: BMJ Books 1997:196.

10. Smith B, Darzins P, Quinn M, Heller R. Modern methods of searching the medical literature. *Med J Aust* 1992;**157**: 603–11.

11. Mulrow C, Oxman A, eds. Cochrane Collaboration Handbook (updated 1 March 1997). In: Cochrane Collaboration. *Cochrane Library* Oxford: Update Software 1997.

7

The hierarchy of evidence

Michael Bigby

Once appropriate questions have been formulated, what are the sources for **the best evidence** to answer these questions? Potential sources include personal experience, colleagues or experts, textbooks, articles published in journals and systematic reviews. An important principle of evidence-based medicine is that the quality (strength) of evidence is based on a concept of a **hierarchy of evidence**. This hierarchy of evidence consists of, in descending order[1,2]:

- results of systematic reviews of well designed studies
- results of one or more well designed studies,
- results of large case series
- expert opinion
- personal experience.

The ordering of the hierarchy of evidence has been widely discussed, actively debated and sometimes hotly contested.[3–7]

Well done systematic reviews of well-performed clinical studies (especially if the studies have results of similar magnitude and direction, and if there is statistical homogeneity) are most likely to have results that are true and useful. A systematic review is an overview that answers a specific clinical question, contains a thorough and unbiased search of the relevant literature, explicit criteria for assessing studies and structured presentation of the results.

A systematic review that uses quantitative methods to summarise results is a meta-analysis.[3,8] Meta-analysis is credited with allowing recognition of important treatment effects by combining the results of small trials that individually lacked the power to demonstrate differences between treatments. For example, the benefits of intravenous streptokinase in acute myocardial infarction was recognised from the results of a cumulative meta-analysis of smaller trials at least a decade before the treatment was recommended by experts and before it was demonstrated to be efficacious in large clinical trials.[3,4] Meta-analysis has been criticised because of discrepancies between the results of meta-analysis and results of large clinical trials.[3,5–7] For example, results of a meta-analysis of 14 small studies of calcium in the treatment of pre-eclampsia showed benefit of treatment, whereas a large trial failed to show a treatment effect.[3] The frequency of discrepancies ranges from 10% to 23%.[3] Discrepancies can often be explained by differences in treatment protocols, heterogeneity of study populations or changes that occur over time.[3] Not all systematic reviews and meta-analyses are equal. Systematic reviews conducted within the Cochrane Collaboration are rated among the best, but even then up to a third may contain significant problems.[9,10] Methods for assessing the quality of each type of analysis are available.[2,11]

The type of clinical study that constitutes best evidence is determined by the category of the question being asked (Table 7.1).[12] Questions about diagnosis are best addressed by comparisons with a reference standard

Table 7.1 Grades of evidence[1,2]

Grade	Level of evidence	Therapy/prevention Harm	Prognosis/aetiology	Diagnosis
A	1a	Systematic review (with homogeneity[a]) of RCTs	Systematic review (with homogeneity) of inception cohort studies, or a CPG validated on a test set	Systematic review (with homogeneity) of Level 1 (see column 2) diagnostic studies, or a CPG validated on a test set
	1b	Individual RCT (with narrow confidence intervals)	Individual inception cohort study with at least 80% follow up	Independent blind comparison of an appropriate spectrum of consecutive patients, all of whom have undergone both the diagnostic test and the reference standard
	1c	All or none[b]	All-or-none case series	Very high sensitivity or specificity
B	2a	Systematic review (with homogeneity) of cohort studies	Systematic review (with homogeneity) of either retrospective cohort studies or untreated control groups in RCTs	Systematic review (with homogeneity) of at least level 2 (see column 2) diagnostic studies
	2b	Individual cohort study (including low quality RCT; for example <80% follow up)	Retrospective cohort study or follow up of untreated control patients in an RCT, or CPG not validated in a test set	Independent blind comparison but either in non-consecutive patients, or confined to a narrow spectrum of study individuals (or both), all of whom have undergone both the diagnostic test and the reference standard, or a diagnostic CPG not validated in a test set
	2c	"Outcomes" research[c]		
	3a	Systematic review (with homogeneity) of case-control studies		Systematic review (with homogeneity) of 3b (see column 2) and better studies
	3b	Individual case-control study		Independent blind comparison of an appropriate spectrum, but the reference standard was not applied to all study patients
C	4	Case series (and poor quality cohort and case-control studies)	Case series (and poor quality prognostic cohort studies)	Reference standard was not applied independently or not applied blindly

(*Continued*)

Table 7.1 (*Continued*)

Grade	Level of evidence	Therapy/prevention Harm	Prognosis/aetiology	Diagnosis
D	5	Expert opinion without explicit critical appraisal, or based on physiology, bench research or "first principles"		

These levels were generated in a series of iterations among members of the NHS R&D Centre for Evidence-based Medicine (Chris Ball, Dave Sackett, Bob Phillips, Brian Haynes and Sharon Straus). For details see http://cebm.jr2.ox.ac.uk/docs/levels.html (accessed 17 Sep 1998). Recommendations based on this approach apply to "average" patients and may need to be modified in light of an individual patient's unique biology (risk, responsiveness etc.) and preferences about the care they receive.

RCT, randomised controlled trial; CPG, clinical practice guideline – a systematically developed statement designed to help practitioners and patients make decisions about appropriate health care for specific clinical circumstances.

[a]Homogeneity: lacking variation in the direction and magnitude of results of individual studies.

[b]All or none: interventions that produced dramatic increases in survival or outcome, for example streptomycin for tuberculosis meningitis.

[c]Outcomes research includes cost-benefit, cost-effectiveness and cost-utility analysis.

evaluated in an appropriate spectrum of patients where the test is likely to be used.[2,11,13,14] Questions about therapy and prevention are best addressed by randomised controlled trials (RCTs).[2,11,15,16] Cohort studies or case-control studies best address questions about prognosis, harm and disease aetiology.[2,11,17,18] Methods for assessing the quality of each type of evidence are available.[2,9]

The RCT has become the gold standard for determining treatment efficacy, following the publication in 1948 of the trial that demonstrated that streptomycin was effective in the treatment of tuberculosis.[19] Over 327 700 RCTs have been recorded in the Cochrane Central Register of Controlled Trials and thousands more probably exist in an unpublished form.[20] Large inclusive fully blinded RCTs are likely to provide the best possible evidence about effectiveness.[21–23] However, this assumption about methods should be tested empirically, just as assumptions about treatment effects need to be substantiated by empirical evidence.[4] Studies have demonstrated that failure to use randomisation or adequate concealment of allocation resulted in larger estimates of treatment effects, caused predominantly by a poorer prognosis in non-randomly selected control groups compared with randomly selected control groups.[23]

Expert opinion can be valuable, particularly for rare conditions in which the expert has the most experience or when other forms of evidence are not available. However, several studies have demonstrated that expert opinion often lags significantly behind conclusive evidence.[1] Experts should be aware of the quality of evidence that exists.

Whereas personal experience is an invaluable part of becoming a competent physician, the pitfalls of relying too heavily on personal experience have been widely documented.[1,24,25] Nisbett and Ross extensively reviewed people's ability to draw inferences from personal experience and documented several pitfalls.[26] They include:

- overemphasis on vivid anecdotal occurrences and underemphasis on significant statistically strong evidence;
- bias in recognising and accepting evidence that supports one's beliefs, and parallel failure to recognise or accept evidence that contradicts one's beliefs;

- persistence of beliefs in spite of overwhelming evidence presented against.

Although textbooks appear to be a valuable source of evidence, they have several well-documented shortcomings. First, by virtue of how they are written, produced and distributed, most are about 2 years out of date at the time of publication. Most textbook chapters are narrative reviews that do not consider the quality of the evidence reported.[1,2] They also tend to reflect the biases and shortcomings of the experts who write them.

More detailed studies of the relationship of study type and the direction and magnitude of purported benefit are needed in dermatology in order to guide dermatologists on the relative merits of different study designs. In the meantime, the hierarchy of evidence should not be conceptualised as a linear phenomenon (i.e. as a scale going from "good" to "bad"). The quality and relevance of evidence should be considered. Thus, a well-conducted large cohort study may be more reliable than a small RCT that has violated most aspects of good RCT design and reporting. Similarly, a small RCT of moderate quality dealing with the exact problem that the patient is complaining about (for example lipodermatosclerosis) is likely to be more useful than a large RCT dealing with a different problem (for example venous stasis ulcer).

References

1. Sackett DL, Haynes RB, Guyatt GH, Tugwell P. *Clinical Epidemiology. A Basic Science for Clinical Medicine.* Boston: Little, Brown and Company, 1991:441.

2. Greenhalgh T. *How to Read a Paper. The Basics of Evidence Based Medicine.* London: BMJ Books, 1997:196.

3. Lau J, Ionnidis JPA, Schmid CH. Summing up evidence: one answer is not always enough. *Lancet* 1998;**351**:123–7.

4. Lau J, Antman EM, Jimenez-Silva J, Kupelnick B, Mosteller F, Chalmers TC. Cumulative meta-analysis of therapeutic trials for myocardial infarction [see comments]. *N Engl J Med* 1992;**327**:248–54.

5. Villar J, Carroli G, Belizan JM. Predictive ability of meta-analyses of randomised controlled trials [see comments]. *Lancet* 1995;**345**:772–6.

6. Cappelleri JC, Ioannidis JP, Schmid CH *et al.* Large trials v meta-analysis of smaller trials: how do their results compare? *JAMA* 1996;**276**:1332–8.

7. LeLorier J, Gregoire G, Benhaddad A, Lapierre J, Derderian F. Discrepancies between meta-analyses and subsequent large randomized, controlled trials. *N Engl J Med* 1997;**337**:536–42.

8. Chalmers I, Altman D, eds. *Systematic Reviews.* London: BMJ Publishing Group, 1995.

9. Jadad AR, Moher M, Browman GP, Booker L, Sigouin C, Fuentes M. Systematic reviews and meta-analyses on treatment of asthma: critical evaluation. *BMJ* 2000;**320**: 537–40.

10. Olsen O, Middleton P, Ezzo J, Gøtzsche PC *et al.* Quality of Cochrane reviews: assessment of sample from 1998. *BMJ* 2001;**323**:829–32.

11. Sackett D, Richardson W, Rosenberg W, Haynes R. *Evidence-Based Medicine: How to Practise and Teach EBM.* Edinburgh: Churchill Livingstone, 1996:250.

12. Ball C, Sackett D, Phillips RBH, Straus S. Levels of evidence and grades of recommendations. http://cebm. jr2.ox.ac.uk/docs/levels.html (accessed 31 July 1999).

13. Jaeschke R, Guyatt G, Sackett DL. Users' guides to the medical literature III. How to use an article about a diagnostic test A. Are the results of the study valid? *JAMA* 1994;**271**:389–91.

14. Jaeschke R, Guyatt GH, Sackett DL. Users' guides to the medical literature III. How to use an article about a diagnostic test B. What are the results and will they help me in caring for my patients? *JAMA* 1994;**271**: 703–7.

15. Guyatt GH, Sackett DL, Cook DJ. Users' guides to the medical literature II. How to use an article about therapy or prevention A. Are the results of the study valid? *JAMA* 1993;**270**:2598–601.

16. Guyatt GH, Sackett DL, Cook DJ. Users' guides to the medical literature II. How to use an article about therapy or prevention B. What were the results and will they help me in caring for my patients? *JAMA* 1994;**271**:59–63.

17. Levine M, Walter S, Lee H, Haines T, Holbrook A, Moyer V. Users' guides to the medical literature IV. How to use an article about harm. *JAMA* 1994;**271**:1615–19.

18. Laupacis A, Wells G, Richardson WS, and Tugwell P. Users' guides to the medical literature V. How to use an article about prognosis. *JAMA* 1994;**272**:234–8.

19. Anonymous. Medical Research Council Streptomycin in Tuberculosis Trials Committee. Streptomycin treatment of pulmonary tuberculosis. *BMJ* 1948;**ii**: 769–82.

20. Cochrane Collaboration. *Cochrane Library*. Issue 4. Oxford: Update Software, 2001.

21. Barton S. Which clinical studies provide the best evidence: the best RCT still trumps the best observational study. *BMJ* 2000;**321**:255–6.

22. Pocock SJ, Elbourne DR. Randomized trials or observational tribulations? *N Engl J Med* 2000;**342**:1907–9.

23. Kunz R, Oxman AD. The unpredictability paradox: review of empirical comparisons of randomised and non-randomised clinical trials. *BMJ* 1998;**317**:1185–90.

24. Bigby M, Gadenne A-S. Understanding and evaluating clinical trials. *J Am Acad Dermatol* 1996;**34**:555–90.

25. Hines DC, Goldheizer JW. Clinical investigation: a guide to its evaluation. *Am J Obstet Gynecol* 1969;**105**:450–87.

26. Nisbett R, Ross L. *Human Inference: Strategies and Shortcomings of Social Judgement*. Englewood Cliffs, NJ: Prentice-Hall Inc.,1980.

8

How to critically appraise systematic reviews and meta-analyses

Michael Bigby and Hywel Williams

A systematic review is an overview that answers a specific clinical question, contains a thorough, unbiased search of the relevant literature, explicit criteria for assessing studies and structured presentation of the results. Many systematic reviews incorporate a meta-analysis, that is, a quantitative pooling of several similar studies to produce one overall summary of treatment effect.[1,2] Meta-analysis provides an objective and quantitative summary of evidence that is amenable to statistical analysis.[1] Meta-analysis allows recognition of important treatment effects by combining the results of small trials that individually might have lacked the power to consistently demonstrate differences among treatments. Meta-analysis has been criticised for the discrepancies between the results of meta-analysis and results from large clinical trials.[3–6] The frequency of discrepancies ranges from 10% to 23%.[3] Discrepancies can often be explained by differences in treatment protocols, differences in study populations or changes that occur over time.[3] Because of the importance of considering the need to have clear objectives, explicit criteria for study selection, an assessment of the quality of included studies and prior consideration of which studies to combine, meta-analyses that are not conducted within the context of a systematic review should be viewed with great caution.[7]

A systematic review can be viewed as a scientific and systematic examination of the available evidence. A good systematic review will have explicitly stated objectives (the focused clinical question), materials (the relevant medical literature) and methods (the way studies are assessed and summarised). The steps taken during a systematic review are shown in Box 8.1.

> **Box 8.1 The six steps of undertaking a systematic review**
>
> - Asking a clearly focused question
> - An explicit and thorough search of the literature
> - Data extraction
> - Critical appraisal of the quality of the primary studies
> - Quantitative pooling of the data if appropriate
> - Interpretation of the data, including implications for clinical practice and further research

Not all systematic reviews and meta-analyses are equal. A systematic review should be conducted in a manner that will include all the relevant trials, minimise the introduction of bias, and synthesise the results to be as truthful and useful to clinicians as possible. A systematic review can only be as good as the clinical trials that it includes. The criteria to critically appraise systematic reviews and meta-analyses are shown in Box 8.2. In general, these criteria are similar to those used to appraise the individual studies that make up the systematic review. Detailed explanations of each criterion are available.[1,7]

Box 8.2 Critical appraisal of a systematic review[7]

Are the results of this systematic review valid?

- Did the review address a focused clinical question?[a]
- Were the criteria used to select articles for inclusion appropriate?[a]
- Is it unlikely that important, relevant studies were missed?[b]
- Was the validity of the included studies appraised?[b]
- Were assessments of studies reproducible?[b]
- Were the results similar from study to study?[b]

Are the valid results of this systematic review important?

- What are the overall results of the review in terms of magnitude of benefit or harm?
- How precise were the results?

Can you apply this valid, important evidence in caring for your patient?

- Can the results be applied to my patient's care?
- Were all clinically important outcomes considered?
- Are the benefits worth the harms and costs?

[a]Primary guides
[b]Secondary guides

Asking a clear question

The validity criteria are designed to ensure that the systematic review is conducted in a manner that minimises the introduction of bias. Like the well-built clinical question for individual studies, a focused clinical question for a systematic review should contain four elements[8]:

1. a patient, group of patients or problem
2. an intervention

3. comparison interventions
4. specific outcomes

The patient groups should be similar to the majority of patients seen in the population to which one wishes to apply the results of the systematic review. The interventions studied should be those commonly available in practice. Outcomes reported should be those that are most relevant to physicians and patients.

Sources of evidence within a systematic review

The overwhelming majority of systematic reviews involve therapy. Therefore, randomised controlled clinical trials should be used for systematic reviews of therapy if they are available because they are generally less susceptible to selection and information bias than are other study designs. The quality of included trials is assessed using the criteria that are used to evaluate individual randomised controlled clinical trials. The quality criteria commonly used include:

- concealed random allocation
- groups similar in terms of known prognostic factors
- equal treatment of groups
- accounting for all patients entered into the trial in analysing results (intent-to-treat design).

These are discussed in more detail in Chapter 9.

Systematic reviews of treatment efficacy should always include an assessment of common and serious adverse events as well as efficacy, in order to come to an informed and balanced decision about the utility of a treatment. Randomised controlled trials are rarely a reliable source of identification of adverse reactions, unless the adverse events are very common. Other sources of evidence such as case–control studies, case reports and post-marketing surveillance studies should therefore be examined, as discussed in Chapter 10.

The hazards of "quick" searches

A sound systematic review can be performed only if most or all of the available data are examined. Simply performing a quick Medline search using "clinical trial" as publication type is rarely adequate because complex and sensitive search strategies are needed to identify all potential trials, and because clinical trials that are published in a journal not listed by Medline will be missed. Potential sources for finding studies about treatment include: The Cochrane Central Register of Controlled Trials (CENTRAL), which is part of the *Cochrane Library*, Medline, Embase, bibliographies of studies, review articles and textbooks, symposia proceedings, pharmaceutical companies and contacting experts in the field. Searching the literature is discussed in more detail in Chapter 6.

The CENTRAL is a database of over 300 000 controlled clinical trials and is now the largest single and most complete database of clinical trials worldwide. The CENTRAL has been compiled through several complex searches of the Medline and Embase databases, and by hand searching many journals, a process that is quality controlled and monitored by the Cochrane Collaboration in Oxford, UK. Hand searching of journals to identify controlled clinical trials and randomised controlled clinical trials was undertaken because members of the Cochrane Collaboration noticed that many trials were incorrectly classified in the Medline database. As an example, Adetugbo *et al.* hand searched the *Archives of Dermatology* from 1990 to 1998 and identified 99 controlled clinical trials. Nineteen of the trials were not classified as controlled clinical trials in Medline and 11 trials that were not controlled clinical trials were misclassified as controlled clinical trials in Medline.[9]

Medline is the National Library of Medicine's (NLM) bibliographic database covering the fields of medicine, nursing, dentistry, veterinary medicine, the healthcare system and the preclinical sciences. The Medline file contains bibliographic citations and author abstracts from approximately 3900 current biomedical journals published in the US and 70 other countries. The file contains approximately 9 million records dating back to 1966.[10]

Medline searches have inherent limitations that make their reliability less than ideal.[11] For example, Spuls *et al.* conducted a systematic review of systemic treatments for psoriasis.[12] Treatments analysed included UVB, PUVA, methotrexate, ciclosporin A and retinoids. The authors used an exhaustive strategy to find relevant references, including Medline searches, contacting pharmaceutical companies, polling leading authorities, reviewing abstract books of symposia and congresses, and reviewing textbooks, reviews, editorials, guideline articles and the reference lists of all papers identified. Of 665 studies found, 356 (54%) were identified by a Medline search (range 30–70% for different treatment modalities).[12]

Embase is Excerpta Medica's database covering drugs, pharmacology and biomedical specialties.[1] Embase has better coverage of European and non-English language sources and may be more up to date than Medline.[1] The overlap in journals covered by Medline and Embase is about 34% (range 10–75% depending on the subject).[1,13,14]

Publication bias

Publication bias – the tendency that studies that are easy to locate are more likely to show "positive" effects – is an important concern for systematic reviews; a useful review of this subject can be found elsewhere.[15] Publication bias results from allowing factors other than the quality of the study to influence its acceptability for publication. Several studies have shown that factors such as sample size, direction and statistical significance of findings, or investigators' perception of whether the findings are "interesting", are related to the likelihood of publication.[16,17] Language bias may also be a problem – studies that are "positive" have a tendency to be published in an English language journal and also more quickly than inconclusive or negative studies.[16,17] A thorough systematic review should therefore include a search for high-quality, unpublished trials and should not be restricted to journals written in English. Studies with small samples are less likely to be published, especially if they have negative results.[16,17] By emphasising only those studies that have positive results, this type of publication bias jeopardises one of the main goals of meta-analysis (i.e. an increase in power when pooling results of small studies). Creation of study registers and advance publication of research designs have been proposed as ways to prevent publication bias.[18,19] Publication bias can be detected by using a simple graphic test (funnel plot) or by calculating the "fail-safe N",[20,21] but these techniques are of limited value when fewer than 10 randomised controlled trials are included. In addition, for many diseases, the studies published are dominated by pharmaceutical-company-sponsored trials of new expensive treatments. This bias in publication can result in data-driven systematic reviews that draw more attention to those medicines. In contrast, question-driven systematic reviews answer the sorts of clinical questions of most concern to practitioners. In many cases, studies that are of most relevance to doctors and patients have not been done in the field of dermatology because of inadequate sources of independent funding. Systematic reviews that have been sponsored directly or indirectly by industry are also prone to bias by over-inclusion of unpublished "positive" studies that are kept "on file" by that company. Until it becomes mandatory to register all clinical trials conducted on human beings in a central register and to make all of the results available in the public

domain, all sorts of distortions may occur as a result of selective withholding or release of data.

Generally reviews that have been conducted by volunteers in the Cochrane Collaboration are of better quality than non-Cochrane reviews, but even despite this, potentially serious errors have been noted in up to a third of such reviews.[1,7]

Data abstraction

In general, the studies included in systematic reviews are reviewed by at least two reviewers. Data such as numbers of people entered into studies, numbers lost to follow up, effects sizes and quality criteria are recorded on predesigned data abstraction forms by at least two reviewers. Differences between reviewers are usually settled by consensus or by a third arbitrator. A systematic review in which there are large areas of disagreement between reviewers should lead the reader to question the validity of the review.

Pooling results

Results in the individual clinical trials that make up a systematic review may be similar in magnitude and direction (for example they may all indicate that treatment A is superior to treatment B by a similar magnitude). Assuming that publication bias can be excluded, systematic reviews with studies that have results that are similar in magnitude and direction provide results that are most likely to be true and useful. It may be impossible to draw firm conclusions from systematic reviews in which studies have results of widely different magnitude and direction.

The magnitude of the difference between the treatment groups in achieving meaningful outcomes is the most useful summary result of a systematic review. The most easily understood measures of the magnitude of the treatment effect are the difference in response rate and its reciprocal, the number needed to treat (NNT).[1,7,11] The NNT represents the number of patients one would need to treat to achieve one additional cure. Whereas the interpretation of NNT might be straightforward within one trial, interpretation of NNT within a systematic review requires some caution as this statistic is highly sensitive to baseline event rates. For example, if treatment A is 30% more effective than treatment B for clearing psoriasis, and 50% of people on treatment B are cleared with therapy, then 65% will be cleared with treatment A. This corresponds to a rate difference of 15% (65–50) and an NNT of 7 (1/0·15). This sounds quite worthwhile clinically. However, if the baseline clearance rate for treatment B in another trial or setting is only 30%, the rate difference will be only 9% and the NNT now becomes 11. If the baseline clearance rate is 10%, then the NNT for treatment A will be 33, which is perhaps less worthwhile. In other words, it rarely makes sense to provide one NNT summary measure within a systematic review because "control" or baseline events rates usually differ considerably between studies because of differences in study populations, interventions and trial conditions.[1,2,7,15] Instead, a range of NNTs for a range of plausible control event rates that occur in different clinical settings should be given, along with their 95% confidence intervals.

The precision of the estimate of the differences among treatments should be estimated. The confidence interval provides a useful measure of the precision of the treatment effect.[1,7,11,22,23] The calculation and interpretation of confidence intervals has been extensively described.[24] In simple terms, the reported result (known as the "point estimate") provides the best estimate of the treatment effect. The population or "true" response to treatment will most likely lie near the middle of the confidence interval and will rarely be found at or near the ends of the interval. The population or true response to treatment has only

a 1 in 20 chance of being outside of the 95% confidence interval.

Certain conditions must be met when meta-analysis is performed to synthesise results from different trials. The trials should have conceptual homogeneity. They must involve similar patient populations, have used similar treatments and have measured results in a similar fashion, at a similar point in time. There are two main statistical methods by which results are combined: using random effects models and fixed effects models.

- Random effects models assume that the results of the different studies may come from different populations with varying responses to treatment.
- Fixed effects models assume that each trial represents a random sample of a single population with a single response to treatment.

In general, random effects models are more conservative (i.e. are less likely to show statistically significant results) than fixed effects models. When the combined studies have statistical homogeneity (i.e. when the studies are reasonably similar), random effects and fixed effects models give similar results.

The key principle when considering combining results from several studies is that conceptual homogeneity precedes statistical homogeneity. In other words, results of several different studies should not be combined if it does not make sense to combine them, for example if the patient groups or interventions studied are not sufficiently similar to each other. Although what constitutes "sufficiently similar" is a matter of judgement, the important thing is to be explicit about one's decision to combine or not combine different studies. Tests for statistical heterogeneity are typically of very low power, so that statistical homogeneity does not mean clinical homogeneity.

When there is evidence of heterogeneity, reasons for heterogeneity between studies such as different disease subgroups, intervention dosage or study quality should be sought.

Sometimes, the robustness of an overall meta-analysis is tested further by means of a sensitivity analysis. In a sensitivity analysis the data are re-analysed, excluding those studies that are suspect because of quality or patient factors, to see whether their exclusion makes a substantial difference to the direction or magnitude of the main original results. In some systematic reviews in which a large number of trials have been included, it is possible to evaluate whether certain subgroups (for example children versus adults) are more likely to benefit than others. Subgroup analysis is rarely possible in dermatology, however, because few trials are available.

The conclusions in the discussion section of a systematic review should closely reflect the data that have been presented within that review. The authors should make it clear which of the treatment recommendations are based on the review data and which reflect their own judgements. In addition to making clinical recommendations of therapies when evidence exists, many reviews in dermatology find little evidence to address the questions posed. This lack of conclusive evidence does not, however, mean that the review is a waste of time, especially if the question addressed appears to be an important one. For example, the systematic review of antistreptococcal therapy for guttate psoriasis provided the authors with an opportunity to call for primary research in this area, and to make recommendations on study design and outcomes that might help future researchers.[14]

Applying evidence summarised in a systematic review to specific patients requires the same processes used to apply the results of individual controlled clinical trials to patients. This process is described in Chapter 12.

References

1. Greenhalgh T. *How to Read a Paper: the Basics of Evidence-based Medicine.* London: BMJ Books, 1997.

2. Chalmers I, Altman D, eds. *Systematic Reviews.* London: BMJ Publishing Group, 1995.

3. Lau J, Ionnidis JPA, Schmid CH. Summing up evidence: one answer is not always enough. *Lancet* 1998;**351**: 123–7.

4. Villar J, Carroli G, Belizan JM. Predictive ability of meta-analyses of randomised controlled trials [see comments]. *Lancet* 1995;**345**:772–6.

5. Cappelleri JC, Ioannidis JP, Schmid CH et al. Large trials v meta-analysis of smaller trials: how do their results compare? *JAMA* 1996;**276**:1332–8.

6. LeLorier J, Gregoire G, Benhaddad A, Lapierre J, Derderian F. Discrepancies between meta-analyses and subsequent large randomised, controlled trials. *N Engl J Med* 1997;**337**:536–42.

7. Sackett D, Richardson W, Rosenberg W, Haynes R. *Evidence-Based Medicine: How to Practise and Teach EBM.* Edinburgh: Churchill Livingstone, 1996.

8. Richardson W, Wilson M, Nishikawa J, Hayward R. The well-built clinical question: a key to evidence-based decisions (editorial). *ACP Journal Club* 1995;**123**: A12–13.

9. Adetugbo K, Williams HC. How can hand searching the dermatological literature benefit people with skin problems? *Arch Dermatol* 2001;**137**:332–5.

10. PubMed Overview. http://www4.ncbi.nlm.nih.gov/PubMed/overview.html (accessed 12 Jan 1998).

11. Bigby M. Evidence-based medicine in a nutshell. A guide to finding and using the best evidence in caring for patients. *Arch Dermatol* 1998;**134**:1609–18.

12. Spuls PI, Witkamp L, Bossuyt PM, Bos JD. A systematic review of five systemic treatments for severe psoriasis. *Br J Dermatol* 1997;**137**:943–9.

13. Haynes RB, Wilczynski N, McKibbon KA, Walker CJ, Sinclair JC. Developing optimal search strategies for detecting clinically sound studies in MEDLINE. *J Am Med Inform Assoc* 1994;**1**:447–58.

14. Chalmers RR, O'Sullivan T, Owen CC, Griffiths CC. A systematic review of treatments for guttate psoriasis. *Br J Dermatol* 2001;**145**:891–4.

15. Mulrow C, Oxman A, eds. Cochrane Collaboration Handbook. In: Cochrane Collaboration. *Cochrane Library*. Oxford: Update Software, 1997.

16. Dickersin K, Min YI, Meinert CL. Factors influencing publication of research results. Follow-up of applications submitted to two institutional review boards. *JAMA* 1992;**267**:374–8.

17. Easterbrook PJ, Berlin JA, Gopalan R, Matthews DR. Publication bias in clinical research. *Lancet* 1991;**337**:867–72.

18. Dickersin K. Report from the panel on the Case for Registers of Clinical Trials at the Eighth Annual Meeting of the Society for Clinical Trials. *Control Clin Trials* 1988;**9**:76–81.

19. Piantadosi S, Byar DP. A proposal for registering clinical trials. *Control Clin Trials* 1988;**9**:82–4.

20. Egger M, Davey Smith G, Schneider M, Minder C. Bias in meta-analysis detected by a simple, graphical test. *BMJ* 1997;**315**:629–34.

21. Abramson J. Making sense of data: a self-instruction manual on the interpretation of epidemiological data. New York: Oxford University Press, 1994.

22. Gardner MJ, Altman DG. Estimating with confidence. In: Gardner MJ, Altman DG, eds. *Statistics with Confidence*. London: BMJ Publishing Group, 1989;3–5.

23. Gardner MJ, Altman DG. Estimation rather than hypothesis testing: confidence intervals rather than P values. In: Gardner MJ, Altman DG, eds. *Statistics with Confidence*. London: BMJ Publishing Group, 1989;6–19.

24. Gardner MJ, Altman DG, eds. *Statistics with Confidence*. London: BMJ Publishing Group 1989;140.

9

How to critically appraise a study reporting effectiveness of an intervention

Hywel Williams

Definitions of quality, validity and bias

Quality, when referring to randomised controlled trials (RCTs), is a multidimensional concept that includes appropriateness of design, conduct, analysis, reporting and its perceived clinical relevance.[1-4] Validity refers to the extent to which the study results relate to the "truth". Validity may be internal (i.e. are the results of *this* trial true?) or external (to what extent do the results of this trial apply to *my* patients?). Factors affecting external validity are discussed further in Chapter 12. Internal validity is a prerequisite for external validity.

In addition to assessing the role of chance, a crucial component in appraising the internal validity of a trial is assessment of its potential for bias. Bias denotes a systematic error resulting in an incorrect estimation of the true effect. With respect to clinical trials, bias may be best understood in terms of:

- selection bias – resulting in an imbalance in treatment groups
- performance bias – treating one group of people differently from the other
- detection bias – biased assessment of outcome resulting from lack of blinding
- attrition bias – biased handling of deviations from the study protocol and those lost to follow up.

This chapter guides the reader on applying the various forms of bias to appraising the internal validity of an RCT.

How does one tell a good RCT from a bad one?
Quality criteria derived from research

Three main factors related to study reporting have been associated with altering the estimation of the risk estimate, usually by inflating the claimed benefit.[3] These are shown in Box 9.1.

Generation and concealment of treatment allocation

Generation and concealment of treatment allocation are two interrelated steps in the crucial process of randomisation. The first refers to the method used to generate the randomisation sequence. The second refers to the subsequent steps taken by the trialists to conceal the allocation of participants to the intervention groups from the people recruiting the participants. Suggestions for adequate and inadequate definitions of generation of randomisation and subsequent concealment are shown in Box 9.2. Studies that do not describe how the randomisation sequence was generated should be viewed with some suspicion, given that humans frequently subvert the intended aims of randomisation.[5]

Box 9.1 Factors to consider when assessing the validity of clinical trials in dermatology

The "big three" that should always be assessed

- Is the method of generating the randomisation sequence and subsequent concealment of allocation of participants described?
- Were participants and study assessors blind to the intervention?
- Were all those who originally entered the study accounted for in the results and analysis (i.e. was an intention-to-treat analysis performed)?

Other factors worth looking for

- Did the study investigators use an adequate disease definition?
- Did they use outcome measures that mean something to you and your patient?
- Were the treatment groups similar with respect to predictors of treatment response at baseline?
- Were the main outcome measures declared a priori or did the investigators "data dredge" amongst many outcomes for a statistically significant result?
- Did the investigators do an appropriate statistical test if the data were skewed?
- Did the investigators test the right thing (i.e. between-group differences rather than just differences from baseline)?
- Have the authors misinterpreted no evidence of an effect as being evidence of no effect?
- Were the groups treated equally except for the interventions studied?
- Who sponsored the study? Could sponsorship have affected the results or the way they were reported?
- Is the trial clearly and completely reported by CONSORT standards?

Box 9.2 Adequacy of generation and concealment of randomisation sequence

Generation of the randomisation code

- Adequate: random numbers generated by computer program, table of random numbers, flipping a coin
- Inadequate: quasi-randomisation methods (for example date of birth, alternate records, date of attendance at clinic)

Concealing the sequence from recruiters

- Adequate: if investigators and patients cannot foresee the assignment to intervention groups (i.e. numbered and coded identical sealed boxes prepared by central pharmacy, sealed opaque envelopes)
- Inadequate: allocation schedule open for recruiting physician to view beforehand, unsealed envelopes

example in a central clinical trials office or pharmacy). Less ideally, sealed opaque envelopes are used – a method that is still susceptible to tampering by opening the envelopes or holding them up against a bright light.[5] Failure to conceal such allocation means that those recruiting patients can foresee which treatment a patient is about to have. Such lack of concealment can result in selective enrolment of patients on the basis of prognostic factors,[6] and loss of the "even playing field" that randomisation was designed to achieve.

Motives for interfering with the randomisation schedule include a desire on the part of investigators to ensure that their new treatment is successful by deliberately allocating patients in a better prognostic group to that treatment. Another reason may be that a doctor wants to ensure that particular patients are not allocated to a control or placebo group. Such selective recruitment is a form of selection bias, resulting in an unfair comparison of the interventions

Concealing the allocation of interventions from those recruiting participants is a crucial step in the progress of an RCT. The randomisation list is usually kept away from enrolment sites (for under evaluation. Trials in which concealment of allocation was judged to have been inadequate were found to have inflated the estimates of benefit by about 30% when compared with studies reporting adequate concealment.[3]

Blinding (masking) the intervention

Blinding or masking is the extent to which trial participants are kept unaware of treatment allocation. Blinding can refer to at least four groups of people: those recruiting patients, the study participants themselves, those assessing the outcomes in study participants, and those analysing the results.[7] The term "double blind" traditionally refers to a study in which both the participants and the investigators are "blind" to the study intervention allocation, but the term is ambiguous unless qualified by a statement as to who exactly was blinded.

Blinding is less of an issue with objective outcomes such as death but is very important with subjective outcomes such as the opinion of participants or assessment of disease activity, as in most dermatology trials. Blinding may be achieved by a range of techniques such as ensuring that placebo tablets look, feel, smell and taste the same as the active tablets,[8] or, in the case of ointments, by using as a placebo the same vehicle or base in which the active ingredient is formulated.[9]

Issues of blinding may seem superficially similar to allocation concealment in that both refer to concealing the interventions. The distinction is important in the sense that failure to conceal the randomisation sequence may result in unequal groups, (i.e. a form of selection bias) whereas failure to mask the intervention once a fair randomisation has taken a place represents a form of detection or information bias. Both can result in an incorrect estimate of the effects of a treatment. Studies that are not double blind typically overestimate treatment effects by about 14% when compared with studies that are double blind.[3]

Accounting for all those randomised

The whole point of randomisation is to create two or more groups that are as similar to each other as possible, the only exception being the intervention under study. In this way the additional effects of the intervention can be assessed.[10] A potentially serious violation of this principle is the failure to take into account all those who were randomised when conducting the final main analysis, for example participants who deviate from the study protocol, those who do not adhere to the interventions and those who subsequently drop out for other reasons. People who drop out of trials differ from those who remain in them in several ways.[11] People may drop out because they die, encounter adverse events, get worse (or no better), or simply because the proposed regimen is too complicated for a busy person to follow. They may even drop out because the treatment works so well. Ignoring participants who have dropped out in the analysis is not acceptable. Excluding participants who drop out after randomisation potentially biases the results. One way to reduce bias is to perform an intention-to-treat (ITT) analysis, in which all those initially randomised in the final analysis are included.[11,12]

Unless one has detailed information on why participants dropped out of a study, it cannot be assumed that an analysis of those remaining in the study to the end are representative of those randomised to the groups at the beginning. Failure to perform an ITT analysis may inflate or deflate estimates of treatment effect.[4] Performing an ITT analysis is often regarded as a major criterion by which the quality of an RCT is assessed.

It is entirely appropriate to conduct an analysis of all those who remained at the end of a study (a "per protocol" analysis) alongside the ITT analysis.[12] Discrepancies between results of ITT and per protocol analyses may indicate the potential benefit of the intervention under ideal compliance conditions and the need to explore ways of reformulating the intervention so that fewer participants drop out of the trial. Discrepancies may also indicate serious flaws in the study design.

Quality scales

Faulty reporting generally reflects faulty trial methods.[3,5] A number of scales have been developed for assessing study trial quality over the past 15 years. These vary in the dimensions covered and complexity.[2] Generally, the recent trend has been to use the few quality criteria given in Box 9.1, plus a few more that the appraiser considers important in relation to the condition being studied.[3] It is now considered unwise to use summary quality scores in an attempt to "adjust" the potentially biased treatment estimate because this varies with the scale used and how the components of each scale are weighted.[13] Instead, greater emphasis is placed on using the components of the scale as a check list and considering how each may affect the results.[3]

Additional empirical criteria
Disease definition

Whilst it may seem simple to apply the three criteria of randomisation generation/concealment, blinding and ITT to judge the quality of RCTs, it is still uncertain how far these factors can reliably discriminate between "good" and "bad" RCTs in dermatology. Other factors that are disease specific and rely on content knowledge/expertise are likely to be equally important in determining the quality of some dermatology trials. The influence of such disease-specific factors in dermatology is an area that requires further systematic research.

Therefore, as someone with an interest in atopic eczema, I would not trust a study that claimed a beneficial effect for a new treatment if the study included both children and adults with diverse eczematous dermatoses,[14] as people with such conditions might respond differently.[15] Similarly, the definitions of disease used may be an important quality criterion. For example, if I were reading the report of an RCT of an intervention for bullous pemphigoid, I would want to know that the diagnosis in study participants was confirmed by immunofluorescence in order to distinguish it from other bullous disorders of diverse aetiologies and with differing treatment responsiveness.

"Sensible" outcome measures

In evaluating a clinical trial, look for clinical outcome measures that are clear cut and clinically meaningful to you and your patients.[16] For example, in a study of a systemic treatment for warts, complete disappearance of warts is a meaningful outcome, whereas a decrease in the volume of warts is not. The development of scales and indices for cutaneous diseases and testing their validity, reproducibility and responsiveness has been inadequate.[16,17] A lack of clearly defined and useful outcome variables remains a major problem in interpreting clinical trials in dermatology.

Until better scales are developed, trials with the simplest and most objective outcome variables are the best. Categorical outcomes lead to the least amount of confusion and have the strongest conclusions. Thus, trials in which a comparison is made between death and survival, patients with recurrence of disease and those without recurrence, or patients who are cured and those who are not cured are studies whose outcome variables are easily understood and verified. For trials in which the outcomes are less clear cut and more subjective, a simple ordinal scale is probably the best choice. The best ordinal scales involve a minimum of human judgement, have a precision that is much smaller than the differences being sought, and are sufficiently standardised to enable others to use them and produce similar results.[16,17]

Similarity of groups for baseline differences

In addition to helping to balance known predictors of treatment response such as baseline disease severity (which could serve as confounders when evaluating treatment efficacy between groups), it has also been suggested that randomisation will balance against unknown confounders.[3] This statement is superficially appealing, but is difficult to verify if these confounders are indeed unknown. Even so, randomisation, especially when implemented on small sample sizes, may result in imbalances in possible cofactors that can affect treatment response. In other words, randomisation is not a guarantee against imbalance, although more sophisticated methods of randomisation such as blocking and stratification can help to minimise this.[7]

It is quite common to see as the first table in the results section of an RCT report a long list of demographic characteristics of the participants in the different treatment groups and a statement to the effect that "the two groups did not differ statistically at baseline". This statement is problematic for two reasons.

- It is inappropriate to perform such multiple statistic tests without prior hypotheses – indeed many of the variables recorded may be totally irrelevant to predicting treatment response.
- There may still be no arbitrary 5% statistical significance even for gross imbalances in treatment groups simply because the groups are so small.

Before reading such tables, the most important thing to do is to ask oneself, "What are the most important factors which may predict treatment response?" and then to "eyeball" these in the table of baseline characteristics, if they have been recorded. If there are major imbalances such as baseline severity score, then these can and should be allowed for in a number of ways during analysis, for example a multivariate analysis adjusting for baseline severity as a covariate.[7]

Data dredging

Many dermatology trials report as many as 10 different outcome measures recorded at several different time points. Even by chance, at least 1 in 20 of such outcomes will be "significant" at the 5% level. Therefore, it is important in studies that use multiple outcomes to ensure that the trialists are not data dredging, that is performing repeated statistical tests for a range of outcome measures and then emphasising only the one that is "significant" at the "magic" 5% level. Such practice is akin to throwing a dart and drawing a dartboard around it. Instead, trialists should declare up front what they would regard as a single "success criterion" for a particular trial. This way it is more credible if that main success criterion is indeed fulfilled – as opposed to some secondary or tertiary outcome measure that turns out to be "significant". Sometimes, trialists will try to save face by emphasising a range of less clinically significant biological markers of success when in fact the main clinical comparisons look disappointing.

Doing the wrong tests

It is quite common for continuous data such as acne spot counts to have a skewed frequency distribution. It may then be inappropriate to use parametric tests such as the Student *t*-test without first transforming the data. Alternatively, non-parametric tests that do not rely on the assumption of a normal distribution can be used. A quick way to check whether a continuous variable is normally distributed is to determine whether the mean minus two standard deviations is less than zero. If it is, the data are likely to be skewed.

Testing the wrong thing

Performing a statistical test on something other than the main outcome of interest is a subtle but not uncommon error in dermatology trials.[18,19] When comparing a continuous outcome measure such as decrease in acne spots between treatment A and treatment B, the correct summary statistic to challenge the null hypothesis of no difference between the treatment is to examine the *difference between the two treatments* in terms of change of spot count from baseline. Sometimes the investigators simply perform a statistical test on whether the acne lesion count falls from baseline in the two groups independently. If the fall in spot count reaches the 5% level in one group but not in the other, then the authors may conclude that "therefore treatment A is more effective than treatment B". Perhaps the *P* value for change in spot count from baseline is 0·04 in one group (i.e. significant) and 0·06 in the other (i.e. conventionally non-significant). This practice is clearly inappropriate since the difference between the two treatments has not been tested.

Interpreting trials with negative results

Misinterpreting trials with negative results is a common error in dermatology clinical trials.[20] Failure to find a statistically significant difference between treatments should not be interpreted that "treatment is ineffective". Put another way, no evidence of effect is not the same as evidence of no effect.[21] In many dermatology trials the sample sizes are too small to detect clinically important differences. Providing 95% confidence intervals around the main response estimates allows readers to see what kind of effects might have been missed. For example, in an RCT of famotidine versus diphenhydramine for acute urticaria, itch as measured by a 100 mm visual analogue scale decreased by 36 mm in the famotidine group and by 54 mm in the diphenhydramine group, a difference of 18 mm (54 − 36) in favour of diphenhydramine. Although the statistical test for this difference of 18 mm between the two treatment groups was not significant at the 5% level, there was a trend towards to greater reduction in itch in the diphenhydramine group. The 95% confidence interval around the 18 mm difference between the groups was from −3 to 38. In other words, the results were compatible with a difference of as little as 3 mm in favour of famotidine and as much as 38 mm in favour of diphenhydramine.[22]

The trial environment

Once randomised, it is important that the two intervention groups are followed up in similar ways. Previous studies have shown the non-specific benefits of being included in a clinical trial, even in placebo groups.[23] Part of the benefit might be the result of better ancillary care prompted by frequent follow ups and being "fussed over" by study assessors.' It is important therefore to scrutinise whether the treatment groups have been treated equally in terms of frequency and duration of follow up and whether they have been afforded identical privileges except for the treatment under investigation.

Sponsorship issues

It is natural to assume that a clinical trial of a drug that has taken years of investment by a drug company and that is sponsored by that same company will strive to demonstrate that the drug is successful. Indeed, millions of dollars of profit may rely on convincing opinion leaders in dermatology of a new drug's worth. Yet the influence of sponsorship on efficacy claims has not been tested in dermatology RCTs. Drug companies and trialists have many opportunities to influence journal readers when the results of their trial are published (Box 9.3).

It should not be assumed that biases in relation to sponsorship are confined to the pharmaceutical industry. Those conducting trials for government agencies might hope to show that a new drug is less cost-effective than standard therapy. Some independent clinicians with preformed

Box 9.3 Ways to enhance the impact of positive studies or reduce the impact of negative studies

- Withhold "negative" trials from being published at all by keeping them as "data on file"
- Delay release of such "negative" studies into the public domain
- Publish negative studies in an obscure or non-English language journal
- Select outcome measures that show the treatment in a better light
- "Torture" the data by performing multiple statistical tests on subgroups
- Select one of many statistical techniques to show the results in the best light
- Divert attention from the main "negative" findings by emphasising biomedical markers and "mechanism of action"
- Incorrectly interpret equivalence studies, for example by suggesting that two drugs are the same when the confidence intervals surrounding their differences are large
- Use a comparator that other studies have not used in order to avoid a head-to-head comparison with a current established treatment
- Do not highlight adverse events in the abstract and discussion sections
- Use optimistic language and writing styles when discussing essentially negative studies – for example repetition for positive results
- Publish positive study results in duplicate or triplicate – overtly or even covertly

conclusions about an existing treatment may be equally susceptible to being influenced by their own prejudices when testing and writing up the results for that treatment. In assessing a study, readers should always consider who sponsored the study, and ask themselves whether such sponsorship could have influenced the results or the way that they are presented. Absence of declared sponsorship may not mean absence of sponsorship.[24]

Attempts to overcome limitations in the conduct, reporting and publication of clinical trials

To overcome many of the difficulties discussed in this section, calls for better standards of reporting of trials have led to the CONSORT statement.[25] This contains a structured checklist for reporting the details of clinical trials, including methods of randomisation and concealment, blinding, ITT analysis and a flow diagram to illustrate the progress of trial participants. Several dermatology journals now require that submitted clinical trial reports meet CONSORT standards to be published.[26]

Whereas CONSORT may help with better reporting of trials, the creation of prospective clinical trial registers has been seen as one possible way of ensuring that the trial results eventually reach the public domain, and for checking that the investigators adhered to their original protocol.[27]

References

1. Jadad AR, Cook DJ, Jones A *et al*. Methodology and reports of systematic reviews and meta-analyses: a comparison of Cochrane reviews with articles published in paper-based journals. *JAMA* 1998;**280**:278–80.
2. Moher D, Jadad AR, Nichol G, Penman M, Tugwell P, Walsh S. Assessing the quality of randomized controlled trials: an annotated bibliography of scales and checklists. *Control Clin Trials* 1995;**16**:62–73.
3. Juni P, Altman DG, Egger M. Systematic reviews in health care: Assessing the quality of controlled clinical trials. *BMJ* 2001;**323**:42–6.
4. Juni P, Altman DG, Egger M. Assessing the quality of controlled clinical trials. In: Egger M, Davey Smith G, Altman DG, eds. *Systematic reviews in health care: meta-analysis in context, 2nd ed*. London: BMJ Books, 2001.
5. Schulz KF. Subverting randomization in controlled trials. *JAMA* 1995;**274**:1456–8.
6. Schulz KF. Randomised trials, human nature, and reporting guidelines. *Lancet* 1996;**348**:596–8.

7. Pocock SJ. *Clinical Trials: a Practical Approach.* New York: John Wiley & Sons, 1983.

8. Karlowski TR, Chalmers TC, Frenkel LD, Kapikian AZ, Lewis TL, Lynch JM. Ascorbic acid for the common cold. A prophylactic and therapeutic trial. *JAMA* 1975; **231**:1038–42.

9. Thomas KS, Armstrong S, Avery A, Li Wan Po A, O'Neill C, Williams HC. Randomised controlled trial of short bursts of a potent topical corticosteroid versus more prolonged use of a mild preparation, for children with mild or moderate atopic eczema. *BMJ* 2002;**324**:768–71.

10. Altman DG, Bland JM. Statistics notes. Treatment allocation in controlled trials: why randomise? *BMJ* 1999;**318**:1209.

11. Hollis S, Campbell F. What is meant by intention to treat analysis? Survey of published randomised controlled trials. *BMJ* 1999;**319**:670–4.

12. Williams HC. Are we going OTT about ITT? *Br J Dermatol* 2001;**144**:1101–2.

13. Juni P, Witschi A, Bloch R, Egger M. The hazards of scoring the quality of clinical trials for meta-analysis. *JAMA* 1999;**282**:1054–60.

14. English JS, Bunker CB, Ruthven K, Dowd PM, Greaves MW. A double-blind comparison of the efficacy of betamethasone dipropionate cream twice daily versus once daily in the treatment of steroid responsive dermatoses. *Clin Exp Dermatol* 1989;**14**:32–4.

15. Hoare C, Li Wan Po A, Williams H. Systematic review of treatments for atopic eczema. *Health Technol Assess* 2000;**4**:1–191.

16. Bigby M, Gadenne A-S. Understanding and evaluating clinical trials. *J Am Acad Dermatol* 1996;**34**:555–90.

17. Allen AM. Clinical trials in dermatology, part 3: Measuring responses to treatment. *Int J Dermatol* 1980;**19**:1–6.

18. Williams HC. Hywel Williams. Top 10 deadly sins of clinical trial reporting. *Ned Tijd Derm Venereol* 1999; **9**:372–3.

19. Harper J. Double-blind comparison of an antiseptic oil-based bath additive (Oilatum Plus) with regular Oilatum (Oilatum Emollient) for the treatment of atopic eczema. In: Lever R, Levy J, eds. *The Bacteriology of Eczema.* London: The Royal Society of Medicine Press, 1995.

20. Williams HC, Seed P. Inadequate size of 'negative' clinical trials in dermatology. *Br J Dermatol* 1993;**128**: 317–26.

21. Altman DG, Bland JM. Absence of evidence is not evidence of absence. *BMJ* 1995;**311**:485.

22. Watson NT, Weiss EL, Harter PM. Famotidine in the treatment of acute urticaria. *Clin Exp Dermatol* 2000; **25**:186–9.

23. Braunholtz DA, Edwards SJ, Lilford RJ. Are randomized clinical trials good for us (in the short term)? Evidence for a "trial effect". *J Clin Epidemiol* 2001;**54**:217–24.

24. Davidoff F, DeAngelis CD, Drazen JM *et al.* Sponsorship, authorship, and accountability. *Lancet* 2001;**358**:854–6.

25. Moher D, Schulz KF, Altman DG, Lepage L. The CONSORT statement: revised recommendations for improving the quality of reports of parallel-group randomised trials. *Lancet* 2001;**357**:1191–4.

26. Cox NH, Williams HC. Can you COPE with CONSORT? *Br J Dermatol* 2000;**142**:1–3.

27. Stern JM, Simes RJ. Publication bias: evidence of delayed publication in a cohort study of clinical research projects. *BMJ* 1997;**315**:640–5.

10

How to assess the evidence for the safety of medical interventions

Luigi Naldi

Introduction

As for any other human activities, medical interventions may carry a risk of unintended adverse events. Whenever a physician prescribes a drug, there is the potential for an adverse reaction connected with drug use. Despite limited accurate data, a widely cited meta-analysis of 39 prospective studies performed in US hospitals from 1966 to 1996 found that the incidence of severe adverse drug reactions (i.e. life-threatening reactions and reactions that prolonged hospitalisation) among inpatients was 6·7%, with 0·32% being fatal.[1] Despite these impressive figures, the rate of severe adverse reactions for any given drug is usually very low. However, the system works in such a way that even a small increase in the incidence of a clinically severe reaction may prompt the withdrawal of the implicated drug from the market.

It is commonly stated that clinical decisions should balance the benefit of the available options with the risk. A difficulty stems from the fact that data on benefits and risks of medical interventions are usually derived from different study designs and information sources. A large part of our discussion will be focused on the safety of drug use. While systems to survey the safety of medications are well established, they are not for other medical interventions such as surgical procedures and invasive diagnostic tests. It is well accepted that no *in vitro* or animal models can accurately predict adverse events

associated with drug use before the drug is employed in humans. Advances in understanding the causes of adverse reactions (for example pharmacogenomics) may, in the future, enable the risk in individual patients to be predicted in a more reliable way.[2–4]

Data sources for determining the safety of medical interventions
The limitation of randomised controlled trials (RCTs)

The great strength of RCTs is the ability to provide an unbiased estimate of treatment effect by controlling not only for determinants of outcome we know about, but also for those we do not know about. If RCTs demonstrate an important relationship between an agent and an adverse event, then we can be confident of the results. However, RCTs are usually designed to document frequent events, that is, those associated with the intended effect of a treatment. With the usual sample size, which rarely exceeds a few thousand people, RCTs are not suited to accurate documentation of the safety of medical intervention for uncommon events.[5,6] Besides the issue of statistical power, additional limitations include the usual short duration of most clinical trials and the careful selection of the eligible population (restriction in patient selection according to age, comorbidity, etc.). All in all, when an intervention has been proved to be effective in an RCT, the safety issue still remains to be well established. Pharmaceutical companies may strive to work out the adverse effect profile of a drug before licensing, but because only a limited number of selected individuals can be exposed to the drug before it is released, only common adverse events can be accurately documented and the complete range of adverse events remains to be elucidated in the post-marketing phase. This limitation is particularly true for delayed reactions and rare but severe acute events.

The value of suspicion: case reports and case series

In contrast to RCTs, individual cases or case series do not provide a comparison with a control group and are unable to produce reliable risk estimates. In spite of their limitations, astute clinical observations are still fundamental to the description of new disease entities and the raising of new hypotheses concerning disease causation, including the effects of medical interventions. Case reports still represent a first-line modality to detect new adverse reactions once a drug is marketed.[7] Spontaneous surveillance systems such as the International Drug Monitoring Program of the World Health Organization (WHO) capitalise on the collection and periodical analysis of spontaneous reports of suspected adverse drug reactions.[8] All physicians are expected to take an active part in promoting the safety of medical interventions and to contribute by reporting any suspected adverse events they observe in association with drug use.[9] Such a collection of reported adverse events may be explored to raise signals (Box 10.1) to be validated by more formal study designs, that is, studies providing estimates of incidence rates and quantifying risks.[10,11] Spontaneous reporting should be seen as an early warning system for possible unknown adverse events and may be prone to all sorts of bias.[12] Case reports may be more effective in revealing unusual or rare acute adverse events. In general, however, they do not reliably detect adverse drug reactions that occur widely separated in time from the original use of the drug or represent an increased risk of an adverse event that occurs commonly in populations not exposed to the drug.

Box 10.1 Criteria for signal assessment in spontaneous surveillance systems

- Number of case reports
- Presence of a characteristic feature or pattern and absence or rarity of converse findings
- Site, timing, dosage–response relationship, reversibility
- Rechallenge
- Biological plausibility
- Laboratory findings (for example drug-dependent antibodies)
- Previous experience with related drugs

Epidemiological studies: the most comprehensive source of data

Quantitative estimates of risks associated with drug use may be obtained from analytic epidemiology studies (i.e. cohort and case-control studies),[13] and from a number of modifications of these traditional study designs pertaining to the broad area of pharmacoepidemiology (Box 10.2). These observational (non-randomised) studies produce less stringent results than RCTs, being prone to unmeasured confounders and biases. On the other hand, these study designs may represent in the "real world" the only practical option to obtain risk estimates once a new drug has entered the market.

Box 10.2 Examples of pharmacoepidemiological methods

- Intensive hospital monitoring
- Prescription event monitoring (PEM)
- Cohort studies
- Case-control studies and case-control surveillance
- Case-crossover design
- Record linkage

Cohort studies are studies where groups are defined according to the exposure status (for example users and non-users of a drug) and are followed up, with subsequent events being recorded and compared.[14,15] By contrast, case-control studies are studies where a group is defined according to its experience of an outcome of interest (for example cases of toxic epidermal necrolysis) and is compared with a control group that has not experienced the outcome. Prior exposures are ascertained for each group retrospectively and are compared.[16] A crucial point for the validity of a case-control study is the choice of appropriate controls. In principle, controls should be an unbiased sample of those individuals composing the so-called "study base". Controls for cases arising in the ambulatory population with resultant hospitalisation (community cases) may be represented by patients admitted to the same hospital for an acute condition or for an elective procedure not suspected of being related to drugs.[17]

Generally speaking, cohort studies are better suited to the study of rare exposures and common events, and case-control studies to the assessment of rare outcomes and relatively common exposures. Cohort studies allow the assessment of several outcomes for one specific exposure. Case-control studies allow the assessment of the role of a range of different exposures on the development of a single specific outcome. Cohort studies are not feasible when dealing with rare events, because millions of drug users have to be observed for years. In this situation, case-control studies with a very large population base are the most feasible method. For example, it is intuitive that only a case-control study would be feasible to assess the pharmacological risk for a disease like toxic epidermal necrolysis, with an expected rate in the general population of one case per million people per year.[18,19]

It is important that outcome and exposure are measured in the same way in the groups being compared in observational studies. However, even if investigators document the comparability of potential confounding variables in the groups being analysed (exposed and non-exposed cohorts, or cases and controls) or use statistical techniques to adjust for them, there may be an important imbalance that the investigators do not know about or simply have not measured that may be responsible for any observed difference.

Case-control and cohort studies should be developed with the aim of testing a specific predefined hypothesis. In the past few decades, modifications of traditional cohort and case-control studies have been developed to explore new associations and to raise signals. Record linkage is based on linkage of data from large electronic databanks on exposure and outcome. Case-control surveillance is the ongoing collection of cases of prespecified rare and severe acute events and of suitable controls, looking for new associations of the events with drug exposure.[20]

The association of an exposure with a given event is usually expressed in terms of a relative risk or odds ratio (an estimate of the relative risk obtained from case-control sudies) (Table 10.1). The relative risk is a measure of the size of an association in relative terms. It refers to the ratio of the incidence of the outcome among exposed individuals to that among non-exposed individuals. Values greater than 1 represent an increase in risk associated with the exposure; values less than 1 represent a reduction in risk. A relative risk of 2, for example, tells us that the event under study occurs twice as often in the exposed people as in the non-exposed. For rare events, even a large relative risk may translate to the occurrence of a few additional drug reactions. The total incidence of an outcome among exposed individuals is a combination of the baseline incidence plus the excess of incidence due to the exposure.

Table 10.1   Measures of association

Patients	Adverse event (cases)	No adverse event (controls)
Exposed	a	b
Not exposed	c	d

Relative risk = [a/(a + b)] / [c/(c + d)]

Odds ratio = (a/c) / (b/d)

Excess risk* = [a/(a + b)] − [c/(c + d)]

NNT or NNH = 1/excess risk

NNH from case-control studies = 1/[(odds ratio − 1) (unexposed event rate)]

*The excess risk may be also referred to as the "risk difference" or the "absolute risk reduction"

The excess risk (or risk difference or absolute risk reduction) is calculated as the difference between the incidence among exposed individuals and the incidence among non-exposed individuals. It measures the occurrence of an outcome among exposed individuals that can be attributed to the exposure. As such, it is a better measure of the impact of different outcomes than the relative risk, and a more informative measure from the points of view of an individual physician and public health. Measures of excess risk are directly calculated in cohort studies and, provided that data on the incidence of the outcome are available in the underlying unexposed population, they can also be derived from case-control studies.

Back to the individual patient

What is the risk of extraspinal hyperostosis in a patient with psoriasis treated for several months with acitretin? Does PUVA therapy increase the risk of non-melanoma skin cancer in a patient being treated for mycosis fungoides? What is the chance of severe depression in an adolescent taking 13-*cis*-retinoic acid for acne? To address these questions, physicians must effectively search for evidence and must be able to assess

the validity of the available data, and consider the strength of any documented association, and the relevance when the issue is applied back to an individual patient.[21]

We have already considered that many different sources of information should be sought and the search should not be limited to RCTs.[22] When data from RCTs are scrutinised, the statistical power to detect an important adverse event should be taken into account. When dealing with observational studies, it should be carefully considered if the studies provide reliable quantitative risk estimates or simply generate signals needing further validation. The optimal study design should be one assuring unbiased comparison between exposed and unexposed groups. Comparison groups should be similar with respect to important determinants of outcome. Outcome and exposure should be measured in the same way in the groups being compared, and the exposure should clearly precede the adverse outcome. In addition, follow up should be sufficiently long and complete and the study should have enough statistical power to document the association of interest.

When risk estimates from several studies are available, one should evaluate whether these are roughly in the same direction or if there are discrepancies between the studies. If there are discrepancies between studies, reasons for the discrepancies should be considered. Systematic reviews may help in summarising the study results.[23] Unfortunately, the criteria for assessing the quality of meta-analyses of observational studies are not as well established as those concerning RCTs.[24]

Once an association has been established, the magnitude of the risk should be taken into account and expressed in understandable terms if it is to be of practical use to clinicians. We have already considered that, from the perspective of a physician deciding about the risk of prescribing a particular drug, the excess risk (or risk difference) is a more informative measure than is the relative risk. In the context of RCTs, Sackett *et al.* proposed a method for converting risk differences into a more intuitive quantity. This quantity was named the number needed to treat (NNT = 1/excess risk).[25] It is the number of people who must be treated in order that one clinical event is prevented by the treatment at issue (for example the number of people to be treated to avoid one patient experiencing a relapse of psoriasis) or one additional beneficial outcome is achieved. By analogy, the "number needed to harm" (NNH) or "number of patients needed to be treated for one additional patient to be harmed"[26] is the number of people exposed to a given treatment such that on average and over a given follow up period, one additional person experiences an adverse effect of interest because of the treatment. In RCTs and cohort studies, NNH is directly calculated as the reciprocal of the excess risk. Recently, a formula has been proposed using odds ratios from case-control studies and data on the event rate in the unexposed population (Table 10.1).[27] According to the formula, given an odds ratio of 3 and unexposed event rate of 1 per 1 000 000 people, the NNTH can be calculated as 500 000 (i.e. 500 000 people to be treated to experience one additional adverse effect with the treatment).

After deriving estimates for the potential harm of an intervention, the estimates should be weighted against the expected benefits of the same intervention. The adverse consequence of withholding the intervention should be carefully considered. A final decision should try to integrate probability issues with the patient's values and preferences about therapy. This requires patient education about the benefits and risks of alternatives, tailored to the particular patient's risk profile.

To conclude, not only should physicians be able to retrieve and critically assess the evidence concerning the safety of any given intervention, they should also take an active part in promoting safety by contributing to surveillance programmes once an intervention is proposed to the medical community.

References

1. Lazarou J, Pomeranz B, Corey D *et al.* Incidence of adverse drug reactions in hospitalized patients: a meta-analysis of prospective studies. *JAMA* 1998;**279**:1200–5.

2. Phillips KA, Veenstra DL, Oren E, Lee JK, Sadee W. Potential role of pharmacogenomics in reducing adverse drug reactions. A systematic review. *JAMA* 2001;**286**: 2270–9.

3. Knowles SR, Uetrecht J, Shear NH. Idiosyncratic drug reactions: the reactive metabolite syndromes. *Lancet* 2000;**356**:1587–91.

4. Meyer UA. Pharmacogenetics and adverse drug reactions. *Lancet* 2000;**356**:1667–71.

5. Eypasch E, Lefering R, Kum CK, Troidl H. Probability of adverse events that have not yet occurred: a statistical reminder. *BMJ* 1995;**311**:619–20.

6. Hanley JA, Lippman-Hand A. If nothing goes wrong, is everything all right? Interpreting zero numerators. *JAMA* 1983;**249**:1743–5.

7. Brewer T, Colditz GA. Postmarketing surveillance and adverse drug reactions: current perspectives and future trends. *JAMA* 1999;**281**:824–9.

8. Venning GR. Identification of adverse reactions to new drugs. II. How were 18 important adverse reactions discovered and with what delays? *BMJ* 1983;**286**: 289–92;365–8.

9. Gruchalla RS. Clinical assessment of drug-induced disease. *Lancet* 2000;**356**:1505–11.

10. Edwards R, Lindquist M, Wiholm BE *et al.* Quality criteria for early signals of possible adverse drug reactions. *Lancet* 1990;**336**:156–8.

11. Meyboom RHB, Egherts ACG, Edwards JR *et al.* Principles of signal detection in pharmacovigilance. *Drug Saf* 1997;**16**:355–65.

12. Belton KJ, Lewis SC, Payne S, Rawlins MD, Wood SM. Attitudinal survey of adverse reaction reporting by medical practitioners in the United Kingdom. *Br J Pharmacol* 1995;**39**:223–6.

13. Kaufman DW, Shapiro S. Epidemiological assessment of drug-induced disease. *Lancet* 2000;**356**:1339–43.

14. Van der Linden PD, van der Lei J, Vlug AE, Stricker BH. Skin reactions to antibacterial agents in general practice. *J Clin Epidemiol* 1998;**51**:703–8.

15. Fellay J, Boubaker K, Ledergerber B *et al.* Prevalence of adverse events associated with potent antiretroviral treatment: Swiss HIV Cohort Study. *Lancet* 2001;**358**:1322–7.

16. Roujeau JC, Kelly JP, Naldi L *et al.* Medication use and the risk of Stevens–Johnson syndrome or toxic epidermal necrolysis. *N Engl J Med* 1995;**333**:1600–7.

17. Kelly JP, Auqier A, Rzany B *et al.* An international collaborative case-control study of severe cutaneous adverse reactions (SCAR). Design and methods. *J Clin Epidemiol* 1995;**48**:1099–108.

18. Roujeau JC, Guillaume JC, Fabre JP, Penso D, Flechet ML, Girre JP. Toxic epidermal necrolysis (Lyell's syndrome): incidence and drug etiology in France 1981–1985. *Arch Dermatol* 1990;**126**:37–42.

19. Schöpf E, Stühmer A, Rzany B, Victor N, Zentgraf R, Kapp JF. Toxic epidermal necrolysis and Stevens–Johnson syndrome: an epidemiologic study from West Germany. *Arch Dermatol* 1991;**127**:839–42.

20. Kaufman DW, Rosenberg L, Mitchell AA. Signal generation and clarification: use of case-control data. *Pharmacoepidemiol Drug Saf* 2001;**10**:197–203.

21. Levine M, Walter S, Lee H, et al. Users' guides to the medical literature. IV. How to use an article about harm. *JAMA* 1994;**271**:1615–19.

22. Maistrello M, Morgutti M, Rossignoli A, Posca M. A selective guide to pharmacovigilance resources on the internet. *Pharmacoepidemiol Drug Saf* 1998;**7**:183–8.

23. Bigby M. Rates of cutaneous reactions to drugs. *Arch Dermatol* 2001;**137**:765–70.

24. Temple R. Meta-analysis and epidemiologic studies in drug development and postmarketing surveillance. *JAMA* 1999;**281**:841–4.

25. Laupacis A, Sackett DL, Roberts RS. An assessment of clinically useful measures of the consequences of treatment. *N Engl J Med* 1998;**318**:1728–33.

26. Altman DG. Confidence intervals for the number needed to treat. *BMJ* 1998;**317**:1309–12.

27. Bjerre LM, LeLorier J. Expressing the magnitude of adverse effects in case-control studies: "the number of patients needed to treat for one additional patient to be harmed". *BMJ* 2000;**320**:503–6.

11
How to critically appraise pharmacoeconomic studies

Suephy C Chen

Dermatologists are increasingly interested in pharmacoeconomic studies because of the realisation that funds for health care are limited. There are four fundamental types of pharmacoeconomic studies (Table 11.1). This chapter outlines the types of studies, gives dermatological examples, and concludes with a discussion of the necessary items for pharmacoeconomic studies. Readers can then critically appraise these studies.

Cost analysis

Cost analysis is the most fundamental pharmacoeconomic study. This type of analysis deals solely in costs and does not directly account for the outcome of the therapy. Researchers can report their results from either micro-costing or macro-costing. Micro-costing involves enumerating each component of a therapeutic strategy and then determining the cost of each component. Tsao et al.[1] used micro-costing methods to determine the annual direct cost of diagnosing and treating melanoma. The authors systematically itemised the components of direct healthcare costs for melanoma care such as excisional biopsies, excision with primary closure, encounters with physicians, lymph node biopsy and interferon alpha. They estimated the annual direct cost of treating newly diagnosed melanoma in 1997 to be US$563 million.

Macro-costing determines the overall cost to care for a particular disease, usually with a population-based approach. Kirsner et al.[2] used a macro-costing approach to evaluate the cost of hospitalisation for dermatology-specific and diagnosis-related groups (DRGs) using data from the Medicare Provider Analysis and Review (MEDPAR) 1990–1996 database, which contains information for all Medicare beneficiaries using hospital inpatient services. The authors used codes for "major skin disorders", "minor skin disorders", "skin grafting/debridement for ulcer and cellulites", "skin ulcer" and "cellulitis", and found that in 1996, Medicare reimbursement was US$52 million for dermatology-specific DRGs and US$840 million for dermatology-related DRGs, a combined total of US$892 million.

Cost analysis is useful as a source of rigorous cost accounting and as the basis for other pharmacoeconomic studies. However, cost analyses do not account for outcomes and potential side-effects. Without accounting for the outcomes, the value of the therapeutic intervention cannot be easily measured. A costly medication that does not work well and does not provide quality outcomes has very little value. On the other hand, a costly medication that routinely improves lives may have very high value.

Cost-effectiveness analysis

Cost-effectiveness analysis (CEA) is one form of pharmacoeconomic analysis that incorporates both costs and outcome. The results of CEAs are

Table 11.1 Summary of the advantages and disadvantages of different types of pharmacoeconomic analyses

Type of pharmacoeconomic analysis	Advantages	Disadvantages
Cost analysis	Sources of rigorous cost accounting Basis of other pharmacoeconomic studies	Does not account for outcomes and side-effects Does not measure the value of the therapy
Cost-effectiveness analysis (CEA)	Accounts for outcomes and side-effects Measures value of the therapy	Outcomes are not standardised across disease processes Results are not weighted according to importance
Cost-utility analysis (CUA)*	Accounts for outcomes and measures value of therapy Results are standardised Accounts for importance	Need to invoke some external criterion of value to interpret results
Cost-benefit analysis (CBA)	Accounts for outcomes and measures value of therapy Does not need external criterion of value to interpret results	Assigning monetary value to health may be offensive May be difficult to measure benefits in monetary terms for expensive and complex therapies

*Often called cost-effectiveness analysis by health services researchers

presented as a cost-effectiveness ratio (CE ratio), with costs in the numerator and health outcomes in the denominator. The ratio is a measure of value; the smaller the ratio, the fewer the resources required for a given unit of health outcome. Costs are determined in the same manner as for cost analysis, as discussed above. The health outcomes are generally measured by some biological unit, such as intra-ocular pressure for glaucoma interventions, or by life-years saved for cancer chemotherapy.

CEAs generally compare at least two therapies – usually a new therapy is compared with a currently available therapy. A CEA that compares two therapies is called an incremental CEA; the additional costs that one therapy would entail are compared with the additional benefits that it provides. This is in contrast to an average CEA in which the therapy in question is not

compared with anything. However, this approach does not provide useful information to the policymaker or the clinician unless the currently available therapy is to do nothing.

CEAs provide information about the value of the therapeutic intervention in question by accounting for the outcomes of the therapy. However, the outcome measure is not standardised and therefore cannot be used to make comparisons with other disease processes. For example, even if a reasonable outcome measure for a new therapy for seborrhoeic dermatitis may be dollars per clear scalp, this measure cannot be used when the policymaker wants to compare the CE ratio with analyses of new therapies for disparate diseases such as onychomycosis, venous ulcers or acne. Even if "clear skin" is used as the outcome measure, it cannot be used to make comparisons with non-dermatological problems. Another problem with CEA is that the outcomes are not weighted according to their importance. For instance, assume that new therapies for scalp psoriasis, onychomycosis and venous ulcers were cost-effective compared with their respective current therapies. Policymakers may not be able to incorporate all the therapies into their formulary because of budgetary constraints. They would need to decide which is the most important outcome: clear scalp, smooth nails or healed ulcer. A better situation would be to have the outcomes standardised and weighted according to value so that policymakers could compare CEAs results across disease processes.

Stern et al.[3] published a CEA comparing topical versus systemic therapy for acne. Because of the lack of efficacy data, they had to rely on expert impressions. They calculated an incremental cost-effectiveness ratio, but used "side-effect averted" as their outcome measure. While this outcome may be useful for making comparisons with other acne therapies, the definition and magnitude of the side-effect episodes are hard to standardise across other diseases.

Cost-utility analysis

Cost-utility analysis (CUA) provides outcomes that are standardised and weighted. The CUA gives rise to a ratio similar to that of a CEA except that the outcomes are measured in quality-adjusted life-years (QALYs). Note that many health services researchers use the two terms CUA and CEA synonymously.[4] QALYs reflect both the additional quantity of life that a therapy extends and also the quality of that additional amount of life. The latter measurement is particularly important in fields like dermatology in which therapeutic interventions rarely save lives but often improve qualify of life. In the QALY approach,

quality of life is measured by a set of weights called utilities, one for each possible health state, that reflect the relative desirability of the health state. The reader is encouraged to consult other references for a detail explanation of utilities.[4,5] By incorporating quality of life and by standardising the outcome measure with QALYs, a dermatology CUA such as acne therapy can be compared with a mortality-impacting CUA such as breast cancer therapy.

Freedberg et al.[6] published a CUA comparing a one-time screening strategy for melanoma with a no-screening strategy. They primarily used life-year saved as their outcome measure, but they also used an estimate of utilities to estimate a QALY outcome. They found the CE ratio for the screening programme to be US$29 170 per life-year saved and US$30 360 per QALY. While the strategy of screening once in a lifetime may not mimic reality, the analysis was a good beginning for investigating the cost-effectiveness of melanoma screening. Before interpreting the QALY result (US$30 360 per QALY), readers should realise that the criterion for cost-effectiveness, called the CE threshold, is arbitrary and open to debate. A cost-effective therapy is one that delivers more QALYs per dollar (or costs fewer dollars per QALY) compared with some benchmark. Researchers consider therapies less than US$50 000 per QALY to be relatively cost-effective whereas those greater than US$175 000 per QALY are not.[7–9]

Cost-benefit analysis

Cost-benefit analysis (CBA) differs from CEA and CUA in that the results are reported as differences between the costs and health benefits of the therapeutic programme. The health benefits are represented in monetary terms, usually by asking subjects how much they would be willing to pay for the therapy. The interpretation of a CBA is also different from that of a CEA or CUA. The CEA/CUA results give the value of a particular therapy relative to a standard therapy. However, in order to decide whether the new therapy is worth adapting at the expense of forgoing a different therapy, the reader must invoke some external criterion of value, such as the CE threshold. The CBA, in contrast, allows the investigator to determine whether the therapy is worth the costs without an external criterion since all benefits in CBA are valued in monetary terms.

We[10] compared Goeckerman therapy with methotrexate for psoriasis using CBA in addition to the CUA described above. We queried a sample of "society" for the amount that they would be willing to pay for each therapy if their insurance company did not provide cover for it. We found that there was no net benefit of Goeckerman therapy over methotrexate for mild, moderate and severe psoriasis. When we compared each therapy with a "do nothing" approach for all three severity levels of psoriasis, only methotrexate produced net benefits for severe psoriasis.

Detractors of CBA cite a wariness of assigning monetary value to health because of moral and ethical issues.[5] However, proponents of the method point out that decision-makers who use the CEA/CUA must either implicitly or explicitly place a monetary value on the health outcome since they will need to choose some threshold below which they consider that the outcome is worth the cost.[4] Another disadvantage to the CBA method lies in the validity of the "willingness to pay" estimate of the value of the health benefits. Fortunately, many dermatological therapeutic programmes are neither overly expensive nor complex, and thus it is reasonable to expect subjects to be able to conceptualise how much they would be willing to pay for a dermatological therapy.

Guidelines for critical appraisal of pharmacoeconomic studies (Box 11.1)

Box 11.1 Checklist for readers of pharmacoeconomic analyses (adapted from Siegel et al.[11]).

Framework

- Perspective of analysis
- Target population for intervention
- Description of comparator programmes

Data and methods

- Diagram of pathway of health intervention
- Type of outcome used in analysis
- Methods for obtaining cost, effectiveness and quality of life
- Costs are market rates and not charges
- Critique of data quality
- Assumptions for input data are tested with sensitivity analysis
- Inflation and discount rates noted

Results

- Reference case
- Sensitivity analysis

Discussion

- Summary of reference case
- Discussion of sensitivity analysis
- Limitations of study pointed out
- Discussion of relevance to health policy decisions

Framework

To evaluate any pharmacoeconomic analysis, the reader must bear in mind several points about the framework of the study. First, the study needs to be clear about the perspective of the analysis. Three main perspectives of a pharmacoeconomic analysis include the individual patient, the third-party payer and society. The perspective dictates the cost used in the analysis (see below). The Panel on Cost-effectiveness in Health and Medicine has recommended including an analysis from the societal perspective, called the reference case.[11] Second, along with perspective, the target population to which the intervention is directed should be explicitly stated. Lastly, all pharmacoeconomic studies should be incremental analyses, comparing at least two therapies unless no standard of care exists. Pure cost analyses can be an exception to this guideline since they can be used purely to account for cost.

Data and methods

Authors of pharmacoeconomic studies should detail the pathway of the health intervention being analysed, preferably with diagrams. In this way, readers can determine whether the proposed flow of health care is comparable to their own method of health care. If not, then the analysis may not be relevant to the reader. The study should be explicit in the types of outcomes used in the analysis, whether it is QALYs, life-years saved, or disease-specific outcomes such as clear scalp. The methods for obtaining cost, effectiveness, and quality-of-life measures should also be clear. If primary data are not available, the assumptions must be clearly stated and a sensitivity analysis performed to make sure that the results of the analysis are robust to these assumptions (see below). A critique of the quality of the input data should also be explicit.

Several general points about cost should be mentioned at this point. The perspective of the study influences the costs used in the analysis. If an analysis is performed from the perspective of the individual patient, then only the costs relevant to the patient should be considered. These costs would include the copay that is involved with the physician visit and the drug, and the time off from work that is needed to see the doctor. Assuming that the drug is covered by insurance, the actual cost of the drug would not be factored since it is irrelevant from the perspective of the patient. On the other hand, third-party payers would be concerned about the cost of the drug as well as the cost of the physician, but not the copay or the time off from work. The analysis performed from the societal perspective would factor in costs that affect all members of society: the cost of the drug, the physician, and the time off from work, as well as any impact on family members.

It is also useful to consider the categories of cost when evaluating a pharmacoeconomic analysis.

Direct healthcare costs are the cost of the resources that directly provide the therapy. These include physicians, medications, laboratory monitoring, radiography, for example.

Indirect costs are those resources that related to time and productivity. Indirect costs include the cost of the consumption of the time that the patient took from work, volunteer time and family-leisure time. It can also include costs associated with the loss of or impaired ability to work secondary to illness.

The theoretically correct manner to estimate cost is by determining the opportunity cost. Opportunity costs consist of the value of forgone benefits; some other programme must have been forsaken in order to pay for a particular therapeutic regimen. For instance, in a hypothetical developing country, it might be necessary to sacrifice an education programme in order to implement a vaccination programme. However, sometimes one cannot assume perfect competition between two competing programmes, so healthcare prices may not approximate true opportunity costs. Instead, health economists use existing market prices to estimate costs. The reader should be wary of analyses that use charges to estimate costs, since charges rarely approximate the market prices of services.

In general, analyses performed from the societal perspective approximate the cost of physician and hospital services by using the Medicare reimbursement rate and estimate the cost of medication using the average wholesale price.

If the study analyses the therapy over a long time course, such as the 10-year outcome of a vaccination programme, then the study needs to outline methods to account for inflation. Also, because, in general, people prefer to have money and benefits now rather than in the future, future costs and benefits in the analysis must be discounted. The Panel on Cost-effectiveness in Health and Medicine has recommended using a 3% discount rate.[11]

Results and discussion

The authors should report and discuss their findings for the reference case, the analysis performed from the societal perspective. They should also report and discuss the results of their sensitivity analysis. When assumptions have been made for the input data, those variables should be varied within reasonable clinical parameters. If the results are sensitive to those variables change substantially, then readers should be wary of drawing firm conclusions and the authors should point out the limitations of the robustness of the results. Finally, the authors should discuss the relevance and limitations of their analysis to health policy questions and decisions.

References

1. Tsao H, Rogers G, Sober A. An estimate of the annual direct cost of treating cutaneous melanoma. *J Am Acad Dermatol* 1998;**38**:669–80.

2. Kirsner R, Yang D, Kerdel F. Dermatologic disease accounts for a large number of hospital admissions annually. *J Am Acad Dermatol* 1999;**41**:970–3.

3. Stern R, Pass T, Komaroff A. Topical v systemic agent treatment: A cost-effectiveness analysis. *Arch Dermatol* 1984;**120**:1571–8.

4. Drummond M, O'Brien B, Stoddart G, Torrance G. *Methods for the Economic Evaluation of Health Care Programmes, 2nd ed.* Toronto: Oxford Medical Publishers, 1990.

5. Gold M, Siegel J, Russell L, Weinstein M, eds. *Cost-Effectiveness in Health and Medicine.* New York: Oxford University Press, 1996.

6. Freedberg K, Geller G, Miller D, Lew R, Koh H. Screening for malignant melanoma: A cost-effectiveness analysis *J Am Acad Dermatol* 1999;**41**:738–45.

7. Owens D. Interpretation of cost-effectiveness analyses. *J Gen Intern Med* 1998;**13**:716–17.

8. Hlatky M, Owens D. Cost-effectiveness of tests to assess the risk of sudden death after acute myocardial infarction. *J Am Coll Cardiol* 1998;**31**:1490–2.

9. Goldman L, Garber A, Grover S, Hlatky M. Cost-effectiveness of assessment and management of risk factors. *J Am Coll Cardiol* 1996;**27**:1020–30.

10. Chen S, Shaheen A, Garber A. Cost-effectiveness and cost-benefit analysis of using methotrexate v Goeckerman therapy for psoriasis: A pilot study. *Arch Dermatol* 1998;**134**:1602–8.

11. Siegel J, Weinstein M, Russell L, Gold M. Recommendations for reporting cost-effectiveness analyses. *JAMA* 1996;**276**:1339–41.

12

Applying the evidence back to the patient

Hywel Williams

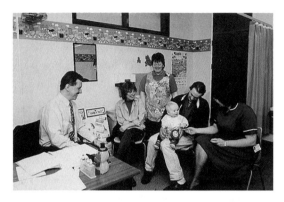

Figure 12.1   Clinical trial evidence is all very well, but if the patient in front of you tells you "I don't want that treatment", what then?

Applying the external evidence back to the patient sitting in front of you is perhaps one of the most difficult and least discussed steps of evidence-based medicine.[1,2] Having unearthed some relevant, high-quality and valid information from clinical trials in relation to a clinical question generated by a patient encounter, five questions now need to be asked in order to guide the application of such information to that patient.[3] These are listed in Box 12.1 and discussed in turn below.

1. How similar are the study participants to my patient?
Trial participants are sometimes atypical

Participants in clinical trials may be different from the patient who originally prompted you to

Box 12.1 (continued)

its comparator, is the magnitude of that gain clinically worthwhile?

- Is your patient as impressed as you are by such a potential magnitude of gain?
- Have you translated the magnitude of benefit into the number needed to treat for that patient's baseline risk – do you still think it is worthwhile?

4. What are the adverse effects?

- Why did the patients drop out of the studies?
- Have you considered rare side-effects that might not show up in the trials?
- How will you communicate this risk of adverse events to your patient?
- How will you involve your patient in weighing up the pros and cons of the treatment choices?

5. Does the treatment fit in with my patient's values and beliefs?

- What is their prior belief about the proposed intervention?
- Do they prefer a topical or systemic medication?
- Would they prefer no pharmacological treatment at all?
- What treatments have they had before?

ask an evidence-based question in obvious biological ways such as age, sex and clinical disease type.[4] In most circumstances, these differences do not prevent you from making some useful generalisations from the literature. For example, I would be quite happy to generalise from a randomised controlled trial (RCT) of topical steroids for atopic eczema in the absence of strict diagnostic criteria, provided that the description of that disease made sense to me, for example phrases such as "itchy red flexural eczema".

Occasionally, the description of the clinical trial participants may render it difficult to extrapolate study results to the patient in front of you. For example, it may be unrealistic to generalise the results of an RCT dealing with high-dose UVA in

the treatment of German women with an acute flare of atopic eczema to a South African man with chronic lichenified atopic eczema. In such circumstances, perhaps more weight is then given to one trial of chronic eczema in adult men than to several trials conducted in younger women.

Perhaps one of the most frequent problems encountered here is that of having to generalise trials of adult therapy to children, in whom RCTs are rarely performed. Yet, children can suffer almost all of the "adult" skin diseases, and practitioners frequently have no choice but to use adult-based data as a guide.

Another difficulty is that treatments that appear promising when tested in enthusiastic and healthy "atypical" clinical trial volunteers often turn out to be less effective when applied to a wider group of patients with other co-morbidities and levels of compliance. Such a divergence between study participants and real patients has been termed the difference between efficacy and effectiveness.[5] A regimen that involves fiddling around with creams three times a day may be just maintained under the special conditions of a clinical trial with continuous encouragement by the study assessors (and sometimes financial inducements), but when it comes to trying it in everyday life it may simply be too much trouble. These effects can often be explored by looking at the dropout rate for different interventions and reasons for such dropouts. Finding such effects should not deter the reader from using the evidence, but rather make him/her more aware of the factors that need to be taken into account when describing the potential efficacy of a treatment to the patient. One type of trial design, namely the pragmatic clinical trial, overcomes the "ideal patient" effect by recruiting as wide a mix of patients as possible and by capturing the effects of poor compliance in the final analysis.[6]

Groups are different from individuals

Even if the person in front of you is a German woman with acute atopic eczema, the results of the trial may not translate to real clinical benefit to her for several reasons. First, because the treatment effects reported in clinical trials, whether this is a mean change in severity score or proportion of people cleared, refers to *groups* of people. In a group of patients with a summary treatment effect such as a mean change in SCORAD (SCORing Atopic Dermatitis) of 5 points, there will be some individuals with score changes of 10 or 15 points, some with changes of 3 or 4, some with no change, and possibly some whose disease worsened. For example, closer inspection of the trial data on sildenafil (Viagra) for the treatment of erectile dysfunction[7] suggested that some men had all the fun! It follows that the patient sitting in front of you might benefit a lot or very little from the proposed treatment, and one has little way of knowing, apart from trying the treatment and seeing what happens. Similarly, telling your patient that "on average 60% of patients clear with this treatment" may not be very helpful if the patient then wants to know, "Am I in that 60%, Doctor?".

One way forward is to see whether treatment response varies according to different study subgroups, although it is unusual for dermatology RCTs to be large enough to include such subgroup analysis, and care has to be taken in "data dredging" in such studies. Conducting a series of n of 1 trials on that patient may appear one way forward,[8] but such an approach is only suitable for stable chronic diseases and for treatments that do not affect the response to subsequent treatments. Pharmacogenetic testing offers one way of predicting whether an individual will respond to a drug. For example, measurement of thiopurine methyl tranferase levels predicts who will develop serious bone marrow suppression from oral azathioprine.[9]

Triumph of the aggregate

It is easy to misinterpret the application of aggregate data to individuals by equating group probabilities to individuals.[10] Thus, if a trial of excisional surgery for melanoma showed that 95% of participants (similar to your patient) were clear from disease at 5 years, one cannot then tell your patient "You have a 95% chance of being clear at 5 years with this treatment" since this 95% refers to the group and not the individual. The patient in front of you will either clear or not clear – the patient's fate or response is already determined at that moment by that patient's microdisease and other cofactors such as immunological status, much of which may be under genetic influence. However, it is correct to tell that patient that "95% of people similar to you are clear at 5 years".

This inability to directly map aggregate data directly to individuals is not unique to RCTs – it applies to most basic science.[11] Our everyday "clinical experience" with a particular drug is, after all, a form of aggregation of data based on recollection of treatment responses amongst *groups* of previous patients. The same difficulties in predicting whether the next patient will respond to that drug and by how much exists more in anecdote-based clinical practice than in an RCT-based approach.

Conclusions

Thus, it is important to consider a number of factors when thinking about study participants and the patient in front of you.[4] There may be pathophysiological differences that could lead to diminished treatment response. For example, people with atopic eczema may not respond well to reduction to house dust mite if they were not allergic to house dust mite in the first place. There may be important social and economic differences that may diminish treatment compliance and hence response. For example a single parent with four children and a full-time job may not have the time to diligently apply short-contact dithranol to his/her widespread plaque psoriasis every day. Comorbidities such as renal disease might also affect treatment response either directly by affecting drug metabolism and clearance or indirectly through drug interaction and compliance. Many doctors practise this process "automatically" without labelling it as "evidence-based medicine". Sometimes, the patient's baseline risk of adverse events also profoundly affects the effectiveness of the treatment being contemplated. These factors do not mean that it is impossible to apply the results of RCTs to your patient – they are simply prompts to think about when generalising from a published study.

2. Do the outcomes make sense to me?

First, some things to watch out for. Even though you might have specified which outcomes would change your practice in your structured evidence-based question, for example "proportion of patients cleared at 6 months", very often the studies will contain a number of other short-term outcomes.[12] You then have to decide whether these outcomes provide useful clinical information. In most circumstances, there will be at least some information that makes some clinical sense to you.

Does PASI mean anything to you?

Particular care should be taken not to accept quantitative scales at face value. Scales that combine several objective clinical signs mixed up with symptoms into an overall scoring system have been very fashionable in dermatology RCTs in the past 30 years yet, despite their objective ring, they have rarely been tested for validity.[13] More importantly, such composite scales are often difficult to translate into clinical practice. What, for instance, does a difference of 8 units ($P<0.05$) in mean change of PASI score from baseline between two treatments mean to

you? Is the scale linear (i.e. does a PASI score of 30 mean "twice as bad" as a score of 15) as in other continuous variables such as height and weight? Should different components of these scales be added or multiplied by extent? Does a lot of psoriasis over the covered areas of the body mean more distress than a little bit of psoriasis on the backs of the hands and face?

Sensitive scales to amplify effects

There is a tendency for scales that are very sensitive to change to amplify statistically significant changes that may be clinically irrelevant. Take for example the trial of 2% minoxidil against placebo for androgenetic alopecia in women.[14] This study found a statistically significant increase in non-vellus target area hairs in the minoxidil-treated group versus the vehicle-treated group after 32 weeks ($P = 0.006$), although the "subjects discerned no difference". The study, which was otherwise well conducted, should have concluded something along the lines of, "something seems to be happening, but it is not clinically useful yet". However, the authors' conclusion was that, "Two per cent minoxidil appears to be effective in the treatment of female androgenetic alopecia". Effective for whom?

Too many scales, and too many short-term studies

Given the profusion of scales used in dermatology (there are at least 13 named and at least 30 unnamed scales in atopic eczema alone[15]), it is quite easy to introduce bias by choosing a scale which contains features that will enhance your product when compared with competing products. Introduction of a new scale is another potential source of bias since they can increase the likelihood of showing a treatment benefit.[16] Lack of suitable long-term outcomes is another problem frequently encountered in dermatology clinical trials. For example, atopic eczema is a long-term condition for most sufferers, yet of the 272 RCTs conducted to date, most have been less than 6 weeks' duration.[12] Other factors such as frequency and duration of the remission are key components in evaluating the value of therapy. It is therefore important when reading a trial report to think of the time frame for outcomes as well as the type of outcome.

So what would I go for?

Although composite scales may be useful in the early development of a drug in that they may show that something is happening, the key question within the framework of pursuing an evidence-based prescription is whether something *useful* is happening. Given the limitations of quantitative composite scales in dermatology, what should one look for in terms of outcomes that can best inform practice? My starting position would be to see what the patients who participated in the trials thought of their treatment, using simple measures such as proportion of participants with "good or excellent" response or other categorical measures such as percentage cleared. Did the quality of life of the patients improve? Although such measures are subjective, is not such subjective distress the precise treatment goal for many chronic skin diseases with significant psychological effects? Objective measures are of course also needed alongside measures that help to generalise the meaning of such subjective responses across cultures, since it is possible that some cultural groups may complain less about symptoms. Objective measures are also more useful in some diseases (for example to assess the response of treatments for basal cell carcinoma). Again, these need to be simple enough for most physicians and their patients to understand, for example the proportion of recurrences within 5 years rather than hazard ratios for first recurrence.

3. Magnitude of treatment effects
How big?

Even if a trial yields a result which is clinically meaningful, it is important to take the results of that study one step further by asking yourself, "Is the *size* of that benefit likely to be helpful for *my patient*?". Many trials report significant differences in treatment responses that might sound impressive at face value, yet when one considers the magnitude of such benefits, they are less exciting. Even when the study benefits are of large magnitude, they may still not be enough. Consider a patient with a facial port wine stain who is treated by pulsed tunable dye laser, and who achieves a 70% reduction in total surface area involved. We might be impressed by such a magnitude of gain, but if the patient is still unhappy because he or she feels that the stigma associated with the residual lesion is just as disabling, or that the odd pattern of circular pale holes left by the laser within the lesion draws even more attention to it, then this is a treatment failure.

Thus, it is crucial to consider not only if a treatment is effective in a published report, but to follow with the additional question of *how* effective. It follows that an important part of the discussion with the patient is to agree on what is possible or not possible in terms of realistic treatment objectives.

Number needed to treat

Because many interventions in medicine are of only modest effect, their apparent benefit may not be that noticeable after one has tried the intervention on a few patients. One way to understand the magnitude of benefit in relation to baseline risk is to use the concept of "number needed to treat" (NNT).[17] This refers to the number of patients that on average you would need to treat in order to see one additional success in the new treatment when compared with standard treatment. NNT is calculated simply as the reciprocal of the difference in success rates between the treatments being compared. Thus, a new treatment that results in clearing of psoriasis in 40% of patients compared with 30% for the conventional treatment translates to a risk difference of 10% (40 – 30) and an NNT of 1/0·10 which equals 10. In other words, one needs to treat 10 patients on average in order to see on extra gain in terms of clearance for the new treatment.

Patients' versus physicians' views regarding the threshold for what might constitute a useful NNT may differ significantly. Thus, in a study of perspectives of physicians and patients on anticoagulation for atrial fibrillation, patients placed significantly more value on the avoidance of bleeding than did doctors.[18] Again, the message here is not to think of NNT as belonging exclusively to doctors – patients too need to be incorporated into the decision-making process of determining what is useful and important.

It is also important that the dermatologist and patient decide for themselves as to what might constitute a useful NNT, rather than blindly accepting the sort of conventions that have been derived from acute medicine where the stakes are perhaps higher. So, although it may be perfectly justifiable to treat 200 patients with a low dose, aspiring to prevent one stroke, I would certainly not be willing to work with such an NNT for a new antibiotic if the gain was just one extra short-term remission of acne. In a pressurised health service I might even question the value of a new treatment for plaque psoriasis with an NNT of 20. Perhaps the opportunity costs associated with seeing the extra 20 patients needed in order to achieve one extra response from the new treatment could be better spent discussing other treatment options with them or assessing other new patients. Despite these caveats, the NNT is a more useful tool than measures of relative risk such as odds ratios to translate the evidence back to the patient.

4. Adverse events
Trials are not a useful source of rare but serious side-effects
As highlighted in Chapter 10, adverse events are often overshadowed by emphasis of the positive treatment benefits in clinical trials. Details of reasons for withdrawals are frequently missing altogether in trial reports, and failure to perform an intention-to-treat analysis may compound this because dropouts may be related to lack of efficacy or to adverse events which are not obviously related to the trial medication.[19] Rare side-effects are unlikely to show up in small clinical trials and often emerge as subsequent case reports or during post-marketing surveillance. Simply stating that no serious liver problems occurred in 100 patients taking traditional Chinese herbs for atopic eczema is still compatible with an upper 95% confidence limit of 3% if a larger population were tested.[20]

Particular efforts should therefore be made to scrutinise trials for a list of the frequency and severity of adverse events, as discussed in Chapter 10. As the events surrounding the thalidomide tragedy remind us, caution should be exercised when using new treatments that have not been tested on thousands of patients. Additional literature sources and post-marketing surveillance studies need to be scrutinised before one can reassure patients on side-effect issues within a reasonable degree of certainty.

Limitations of aggregate data
Just as for assessing treatment benefits, aggregate data on side-effects can be misleading. Thus, when comparing two types of corticosteroids, one may find that the mean decrease in skin thickness is similar in the two groups. Yet, if by further scrutiny of the individual data, one finds that two children in one group developed skin thinning with noticeable visible striae, then that might influence your decision to use such treatment despite the relative reassurance of the group means. Even when such adverse events are very rare, this may be of little comfort to the patient in the sense that it is an all-or-nothing predetermined event.

Communicating risks

How to communicate risk presents its own problems, with different conclusions being reached by doctors and their patients depending on how the information is presented in terms of relative or absolute risk.[21] Even when the risks are understood, weighing up the pros and cons of an intervention is a highly variable affair. Not only does this depend on the type of information presented to the patient, but also on the way the information is presented. Thus, a doctor who believes that a patient with psoriasis needs ciclosporin A may play down the possibility of permanent kidney damage by his or her body language and by saying that he or she has treated hundreds of patients without any problem. However, for another patient who has requested the same treatment, but for whom the doctor considers ciclosporin A inappropriate, he or she may use the very same potential adverse event as a "threat" to dissuade the patient.

Weighing up risks and benefits

Combining the values of treatment benefits versus risks for individual patients has been tackled using approaches such as decision analysis – a process whereby the sequential choices faced by patents are made explicit.[22] Patients are then invited to place their own values on the various potential gains and losses. These methods have been used extensively in areas such as amniocentesis for detecting fetal abnormalities, but less so in dermatology.[23] Simplifications of a decision analysis approach such as the likelihood of being helped or harmed have been advocated by others.[24]

5. What are the patient's values?
Values and belief models

Even if the external evidence suggests a good treatment for your patient, he or she might have a number of unforeseen reasons for choosing or not choosing that treatment. Therefore, a teenager who consults you with acne, whose friend developed pigmentation of the gums whilst taking minocycline, might initially refuse that treatment option. This does not mean that, if that drug is deemed to be the best choice in those circumstances, the dermatologist does not then go on to explain how rare such an event really is in order to reach a joint decision with the patient. Another patient with acne might come back demanding treatment with isotretinoin simply because his or her friend at school had similar treatment with excellent long-term results and tolerable side-effects. Again, although such a declaration might influence the consultation, this does not automatically mean that the dermatologist will concede to such a request if he or she feels that the treatment is not in the patient's best interest (for example very mild disease or a history of several unplanned pregnancies). The point here is that application of the best external evidence requires a dialogue with the patient to explore their values and expectations.

Sometimes, patients prefer to use something that they perceive to be more "natural", for example evening primrose oil rather than synthetic topical corticosteroids for atopic eczema. Sometimes patients prefer to forgo pharmacological treatment and instead undertake various measures to manipulate their environment. Others just prefer to take a few pills and forget about it. Some like creams, others like ointments. Some people do not wish to be involved in lengthy discussions of treatment options if indeed they believe that their doctor is the best person to help them choose a treatment option. For example, a person with a basal cell carcinoma may be happy to be recommended surgical excision rather than debate the 10 or so treatment options available to treat such lesions.

These issues of personal perception, belief models, locus of control, and personal experience only reveal themselves at the follow up consultation with the patient. Although patients' treatment choices may at times appear to be at odds with the external trial reports, patients are human beings who have their own set of preferences and values, and these need to be respected and understood. Like the first patient encounter, this area is where the art of healing and science of medicine meet.[25] Both the doctor and their patient may indeed resort to various "games" in order to achieve each other's ulterior motives.[26]

And if the treatment still does not work?

After agreeing on a treatment, a patient may return saying that the treatment does not work. Having explored obvious issues such as whether the ointment ever reached the skin, and whether the "allergic reaction" from topical benzoyl peroxide was in fact a predictable irritant reaction which could be circumvented by less frequent or vigorous application, other treatment options are often explored. If several treatments fail in a particular patient, the patient may belong to a subset with refractory disease, making it even more difficult to generalise from clinical trials of people with more responsive forms of the disease. Dermatologists frequently face the problem of trying several drugs in succession. External trial evidence could be improved by better descriptions of study participants in terms of previous treatments and by means of sequential RCTs that try different treatment approaches following failure of a treatment.

Conclusions

Applying evidence back to patient is often the most difficult and neglected step in the practice of evidence-based dermatology. This step requires consideration of several factors, including an appraisal of the magnitude and meaning of the treatment benefit and adverse events in relation to the patient's values and preferences.[27] Presenting the evidence back to the patient is a complex process requiring good communication skills and an appreciation of the limitations of the generalisability of trial data in terms of trial participants, relevance and size of benefits.

Having illustrated the chapter with examples of some of the difficulties in applying evidence to individual patients, I would like to close with an example of how easy and fruitful practising evidence-based dermatology can be. I was recently called to see a young woman with cutaneous larva migrans that was causing intense itching on her feet. My first-line treatment would have been oral albendazole, probably because I had been involved in writing up a case series several years earlier.[28] I was just about to recommend this when I reminded myself to practise what I preached by conducting a search of Medline using the term "cutaneous larva migrans" as a sensitive textword search. To my surprise, I quickly found a small but good RCT published in the *American Journal of Tropical Medicine and Hygiene* (not a journal I read every week) suggesting that a single 12 mg dose of ivermectin was more effective than albendazole.[29] And so that is what I recommended. The itching stopped within 24 hours and the visible eruption was cleared within a few days.

References

1. Mant D. Can randomised trials inform clinical decisions about individual patients? *Lancet* 1999;**353**:743–6.
2. Eypasch E. The individual patient and evidence-based medicine – a conflict? *Langenbecks Arch Surg* 1999;**384**:417–22.
3. Williams H. Dowling Oration 2001. Evidence-based dermatology – a bridge too far? *Clin Exp Dermatol* 2001;**26**:714–24.
4. Dans AL, Dans LF, Guyatt GH, Richardson S. Users' guides to the medical literature: XIV. How to decide on the applicability of clinical trial results to your patient. Evidence-Based Medicine Working Group. *JAMA* 1998;**279**:545–9.
5. Li Wan Po, A. *Dictionary of Evidence-based Medicine* Oxford: Radcliffe Medical Press, 1998:52.

6. Roberts RJ, Casey D, Morgan DA, Petrovic M. Comparison of wet combing with malathion for treatment of head lice in the UK: a pragmatic randomised controlled trial. *Lancet* 2000;**356**:540–4.

7. Virag R. Indications and early results of sildenafil (Viagra) in erectile dysfunction. *Urology* 1999;**54**:1073–7.

8. Nikles CJ, Glasziou PP, Del Mar CB, Duggan CM. Mitchell G. N of 1 trials. Practical tools for medication management. *Aust Fam Physician* 2000;**29**:1108–12.

9. Lennard L. Therapeutic drug monitoring of cytotoxic drugs. *Br J Clin Pharmacol* 2001;**52** (Suppl 1):75S–87S.

10. Bakan D. The general and the aggregate: a methodological distinction. *Percept Mot Skills* 1955;**5**: 211–12.

11. Straus SE, McAlister FA. Evidence-based medicine: a commentary on common criticisms. *Can Med Assoc J* 2000;**163**:837–41.

12. Hoare C, Li Wan Po A, Williams H. Systematic review of treatments for atopic eczema. *Health Technol Assess* 2000;**4**(37).

13. Charman C, Williams H. Outcome measures of disease severity in atopic eczema. *Arch Dermatol* 2000;**136**: 763–9.

14. Olsen EA. Topical minoxidil in the treatment of androgenetic alopecia in women. *Cutis* 1991;**48**:243–8.

15. Charman C, Williams HC. The problem of un-named scales for measuring atopic eczema. *J Invest Dermatol* in press).

16. Marshall M, Lockwood A, Bradley C, Adams C, Joy C, Fenton M. Unpublished rating scales: a major source of bias in randomised controlled trials of treatments for schizophrenia. *Br J Psychiatry* 2000;**176**:249–52.

17. Cook RJ, Sackett DL. The number needed to treat: a clinically useful measure of treatment effect. *BMJ* 1995;**310**:452–4.

18. Devereaux PJ, Anderson DJ, Gardner MJ *et al.* Differences between perspectives of physicians and patients on anticoagulation in patients with atrial fibrillation: an observational study. *BMJ* 2001;**323**:1218–22.

19. Hollis S, Campbell F. What is meant by intention to treat analysis? Survey of published randomised controlled trials. *BMJ* 1999;**319**:670–4.

20. Eypasch E, Lefering R, Kum CK, Troidl H. Probability of adverse events that have not yet occurred: a statistical reminder. *BMJ* 1995;**311**:619–20.

21. Levine M, Whelan T. Decision-making process-communicating risk/benefits: is there an ideal technique? *J Natl Cancer Inst Monogr* 2001;**30**:143–5.

22. Thornton JG, Lilford RJ, Johnson N. Decision analysis in medicine. *BMJ* 1992;**304**:1099–103.

23. Ashcroft DM, Li Wan Po A, Williams HC, Griffiths CE. Cost-effectiveness analysis of topical calcipotriol versus short-contact dithranol in the treatment of mild to moderate plaque psoriasis. *Pharmacoeconomics* 2000;**18**:469–76.

24. McAlister FA, Straus SE, Guyatt GH, Haynes RB. Users' guides to the medical literature: XX. Integrating research evidence with the care of the individual patient. Evidence-Based Medicine Working Group. *JAMA* 2000;**283**:2829–36.

25. Gibbs S. Losing touch with the healing art: dermatology and the decline of pastoral doctoring. *J Am Acad Dermatol* 2000;**43**:875–8.

26. Cotterill JA. Dermatological games. *Br J Dermatol* 1981;**105**:311–20.

27. Johnson SR, Dunn BK, Anthony M. Defining benefits and risks for SERMs in clinical trials and clinical practice. *Ann NY Acad Sci* 2001;**949**:304–14.

28. Williams HC, Monk B. Creeping eruption stopped in its tracks by albendazole. *Clin Exp Derm* 1989;**14**:355–6.

29. Caumes E, Carriere J, Datry A, Gaxotte P, Danis M, Gentilini M. A randomized trial of ivermectin versus albendazole for the treatment of cutaneous larva migrans. *Am J Trop Med Hygiene* 1993;**49**:641–4.

Part 3: The evidence

Section A: Common inflammatory skin diseases

Editor: Luigi Naldi

Additional chapters including *Chronic urticaria*, *Cicatrical pemphigoid* and *Epidermolysis bullosa acquisita* are published on the book website http://www.evidbasedderm.com.

13
Acne vulgaris

Sarah E Garner

Web tables referred to in this chapter are published on the book website http://www.evidbasedderm.com.

Background
Definition

Acne vulgaris is a pervasive disease of the pilosebaceous follicles of the skin, which are located on the face, back and chest. The disease has a range of clinical expression and can be classified according to the predominant lesion type.

- Non-inflammatory or comedonal acne is primarily composed of open comedones (blackheads) and closed comedones (whiteheads) with little or no inflammatory involvement.
- Inflammatory acne is characterised by inflamed lesions (pustules, papules and nodules) and can be further subdivided into papulopustular, nodular and conglobate depending on the predominant lesion type.
- Conglobate acne is characterised by clusters of lesions joined by sinus tracts. The older term nodulo-cystic acne is less used as it is accepted that the cysts are actually abscesses or granulomas.[1]

Incidence/prevalence

Estimates of the overall prevalence vary considerably and depend on the study populations and epidemiological methodology used. The disease is probably best defined by a continuum of severity, along which all members of the adolescent population are placed; it is estimated that up to 30% of teenagers have acne of sufficient severity to warrant medical treatment.[1] An increasing number of women in their twenties develop late-onset acne and surveys of adults over the age of 25 years have reported prevalence of 22% in males and 40% in females.[2,3]

Aetiology/risk factors

Although the exact aetiological mechanism is unknown, it is accepted that acne is the result of the interaction of several processes, which centre on pathological changes in the pilosebaceous duct (PSD) in response to an as yet unidentified trigger mechanism. Thickening of the follicular stratum corneum (hypercornification) leads to blockage and accumulation of sebum, which is produced in large quantities in response to the androgen surges that accompany puberty. The resident skin commensal *Propionibacterium acnes* then proliferates in the lipid-rich sebaceous follicles and there is a build up of bacteria and their metabolites, sebum and dead cellular material. This cannot be discharged because of the blockage at the follicle opening and there is therefore an inflammatory response. The extent and duration of the inflammation, and hence the severity of the acne, may be determined by individual variation in the immune response to *P. acnes*, its metabolic products or any component of the blocked PSD contents. The relative roles of the various contributory factors will also differ between individuals and possibly between sites in any individual.

The onset of acne is generally associated with adrenarche, although androgen markers and mild comedonal acne have been detected in children under 10 years of age,[4,5] particularly in girls who have an earlier onset of puberty.[6] Although the overall incidence tends to be equivalent in both sexes, with the peak rates occurring at 17 years of age,[7] boys tend to have more severe disease.[8] There is no evidence that ethnic or racial differences influence the development of acne, although Caucasians have been reported to have a higher incidence of disease.[9] Whilst genetic factors are also thought to influence susceptibility to acne,[10,11] the mode of inheritance has not been determined.

Prognosis

Most cases of acne clear spontaneously as an individual passes through adolescence and into their twenties. The reason for this is as yet undetermined, as there is no concurrent reduction in sebum production or change in its lipid composition. There are, however, two forms of post-adolescent acne in which the disease is evident in adulthood. Persistent acne commences in adolescence but does not resolve and is generally resistant to antibiotic therapy. Conversely, late-onset acne is generally less severe, evolves more commonly in women after 25 years of age, and has been linked to abnormalities in plasma androgens.[11,12]

The total burden of acne extends beyond financial costs; the impact on the individual can be devastating as the disease occurs at an age when its effects are acutely felt. Depression and anxiety are clearly linked to severe acne, and personality and self-esteem issues may arise that can have long-lasting effects on functioning as an adult. It has also been reported that acne patients have higher rates of unemployment, and the disease has been linked to suicide.[13]

Aims of treatment

Treatment aims to alleviate symptoms and accelerate healing of lesions in the short term and in the longer term to limit disease activity, scarring and the impact of the disease on quality of life.

The large number of treatment options available act by correcting one or more of the mediating factors that have been implicated in the pathogenesis of acne, and are commonly classified according to their route of delivery and mode of action. It is difficult to define an optimum treatment strategy because there is wide variation between individuals in response; finding the most suitable treatment is therefore a matter of trial and error. The comparative data on various therapies are limited and individual trials have obtained contradictory results, largely because of inadequate trial design and unfair comparisons in terms of dosage. Isotretinoin is the only acne treatment that can induce persistent remissions, but it is often unacceptable to patients because it has severe adverse effects. All other acne treatments are palliative and whilst improvement of symptoms and control of disease progression is possible, they need to be taken for prolonged periods.

Relevant outcomes

Disease severity is assessed by a visual assessment of the number of lesions and extent of disease. Although numerous visual assessment methods of varying complexity exist, at the basic level they can be subdivided into grades or counts. In both cases, there are three levels at which assessment can be made:

1. an overall or 'global' evaluation
2. subdivision according to the predominant morphological component (i.e. inflammatory or non-inflammatory)
3. separate evaluations of each individual lesion type, for example comedones, papules and pustules.

Results are generally expressed as an absolute or percentage change from onset of therapy and are commonly transformed to give the numbers of individuals attaining a given level of improvement, for example 50%.

Other important outcomes for the evaluation of therapy are changes in quality of life, scarring, patient satisfaction, tolerability and adverse events, speed of action and treatment-free interval.

Search methods

Evidence was reviewed according to the hierarchy of evidence whereby systematic reviews of randomised controlled trials (RCTs) are accepted as the most robust evidence, followed by individual RCTs. The primary source of evidence was therefore a recent systematic review of all acne therapies, prepared for the Agency for Healthcare Research and Quality (AHRQ).[14] This was supplemented by evidence located by searches in the following databases: *Cochrane Library* (Issue 1 2002), Cochrane Skin Group Specialist Trial Register, Medline (1966 to February 2002) and Embase (1980 to February 2002). An initial filter was applied to locate all acne trials [((study or trial) and acne).mp] and then more specific terms were applied within this set for individual interventions. No exclusions on the basis of language or study type were made.

QUESTIONS

Is there any evidence to support the routine use of skin cleansers and/or abrasives in the management of mild-to-moderate acne?

The impact of detergent bases on the control of sebum has not been ascertained, although it has been hypothesised that removal of sebum may enhance the activity of topically applied antibacterials. There is also controversy as to whether exfoliation using abrasives clears blocked PSDs and speeds up lesion healing, or whether associated irritancy and drying may

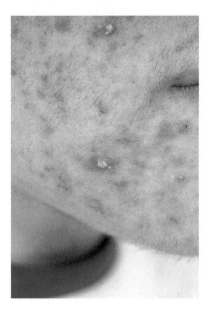

Figure 13.1 Mild-to-moderate acne

aggravate inflamed skin. Antibacterial agents reduce surface bacteria, but there is little evidence to suggest that they penetrate the PSD.

Efficacy

The AHRQ review included four relevant RCTs[15–17] and additional searches provided three others.[18–20] Five of the studies were double blind (Table 13.1); only two studies enrolled more than 100 patients.

The largest RCT showed that an acidic soap-free syndet was less irritant than soap and reduced both inflamed lesions (IL) and non-inflamed lesions (NIL) in 120 patients with mild acne who were not taking any other anti-acne medication.[16] There were no significant differences between the groups, although the individuals using soap experienced a mean increase in both NIL and IL over 12 weeks and 23/57 experienced irritation, compared with 1/57 in the soap-free group.

Cleansers containing the antibacterial hexachlorophene produced improvement in

Table 13.1 Randomised controlled trials of skin cleansers and abrasives

Author	Comparators	Number	Severity	Duration	Blinding	Results	Comments
Bettley and Dale 1976[15]	1. Hexachlorophene 2. Triclosan	34	1/2/3	6/6	0	No significant differences; drug improved: 21/28 v 22/28; local reaction: 11 v 9	6 LTF; not ITT; crossover study; no wash-out period
Fulghum et al. 1982[18]	1. Sulphur/salicylic acid cleanser with polyethylene granules 2. Sulphur/salicylic acid cleanser	53	1/2	8	0	Both reduced IL and NIL; no significant differences; equal sensitivity	7 LTF; not ITT; split half-face study; no concomitant therapy
Kanof 1971 (Part 2)[19]	1. Antibacterial soap 2. Soap	51	3	>12	A, P	Flare 13/30 v 22/31	Tetracycline responders: no details on concomitant therapy
Kanof 1971 (Part 1)[19]	1. Antibacterial soap 2. Soap	86	3	4	A, P	Response 30/44 v 31/42	All tetracycline 250 mg 2 or 3 times daily; no details on concomitant therapy; not ITT
Korting et al. 1995[16]	1. Acidic syndet bar 2. Soap	120	1	12	0	1 reduced IL and NIL; 2 increased IL and NIL; no intergroup comparison	2-week wash-out; 6 LTF; ITT analysis; Soap 5 dropouts exacerbation; no concomitant therapy
Milikan 1976 (A)[17]	1. Povidone-iodine cleanser 2. Vehicle	30	1	12–16	A, P	Improved 9/10 v 3/7; intolerance 1 = 2	13 LTF; not ITT
Milikan 1976 (B)[17]	1. Povidone-iodine cleanser 2. Vehicle	30	2	12–16	A, P	10/13 v 12/14 improved; 0 intolerance	3 LTF; all tetracycline 250 mg 1 or 2 times daily

(Continued)

Table 13.1 (*Continued*)

Author	Comparators	Number	Severity	Duration	Blinding	Results	Comments
Stoughton 1987 (A)[20]	1. Chlorhexidine gluconate cleanser 4% Benzoyl peroxide 5%	50	2	12	A	No significant differences IL or NIL	3 LTF; not ITT; no concomitant therapy twice-daily application
Stoughton and Leyden 1987 (B)[20]	1. Chlorhexidine gluconate cleanser 1·4% 2. Vehicle	110	2	12	A	1 > 2 IL and NIL; dry skin: 3 v 1	17 LTF; not ITT; no concomitant therapy twice-daily application
Millikan 1981[203]	1. Buff-puff 2. No abrasion	50	2	12	A	No intergroup comparisons: suggestion that abrasion better but no data	2 LTF; not ITT; all patients received 5% benzoyl peroxide; split-face study

Number, number of patients enrolled; severity (1 = mild; 2 = moderate; 3 = severe); duration (weeks); blinding (0 = open; A = assessor; P = patient); LTF, lost to follow up; ITT, intention-to-treat; NIL, non-inflamed lesions; IL, inflamed lesions equivalent numbers of patients to triclosan in a 12-week crossover trial with 34 patients,[15] although no wash-out period was permitted. Eleven patients experienced local reactions to triclosan and nine to hexachlorophene; hexachlorophene is now not recommended. Chlorhexidine was shown to produce equivalent significant reductions in NIL and IL in 50 patients with moderate acne when compared with 5% benzoyl peroxide at 12 weeks. It also produced significantly greater reductions in IL and NIL than those treated with the vehicle alone in 110 individuals, again at 12 weeks.[20]

In individuals treated with tetracycline, 500 mg twice daily, additional use of antibacterial soap in a 4-week period offered no benefit over use of normal soap. However, it was shown to significantly reduce the incidence of acne flare in responders to 4-week tetracycline therapy in a 90-day follow up (13/30 flared v 22/31).[19]

After 12–14 weeks' use in a double-blind RCT, povidone-iodine skin cleanser improved 9/10 patients with mild acne, compared with 3/7 in the vehicle group. The results are invalidated however by the high losses to follow up.[17] The results in a second group of patients with more severe acne who also received tetracycline, 250 mg once or twice daily, were equivocal (10/13 compared with 12/14).[17] Only one case of mild itching was experienced.

The addition of abrasives to a combination of sulphur and salicylic acid in a split-half-face study in 44 patients did not show any difference in either efficacy or tolerability after 8 weeks. The potential for the effects of the active ingredients to mask all other effects must be considered.[18] One split-face study evaluated the use of additional abrasion to 5% benzoyl peroxide therapy but there were no intergroup comparisons to validate the authors' claim that the side of the face treated with abrasion showed better results.[21]

Adverse effects

Soaps are of alkaline pH and are known irritants, causing itching, dryness and redness; acidic soap-free cleansers may therefore be preferential. Aggressive use of abrasives may irritate skin and for that reason common sense suggests that they should not be used in conjunction with topical agents such as benzoyl peroxide, which sensitise the skin, unless tolerance has initially been demonstrated. Dermatological reactions are idiosyncratic and cannot be predicted and the patient should be advised to discontinue use immediately if irritation develops. Like any topical agent, it is possible that antibacterial cleansers and abrasives are less suitable in individuals with sensitive skin. The literature does not support a link between the use of topical antimicrobials and the emergence of antiseptic or antibiotic resistance.[22]

Comment

The number of propionibacteria on the skin surface is increased by soap and decreased by synthetic detergents.[23] This may be due to the changes in skin pH, which is increased by soap.[23] There is no evidence either for or against the use of abrasive agents either alone or in combination with topical treatments. There is evidence to suggest that antibacterial skin cleansers may be effective in the management of mild acne,[17] and may produce similar outcomes to benzoyl peroxide in moderate acne.[20] However, the long-term benefits of "step-up" management strategies versus aggressive therapy from onset have not been examined. There is no evidence that antibacterial cleansers offer additional benefits when used in conjunction with oral antibiotics in individuals with more severe acne, but they may help maintain improvement following termination of antibiotic therapy.[19] The impact of increased contact time during washing has not been examined.

Implications for clinical practice

In individuals with mild acne whose disease is not adversely affecting their quality of life, antibacterial washes should be considered in the choice of first-line management strategies in step-up approaches. They should also be considered in the maintenance of patients who have ceased therapy following response. They should not be prescribed routinely in patients who are receiving more aggressive therapy as there is no evidence of any additional benefit. Alkaline syndet bars may be preferential to soap in skin care routines.

What is the role of topical non-antibiotic agents in the treatment of mild primarily non-inflammatory acne?

Mild acne consisting of open and closed comedones with a few inflammatory lesions is commonly treated with topical agents. A number of options have been shown to be effective in placebo-controlled RCTs, and all can be used either alone or in combination. Options include the topical retinoids (isotretinoin, tretinoin and adapalene), benzoyl peroxide, salicylic acid and azelaic acid. Topical antibiotic agents are discussed in the next question.

Topical retinoids

Topical retinoids reduce abnormal growth and development of keratinocytes within the PSD. This inhibits microcomedone formation and therefore subsequently reduces the number of comedones and inflamed lesions.

Efficacy

Evidence for the efficacy of topical retinoids was available from two systematic reviews,[14,24] which examined 20 RCTs and split-face studies.[25–43] Two further studies were located through searching[44,45] (See Web Table 13.1). Focusing

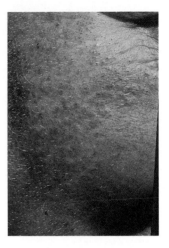

Figure 13.2   Non-inflammatory lesions. By kind permission of Dr Carolyn Charman

only on comparisons that had at least two RCTs of acceptable quality showing moderate-to-strong statistical evidence, the authors of the AHRQ review concluded that 0·1% adapalene and 0·025% tretinoin were equally efficacious and that motretinide and tretinoin were equally effective. The second review[24] evaluated five RCTs of 0·1% adapalene gel versus 0·025% tretinoin.[29–31,34,46] All RCTs were investigator blind and a total of 900 individuals with mild-to-moderate acne were enrolled. Using data collected from intention-to-treat (ITT) analyses, equivalent efficacy against total lesion counts was demonstrated, with adapalene showing greater activity at 1 week.

Further examination of the results show that of the six RCTs that presented data,[29,30,33,34,46] mean percentage reductions in NIL ranged from 46% to 83% in the 0·1% adapalene group and from 33% to 83% in the 0·025% tretinoin group at 12 weeks. Percentage reductions in IL were 48–69% and 38–71%, respectively. Higher-strength adapalene (0·5%) was investigated in one 25-patient split-face study and was shown to have greater activity than 0·1% adapalene against both IL and NIL, but was associated with more erythema.[45] Two strengths of adapalene (0·1% and 0·03%) were evaluated in three studies enrolling a total of 186 patients with mild-to-severe acne.[28,29,47] The higher strength produced greater reductions in IL and NIL counts but was associated with more irritation.

Little comparative data for retinoids against other agents were retrieved. In 77 patients with mild-to-moderate acne, 0·05% isotretinoin applied twice daily was slightly less effective than 5% benzoyl peroxide against IL and NIL and was slower to resolve IL.[42] The results for tretinoin against benzoyl peroxide[48–50] were equivocal and there were no differences in the rate of adverse events.

Adverse effects

Topical retinoids induce local reactions and should be discontinued if the reaction is severe. All studies presenting data suggested that 0·1% adapalene causes less local irritation than 0·025% tretinoin[45] and that the rate of local reactions of both agents increases with concentration.[28,29,45,47,51] Retinoids increase the sensitivity of skin to UV light and should therefore be applied at night and washed off in the morning. Rarely eye irritation, oedema and blistering of the skin occur, and hypopigmentation may result from tretinoin use.

Comment

There remains uncertainty as to whether retinoids applied topically cause birth defects, and whilst minimal absorption has been demonstrated following topical application,[52] it is recommended that they are not used during pregnancy or by women of child-bearing age who are not taking adequate contraceptive precautions.

Implications for practice

The comoedolytic action of topical retinoids suggests that they should be used in the treatment of mild acne. However, as this activity halts subsequent lesion formation, they are also suitable for moderate-to-severe acne and can be used in conjunction with topical and oral antibiotics. Benzoyl peroxide inactivates tretinoin, so the two agents should not be applied simultaneously; if used in combination, one should be applied in the morning and one at night. All topical retinoids cause local sensitivity reactions that appear to be less common with adapalene. To limit local sensitivity, topical retinoid therapy should start at a lower strength applied every third night and increase gradually.

Benzoyl peroxide

The lipid solubility of benzoyl peroxide allows it to penetrate the PSD. It has comoedolytic, anti-inflammatory and bactericidal activity and is therefore suitable for management of individuals with mild inflammatory or mixed acne. It can be bought over the counter from pharmacies and is available in a number of formulations, in strengths of 2·5–10%.

Efficacy

The AHRQ systematic review[14] examined seven placebo-controlled RCTs in patients with mild-to-severe acne[42,53–58] (see Web Table 13.2). Changes in both NIL and IL were consistently significantly superior in the active group. Two RCTs reported mean reductions in lesion counts with 5% benzoyl peroxide: 52% and 60% for IL and 30% and 52% for NIL.[42,55] The reductions in the vehicle comparator arms were less than 10% in each case. Four RCTs compared different dosages of benzoyl peroxide[48,53,59] and no evidence was located to support a dose–response effect (Table 13.2).

Three RCTs compared topical tretinoin with 5% benzoyl peroxide.[49,50,60] Tretinoin was shown to be more effective against NIL up to 12 weeks, but benzoyl peroxide had a greater impact on IL.

Table 13.2 Benzoyl peroxide (BP) dose response randomised controlled trials

Author	Comparators	Number	Severity	Duration	Blinding	Outcomes	Comments
Mills et al. 1986(2)[53]	1. BP 2·5% 2. BP 5%	53	1/2	8	P, A	Equivalent efficacy and burning, peeling and erythema IL: 56% v 58% reduction	2 LTF; not clear if randomised
Mills et al. 1986(3)[53]	1. BP 10% 2. BP 2·5%	50	1/2	8	P, A	Equivalent efficacy but 10% more burning, erythema and peeling IL: 45% v 47% reduction	No LTF; not clear if randomised
Yong 1979[59]	1. BP 2·5% 2. BP 5 %	200	1/2/3	4–18	0	>50% reduction in lesion counts 64/96 v 74/98 (no SSD); erythema 45 v 50; desquamation 22 v 28; itching/burning 16 v 10; no SSD overall	6 LTF, arms not comparable; Asian population; twice-daily application; Variable duration of treatment
Handojo 1979[48]	1. Tretinoin 0·05% 2. BP 5% 3. BP 10% 4. Tretinoin 0·05%/ BP 5 % 5. Tretinoin 0·05%/ BP 10%	250	1/2/3	10	0	Overall change greater in 5% combination group; rate of local intolerance 20% both groups but greater in 10% group; >50% reduction in NIL: 34/47 v 37/45 v 33/47 v 45/50 v 44/50 >50% reduction in IL: 27/36 v 34/42 v 28/41 v 34/44 v 39/49; no SSD between BP concentrations	11 LTF; not ITT; 47 patients needed alterations due to adverse reactions
Marsden 1985[174]	1. BP 5% 2. BP 5%/0·5 g OT 3. BP 5%/1 g OT 4. BP 5%/1·5 g OT	82	1/2/3	16	A	Patient adequate response: 2/23 v 6/24 v 8/19 v 12/17; 10 BP patients local intolerance; IL: 56 v 70 v 75% v 78% reduction	Assume randomised but not stated; previous failure to treatment; 10 LTF; not ITT
Fryand and Jakobsen 1986[202]	1. BP 5% (alcohol) 2. BP 5% (water)	48	–	8	P, A	No difference in clinical effect but less irritation in water-based preparation	Abstract only

Number, number of patients enrolled; severity (1 = mild; 2 = moderate; 3 = severe); duration (weeks); blinding (0 = open; A = assessor; P = patient); LTF, lost to follow up; ITT, intention-to-treat; (N)IL, (non)-inflamed lesions; SSD, statistically significant difference

Compared with topical 0·05% isotretinoin, 5% benzoyl peroxide had a greater effect on IL at 8 weeks but not 12 weeks and a similar effect on NIL at all time points in 77 patients with mild-to-moderate acne[42]; 5% benzoyl peroxide has similar efficacy to 20% azelaic acid in mild acne.[61]

Adverse effects

Benzoyl peroxide is commonly associated with local irritation that presents as erythema, peeling, dryness, burning, stinging, itching and soreness. Use of an emollient or water-based gel may reduce these reactions. Allergic contact dermatitis, characterised by erythema, small papules and pruritus, may occur rarely. RCT evidence shows that the side-effect profile of a 2·5% preparation is similar to that of 5%[53,59] and less than 10% preparations.[53] Combinations of benzoyl peroxide with antibiotics are unstable because of degradation of the antibiotic by benzoyl peroxide. Benzoyl peroxide will bleach hair and fabrics and patients should therefore be counselled accordingly. It is safe for use during pregnancy. There have been concerns that benzoyl peroxide may promote skin cancer[62,63] but these have been refuted.[64]

Comment

A major concern with the continued use of antibiotics, topical and oral, is the promotion of *P. acnes* resistance. Benzoyl peroxide has a broad-spectrum bactericidal action, which does not select for resistance during long-term use. It is therefore recommended that it is used intermittently during courses of antibiotics to eliminate any resistant propionibacteria.[65,66]

Implications for practice

Benzoyl peroxide is an effective treatment for mild-to-moderate acne vulgaris as a result of its activity against both IL and NIL. Some individuals find benzoyl peroxide to be highly irritant on initial application. Tolerance is generally developed with prolonged exposure and individuals should be counselled accordingly. Low-strength benzoyl peroxide is recommended as higher strengths are more irritant and there is no evidence to suggest that 10% in general is more effective than 5%. It is common practice for patients to apply benzoyl peroxide to individual lesions alone; clinicians should advise patients to apply it in a thin layer to all areas to prevent the formation of new lesions.

Salicylic acid

Salicylic acid is an exfoliant and chemical irritant.

Efficacy

The AHRQ review[14] located three RCTs (Table 13.3).[66–68] The largest study found 2% salicylic acid to be more effective against all lesion types than the alcoholic lotion vehicle at 12 weeks in 114 paired individuals with mild-to-moderate acne.[66] The second study enrolled 30 individuals and had major losses to follow up;[68] 1·5 % salicylic acid was more beneficial than placebo. One further cross-over RCT in 30 individuals with mild acne compared a 2% cleanser with 10% benzoyl peroxide facial wash; neither product was therefore in prolonged contact with the skin.[67] The results of the study cannot be considered as valid evidence, however, because the trial was only 4 weeks in total and there was no wash-out period between the 2-week treatment periods.

Adverse effects

Salicylic acid is known to cause skin irritation that presents as erythema, dryness and peeling; this was evident in the RCT evidence located.

Table 13.3 Randomised controlled trials of salicylic acid

Author	Comparators	Number	Duration	Severity	Blinding	NIL	IL	Outcomes	Comments
Shalita 1989[67]	1. Salicylic acid 2% cleanser 2. BP 10% wash	30	2 + 2	1/2	0	34 20		No side-effects reported	Crossover; no wash-out period; no LTF; results not valid as phase 1 only 2 weeks and no wash-out period; BP group higher NIL count at baseline; short contact
Eady et al. 1996[66]	1. Salicylic acid 2% 2. Vehicle	114	12	1/2	2	46* 26	28* 9	1>2 all lesions; irritant dermatitis both groups but greater incidence in 1, % decrease total lesions: 40 v 16*	15 LTF; not ITT; both in alcoholic lotion
Roth 1964[68]	1. Salicylic acid 1·5% 2. Placebo	30	10	1/2	0			Salicylic acid reported as greater reduction but no intergroup comparison; burning in 10/15 salicylic acid group	

Number, number patients enrolled; severity (1 = mild; 2 = moderate; 3 = severe); duration (weeks); blinding (0 = open; A = assessor; P = patient); (N)IL, (non)-inflammatory lesions; decrease from baseline;*, statistically significantly superior ($P<0.05$); LTF, lost to follow up; ITT, intention-to-treat

Implications for practice

There is no evidence to support the routine use of salicylic acid in preference to other topical therapies.

Azelaic acid

Azelaic acid has been shown to normalise the increased keratinocyte production and keratinisation associated with acne and to inhibit *P. acnes*.[69] A direct anti-inflammatory effect has also been demonstrated.[70]

Efficacy

The AHRQ review[14] located eight RCTs of azelaic acid in mild-to-moderate acne (see Web Table 13.3). The comparators used were placebo,[71] vehicle,[72] benzoyl peroxide,[61] tretinoin,[72] oral tetracycline[73,74] and in combination with glycolic acid versus tretinoin.[75] One further RCT published in German evaluated its efficacy against 2% erythromycin.[76,77]

In papulopustular acne 20% azelaic acid has similar efficacy at 5 or 6 months to 0·05% tretinoin,[72] 5% benzoyl peroxide,[61] 2% topical erythromycin[77] and oral tetracycline 1 g/day,[73,74] with consistent percentage reductions in median IL of 80–84%. Across the studies, good-to-excellent improvement occurred in 71–82% of individuals. In comedonal acne 20% azelaic acid has similar activity to 0·05% topical isotretinoin, with 79% and 82% reduction in comedonal counts, respectively, and good or excellent improvement in 59% and 63% of the 289 patients at 6 months.[72]

Adverse effects

In common with other topical agents, azelaic acid induces cutaneous reactions, which occur in approximately one-third of individuals.[77] The incidence is highest in the first four weeks of therapy and, in the RCTs examined, only 5–10%

of reactions were categorised as "marked". In the clinical studies, which also included post-marketing evaluations, 0–5% of individuals experienced scaling, 5–23% burning and 13–29% itching. Azelaic acid is not known to cause photosensitivity and sublethal doses do not promote *P. acnes* resistance.[78] Azelaic acid is better tolerated than benzoyl peroxide,[61] and tretinoin[72,75] and it does not bleach clothing or hair. It is used in hyperpigmentary skin disorders, but has not been shown to have depigmentatory effects in acne patients[77] suggesting that it preferentially targets abnormal melanocytes.

Comments

There are no known incompatibilities between azelaic acid and other topical anti-acne agents.

Implications for practice

Azelaic acid has been shown to be an effective therapy in mild-to-moderate papulopustular acne and to be as effective as 0·05% isotretinoin in comedonal acne. The onset of action is slower than that seen with benzoyl peroxide. Azelaic acid can be used less sparingly than isotretinoin – 2·5 cm of cream should be applied to the face. Patients should be counselled to expect a delayed response. Anecdotal reports have suggested that azelaic acid may reduce the incidence of post-inflammatory hyperpigmentation, which is possibly attributable to its activity on abnormal melanocytes.[79] Darker skinned patients should be monitored for signs of hypopigmentation.

Summary

All of the agents reviewed have been shown to be effective in the treatment of mild and moderate acne vulgaris. There is very little data to support the use of one agent over another and there has only been one RCT of use of the agents in combination, which showed that benzoyl peroxide and tretinoin in combination are superior to either agent alone.[48] Adapalene has been shown to be better tolerated than tretinoin, and the RCT evidence reviewed suggests that azelaic acid may be better tolerated overall than other agents, but there will be considerable variation between individual patients. A number of RCTs compare these agents against and in combination with topical antibiotics; these are considered in the next section.

What is the role of antibiotics in the management of acne vulgaris?

The role of antibiotics in the management of acne is still debated, and although much evidence has been collected on the efficacy of individual agents, there is very little good-quality comparative data. Oral antibiotics were used initially in the 1950s because it was assumed that acne occurred as a result of bacterial infection. Whilst activity against *P. acnes* has been clearly demonstrated, there is evidence of an anti-inflammatory effect,[80] which is still being investigated.

A number of oral antibiotics have been used to treat acne but are no longer used because of their side-effects; clindamycin and lincomycin are associated with an increased risk of pseudomembranous colitis; dimethylchlortetracycline (demeclocycline) induces phototoxic skin reactions and causes dose-dependent nephrogenic diabetes insipidus; and co-trimoxazole is associated with blood dyscrasias. This section therefore focuses on erythromycin, tetracycline, oxytetracycline, minocycline, doxycycline, lymecycline and trimethoprim.

Two systematic reviews provided evidence on the role of antibiotics.[14,81] The conclusions of the AHRQ review are based only on comparisons, where there are at least two trials of acceptable quality showing moderate-to-strong statistical evidence for a clinically meaningful endpoint and effect. Of the oral antibiotics, only clear evidence was located for tetracycline. Topical clindamycin and erythromycin were shown to be superior to vehicle in the treatment of mild-to-moderate acne and topical tetracycline was shown to be of no benefit. The Cochrane Review[81] of minocycline examined 27 RCTs and concluded that whilst minocycline is likely to produce similar outcomes to other first- and second-generation tetracyclines, it should not be used as a first-line agent because of uncertainty over its safety and higher cost compared with older tetracyclines. There was no evidence to suggest that it is superior to other tetracyclines and its efficacy relative to other acne therapies could not be reliably determined because of inadequacies in the studies examined.

Oral antibiotics

The AHRQ report reviewed 11 placebo-controlled trials of oral antibiotics[82–92] and two others were located by searches[93,94] (see Web Table 13.4). All but two RCTs investigated tetracycline; one evaluated minocycline[83] and one doxycycline.[95] All were double blind and most included patients with moderate-to-severe acne. Only three provided data at 12 weeks or more[85,88,89] and only three included more than 50 patients in each arm.[89,91,93] Tetracycline at total daily doses of 500 mg and 1 g was consistently superior to placebo in terms of overall grade and reduction in IL. The only data on NIL was from the doxycycline RCT,[95] which indicated comparable efficacy at 4 weeks, but this is to be expected given the delayed onset of activity associated with oral antibiotics.

Nine head-to-head RCTs of the currently used oral antibiotics were included in the AHRQ review[96–104] and the Cochrane review located a further nine[105–113] (see Web Table 13.5). The majority of the trials had problems with design and execution. No oral antibiotic was demonstrated to be superior to another, although equivalence cannot be conclusively stated as no study was adequately powered to demonstrate it. Percentage reductions in IL were consistently greater than 50% at 12 weeks. Percentage reductions in NIL were more variable, with only two RCTs showing more than 50% reductions at 12 weeks.[110,113] The results consistently showed an improvement in 70–90% of individuals at 12 weeks.

Topical antibiotics

The AHRQ review located 31 RCTs comparing a topical antibiotic with its vehicle and a further six RCTs were located by independent searches (see Web Table 13.6). Nine of the RCTs also included other comparators. The antibiotics investigated were clindamycin (12 RCTs),[58,90,91,114–122] erythromycin (13 RCTs),[123–130] erythromycin/zinc (three RCTs),[92,131,132] 2% fusidic acid (two RCTs),[133,134] meclocycline,[135] metronidazole,[136] triclosan[137] and tetracycline (three RCTs).[87–89] In the studies for which details were available, all but one study used twice-daily application.[58] Many of the studies were underpowered to conclusively state that there were no significant differences between the comparators.

The AHRQ review concluded that although clindamycin tended to produce greater reductions in IL than its vehicle, the results were rarely statistically significant; global measures more consistently indicated superiority to placebo. The evidence available does not support the effectiveness of clindamycin against NIL. Erythromycin similarly had a greater impact on IL. Fusidic acid was shown to be more active than vehicle against IL at 6 weeks in one study but not at 12 weeks in a second study, which also did not show any difference in its activity against NIL. The two meclocycline studies also showed decreases in IL, with no data for NIL. The 0·75% metronidazole RCT showed that it

was no more active than placebo in mild-to-moderate acne, neither producing statistically significant reductions in IL or NIL. The three tetracycline RCTs demonstrated that 0·5% tetracycline was approximately 50% more active than vehicle in terms of change in acne grade from baseline, although no intergroup statistical analyses were performed. Only one trial provided data on differential lesion counts; the results suggested that again tetracycline was active against IL but not NIL. In the larger RCTs a 55–60% mean reduction in IL was consistently seen at 12 weeks.[14]

The AHRQ review located 14 head-to-head trials of topical antibiotics (see Web Table 13.7). There were no differences in efficacy between clindamycin hydrochloride and phosphate,[117,118,122] or between different formulations[121,138,139] in the six RCTs examined. Four large RCTS[132,140–142] and one smaller study[143] compared clindamycin and erythromycin; all enrolled subjects had mild-to-severe acne. Several of the trials reported differences between the topical antibiotics for certain outcomes at certain time points, but there were no overall consistent differences. In comparison with tetracycline of unspecified concentration, the two located studies[144,145] reported insignificant or inconsistent differences in lesion counts. However, both trials demonstrated a significant difference in favour of clindamycin in the overall measures of acne severity or improvement. No difference between clindamycin and nicotinamide was shown in the RCT located, but it was underpowered to conclusively state equivalence.[146]

Oral versus topical antibiotics

The two systematic reviews located also provided comparative data on the use of oral versus topical antibiotics.[14,81] A number of other non-systematic reviews and individual RCTs were also located, giving a total of 20 studies,[127,147–159] six of which also included a placebo control arm.[87–92] (see Web Table 13.8). Twelve used double-dummy designs to maintain blinding. Oral antibiotics have a delayed onset of activity; therefore studies of shorter duration may be biased in favour of the topical agent.

The evidence from three RCTs suggests that minocycline, 50 mg twice daily, produces comparable results against both NIL and IL as 1% clindamycin applied twice daily.[153–155] The trials enrolled fewer than 100 patients and were therefore underpowered to conclusively state equivalence.

Six RCTs compared oral tetracycline 250 mg twice daily with 1% clindamycin twice daily.[90,91,127,147–149] Only one RCT was longer than 8 weeks duration[149] and only one study was adequately powered (305 patients) but was of inadequate duration.[91] This study found that at 8 weeks there was no significant difference in the percentage reductions obtained with either tetracycline 250 mg twice daily or 1% clindamycin applied twice daily in pustules (68% versus 76%) and papules (63% versus 68%) in patients with moderate-to-severe acne. However, the physician rated the clindamycin therapy as good to excellent in a greater number of cases – 86/105 compared with 66/103 ($P<0.05$). Four of the other studies failed to detect any significant differences between the therapies, with the fifth finding that clindamycin caused a significantly greater percentage reductions in IL (57% versus

72% ($P<0.001$)) at 8 weeks in patients with mild acne.[90] The 12-week study found no difference.[149]

Tetracycline, 250 mg twice daily, produced similar changes in lesion counts at 12 weeks to topically applied 1·5% erythromycin in a single RCT of 54 patients with moderate-to-severe acne.[152] Although numerically erythromycin produced greater percentage changes, these were not significant. None of the four RCTs located found any differences in overall grade between oral tetracycline, 250 mg twice daily, and topically applied 1·5% meclcocycline twice daily; both were superior to placebo in the three studies that also used a placebo control.[151] None of the studies used ITT analysis. At 8–12 weeks, oral tetracycline 250 mg twice daily was found to produce similar reductions in overall grade to topical 0·5% tetracycline, with one trial finding no effect on comedones.[87–89]

Combination therapy

A number of RCTs have investigated oral and topical antibiotics either against or in combination with other agents, (see Web Table 13.9) the rationale for this being that treatments that attack more than one factor implicated in the pathogenesis of acne will be more effective. The different mechanisms of action are summarised in Table 13.4.

Table 13.4 Targets of acne therapies (adapted from Gollnick[160])

	Sebum excretion	Keratinisation	Follicular *P. acnes*	Inflammation
Benzoyl peroxide	–	(+)	+++	(+)
Tretinoin	–	++	(+)	–
Clindamycin	–	–	++	–
Antiandrogens	++	–	–	–
Azelaic acid	–	++	++	+
Tetracyclines	–	–	++	+
Erythromycin	–	–	++	–
Isotretinoin	+++	++	(+)	++

+++, very strong effect; ++ strong effect; + moderate effect; (+) indirect/weak effect; – no effect

Efficacy

Only one RCT was located that compared an oral antibiotic with benzoyl peroxide.[158] Although the study was underpowered to conclusively state equivalence, similar efficacy was found between 5% benzoyl peroxide and oral oxytetracycline, 250 mg twice daily, at 6 weeks. The oral agent was more effective against acne of the trunk. The AHRQ review located eight RCTs that compared topical antibiotics with 5% benzoyl peroxide and searches found one additional trial.[58,130,158,161–165] In the three RCTs located, 5% benzoyl peroxide was found to be more active against NIL in moderate acne than 1% clindamycin[58,161,162] over 10–12 weeks. Two studies also found it to be more active against IL,[161,162] although the third found no difference.[58] Benzoyl peroxide was also more active against both NIL and IL than 1% meclocycline.[164] Compared with erythromycin, benzoyl peroxide was more active against NIL and similarly active against IL.[130,163] All RCTs providing data showed benzoyl peroxide to cause more local irritation.

Three RCTs compared 20% azelaic acid with oral tetracycline (variable dose)[73,74] in patients with mild-to-severe acne. No significant differences were reported in any lesion counts except in the smallest trial, which was very small and suffered from high dropouts in the azelaic acid group. A 20-week RCT of 20% azelaic acid compared with 2% topical erythromycin was located through additional searches.[76] No differences between the comparators were found.

Use of combination therapies

Nine RCTs were located examining combinations of 0·025% tretinoin and 1% clindamycin against either tretinoin,[166] clindamycin,[166,167] or both[168,169] (see Web Table 13.10). One additional RCT compared 2% erythromycin/0·05% tretinoin against both agents individually.[170] Numerically, the combination produced greater mean percentage reductions in NIL than either agent alone, but the only statistically significant results were against clindamycin in two studies.[166,167] Against IL, the combination shows greater activity numerically than either agent, but it reached significance only against tretinoin.[166]

Combinations of antibiotics and benzoyl peroxide were examined in nine RCTS (see Web Table 13.11); the antibiotics were clindamycin,[58,161] erythromycin,[130,171–173] meclocycline[164] and metronidazole.[165] In the five studies that used an antibiotic alone as a comparator, the combination was shown to be more active against both IL and NIL.[58,130,161,171] Six studies used benzoyl peroxide alone as a comparator.[58,130,161,164,165] The data were equivocal, with some studies showing a greater effect for the combination and others showing no difference. Combinations of 5% benzoyl peroxide with 3% erythromycin has greater activity against *P. acnes* than 3% erythromycin and results in significantly greater clinical improvement.[66] One study compared 5% benzoyl peroxide plus 2% metronidazole against an oral antibiotic (oxytetracycline), but, because it was of only 6 weeks duration, unfairly biased the results against the oral antibiotic.[165] A 16-week study was the only one that compared concomitant use of 5% benzoyl peroxide with an oral antibiotic (oxytetracycline 0·5 g, 1 g and 1·5 g) but did not clearly state whether patients were randomly allocated to treatment.[174] The response was considered to be adequate in 2/23 patients with 5% benzoyl peroxide alone and in 6/24, 8/19 and 12/17 of patients using 5% benzoyl peroxide plus oxytetracycline 0·5 g, 1 g and 1·5 g, respectively.

Harms

All antibiotics are associated with individual side-effects that are well documented and must be considered. The potential systemic side-effects are theoretically reduced by topical application as usually less than 10% absorption occurs.[175] However, prolonged and extensive application to the skin, which is a good medium for gene exchange amongst bacteria,[176] may facilitate the spread of resistance.[177] This has implications for clinical practice as *P. acnes* resistance is associated with poor therapeutic response to antibiotics. Of greater importance, however, is the spread of resistance to other microorganisms and there have been calls for policies to restrict the prescribing of antibiotics in acne.[65,178] One systematic review examined *P. acnes* resistance to systematic antibiotics.[179] The 12 articles examined demonstrated an overall increase in *P. acnes* resistance from 20% in 1978 to 62% in 1996. Resistance was most commonly reported to erythromycin, clindamycin, tetracycline, doxycycline and trimethoprim; resistance to minocycline was rare. The authors concluded that long-term rotational antibiotics are inappropriate and that treatment should be adjusted when therapeutic failure becomes evident.

Comment

A proportion of individuals fail to respond to antibiotics - epidemiological studies estimated that this is between 10%[180] and 17%[181] of individuals. Theories that have been proposed include individual differences in the absorption, distribution and elimination of the antibiotic as well as poor compliance, the follicular micro-environment and *P. acnes* resistance.[180] The underlying severity of the disease may also determine response to antibiotics, as severe acne and acne of the trunk has been shown to respond less well than moderate acne,[182,183] possibly as a result of the higher sebum excretion rate[184] diluting follicular drug concentrations.[180] Clinically another important impact of alteration in cutaneous microflora is the possibility of the development of gram-negative folliculitis, which presents with profuse

superficial pustules around the nose and deep cystic lesions on the face and neck, usually colonised by *Proteus*, *Enterobacter* or *Klebsiella* species.[185]

Implications for practice

There is no conclusive evidence of the superiority of one antibiotic over another or between oral or topical application. Choice of agent should therefore be based on patient preference, with consideration of the individual side-effects of the antibiotics and the cost. The formulation of the topical antibiotic may also be important, for example alcohol bases are likely to be more drying and therefore more suitable for oilier skins. Patients with more extensive disease, particularly those with acne of the trunk, may prefer oral treatment rather than having to apply topical agents to extensive areas. It is vital that patients are properly counselled on how to use their medication as inappropriate use has been shown to reduce effectiveness.[174]

Second-generation tetracyclines such as minocycline, doxycycline and lymecycline are widely perceived to be more active in the belief that their greater lipophilicity results in greater sebum penetration and PSD concentration. This review has not found any evidence to support this and superiority has not been demonstrated. These agents are easier for patients to take, however, as they can be taken once daily and the absorption may be less affected by food.[186–188] However, there is no evidence to support the view that tetracycline needs to be taken four times a day: its half-life of approximately 9 hours in plasma is likely to be increased in the skin. There is also no evidence to suggest that maintaining serum antibiotic concentrations at steady state is necessary for clinical efficacy or moderates anti-inflammatory effects.

It is recognised that antibiotics have less activity than other agents against NIL, which makes them less suitable for use in patients with primarily non-inflammatory acne. The evidence for the comparative efficacy of antibiotics and benzoyl peroxide against IL is equivocal and further research is required to establish their relative place in acne therapy. The studies reviewed found that combinations of antibiotics with benzoyl peroxide were more effective than antibiotics alone, which can probably be attributed in part to the lack of activity of antibiotics against NIL. However, the irritancy of benzoyl peroxide may make it unacceptable to some patients. There is no compelling evidence for the combined use of antibiotics and retinoids. There is no benefit in concomitant use of oral and topical antibiotics and this practice may select for resistant strains. Intermittent use of benzoyl peroxide is recommended during extended antibiotic therapy to eliminate any resistant strains.[189]

What dose of oral antibiotics should be prescribed?

Historically, antibiotics have been used for the treatment of acne vulgaris at doses that are lower than those used for other infections. Although, the exact origin and rationale of this convention is not known, the most likely explanation is that doses were reduced initially in response to concerns over maintaining patients on high-dose antibiotics for long periods of time. When it was subsequently observed that lesions did not recur when the dose was reduced and that patients relapsed as soon as therapy was discontinued, dose reduction would have become standard practice.[190] Low doses of antibiotics were therefore used in early trials.[85,94,191,192] Guidelines recommended that full antibiotic doses should be used initially for 3–4 weeks and then reduced gradually until the patient can be maintained on the lowest possible dose.[193,194] Despite the fact that there are no adequate dose–response studies to support it, this use of low-dose antibiotics has remained standard practice for many years.

Only two RCTs were located that investigated the use of different doses of antibiotics: one failed to find any clinical difference after 8 weeks of therapy between patients maintained on an initial starting dose of minocycline 100 mg daily and those in whom the initial dosage was reduced to 50 mg daily after 4 weeks.[195] Minocycline may not be typical of all antibiotics, however, because there is considerable variation between individuals in the serum levels attained after oral administration.[196] Eight weeks may also be an inadequate period to examine comparative efficacy. In the second study, roxithromycin 300 mg was found to be more effective than 150 mg over 8 weeks in 30 patients with severe acne.[197]

Other evidence located comprised a series of non-randomised studies in 420 individuals with moderate-to-severe acne. In a non-randomised controlled study of 152 patients matched for age, sex, site of involvement and severity, those maintained on erythromycin, 1 g daily, and 5% benzoyl peroxide showed a significantly greater response than those receiving 0·5 g and 5% benzoyl peroxide. The improvements in acne grade at 6 months were 35% and 79% in men and 59% and 79% in women. The relapse rates within 1 year were also significantly lower in the high-dose group: 31% versus 60% in women and 82% versus 39% in men. A similar group of 296 patients did not show higher rates of gastrointestinal side-effects on the higher dose.[182] Individuals with severe acne, acne of the trunk and high sebum excretion rates responded less well to combined treatment with 5% benzoyl peroxide and erythromycin 250 mg twice daily over 6 months.[182]

There are also reports in the literature that higher daily doses of tetracycline[198] and oxytetracycline,[174] are more effective in patients with severe acne or acne that is recalcitrant to standard therapy. The results of these studies are questionable, however, as both have serious methodological flaws and used concomitant topical therapy. A cohort of 80 patients with nodulocystic and conglobate acne who had not responded to standard antibiotic doses showed improvement with 1·5–3 g tetracycline.[199] A second similar cohort of 31 patients with severe acne or acne resistant to standard-dose antibiotics received up to 3·5 g with concomitant topicals, 27 of whom showed great improvement. Fifteen individuals suffered adverse events and two had to discontinue therapy because of raised serum creatinine phosphokinase, emphasising the need for ongoing renal and hepatic monitoring. Onset of improvement ranged from 1 to 6 months. Flare occurred in nine patients on reduced dose, despite use of topicals.[198]

A prospective case series of 68 patients with moderate-to-"cystic" acne, in whom dose was titrated according to response, found that in a period of up to 2·5 years of the 58 patients who improved 51 required only 250 mg tetracycline daily.[192] Increased severity of acne was an indicator for higher dose and non-response. In 10 cases, tetracycline had no effect, regardless of dose.

For how long should antibiotic therapy be continued?

This question was not addressed in either of the systematic reviews and no specific RCT evidence was located. The literature contains a number of recommendations, few of which are backed by hard evidence. The consensus of opinion is that although the effects of antibiotics

Key points

- Antibacterial washes should be considered in the first-line management of mild acne and in the maintenance of individuals who have improved following other therapy. They should not be used routinely in conjunction with other therapies. There is no evidence to support the use of abrasives, which may further irritate already sensitised skin. Alkaline syndet bars are less irritant than soap for cleansing.
- Topical retinoids can be used in both non-inflammatory and inflammatory acne and in conjunction with oral and topical antibiotics. The evidence suggests that adapalene is less irritant than other retinoids.
- Azelaic acid is effective in mild to moderate acne and may be less irritant than topical retinoids, but has a slower onset of response.
- Benzoyl peroxide is an effective treatment in mild to moderate acne but causes an initial sensitisation that may persist in some individuals. Higher strength benzoyl peroxide is in general no more effective than lower strength but is associated with more irritation.
- Antibiotics are more effective against inflamed lesions than non-inflamed lesions. There is no evidence to support a difference in efficacy between any of the agents, either oral or topical.
- There is no good quality evidence to support recommendations about either the dose of antibiotics to be used or the duration of therapy; further research is urgently required.
- Benzoyl peroxide appears to have similar activity to antibiotics against inflamed lesions and greater activity against non-inflamed lesions, but causes local irritation. The evidence suggests that combined use of antibiotics with retinoids is more active than either agent alone, and whilst benzoyl peroxide combinations are more effective than antibiotics alone, the data against benzoyl peroxide alone are equivocal.
- Given concerns about the development of resistance, further research is urgently required to assess the efficacy of antibiotics relative to other agents and to provide data for an appropriate assessment of the risks and benefits associated with their continued use.
- Benzoyl peroxide should be used intermittently during extended antibiotic therapy to eliminate any resistant strains.

on inflammatory lesions are visible after a few days, a minimum of 3 weeks is required before any improvement can be categorically stated[89,194] and therapy should therefore be continued for a minimum of 3 months, and 6 months for maximum benefit.[1] As antibiotics do not expel existing comedones, the effect on these lesions only becomes evident after a few months of continual use; it takes approximately 8 weeks for a micro-comedone to develop into a visible lesion. Relapse occurs in nearly half of all patients up to 8 weeks after stopping therapy,[200] necessitating additional courses.[181] In patients who relapse immediately, the antibiotic used should be rotated every 6 months.[201] Two RCTs that included intermediate assessments showed that improvement continued beyond 4–6 weeks to 3 months.[85,100]

An observational cohort study of 543 patients with moderate acne treated with erythromycin, 1 g/day, combined with 5% benzoyl peroxide suggested that the median percentage improvement at 6 months was 78% (interquartile range 67–90%); 408/492 individuals showed over 50% reduction in acne grade; 247/279 who continued with benzoyl peroxide alone maintained improvement; 174 individuals who continued with combination for a further 6 months showed no additional benefit but this group also included a subgroup of responders, non-responders and those switched to alternative antibiotics. Therapy was continued in 31 patients who had not shown 50% improvement within the 6 month period: the percentage improvement was greater in the 29 individuals treated with minocycline.

References

1. Cunliffe WJ. *Acne*. London: Martin Dunitz Ltd, 1989.
2. Newton JN, Edwards C. Epidemiology and treatment of acne in primary care. *J Eur Acad Dermatol Venereol* 1997; 9(suppl.1):581.
3. Poli F, Dreno B, Verschoore M. An epidemiological study of acne in female adults: Results of a survey conducted in France. *J Eur Acad Dermatol Venereol* 2001;15:541–5.
4. Lucky AW, Biro FM, Huster GA, Leach AD, Morrison JA, Ratterman J. Acne vulgaris in premenarchal girls: An early sign of puberty associated with rising levels of dehydroepiandrosterone. *Arch Dermatol* 1994;130:308–14.
5. Lucky AW, Biro FM, Simbarti LA, Morrison JA, Sorg NW. Predictors of severity of acne vulgaris in young adolescent girls: Results of a five-year longitudinal study. *J Pediatr* 1997;130:30–9.
6. Stewart ME, Downing DT, Cook JS, Hansen JR, Strauss JS. Sebaceous gland activity and serum dehydroepiandrosterone sulfate levels in boys and girls. *Arch Dermatol* 1992;128:1345–8.
7. Burton JL, Cunliffe WJ, Stafford I, Shuster S. The prevalence of acne vulgaris in adolescence. *Br J Dermatol* 1971;85:119–26.
8. Cunliffe WJ, Gould DJ. Prevalence of facial acne vulgaris in late adolescence and in adults. *BMJ* 1979;1:1109–10.
9. Siemens HW. [The treatment and control of patients with acne]. [German]. *Munchener Medizinische Wochenschrift* 1965;107:1652–5.
10. Walton S, Wyatt R, Cunliffe WJ. Genetic control of sebum excretion and acne. A twin study. *Br J Dermatol* 1988;18:393–6.
11. Goulden V, McGeown CH, Cunliffe WJ. The familial risk of adult acne: a comparison between first-degree relatives of affected and unaffected individuals. *Br J Dermatol* 1999;141:297–300.
12. Goulden V, Clark SM, Cunliffe WJ. Post-adolescent acne: a review of clinical features. *Br J Dermatol* 1997;136: 66–70.
13. Cunliffe WJ. Acne and unemployment. *Br J Dermatol* 1986;115:386.
14. Lehmann HP, Andrews JS, Robinson KA *et al.* Management of Acne (Evidence Report/Technology Assessment No. 17 (Prepared by Johns Hopkins Evidence-based Practice Center under Contract No. 290–97–006). AHRQ Publication No. 01–E019. Rockville, MD: Agency for Healthcare Research and Quality, September 2001.
15. Bettley FR, Dale TL. The local treatment of acne. *Br J Clin Pract* 1976;30:67–9.
16. Korting HC, Ponce-Poschl E, Klovekorn W, Schmotzer G, Arens-Corell M, Braun-Falco O. The influence of the regular use of a soap or an acidic syndet bar on pre-acne. *Infection* 1995;23:89–93.

17. Milikan LE. A double-blind study of Betadine skin cleanser in acne vulgaris. *Cutis* 1976;**17**:394–8.

18. Fulghum DD, Catalano PM, Childers RC, Cullen SI, Engel MF. Abrasive cleansing in the management of acne vulgaris. *Arch Dermatol* 1982;**118**:658–9.

19. Kanof NB. Acne control with an antibacterial soap bar – a double-blind study. *Cutis* 1971;**7**:57–61.

20. Stoughton RB, Leyden JJ. Efficacy of 4 percent chlorhexidine gluconate skin cleanser in the treatment of acne vulgaris. *Cutis* 1987;**39**:551–3.

21. Millikan LE, Ameln R. Use of Buf-Puf(TM) and benzoyl peroxide in the treatment of acne. *Cutis* 1981;**28**:201–5.

22. Vaughan Jones SA, Hern S, Black MM. Neutrophil folliculitis and serum androgen levels. *Clin Exp Dermatol* 1999;**24**:392–5.

23. Korting HC, Kober M, Mueller M, Braun-Falco O. Influence of repeated washings with soap and synthetic detergents on pH and resident flora of the skin of forehead and forearm. *Acta Derm Venereol* 1987;**67**:41–7.

24. Cunliffe WJ, Poncet M, Loesche C, Verschoore M. A comparison of the efficacy and tolerability of adapalene 0·1% gel versus tretinoin 0·025% gel in patients with acne vulgaris: A meta-analysis of five randomized trials. *Br J Dermatol* 1998;**139**(Suppl. 52):48–56.

25. Caron D, Sorba V, Kerrouche N, Clucas A. Split-face comparison of adapalene 0·1% gel and tretinoin 0·025% gel in acne patients. *J Am Acad Dermatol* 1997;**36**(6 II Suppl):S110–S112.

26. Dunlap FE, Mills OH, Tuley MR, Baker MD, Plott RT. Adapalene 0·1% gel for the treatment of acne vulgaris: Its superiority compared to tretinoin 0·025% cream in skin tolerance and patient preference. *Br J Dermatol* 1998;**139**(Suppl. 52):17–22.

27. Galvin SA, Gilbert R, Baker M, Guibal F, Tuley MR. Comparative tolerance of adapalene 0·1% gel and six different tretinoin formulations. *Br J Dermatol* 1998;**139**(Suppl. 52):34–40.

28. Verschoore M, Langner A, Wolska H, Jablonska S, Czernielewski J, Schaefer H. Efficacy and safety of CD 271 alcoholic gels in the topical treatment of acne vulgaris. *Br J Dermatol* 1991;**124**:368–71.

29. Alirezai M, Meynadier J, Jablonska S, Czernielewski J, Verschoore M. [Comparative study of the efficacy and tolerability of 0·1 and 0·03 p.100 adapalene gel and 0·025

p.100 tretinoin gel in the treatment of acne]. [French]. *Ann Dermatol Venereol* 1996;**123**:165–70.

30. Grosshans E, Marks R, Mascaro JM *et al*. Evaluation of clinical efficacy and safety of adapalene 0·1% gel versus tretinoin 0·025% gel in the treatment of acne vulgaris, with particular reference to the onset of action and impact on quality of life. *Br J Dermatol* 1998;**139**(Suppl 52):26–33.

31. Berger RS, Griffin E, Jones L *et al*. Clinical safety and efficacy evaluation of 0·1% CD271 gel versus 0·025% Retin A gel and CD271 gel vehicle. 2002. Unpublished data (CIRD Galderma).

32. Clucas A, Verschoore M, Sorba V, Poncet M, Baker M, Czernielewski J. Adapalene 0·1% gel is better tolerated than tretinoin 0·025% gel in acne patients. *J Am Acad Dermatol* 1997;**36**(6 Pt 2):S116–18.

33. Ellis CN, Millikan LE, Smith EB *et al*. Comparison of adapalene 0·1% solution and tretinoin 0·025% gel in the topical treatment of acne vulgaris. *Br J Dermatol* 1998;**139**(Suppl. 35):41–7.

34. Shalita A, Weiss JS, Chalker DK *et al*. A comparison of the efficacy and safety of adapalene gel 0·1% and tretinoin gel 0·025% in the treatment of acne vulgaris: a multicenter trial. *J Am Acad Dermatol* 1996;**34**:482–5.

35. Christiansen JV, Gadborg E, Ludvigsen K *et al*. Topical vitamin A acid (Airol) and systemic oxytetracycline in the treatment of acne vulgaris. A controlled clinical trial. *Dermatologica* 1974;**149**:121–8.

36. Krishnan G. Comparison of two concentrations of tretinoin solution in the topical treatment of acne vulgaris. *Practitioner* 1976;**216**:106–9.

37. Schafer-Korting M, Korting HC, Ponce-Poschl E. Liposomal tretinoin for uncomplicated acne vulgaris. *Clin Invest* 1994;**72**:1086–91.

38. Dominguez J, Hojyo MT, Celayo JL, Dominguez-Soto L, Teixeira F. Topical isotretinoin *v.* topical retinoic acid in the treatment of acne vulgaris. *Int J Dermatol* 1998;**37**:54–5.

39. Elbaum DJ. Comparison of the stability of topical isotretinoin and topical tretinoin and their efficacy in acne. *J Am Acad Dermatol* 1988;**19**(3):486–91.

40. Christiansen J, Holm P, Reymann F. Treatment of acne vulgaris with the retinoic acid derivative Ro 11–1430. A controlled clinical trial against retinoic acid. *Dermatologica* 1976;**153**:172–6.

41. Christiansen J, Holm P, Reymann F. The retinoic acid derivative Ro 11–1430 in Acne vulgaris. A controlled multicenter trial against retinoic acid. *Dermatologica* 1977;**154**:219–27.

42. Hughes BR, Norris JF, Cunliffe WJ. A double-blind evaluation of topical isotretinoin 0·05%, benzoyl peroxide gel 5% and placebo in patients with acne. *Clin Exp Dermatol* 1992;**17**:165–8.

43. Nordin K, Fredriksson T, Rylander C. Ro 11–1430, a new retinoic acid derivative for the topical treatment of acne. *Dermatologica* 1981;**162**:104–11.

44. Shalita AR, Chalker DK, Griffith RF *et al.* Tazarotene gel is safe and effective in the treatment of acne vulgaris: a multicenter, double-blind, vehicle-controlled study. *Cutis* 1999;**63**:349–54.

45. Pierard-Franchimont C, Henry F, Fraiture AL, Fumal I, Pierard GE. Split-face clinical and bio-instrumental comparison of 0·1% adapalene and 0·05% tretinoin in facial acne. *Dermatology* 1999;**198**:218–22.

46. Cunliffe WJ, Caputo R, Dreno B *et al.* Efficacy and safety comparison of adapalene (CD271) gel and tretinoin gel in the topical treatment of acne vulgaris. A European multicentre trial. *J Dermatol Treat* 1997;**8**:173–8.

47. Dunlap FE, Baker MD, Plott RT, Verschoore M. Adapalene 0·1% gel has low skin irritation potential even when applied immediately after washing. *Br J Dermatol* 1998;**139**(Suppl. 35):23–5.

48. Handojo I. The combined use of topical benzoyl peroxide and tretinoin in the treatment of acne vulgaris. *Int J Dermatol* 1979;**18**:489–96.

49. Lyons RE. Comparative effectiveness of benzoyl peroxide and tretinoin in acne vulgaris. *Int J Dermatol* 1978;**17**:246–51.

50. Bucknall JH, Murdoch PN. Comparison of tretinoin solution and benzoyl peroxide lotion in the treatment of acne vulgaris. *Curr Med Res Opin* 1977;**5**:266–8.

51. Christiansen JV, Gadborg E, Ludvigsen K *et al.* Topical tretinoin, vitamin A acid (Airol) in acne vulgaris. A controlled clinical trial. *Dermatologica* 1974;**148**:82–9.

52. Van Hoogdalem EJ, Baven TL, Spiegel-Melsen I, Terpstra IJ. Transdermal absorption of clindamycin and tretinoin from topically applied anti-acne formulations in man. *Biopharmaceutics Drug Disposition* 1998;**19**:563–9.

53. Mills OH, Jr., Kligman AM, Pochi P, Comite H. Comparing 2·5%, 5%, and 10% benzoyl peroxide on inflammatory acne vulgaris. *Int J Dermatol* 1986;**25**:664–7.

54. Smith EB, Padilla RS, McCabe JM, Becker LE. Benzoyl peroxide lotion (20%) in acne. *Cutis* 1980;**25**:90–2.

55. Hunt MJ, Barnetson RS. A comparative study of gluconolactone versus benzoyl peroxide in the treatment of acne. *Australasian J Dermatology* 1992;**33**:131–4.

56. Jaffe GV, Grimshaw JJ, Constad D. Benzoyl peroxide in the treatment of acne vulgaris: a double-blind, multi-centre comparative study of "Quinoderm" cream and "Quinoderm" cream with hydrocortisone versus their base vehicle alone and a benzoyl peroxide only gel preparation. *Curr Med Res Opin* 1989;**11**:453–62.

57. Ede M. A double-blind, comparative study of benzoyl peroxide, benzoyl peroxide-chlorhydroxyquinoline, benzoyl peroxide-chlorhydroxyquinoline-hydrocortisone, and placebo lotions in acne. *Curr Ther Res Clin Exp* 1973;**15**:624–9.

58. Lookingbill DP, Chalker DK, Lindholm JS *et al.* Treatment of acne with a combination clindamycin/benzoyl peroxide gel compared with clindamycin gel, benzoyl peroxide gel and vehicle gel: Combined results of two double-blind investigations. *J Am Acad Dermatol* 1997;**37**:590–5.

59. Yong CC. Benzoyl peroxide gel therapy in acne in Singapore. *Int J Dermatol* 1979;**18**:485–8.

60. Handojo I. Retinoic acid cream (Airol cream) and benzoyl-peroxide in the treatment of acne vulgaris. *Southeast Asian J Trop Med Public Health* 1979;**10**:548–51.

61. Cavicchini S, Caputo R. Long-term treatment of acne with 20% azelaic acid cream. *Acta Derm Venereol Suppl* 1989;**143**:40–4.

62. Cartwright RA, Hughes BR, Cunliffe WJ. Malignant melanoma, benzoyl peroxide and acne: a pilot epidemiological case-control investigation. *Br J Dermatol* 1988;**118**:239–42.

63. Liden S, Iindelof B, Sparen P. Is benzoyl peroxide carcinogenic. *Br J Dermatol* 1990;**123**:129.

64. Kraus AL, Munro IC, Orr JC, Binder RL, LeBoeuf RA, Williams GM. Benzoyl peroxide: An integrated human safety assessment for carcinogenicity. *Regul Toxicol Pharmacol* 1995;**21**:87–107.

65. Eady EA, Jones CE, Tipper JL *et al.* Antibiotic resistant propionibacteria in acne; need for policies to modify antibiotic usage. *BMJ* 1993;**306**:555–6.

66. Eady EA, Bojar RA, Jones CE, Cove JH, Holland KT, Cunliffe WJ. The effects of acne treatment with a combination of benzoyl peroxide and erythromycin on

skin carriage of erythromycin-resistant propionibacteria. *Br J Dermatol* 1996;**134**:107–13.

67. Shalita AR. Treatment of mild and moderate acne vulgaris with salicylic acid in an alcohol-detergent vehicle. *Cutis* 1981;**28**:556–8.

68. Roth HL. Acne vulgaris: evaluation of a medicated cleansing pad. *Calif Med* 1964;**100**:167.

69. Gibson JR. Azelaic acid 20% cream (AZELEX) and the medical management of acne vulgaris. [Review] [30 refs]. *Dermatol Nurs* 1997;**9**(5):339–44.

70. Kurokawa I, Akamatsu H, Nishijima S, Asada Y, Kawabata S. Clinical and bacteriologic evaluation of OPC-7251 in patients with acne: a double-blind group comparison study versus cream base. *J Am Acad Dermatol* 1991;**25**:674–81.

71. Cunliffe WJ, Holland KT. Clinical and laboratory studies on treatment with 20% azelaic acid cream for acne. *Acta Derm Venereol Suppl* 1989;**143**:31–4.

72. Katsambas A, Graupe K, Stratigos J. Clinical studies of 20% azelaic acid cream in the treatment of acne vulgaris. Comparison with vehicle and topical tretinoin. *Acta Derm Venereol Suppl* 1989;**143**:35–9.

73. Bladon PT, Burke BM, Cunliffe WJ, Forster RA, Holland KT, King K. Topical azelaic acid and the treatment of acne: a clinical and laboratory comparison with oral tetracycline. *Br J Dermatol* 1986;**114**:493–9.

74. Hjorth N, Graupe K. Azelaic acid for the treatment of acne. A clinical comparison with oral tetracycline. *Acta Derm Venereol Suppl* 1989;**143**:45–8.

75. Spellman MC, Pincus SH. Efficacy and safety of azelaic acid and glycolic acid combination therapy compared with tretinoin therapy for acne. *Clin Ther* 1998;**20**:711–21.

76. Graupe K, Zaumseil RP. Skinoren – a new local therapeutic agent for the treatment of acne vulgaris. In: *Jahrbuch de Dermatologie*. Macher E, Kolde G, Bröcker EB eds. Zülpich: Biermann, 1991:159–69.

77. Graupe K, Cunliffe WJ, Gollnick HP, Zaumseil RP. Efficacy and safety of topical azelaic acid (20 percent cream): an overview of results from European clinical trials and experimental reports. [Review] [53 refs]. *Cutis* 1996;**57**(Suppl.1):S20–35.

78. Holland KT, Bojar RA. The effect of azelaic acid on cutaneous bacteria. *J Dermatol Treat* 1989;**1**:17–19.

79. Breathnach AS. Melanin hyperpigmentation of skin: melasma, topical treatment with azelaic acid and other therapies. *Cutis* 1996;**57**(Suppl. 1):36–45.

80. Eady EA, Ingham E, Walters CE, Cove JH, Cunliffe WJ. Modulation of comedonal levels of interleukin-1 in acne patients treated with tetracyclines. *J Invest Dermatol* 1993;**101**:86–91.

81. Garner SE, Eady EA, Popescu C, Newton J, Li Wan PA. Minocycline for acne vulgaris: efficacy and safety. In: Cochrane Collaboration. *Cochrane Library*. Issue 2. Oxford: Update Software, 2000.

82. Plewig G, Petrozzi JW, Berendes U. Double-blind study of doxycycline in acne vulgaris. *Arch Dermatol* 1970;**101**: 435–8.

83. Hersle K, Gisslen H. Minocycline in acne vulgaris: a double-blind study. *Curr Ther Res Clin Exp* 1976;**19**: 339–42.

84. Crounse RG. The response of acne to placebos and antibiotics. *JAMA* 1965;**193**:906–10.

85. Lane P, Williamson DM. Treatment of acne vulgaris with tetracycline hydrochloride: a double-blind trial with 51 patients. *BMJ* 1969;**2**:76–9.

86. Wong RC, Kang S, Heezen JL. Oral ibuprofen and tetracycline for the treatment of acne vulgaris. *J Am Acad Dermatol* 1984;**11**:1076–81.

87. Anderson RL, Cook CH, Smith DE. The effect of oral and topical tetracycline on acne severity and on surface lipid composition. *J Invest Dermatol* 1976;**66**: 172–7.

88. Blaney DJ, Cook CH. Topical use of tetracycline in the treatment of acne: a double-blind study comparing topical and oral tetracycline therapy and placebo. *Arch Dermatol* 1976;**112**:971–3.

89. Smith JG, Jr., Chalker DK, Wehr RF. The effectiveness of topical and oral tetracycline for acne. *Southern Med J* 1976;**69**:695–7.

90. Braathen LR. Topical clindamycin versus oral tetracycline and placebo in acne vulgaris. *Scand J Infect Dis* 1984; **16**(Suppl. 43):71–5.

91. Gratton D, Raymond GP, Guertin-Larochelle S *et al*. Topical clindamycin versus systemic tetracycline in the treatment of acne. Results of a multiclinic trial. *J Am Acad Dermatol* 1982;**7**:50–3.

92. Feucht CL, Allen BS, Chalker DK, Smith JG, Jr. Topical erythromycin with zinc in acne. A double-blind controlled study. *J Am Acad Dermatol* 1980;**3**:483–91.

93. Stewart WD, Maddin SW, Nelson AJ *et al*. Therapeutic agents in acne vulgaris: I Tetracycline. *Can Med Assoc J* 1963;**89**:1096–7.

94. Ashurst PJ. Tetracycline in acne vulgaris. *Practitioner* 1968;**200**:539–41.

95. Plewig G. Vitamin A acid. Topical treatment in acne vulgaris. *Pennsylvania Med* 1969;**72**:33–5.

96. Al Mishari MA. Clinical and bacteriological evaluation of tetracycline and erythromycin in acne vulgaris. *Clin Ther* 1987;**9**:273–80.

97. Bleeker J. Tolerance and efficacy of erythromycin stearate tablets versus enteric-coated erythromycin base capsules in the treatment of patients with acne vulgaris. *J Int Med Res* 1983;**11**:38–41.

98. Brandt H, Attila P, Ahokas T *et al.* Erythromycin acistrate – an alternative oral treatment for acne. *J Dermatol Treat* 1994;**5**:3–5.

99. Cullen SI, Cohan RH. Minocycline therapy in acne vulgaris. *Cutis* 1976;**17**:1208–10.

100. Gammon WR, Meyer C, Lantis S, Shenefelt P, Reizner G, Cripps DJ. Comparative efficacy of oral erythromycin versus oral tetracycline in the treatment of acne vulgaris. A double-blind study. *J Am Acad Dermatol* 1986;**14** (2Pt 1):183-6.

101. Gibson JR, Darley CR, Harvey SG, Barth J. Oral trimethoprim versus oxytetracycline in the treatment of inflammatory acne vulgaris. *Br J Dermatol* 1982;**107**: 221–4.

102. Hubbell CG, Hobbs ER, Rist T, White JW, Jr. Efficacy of minocycline compared with tetracycline in treatment of acne vulgaris. *Arch Dermatol* 1982;**118**:989–92.

103. Olafsson JH, Gudgeirsson J, Eggertsdottir GE, Kristjansson F. Doxycycline versus minocycline in the treatment of acne vulgaris: A double-blind study. *J Dermatol Treat* 1989;**1**:15–17.

104. Samuelson JS. An accurate photographic method for grading acne: initial use in a double-blind clinical comparison of minocycline and tetracycline. *J Am Acad Dermatol* 1985;**12**:461–7.

105. Blechschmidt J, Engst R, Hoting E *et al.* Behandlung der acne papulopustulosa-vergleich der wirksmkeit und vertraglichkeit von minocyclin und oxytetracyclin. *Munchener Medizinische Wochenschrift* 1987;**129**:562–4.

106. Cunliffe WJ, Grosshans E, Belaich S, Meynadier J, Alirezai M, Thomas L. A comparison of the efficacy and safety of lymecycline and minocycline in patients with moderately severe acne vulgaris. *Eur J Dermatol* 1998;**8**:161–6.

107. Fallica L, Vignini M, Rodeghiero R *et al.* La minociclina e la tetracicline chloridrato nel trattamento del'acne vogare. *Dermatol Clin* 1985;**5**:145–50.

108. Khanna N. Treatment of acne vulgaris with oral tetracyclines. *Indian J Dermatol Venereol Leprol* 1993;**59**:74–6.

109. Laux B. Treatment of acne vulgaris. A comparison of doxycycline versus minocycline. [German]. *Hautarzt* 1989;**40**:577–81.

110. Lorette G, Belaich S, Beylot MC, Ortonne JP. Doxycycline (Tolexine(TM)) 50 mg/day versus minocycline 100 mg/day in the treatment of acne vulgaris. Evaluation on four months of treatment. [French]. *Nouv Dermatol* 1994; **13**:662–5.

111. Ruping KW, Tronnier H. Acne therapy: results of a multicentre study with minocycline. Royal Society of Medicine Services International Congress and Symposium Series 1985;103–8.

112. Schollhammer M, Alirezai M. Etude comparative de la lymecycline, de la minocycline et de la doxycycline dans la traitement de l'acne vulgaire. *Real Ther Derm Venerol* 1994;**42**:24–6.

113. Waskiewicz W, Grosshans E. Traitement de l'acne juvenile par les cyclines de deuxieme generation. *Nouv Dermatol* 1982;**11**:8–11.

114. Christian GL, Krueger GG. Clindamycin v placebo as adjunctive therapy in moderately severe acne. *Arch Dermatol* 1975;**111**:997–1000.

115. Lucchina LC, Kollias N, Gillies R *et al.* Fluorescence photography in the evaluation of acne. *J Am Acad Dermatol* 1996;**35**:58–63.

116. Thomsen RJ, Stranieri A, Knutson D, Strauss JS. Topical clindamycin treatment of acne. Clinical, surface lipid composition, and quantitative surface microbiology response. *Arch Dermatol* 1980;**116**: 1031–4.

117. Becker LE, Bergstresser PR, Whiting DA *et al.* Topical clindamycin therapy for acne vulgaris. A cooperative clinical study. *Arch Dermatol* 1981;**117**:482–5.

118. Guin JD. Treatment of acne vulgaris with topical clindamycin phosphate: a double-blind study. *Int J Dermatol* 1981;**20**:286–8.

119. Kuhlman DS, Callen JP. A comparison of clindamycin phosphate 1 percent topical lotion and placebo in the treatment of acne vulgaris. *Cutis* 1986;**38**:203–6.

120. Petersen MJ, Krusinski PA, Krueger GG. Evaluation of 1% clindamycin phosphate lotion in the treatment of acne. *Curr Ther Res* 1986;**40**:232–8.

121. Ellis CN, Gammon WR, Stone DZ, Heezen-Wehner JL. A comparison of Cleocin T Solution, Cleocin T Gel, and placebo in the treatment of acne vulgaris. *Cutis* 1988;**42**:245–7.

122. McKenzie MW, Beck DC, Popovich NG. Topical clindamycin formulations for the treatment of acne vulgaris. An evaluation. *Arch Dermatol* 1981;**117**:630–4.

123. Jones EL, Crumley AF. Topical erythromycin v blank vehicle in a multiclinic acne study. *Arch Dermatol* 1981;**117**:551–3.

124. Hellgren L, Vincent J. Entzundungshemmung bei akne vulgaris durich ein erythromycin-externum in alkoholischer losung. *Dermatol Monatsschr* 1983;**169**:705.

125. Lesher Jr JL, Chalker DK, Smith Jr JG. An evaluation of a 2% erythromycin ointment in the topical therapy of acne vulgaris. *J Am Acad Dermatol* 1985;**12**:526–31.

126. LLorca M, Hernandez-Gill A, Ramos M *et al.* Erythromycin laurilsulfate in the topical treatment of acne vulgaris. *Curr Ther Res* 1982;**32**:14–20.

127. Perez M, Aspiolea F, De Moragas JM. [Comparative double-blind study of topical clindamycin phosphate and oral tetracycline in the treatment of acne]. [Spanish]. *Med Cutan Ibero Lat Am* 1987;**15**:173–7.

128. Pochi PE, Bagatell FK, Ellis CN *et al.* Erythromycin 2 percent gel in the treatment of acne vulgaris. *Cutis* 1988;**41**:132–6.

129. Prince RA, Busch DA, Hepler CD, Feldick HG. Clinical trial of topical erythromycin in inflammatory acne. *Drug Intell Clin Pharm* 1981;**15**:372–6.

130. Chalker DK, Shalita A, Smith JG, Jr, Swann RW. A double-blind study of the effectiveness of a 3% erythromycin and 5% benzoyl peroxide combination in the treatment of acne vulgaris. *J Am Acad Dermatol* 1983;**9**:933–6.

131. Schachner L, Pestana A, Kittles C. A clinical trial comparing the safety and efficacy of a topical erythromycin-zinc formulation with a topical clindamycin formulation. [see comments.]. *J Am Acad Dermatol* 1990;**22**:489–95.

132. Strauss JS, Stranieri AM. Acne treatment with topical erythromycin and zinc: effect of *Propionibacterium acnes* and free fatty acid composition. *J Am Acad Dermatol* 1984;**11**:86–9.

133. Hansted B, Jorgensen J, Reymann F, Christiansen J. Fucidin(TM) cream for topical treatment of acne vulgaris. *Curr Ther Res Clin Exp* 1985;**37**:249–53.

134. Sommer S, Bojar R, Cunliffe WJ, Holland D, Holland KT, Naags H. Investigation of the mechanism of action of 2% fusidic acid lotion in the treatment of acne vulgaris. *Clin Exp Dermatol* 1997;**22**:211–15.

135. Knutson DD, Swinyer LJ, Smoot WH. Meclocycline sulfosalicylate. Topical antibiotic agent for the treatment of acne vulgaris. *Cutis* 1981;**27**:203–4.

136. Tong D, Peters W, Barnetson RSC. Evaluation of 0·75% metronidazole gel in acne – a double-blind study. *Clin Exp Dermatol* 1994;**19**:221–3.

137. Franz E, Weidner-Strahl S. The effectiveness of topical antibacterials in acne: a double-blind clinical study. *J Int Med Res* 1978;**6**:72–7.

138. Parker F. A comparison of clindamycin 1% solution versus clindamycin 1% gel in the treatment of acne vulgaris. *Int J Dermatol* 1987;**26**:121–2.

139. Goltz RW, Coryell GM, Schnieders JR, Neidert GL. A comparison of Cleocin T 1 percent solution and Cleocin T 1 percent lotion in the treatment of acne vulgaris. *Cutis* 1985;**36**:265–8.

140. Henderson TA, Olson WH, Leach AD. A single-blind, randomized comparison of erythromycin pledgets and clindamycin lotion in the treatment of mild-to-moderate facial acne vulgaris. *Adv Ther* 1995;**12**:172–7.

141. Leyden JJ, Shalita AR, Saatjian GD, Sefton J. Erythromycin 2% gel in comparison with clindamycin phosphate 1% solution in acne vulgaris. *J Am Acad Dermatol* 1987;**16**:822–7.

142. Mills OH, Berger RS, Kligman AM, McElroy JA, Di Matteo J. A comparative study of Erycette(TM) v Cleocin-T(TM). *Adv Ther* 1992;**9**:14–20.

143. Thomas DR, Raimer S, Smith EB. Comparison of topical erythromycin 1·5 percent solution versus topical clindamycin phosphate 1·0 percent solution in the treatment of acne vulgaris. *Cutis* 1982;**29**:624–5.

144. Padilla RS, McCabe JM, Becker LE. Topical tetracycline hydrochloride *v.* topical clindamycin phosphate in the treatment of acne: a comparative study. *Int J Dermatol* 1981;**20**:445–8.

145. Robledo AA, Lopez BE, del Pino GJ *et al*. Multicentric comparative study of the efficacy and tolerance of clindamycin phosphate 1% topical solution and tetracycline topical solution for the treatment of acne vulgaris. *Curr Ther Res Clin Exp* 1988;**43**:21–6.

146. Shalita AR, Smith JG, Parish LC, Sofman MS, Chalker DK. Topical nicotinamide compared with clindamycin gel in the treatment of inflammatory acne vulgaris. *Int J Dermatol* 1995;**34**:434–7.

147. Borglund E, Hagermark O, Nord CE. Impact of topical clindamycin and systemic tetracycline on the skin and colon microflora in patients with acne vulgaris. *Scand J Infect Dis* 1984;**16**(Suppl. 43):76–81.

148. Stoughton RB, Cornell RC, Gange RW, Walter JF. Double-blind comparison of topical 1 percent clindamycin phosphate (Cleocin T) and oral tetracycline 500 mg/day in the treatment of acne vulgaris. *Cutis* 1980;**26**:424–5.

149. Katsambas A, Towarky AA, Stratigos J. Topical clindamycin phosphate compared with oral tetracycline in the treatment of acne vulgaris. *Br J Dermatol* 1987;**116**:387–91.

150. Cornbleet HA. Long-term therapy of acne with tetracycline. *Arch Dermatol* 1961;**83**:414–16.

151. Hjorth N, Schmidt H, Thomsen K, Dela K. Meclosorb((TM)), a new topical antibiotic agent in the treatment of acne vulgaris: A double-blind clinical study. *Acta Derm Venereol* 1984;**64**:354–7.

152. Rapaport M, Puhvel SM, Reisner RM. Evaluation of topical erythromycin and oral tetracycline in acne vulgaris. *Cutis* 1982;**30**:122–6.

153. Drake LA. Comparative efficacy and tolerance of Cleocin T topical gel (clindamycin phosphate topical gel) versus oral minocycline in the treatment of acne vulgaris. 1980 unpublished data (Pharmacia and Upjohn Ltd).

154. Peacock CE, Price C, Ryan BE, Mitchell AD. Topical clindamycin (Dalacin T(TM)) compared to oral minocycline (Minocin 50(TM)) in treatment of acne vulgaris. A randomized observer-blind controlled trial in three university student health centres. *Clin Trials J* 1990;**27**:219–28.

155. Sheehan-Dare RA, Papworth-Smith J, Cunliffe WJ. A double-blind comparison of topical clindamycin and oral minocycline in the treatment of acne vulgaris. *Acta Derm Venereol* 1990;**70**:534–7.

156. Wethered R. Sodium fusidate in acne. *Practitioner* 1964;**193**:802–4.

157. Darrah AJ, Gray PL. An open multicentre study to compare fusidic acid lotion and oral minocycline in the treatment of mild-to-moderate acne vulgaris of the face. *Eur J Clin Res* 1996;**8**:97–107.

158. Norris JFB, Hughes BR, Basey AJ, Cunliffe WJ. A comparison of the effectiveness of topical tetracycline, benzoyl-peroxide gel and oral oxytetracycline in the treatment of acne. *Clin Exp Dermatol* 1991;**16**:31–3.

159. Stainforth J, Macdonald-Hull S, Papworth-Smith JW *et al*. A single-blind comparison of topical erythromycin/zinc lotion and oral minocycline in the treatment of acne vulgaris. *J Dermatol Treat* 1993;**4**:119–22.

160. Gollnick H. A new therapeutic agent: Azelaic acid in acne treatment. *J Dermatol Treat* 1990;**1**(Suppl. 3):S23–S28.

161. Tucker SB, Tausend R, Cochran R, Flannigan SA. Comparison of topical clindamycin phosphate, benzoyl peroxide, and a combination of the two for the treatment of acne vulgaris. *Br J Dermatol* 1984;**110**:487–92.

162. Swinyer LJS, Baker MD, Swinyer TA, Mills OH, Jr. A comparative study of benzoyl peroxide and clindamycin phosphate for treating acne vulgaris. *Br J Dermatol* 1988;**119**:615–22.

163. Burke B, Eady EA, Cunliffe WJ. Benzoyl peroxide versus topical erythromycin in the treatment of acne vulgaris. *Br J Dermatol* 1983;**108**:199–204.

164. Borglund E, Kristensen B, Larsson-Stymne B, Strand A, Veien NK, Jakobsen HB. Topical meclocycline sulfosalicylate, benzoyl peroxide, and a combination of the two in the treatment of acne vulgaris. *Acta Derm Venereol* 1991;**71**:175–8.

165. Gamborg NP. Topical metronidazole gel. Use in acne vulgaris. *Int J Dermatol* 1991;**30**:662–6.

166. Cambazard F. Clinical efficacy of Velac(TM), a new tretinoin and clindamycin phosphate gel in acne vulgaris. *J Eur Acad Dermatol Venereol* 1998;**11**(Suppl. 1):S20–S27.

167. Zouboulis C, Derumeaux L, Decroix J, Maciejewska-Udziela B, Cambazard F, Stuhlert A. A multicentre, single-blind, randomized comparison of a fixed clindamycin phosphate/tretinoin gel formulation (Velac(TM)) applied once daily and a clindamycin lotion formulation (Dalacin T(TM)) applied twice daily in the

topical treatment of acne vulgaris. *Br J Dermatol* 2000;**143**:498–505.

168. Rietschel RL, Duncan SH. Clindamycin phosphate used in combination with tretinoin in the treatment of acne. *Int J Dermatol* 1983;**22**:41–3.

169. Richter JR, Bousema MT, De Boulle KLV, Degreef HJ, Poli F. Efficacy of a fixed clindamycin phosphate 1·2%, tretinoin 0·025% gel formulation (Velac) in the topical control of facial acne lesions. *J Dermatol Treat* 1998;**9**:81–90.

170. Mills OH, Jr., Kligman AM. Treatment of acne vulgaris with topically applied erythromycin and tretinoin. *Acta Derm Venereol* 1978;**58**:555–7.

171. Packman AM, Brown RH, Dunlap FE, Kraus SJ, Webster GF. Treatment of acne vulgaris: combination of 3% erythromycin and 5% benzoyl peroxide in a gel compared to clindamycin phosphate lotion. *Int J Dermatol* 1996;**35**:209–11.

172. Chu A, Huber FJ, Plott RT. The comparative efficacy of benzoyl peroxide 5%/erythromycin 3% gel and erythromycin 4%/zinc 1·2% solution in the treatment of acne vulgaris. *Br J Dermatol* 1997;**136**:235–8.

173. Sklar JL, Jacobson C, Rizer R, Gans EH. Evaluation of Triaz 10% Gel and Benzamycin in acne vulgaris. *J Dermatol Treat* 1996;**7**:147–52.

174. Marsden J. Evidence that the method of use, dose and duration of treatment with benzoyl peroxide and tetracycline determines response of acne. *J R Soc Med* 1985;**78**(Suppl. 10):25–8.

175. Brooks JS. The use of acmed in acne. *Australasian J Dermatol* 1968;**9**:256–7.

176. Noble W, Naidoo J. Evolution of antibiotic resistance in *Staphylococcus aureus*: the role of the skin. *Br J Dermatol* 1978;**98**:481–9.

177. Eady EA, Holland KT, Cunliffe WJ. Should topical antibiotics be used for the treatment of acne vulgaris?. [Review] [99 refs]. B*r J Dermatol* 1982;**107**:235–46.

178. Editorial. Antimicrobial resistance. *BMJ* 1998;**317**:609–10.

179. Cooper A. Systematic review of *Propionibacterium acnes* resistance to systemic antibiotics. *Med J Aus* 1998;**169**:259–61.

180. Eady EA, Cove JH, Blake J, Holland KT, Cunliffe WJ. Recalcitrant acne vulgaris. Clinical, biochemical and microbiological investigation of patients not responding to antibiotic treatment. *Br J Dermatol* 1988;**118**:415–23.

181. Hughes BR, Murphy CE, Barnett J, Cunliffe WJ. Strategy of acne therapy with long-term antibiotics. *Br J Dermatol* 1989;**121**:623–8.

182. Greenwood R, Burke B, Cunliffe WJ. Evaluation of a therapeutic strategy for the treatment of acne vulgaris with conventional therapy. *Br J Dermatol* 1986;**114**:353–8.

183. Mandy S. Chest and back acne: a retrospective review. *Adv Ther* 1995;**12**:321–32.

184. Layton AM, Hughes BR, Macdonald-Hull S *et al.* Seborrhoea – an indicator for poor clinical response in acne patients treated with antibiotics. *Clin Exp Dermatol* 1992;**17**:173–5.

185. Leyden JJ, Marples RR, Mills OH, Jr, Kligman AM. Gram-negative folliculitis: a complication of antibiotic therapy in acne vulgaris. *Br J Dermatol* 1973;**88**:533–8.

186. Chopra I, Hawkey P, Hinton M. Tetracyclines: molecular and clinical aspects. *J Antimicrob Chemother* 1992;**29**: 245–77.

187. Meyer FP. Minocycline for acne. Food reduces minocycline's availability. *BMJ* 1996;**312**:1101.

188. Lleyden JJ. Absorption of minocycline hydrochloride and tetracycline hydrochloride: effect of food, milk and iron. *J Am Acad Dermatol* 1985;**12**:308–12.

189. Eady EA, Farmery MR, Ross JI, Cove JH, Cunliffe WJ. Effects of benzoyl peroxide and erythromycin alone and in combination against antibiotic-sensitive and -resistant skin bacteria from acne patients. *Br J Dermatol* 1994;**131**:331–6.

190. Becker FT. The acne problem. *Arch Dermatol Syphiol* 1953;**67**:173.

191. Robinson H. Role of antibiotics in therapy of acne. *Arch Dermatol Syphiol* 1954;**69**:414–17.

192. Smith E, Mortimer PS. Tetracycline in acne vulgaris. *Br J Dermatol* 1967;**79**:78–84.

193. Aulzberger M, Witten V, Steagall R. Treatment of acne vulgaris. *JAMA* 1960;**173**:1911–15.

194. Plewig G, Kligman AM. *Acne: Morphogenesis and Treatment*, 1st ed. Berlin: Springer-Verlag, 1975.

195. Dreno B, Bodokh I, Chivot M *et al.* [ECLA grading: a system of acne classification for every day dermatological practice]. [French]. *Ann Dermatol Venereol* 1999;**126**:136–41.

196. Gardner KJ, Eady EA, Cove JH, Taylor JP, Cunliffe WJ. Comparison of serum antibiotic levels in acne patients receiving the standard or a modified release formulation of

minocycline hydrochloride. *Clin Exp Dermatol* 1997;**22**:72–6.

197. Akamatsu H, Nishijima S, Akamatsu M, Kurokawa I, Asada Y. Clinical evaluation of roxithromycin in patients with acne. *J Int Med Res* 1996;**24**:109–14.

198. Baer RL, Leshaw SM, Shalita AR. High-dose tetracycline therapy in severe acne. *Arch Dermatol* 1976;**112**: 479–81.

199. Friedman-Kien A, Shalita AR, Baer RL. Tetracycline therapy in acne vulgaris. *Arch Dermatol* 1972;**105**:608.

200. Burke BM, Cunliffe WJ. The assessment of acne vulgaris – the Leeds technique. *Br J Dermatol* 1984;**111**:83–92.

201. Goolamali S. Management of acne vulgaris. *Prescribers J* 1990;**30**:78–84.

202. Fyrand O, Jakobsen HB. Water-based versus alcohol-based benzoyl peroxide preparations in the treatment of acne vulgaris. *Dermatologica* 1986;**172**: 263–7.

203. Milikan LE, Ameln R. Use of Buf-Puf and benzoyl peroxide in the treatment of acne. *Cutis* 1981;**28**:201–5.

14
Papulopustular rosacea

Alfredo Rebora

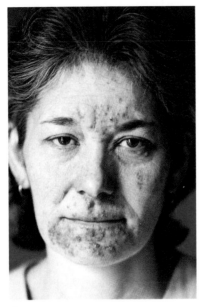
a)

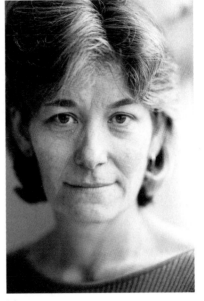
b)

Figure 14.1   Patient with rosacea a) before and b) after treatment. Figures provided by Andrew Herxheimer.

Background
Definition

Papulopustular rosacea is one of the stages of rosacea and concerns only a minority of cases. Papulopustules appear on the nose and cheeks, more rarely on the forehead and chin, and exceptionally on the neck and other body areas, such as the bare skull or the back. The pattern usually consists mainly of papules with a few scattered pustules. In some cases, papules show a granulomatous infiltrate, which is clinically identified from the yellowish colour of the lesions and their duration.

Lymphoedematous rosacea is more rare and is characterised by chronic and persistent oedema in the periocular and perinasal areas. The oedema persists even when inflammation has abated and is probably linked to inflammatory damage to the region's lymphatic vessels. A hyperacute episode with most of the face invaded by papulopustules (facial pyoderma) has also been described as rosacea fulminans. There is no general agreement on its attribution to rosacea.

Incidence/prevalence

Rosacea is a very common disease. In the US, it is the fifth most frequently diagnosed skin condition after acne, atopic dermatitis, psoriasis and actinic keratosis. It affects 10% of the general population in Sweden.

Aetiology/risk factors

Heredity is important. It has been recently shown that 20% of the children with steroid rosacea had at least one close blood relative with rosacea. Fair complexion, blond hair and green/blue eyes are characteristic of patients with rosacea. In England, for example, 48% of patients with rosacea had this skin type. How this frequency compares with that of the general British population is not known. About 0·1% of coloured people are also affected by rosacea, as reported by an old American observation. Rosacea occurs more frequently in women than in men (3:1).

Typically, rosacea is a multistage disease and the prevalence may change according to the stage/s at which the diagnosis is made. The stages are the flushing stage or transitory congestive redness, the erythrosis stage or persistent teleangiectatic redness, the papulopustular stage and the phyma stage. Only a minority of patients with the first two stages of the disease progress to the papulopustular stage and even fewer to the phyma stage. The condition appears more often in middle age, although this varies for the stages of the disease: erythrosis develops earlier (mean age in 1979: 34 years), whilst phymas develops later (mean age 66 years).

The aetiopathogenesis of papulopustular rosacea is controversial and it is unclear why a patient proceeds from stages that are mainly functional to those that are inflammatory. The immune system, with both its cell-mediated and humoral arms, may be involved. Indeed, antibodies directed against collagen VII, the elastotic tissue and the *Demodex folliculorum* mite have been detected. However, the production of antibodies may be a secondary event or the elastotic tissue and *D. folliculorum* may simply represent the structures where antibodies accumulate spontaneously ("beach effect"). In addition, *Helicobacter pylori*, a gram-negative bacterium, has recently been hypothesised to play a role. Opinions diverge on its association with rosacea, but drugs that eradicate *H. pylori* were used to treat papulopustular rosacea long before the issue of *H. pylori* arose.

Prognosis

No long-term prognostic studies are available.

Aims

The aims of treatment are to suppress the symptoms and to maintain such suppression over time.

Outcomes

The following outcome measures are used: state of lesions over time; use of routine treatments; duration of remission; patient satisfaction; disease-related quality of life; adverse effects of treatments and clinical activity scores.

Methods

No Cochrane reviews were found when the *Cochrane Library*, PubMed and Isitrial were searched and appraised in July 2001. I found one systematic review and one partial review. I have checked the data from those reviews and I examined some of the papers they quoted.

Papers dealing with ocular rosacea, granulomatous rosacea and rosacea fulminans were excluded to maintain homogeneity.

Similarly, I did not take into account papers in which erythema and/or telangectasia, steroid-induced rosacea, rosacea-like demodicidosis, rosacea conglobata and rhinophyma were treated.

QUESTIONS

What are the effects of systemic treatments?

Tetracyclines
Efficacy

I found no systematic reviews. I found one randomised controlled trial (RCT) of 78 patients treated with tetracycline, 50 mg/day. Improvement was observed at the end of the first month of treatment in 78% of patients. Improvement was also observed in 45% of patients taking placebo.[1] In another RCT, 56 patients were treated with "three tablets/day" (presumably of 250 mg each) for 6 weeks. Lesions improved by 78%, compared with 10% in the placebo group.[2] In a third RCT, 51 people were treated with tetracycline, 500 mg/day, for 2 months and improved by about 90% (based on scores); similar improvements were seen in the comparison group given 1% metronidazole cream.[3] In a controlled clinical trial (CCT) of 101 patients, tetracycline, 750 mg/day, for 2 months cleared lesions in more than 50% of patients.[4] An uncontrolled trial compared tetracycline, 1 g/day, for 3 weeks with topical clindamycin. No differences were found.[5]

Drawbacks
Diarrhoea occurred at 750 mg/day.

Comment
The second RCT had the smallest placebo effect, contrasting with all other trials in which the placebo effect was very important.

Doxycycline

Doxycycline is perhaps the most popular medication for papulopustular rosacea, but I found no systematic reviews and no RCTs.

Efficacy

In one CCT, 17 patients received doxycycline, 200 mg/day, for 4 weeks then 100 mg/day for 4 weeks. Lesions cleared in 90% of patients in 8 weeks. Comparison with clarithromycin favoured the latter.[6] An anecdotal report of two cases stated that 100 mg/day for 9 weeks and 50 mg/day for 1 month were sufficient to clear the lesions.[7]

Drawbacks
No side-effects have been mentioned.

Comment
Doxycycline is a photosensitising drug in fewer than 1% of patients and the sun sensitivity of rosacea patients should be taken into account.

Ampicillin
Ampicillin is rarely used.

Efficacy

In the only RCT found, 17 patients were treated with ampicillin, 750 mg/day, for 6 weeks. Lesions improved by 55% versus 10% with placebo.[2]

Drawbacks

Two patients developed troublesome diarrhoea after the first few days of treatment and were withdrawn.

Comment
The benefit/harm ratio seems low.

Clarithromycin
I found no systematic reviews and no RCTs.

Efficacy

In the only CCT, 23 patients received clarithromycin, 500 mg/day, for 1 month, then 250 mg/day for a further month. Ninety per cent cleared in 8 weeks; the comparison with doxycycline favoured clarithromycin.[7]

Drawbacks

Clarithromycin was significantly better tolerated than doxycycline.

Comment

Clarithromycin is almost four times more expensive than doxycycline.

Azithromycin

There are no systematic reviews or RCTs.

Efficacy

One uncontrolled study reported that clearing occurred in 9 of 10 cases treated with azithromycin, 500 mg/day for 4 weeks followed by 250 mg/day for 3 months.[8]

Drawbacks

Nausea in one patient resolved without interrupting the treatment.

Comment

A once-daily pulse-dosing regimen may improve compliance.

Metronidazole

Oral metronidazole seems to be effective in papulopustular rosacea. I found no systematic reviews.

Efficacy

In the first of two RCTs, 29 patients received metronidazole, 400 mg/day for 6 weeks. The benefit was significantly superior to placebo.[9] In the second trial, 40 patients received 400 mg/day for 12 weeks. The improvement was similar to that obtained with oxytetracycline.[10] An uncontrolled trial treated 59 patients with 500 mg/day for no more than 6 months, obtaining 90% success.[11] Some trials published in German were not available to me.[12]

Drawbacks

Headache and furred tongue have been noted occasionally.

Comment

Metronidazole has a disulfiram-like effect when alcohol is taken. Metronidazole is half the price of doxycycline.

Eradication of *H. pylori*

H. pylori may be involved in the pathogenesis of rosacea. Even if the issue is still controversial, eradication of *H. pylori* seems to clear rosacea. No systematic reviews are available.

Efficacy

I found no systematic reviews, and only one RCT, in which 44 patients were treated with omeprazole, 40 mg/day, plus clarithromycin, 1500 mg/day, for 2 weeks. Lesions cleared in almost all patients, but there were no differences from the untreated controls.[13] In one CCT, 37 patients received omeprazole, 40 mg/day for 1 month plus clarithromycin, 100 mg/day, plus metronidazole, 2000 mg/day, for 2 weeks. At the twelfth week, 76% of patients had improved compared with no improvement in the 26 untreated patients.[14] In another CCT, 53 patients received omeprazole, 20 mg/day, clarithromycin, 1 g/day) and metronidazole, 1 g/day) for one week. Ninety-six per cent cleared in 2–4 weeks.[15] In an uncontrolled study, 13 patients improved on bismuth, 1200 mg/day, amoxycillin, 500 mg/day, and metronidazole, 1·5 g/day.[16] There is also one anecdotal report.[17]

Drawbacks

Surprisingly, no remarks about side-effects of such a complex therapy are reported.

Comment

The results are homogeneous, with the exception of the RCT. It is very difficult to believe, however, that the placebo-treated patients improved as much as those who received the eradication therapy. It is worth noting that the RCT did not use metronidazole.

Isotretinoin

Isotretinoin is a drug for very severe cases, such as pyoderma faciale.

Efficacy

I found no systematic reviews, but one very small RCT in which eight patients received isotretinoin, 10 mg/day, for 4 months. They improved significantly by 70%.[18] In an uncontrolled study, 22 patients received isotretinoin, 10 mg/day, for 4 months. They improved by 50% in 9 weeks.[19] Two anecdotal reports obtained clearance in 3–6 months.[20,21]

Drawbacks

Most patients complained of dry lips and facial xerosis. A quarter experienced a mild-to-moderate increase in serum triglyceride levels.

Comment

Long-term side-effects have not been reported.

Rilmenidine

Rilmenidine, an antihypertensive drug related to clonidine, does not reduce papules and pustules.

Efficacy

Only one RCT was found, in which 15 patients received 1 mg/day of rilmenidine and 18 received placebo. There was improvement in 69·2% [sic] of the experimental group but there was no difference from the controls.[22]

Drawbacks

Asthenia, xerostomia and palpitations have been reported.

Comment

Rilmenidine may be active against flushes.

What are the effects of topical drugs?

Topical drugs are less likely to cause systemic adverse effects than are systemically administered drugs, and compliance may be better. The drug that has been most widely tested is metronidazole.

Metronidazole

Metronidazole, formulated as either a 1% cream or a 0·75% gel, proved effective in papulopustular rosacea. I found two reviews on the topic.[12,23]

Efficacy

Surprisingly, of the 24 papers that have dealt with this drug, 19 report RCTs (one was an intention-to-treat trial). Of the remaining five, two are definitely CCTs, two were anecdotal reports and I do not have information on the last one. The papers are quite homogeneous. Five of them compared metronidazole with oral tetracycline. One found that azelaic acid was superior and another that permethrin has the same efficacy. Other formulations such as 0·75% lotion, cream and gel have been found to be equivalent. In general, the improvement ranged from 52% to 89% (Table 14.1). In another RCT (not included in Table 14.1), 88 patients successfully treated with oral tetracycline and topical metronidazole, were treated with either 0·76% metronidazole gel or vehicle. Relapses after 6 months of treatment were significantly fewer (23%) with metronidazole than with the vehicle (42%).[45]

Table 14.1   Trials with topical metronidazole

Reference	Design	Number of patients	Dosage and vehicle, duration	Results (% improvement)	Comments
24	RCT	41	1% cream, 8 wks	64% papules improved v 39% P	Dryness
25	?	51	1% cream, 8 wks	Improvement v T	
26	CCT	33	1% cream/day, 16 wks + 1% every other day	Fewer relapses v oral T	
27	RCT	44?	1% cream ?	Non-significant improvement v P	
28	RCT	34	1% cream, 8 wks	89% lesions v 100% T	Dryness and stinging
29	RCT	40	0·75% gel, 9 wks	65% lesions v 15% P	No side-effects
30	RCT	59	0·75% gel, 9 wks	Significant improvement v P	No side-effects
31	RCT	50	1% cream, 8 wks	88% v P	
32	RCT	97	1% cream, 8 wks	Significant improvement v P	No side-effects
33	RCT	42	1% cream, 8 wks	60% v 23% P	
34	RCT	12	0·5% gel, 9 wks	75% v 75% T	
4	CCT	50	1% cream, 8 wks	53% v 61% T	No side-effects
35	RCT	40	0·75% gel, 3 mo	35% v 49% E	No statistical analysis
36	RCT	26	0·75% gel, 6 wks	48% v 17% P	Mediocre tolerability
37	RCT	6	0·75% gel, 7–10 wks	64% v 64% PE	Dryness in one patient
38	RCT	85	0.75% gel, 12 wks	52·1% v 22·4% P	
39	RCT	143[a]	1% cream, 10 wks	62·5% v 42·9% P	
40	RCT	89	1% cream, 10 wks	53% v 17% P	2% had adverse effects
41	RCT	69	1% cream, 10 wks	58% v 30% P	Skin reactions in three patients
42	RCT	100	0·75% gel and cream, 12 wks	61% v 63%	No difference
43	(ITT)	57	0.75% lotion and gel, 12 wks	71% v 63%	No difference
44	RCT	40	0·75% gel, 15 wks	69·4% v 78·5% A	Dryness, burning, stinging

RCT, randomised clinical trial; CCT, controlled non-randomised clinical trial; IIT, intention-to-treat trial; P, placebo; T, tetracycline; E, erythromycin; A, azithromycin; PE, permethrin.

[a]Numbers of individual groups are not reported.

Table 14.2   Trials with topical azelaic acid

Reference	Type of study	Number of patients	Dosage, vehicle, duration	Results (% improvement)	Comments
46	OS	33	20% cream	Reduction of lesions	
47	?	?	20% cream	78% v 31% P	
48	RCT	114	20% cream, 12 wks	73% v 51% P	17% stopped (5 for irritation)
44	RCT	40	20% cream, 15 wks	78% v 69% metronidazole	Stinging

RCT, randomised controlled trial; OS, open study P, placebo

Drawbacks

Side-effects occurred in 2–4% of patients and included dryness, burning and stinging. One paper[36] reported a "mediocre tolerability".

Comment

The majority of papers were RCTs (some even multicentre), mostly comparing drug with the vehicle that must be provided by the manufacturers, and were sponsored by manufacturers. The contrast with the trials of orphan systemic drugs (mostly not RCTs) could not be more striking.

Azelaic acid

Azelaic acid has been found to be effective in rosacea. I found two RCTs.

Efficacy

In one RCT, azelaic acid was compared with its vehicle in 114 patients. Azelaic acid led to a 73% reduction in inflammatory lesions versus 51% with the vehicle. In the second RCT, azelaic acid was compared with 0·75% metronidazole cream. Good results were obtained with both medications, with no significant differences (79% versus 69%) (Table 14.2).

Drawbacks

Burning and stinging were noted in both RCTs.

Sulphur

Sulphur seems to be effective in rosacea. I found two RCTs.

Efficacy

In the first RCT, 20 patients were treated for one month with a 10% sulphur cream plus placebo tablets and compared with 20 patients treated with lymecycline, 150 mg/day, plus placebo cream. Ninety-two per cent of lesions cleared with both treatments.[49] In the second study, a total of 94 patients were treated with a combination of 10% sodium sulfacetamide and 5% sulphur in a lotion for 8 weeks. Inflammatory lesions decreased by 78% versus 36% in the vehicle group.[50]

Drawbacks

There were reactions at the application site, which decreased in frequency over time.

Tretinoin/isotretinoin

Isotretinoin may be effective in rosacea.

Efficacy

In one small RCT, six patients were treated with 0·025% tretinoin cream for 16 weeks. Lesion counts decreased by 42%. Comparison was made with patients treated with either oral isotretinoin or with oral isotretinoin and topical tretinoin. No additive benefit was noted with the combined use.[18] In an uncontrolled small trial, 4 patients were treated with 0·2% isotretinoin cream for 16 days. Inflammatory lesions responded better than non-inflammatory lesions.[51]

Drawbacks

No side-effects were noted in the tretinoin-only arm.

Comment

A drug well-known to produce irritation at the first applications seems likely to cause it in the sensitive skin of rosacea.

Clindamycin
Efficacy

In the only RCT, 43 patients were randomly treated with either 1% clindamycin phosphate lotion for 12 weeks or tetracycline, 1000 mg for 3 weeks then 500 mg for 9 weeks. All inflammatory lesions decreased significantly (by about 60%) in the clindamycin arm, while only papules and nodules decreased significantly in the tetracycline arm.[5]

Drawbacks

No side-effects were noted with clindamycin.

Benzoyl peroxide
Efficacy

In the only CCT, patients were treated with 5% benzoyl peroxide acetone gel for one month and with 10% gel for a further month. Benzoyl peroxide was superior to placebo.[52]

Drawbacks

Twenty-three per cent of the patients treated with benzoyl peroxide dropped out.

Key points

- Only a few RCTs have been conducted on systemic agents. In particular, no RCTs have tested doxycycline, clarithromycin or azithromycin.
- Many RCTs have been performed with topical drugs. In particular, metronidazole has been extensively and thoroughly studied.
- All the drugs examined, except rimelnidine, were found to be effective.
- Side-effects were surprisingly minimal, even for drugs such as tretinoin and benzoyl peroxide that are well-known irritants.
- In most studies, a high rate of response to placebo was found.
- The majority of RCTs have been directly supported by the manufacturer of the drug tested.

Comment

See comment on isotretinoin.

References

1. Sneddon IB. A clinical trial of tetracycline in rosacea. *Br J Dermatol* 1966;**78**:649–52.
2. Marks R, Ellis J. Comparative effectiveness of tetracycline and ampicillin in rosacea. A controlled trial. *Lancet* 1971;**2**:1049–52.
3. Nielsen PG. A double-blind study of 1% metronidazole cream versus systemic oxytetracycline therapy for rosacea. *Br J Dermatol* 1983;**109**:63–5.
4. Schachter D, Schachter RK, Long B *et al.* Comparison of metronidazole 1% cream versus oral tetracycline in patients with rosacea. *Drug Invest* 1991;**3**:220–4.
5. Wilkin JK, Dewitt S. Treatment of rosacea – topical clindamycin versus oral tetracycline. *Int J Dermatol* 1993;**32**:65–7.
6. Bikowski JB. Treatment of rosacea with doxycycline monohydrate. *Cutis* 2000;**66**:149–52.
7. Torresani C, Pavesi A, Manara GC. Clarithromycin versus doxycycline in the treatment of rosacea. *Int J Dermatol* 1997;**36**:942–6.

8. Elewski BE. A novel treatment for acne vulgaris and rosacea. *J Eur Acad Dermatol* 2000;**14**:423–4.

9. Pye RJ, Burton JL. Treatment of rosacea by metronidazole. *Lancet* 1976;(**7971**):1121–2.

10. Saihan EM, Burton JL. A double-blind trial of metronidazole versus oxytetracycline therapy for rosacea. *Br J Dermatol* 1980;**102**:443–5.

11. Guilhou JJ, Guilhou E, Malbos S *et al*. Traitement de la rosacée par le métronidazole. *Ann Dermatol Venereol* 1979;**106**:127–9.

12. Gamborg-Nielsen P. Metronidazole treatment in rosacea. *Int J Dermatol* 1988;**27**:1–5.

13. Bamford JTM, Tilden RL, Blankush JL *et al*. Effect of treatment of *Helicobacter pylori* infection on rosacea. *Arch Dermatol* 1999;**135**:659–63.

14. Hergueta-Delgado P, Rojo JM, Martin-Guerrero JM *et al*. *Helicobacter pylori* in relation with rosacea and chronic urticaria. *Gastroenterology* 1999;**116**:G0808.

15. Szlachcic A, Sliwowski Z, Karczewska E *et al*. *Helicobacter pylori* and its eradication in Rosacea. *J Physiol Pharmacol* 1999;**50**:777–86.

16. Utas S, Ozbakir O, Turasan A *et al*. *Helicobacter pylori* eradication treatment reduces the severity of rosacea. *J Am Acad Dermatol* 1999;**40**:433–5.

17. Kolibasova K, Tothova I, Baumgartner J *et al*. Eradication of *Helicobacter pylori* as the only successful treatment in rosacea. *Arch Dermatol* 1996;**132**:1393.

18. Ertl GA, Levine N, Kligman AM. A comparison of the efficacy of topical tretinoin and low-dose oral isotretinoin in rosacea. *Arch Dermatol* 1994;**130**:319–24.

19. Erdogan FG, Yurtsever P, Aksoy D *et al*. Efficacy of low-dose isotretinoin in patients with treatment-resistant rosacea. *Arch Dermatol* 1998;**134**:884–5.

20. Gajardo J. Treatment of severe rosacea with oral isotretinoin. *Rev Med Chile* 1994;**122**:177–9.

21. Mazzatenta C, Giorgino G, Rubegni P *et al*. Solid persistent facial oedema (Morbihan's disease) following rosacea, successfully treated with isotretinoin and ketotifen. *Br J Dermatol* 1997;**137**:1020–1.

22. Grosshans E, Michel C, Arcade B *et al*. Rilménidine dans la rosacée: étude en double insu contre placebo. *Ann Dermatol Vener* 1997;**124**:687–91.

23. McClellan KJ, Noble S. Topical metronidazole: a review of its use in rosacea. *Am J Clin Dermatol* 2000; 1:191–9.

24. Gamborg Nielsen P. Treatment of rosacea with 1% metronidazole cream: a double blind study. *Br J Dermatol* 1983;**108**:327–32.

25. Holm P. Treatment of rosacea with metronidazole cream 1% versus Oxy-Dumocycline (oxytetracycline) tablets, 0·25 g × 2 (in Swedish):internal report. Copenhagen: Dumex Ltd, 1983. [Cited by Gamborg Nielsen.[12]]

26. Gamborg Nielsen P. The relapse rate for rosacea after treatment with either oral tetracycline or metronidazole cream. *Br J Dermatol* 1983;**109**:122–3.

27. Bang-Pedersen N, Larsson-Stymme B. Metronidazole 1% cream versus placebo in the treatment of rosacea: internal report. Denmark: Dumex Ltd, 1984. [Cited by Gamborg Nielsen.[12]]

28. Veien NK, Munkvad JM, Nielsen AO *et al*. Topical metronidazole in the treatment of perioral dermatitis. *J Am Acad Dermatol* 1991;**24**:258–60.

29. Bleicher PA, Charles JH, Sober AJ. Topical metronidazole therapy for rosacea. *Arch Dermatol* 1987;**123**:609–14.

30. Aronson IK, Rumsfield JA, West DP *et al*. Evaluation of topical metronidazole gel in acne rosacea. *Drug Intell Clin Pharm.* 1987;**213**:46–51.

31. Bjerke JR, Nyfors A, Austad J *et al*. Metronidazole (Elyzol) 1% cream v placebo cream in the treatment of rosacea. *Clin Trials J* 1989;**26**:187–94. [Cited by McClellan and Noble.[23]]

32. Bjerke JR. [Rosacea. Clinical features and treatment]. *Tidsskr Nor Laegeforen* 1989;**109**:2295–7.

33. Bitar A, Bourgouin J, Dore N *et al*. A double-blind randomised study on metronidazole (FlagylRm) 1% cream in the treatment of rosacea. A placebo-controlled study. *Drug Invest* 1990;**2**:242–8. [Cited by McClellan and Noble.[23]]

34. Monk BE, Logan RA, Cook J *et al*. Topical metronidazole in the treatment of rosacea. *J Dermatol Treat* 1991;**2**:91–3.

35. Verea-Hernando M, Margusino Framinàn L, Seco Vilarino C *et al*. Estudio comparativo entre eritromicina tópica y metronidazol tópica en el tratamiento de la rosàcea [in Spanish]. *Farm Clin* 1992;**9**:472–9. [Cited by McClellan and Noble.[23]]

36. Espagne E, Guillaume JC, Archimbaud A *et al*. Étude en double insu contre excipient du métronidazole gel a 0·75 p. 100 dans le traitement de la rosacé. *Ann Dermatol Venereol* 1993;**120**:129–33.

37. Signore RJ. A pilot study of 5 percent permethrin cream versus 0·75 percent metronidazole gel in acne rosacea. *Cutis* 1995;**56**:177–9.

38. Data on file. The safety and efficacy of metronidazole lotion, 0·75% for the treatment of rosacea: a randomised, double blind, vehicle-controlled, parallel comparison. Galderma USA CR, U9418, 29 Mar 1996. [Cited by McClellan and Noble.[23]]

39. Drake L, Leyden J, Lucky A et al. Evaluation of topical metronidazole cream in rosacea. 55th AAD meeting, 1997 Mar 21: abstract P65.

40. Breneman DL, Stewart D, Hevia O, Hino PD et al. A double-blind, multicenter clinical trial comparing efficacy of once-daily metronidazole 1 percent cream to vehicle in patients with rosacea. Cutis 1998;61:44–7.

41. Jorizzo JL, Lebwohl M, Tobey RE. The efficacy of metronidazole 1% cream once daily compared with metronidazole 1% cream twice daily and their vehicles in rosacea: a double-blind clinical trial. J Am Acad Dermatol 1998;39:502–4.

42. Dreno B, Dubertret L, Naeyaert JM et al. Comparison of the clinical efficacy and safety of metronidazole 0·75% cream with metronidazole 0·75% gel in the treatment of rosacea (Abstract). J Eur Acad Dermatol 1998;272–3. [Cited by McClellan and Noble.[23]]

43. Guillet, Rostain, Powell et al. Comparison of clinical efficacy and safety of metronidazole 0·75% lotion with metronidazole 0·75% gel in the treatment of rosacea. Galderma J.CG.03.SRE.2560: 13 Jan 1998. [Cited by McClellan and Noble.[23]]

44. Maddin, S. A comparison of topical azelaic acid 20% cream and topical metronidazole 0·75% cream in the treatment of patients with papulopustular rosacea. J Am Acad Dermatol. 1999;40:961–5.

45. Dahl MV, Katz HI, Krueger GG et al. Topical metronidazole maintains remissions of rosacea. Arch Dermatol 1998;134:679–83.

46. Nazzaro-Porro M, Passi S, Picardo M et al. L'acido azelaico nella rosacea? G Ital Dermatol Vener 1991(Suppl 1)126:19–27.

47. Carmichael AJ, Marks R, Graupe KA et al. Topical azelaic acid in the treatment of rosacea. J Derm Treat 1993;4:S19–S22. [Cited by Bjerke et al.[48]]

48. Bjerke R, Fyrand O, Graupe K. Double-blind comparison of azelaic acid 20% cream and its vehicle in treatment of papulopustular rosacea. Acta Dermatol Venereol 1999; 79:456–9.

49. Blom I, Hornmark AM. Topical treatment with sulfur 10 per cent for rosacea. Acta Dermatol Venereol 1984;64:358–9.

50. Sauder DN, Miller R, Gratton D et al. The treatment of rosacea: The safety and efficacy of sodium sulfacetamide 10% and sulfur 5% lotion (Novacet) is demonstrated in a double-blind study. J Dermatol Treat 1997;8:79–85.

51. Plewig G, Braun-Falco O, Klovekorn W, Luderschmidt C. [Isotretinoin in local treatment of acne and rosacea and animal experimental studies on isotretinoin and arotinoid]. Heautorst 1980;37:138–41. [MEDLINE abstract].

52. Montes LF, Cordero AA, Kriner J et al. Topical treatment of acne rosacea with benzoyl peroxide acetone gel. Cutis 1983;32:185–90.

15
Perioral dermatitis

Aditya K Gupta and Jacqueline E Swan

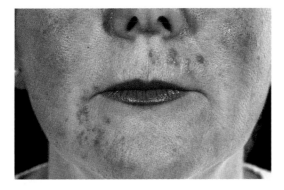

Figure 15.1   Patient with perioral dermatitis

Background
Definition

Perioral dermatitis is a symmetrical eruption involving the area bounded by the alae nasi and the chin, consisting of micropapules, microvesicles or papulopustules of less than 2 mm in diameter, which occur on a diffuse or patchy erythematous base. Some scaling may be present and cropping of the micropapules is usual. A striking and characteristic feature is the sparing of a narrow border around the vermilion of the lips.[1]

Incidence/prevalence

The incidence and prevalence are unknown. Perioral dermatitis predominately affects women aged 15–40 years; the peak incidence is between 25 and 35 years. The condition is occasionally seen in men and children.[1]

Aetiology

The cause of perioral dermatitis is unknown, but some possible aetiological factors include hormonal or emotional factors, cosmetic sensitivity, fluoride dentifrices, infective agents and use of potent topical steroids.[1]

Prognosis

Upon withdrawal of the offending aetiological factor, and with the appropriate treatment, perioral dermatitis generally resolves in a number of weeks. Perioral dermatitis therefore has an excellent prognosis.

Aims of treatment

The aims of treatment are to achieve clinical clearance, to prevent recurrence and to minimise adverse effects of treatment.

Outcomes

The standard outcomes of treatment are clinical clearance, recurrence rates and adverse effects of treatment. We found no standard severity scales in perioral dermatitis.

Methods of search

To identify studies on the treatment of perioral dermatitis, we searched Medline (1966–2000) for publications in English. Since few randomised controlled trials (RCTs) were identified, case series studies were included in this report. Evidence was graded using the quality of evidence scale system reported by Cox *et al.*[2] (Box 15.1). All evidence derived from the literature is presented.

QUESTIONS

What are the effects of metronidazole?

Box 15.1 The quality of evidence rating system reported by Cox et al.[2]

I   Evidence obtained from at least one properly designed randomised control trial
II-i   Evidence obtained from well-designed controlled trials without randomisation
II-ii Evidence obtained from well-designed cohort or case-controlled analytical studies, preferably from more than one centre or research group
II-iii Evidence obtained from multiple time series with or without the intervention. Dramatic results in uncontrolled experiments could also be included
III   Options of respected authorities based on clinical experience, descriptive studies or reports of expert committees
IV   Evidence inadequate owing to problems of methodology (for example sample size, length of comprehensiveness of follow up or conflicts of interest)

Metronidazole 1% cream

Quality of evidence: I

We found no studies comparing metronidazole 1% cream with placebo. One prospective, double-blind, double-dummy, multicentre RCT evaluated the efficacy of metronidazole 1% cream compared with oral tetracycline in the treatment of perioral dermatitis.[3] Tetracycline was statistically more effective in reducing the number of papules associated with perioral dermatitis.

Efficacy

We found one large RCT in which 109 patients were randomised to receive either 1% metronidazole cream (applied twice daily) plus placebo tablets or tetracycline tablets (250 mg twice daily) and a placebo cream.[3] Patients who had been treated with antibiotics or other medications in the 4 weeks before initiation of the trial were not included. In the group of patients given metronidazole the median number of papules was reduced to 33% of the original number after 4 weeks, and to 8% after 8 weeks. The median number of papules in patients given tetracycline reduced to 4% after 4 weeks, and to 0 at 8 weeks. Tetracycline was significantly more effective in reducing the number of papules both after 4 weeks and 8 weeks of treatment ($P<0.01$). No significant differences were noted between the two groups for erythema, and patient and physician assessments, which were the other categories evaluated.

Drawbacks

Seven patients in the metronidazole group and nine patients in the tetracycline group complained of adverse effects, the most common complaint being abdominal discomfort. Pruritus and dryness of the face were reported in a few patients in both groups.

Comment

One RCT was performed to compare the efficacy of metronidazole 1% cream with oral tetracycline. Multiple criteria were evaluated, including papule counts, erythema grading and patient and physician assessments. Tetracycline was more effective than metronidazole 1% cream in reducing the number of papules. No other significant differences were noted.

Metronidazole 0·75% gel

Quality of evidence: III

We found no reliable evidence on the effects of treatment of perioral dermatitis with metronidazole 0·75% gel. Only case reports were available and concerned children under the age of 9 years.[4,5] Studies on adults with perioral dermatitis are needed to justify the use of metronidazole 0·75% gel in older patients.

Efficacy

We found no systematic review or RCTs. We found two case reports which studied 17 children between the ages of 9 months and

9 years with perioral dermatitis.[4,5] Eleven of the 17 children were treated with 0·75% metronidazole gel either once or twice daily. The remaining patients were given metronidazole gel in combination with topical corticosteroids or erythromycin (topical or oral). All patients improved significantly within 8 weeks of therapy. Fourteen patients who were followed up remained lesion-free for up to 16 months.[4]

Drawbacks

None were reported.

Comment

All children included in these case reports had used topical steroids before treatment with metronidazole. Treatment regimens differed: some patients were treated once daily whereas most received twice-daily applications. In the few patients that have been studied, 0·75% metronidazole gel appeared to be effective. Larger studies would help to confirm these preliminary data. We could find no studies conducted in adults.

What are the effects of oral antibiotics?

Tetracycline

Quality of evidence: I

We found no good evidence evaluating tetracycline versus placebo. Our search found one published RCT that evaluated the efficacy of tetracycline, 250 mg twice daily, compared with 1% metronidazole cream in the treatment of perioral dermatitis.[3] In this study, oral tetracyline was found to be significantly more effective than metronidazole cream with 8 weeks of treatment ($P<0.01$). After 4 weeks, the number of papules in the tetracyline group was 4% of the original number, compared with 33% in the metronidazole group. At 8 weeks these numbers were 0% and 4%, respectively.

We also found some case series reporting the efficacy of oral tetracycline.[6-10] Follow up periods for many of the case series ranged from 3 months to 2 years. Tetracycline was found to be effective, but relapse was common after discontinuation of treatment.[6-10]

Efficacy

We found no systematic reviews.

Tetracycline versus placebo

We found no placebo-controlled RCTs of tetracycline. One series involved 29 patients with perioral dermatitis, observed for 3 years.[6] The criteria for inclusion were a diagnosis of perioral dermatitis, based on a clinical appearance of papular erythema involving most of the area bordered by the nasolabial folds and the sides of the chin, and rash of a duration of 3 months or more. Patients were instructed to apply topical 0·5% or 0·25% ichthyol in water, or 0·5% or 1% sulphur in calamine lotion at night, alternating with 1% hydrocortisone cream by day. If no favourable response was seen after 1 or 2 weeks, oral tetracycline was prescribed at a dosage of 250 mg three times daily for 1 week and twice daily thereafter. Four patients responded to topical therapy alone and did not need oral tetracycline. Patients treated with tetracycline usually improved within 10–14 days, and were treated for 2–3 months (mean). They relapsed when treatment was stopped. The tendency to relapse diminished with longer periods of treatment.

Tetracycline plus topical treatments

We found no placebo-controlled RCTs of tetracycline plus topical treatments. One trial followed 95 patients with perioral dermatitis for a period of 42 months.[7] Fifty-six patients were treated with oral tetracycline, 250 mg four times daily, together with a topical sulfacetamide-sulphur-hydrocortisone lotion. The other 25 patients received sodium sulfacetamide-sulfur-hydrocortisone lotion alone. Of the 56 patients treated with oral tetracycline plus sodium sulfacetamide-sulphur-hydrocortisone lotion, 48 (86%) had complete clearing, with a mean treatment duration of 1 month. Fourteen patients (56%) treated with topical sulfacetamide-sulphur-hydrocortisone lotion only had clearing, with a mean treatment duration of 1 month.

In a small subsidiary study, 37 patients received tetracycline 1 g daily, and nine patients received erythromycin 1 g daily.[6] Clearing did not occur in 10 patients, even after 10 weeks of treatment, while patients who did achieve complete clearing needed a mean treatment duration of 4·6 weeks.

In one 6-year case series, 39 patients were treated with either tetracycline or erythromycin, 250 mg twice daily, and with 1% hydrocortisone cream or 0·05% desonide cream, topically twice daily.[8] The mean duration of treatment was 3 months. Twenty-nine (74%) of 39 patients cleared after 2–3 months of therapy and stayed clear. Nine (23%) cleared but relapsed after treatment stopped. One patient did not achieve remission with therapy.

In a separate study, 43 patients previously given potent local steroids were treated with oral tetracycline, 250 mg either once or twice daily, combined with either 1% hydrocortisone ointment or Alphaderm ointment.[9] All patients had improved after 3 months' treatment, and most improved as early as 6 weeks.

Tetracycline with other oral drugs
Nine patients with a 3-year history of perioral dermatitis received oral tetracycline or doxycycline for 2–3 months.[10] Patients with severe disease were treated concurrently with prednisolone, 5–15 mg/day for 2–3 weeks. Topical therapy included precipitated sulphur lotion and methylprednisolone acetate ointment. Seven of nine patients were reported cured after 2 months, the other two patients had symptomatic relief.

Drawbacks
None were reported.

Comment
Most studies did not evaluate the effectiveness of tetracycline alone, but rather in combination with other topical and oral preparations. Much of the available evidence is methodologically flawed. For example, none of the studies adequately defined the term "complete clearing" and results were not evaluated statistically. Before consultation, many of the patients in the case series were treated unsuccessfully with potent topical steroids, therefore allowing for no wash-out period. In addition, some studies did not focus only on perioral dermatitis but included other conditions such as rosacea and rosacea-like dermatitis. Only one double-blind RCT compared oral tetracyline, 250 mg twice daily, with 1% metronidazole cream.

Oxytetracycline
Quality of evidence: III

The only evidence for the treatment of perioral dermatitis with oxytetracycline was a series of case reports. None of the reports were placebo controlled, and many used multiple oral and topical agents in combination with oxytetracycline. For this reason, it is very difficult to compare the results of different case series.

Efficacy
We found no systematic review.

Oxytetracycline versus placebo
We found no placebo-controlled RCTs. The only evidence available were case series. One series involved 116 patients treated with oxytetracycline, 250 mg twice daily for 3 weeks, then once daily for a similar period.[11] Five patients needed two courses and three patients required three courses of treatment. Eighty patients were seen at the end of their course of treatment, 62 patients at 1–3 months post-treatment, 9 patients at 6–12 months, and 9

patients 2–5 years later when they were being treated for another condition. Only five of the returning patients relapsed.

Oxytetracycline plus topical steroids

Another case series evaluated 73 patients (5 men, 68 women) using a combination of 1% hydrocortisone cream and oxytetracycline, 250 mg twice daily.[12] Seventy-one of the patients had used fluorinated topical steroids previously, and after aggravation of the eruption upon discontinuation of the steroids, virtually all of the patients recovered on the regimen of oxytetracycline and 1% hydrocortisone cream. A 6–14 month follow up to the study using a mailed questionnaire revealed that 11 of 13 respondents had remained clear without any further treatment, one had a slight recurrence, and one had a severe recurrence.

In a separate series, 40 patients were assigned to one of three groups: Group 1 – 15 patients treated with topical hydrocortisone and oral oxytetracycline, 250 mg twice daily; Group 2 – 12 patients treated with topical desonide and oxytetracycline, 250 mg twice daily; Group 3 – 7 patients treated with desonide and 6 with hydrocortisone.[13] Groups 1 and 2 were assigned randomly. Group 3 patients were selected according to the mildness of their condition and one patient was included in this group because she was pregnant. In Group 1, 14 of 15 patients improved within 6 weeks and cleared within 3 months. In Group 2, improvement within 6 weeks and clearance within 3 months occurred in 11 of 12 patients. In Group 3, 12 of 13 patients responded completely. The pregnant patient experienced no improvement initially and later dropped out. There was one dropout in each of Groups 1 and 2.

Drawbacks

None were reported.

Comment

We found no RCTs for the treatment of perioral dermatitis with oxytetracycline. Similarly, we found no placebo-controlled trials using oxytetracyclines to treat perioral dermatitis. All the studies looking at the treatment of perioral dermatitis with oxytetracycline were methodologically flawed. For example, in one study patients were randomised to three groups of treatment but only mild cases were assigned to one treatment group. With the lack of quality evidence available, it is difficult to determine the efficacy of oxytetracycline in the treatment of perioral dermatitis.

What are the effects of topical antibiotics?

Topical tetracycline

Quality of evidence: IV

The effects of topical tetracycline were evaluated in the treatment of perioral dermatitis. Because the source of this topical preparation was not disclosed, the dose, potency and efficacy of this type of tetracycline preparation must be questioned.

Efficacy

A series 30 of patients (26 female, 4 male) with clinically typical perioral dermatitis has been reported.[14] Patients were asked to apply topical tetracycline twice daily to all affected areas after gently washing the face. No other treatment was allowed. Twenty-four patients (80%) experienced complete clearing of their condition in 5–28 days; three patients (10%) were at least 50% clear but not totally clear within 28 days, and three (10%) patients discontinued the medication. All patients whose condition cleared were able to maintain clearing with the topical product used on an as-needed basis.

Drawbacks

Two patients discontinued therapy because of stinging and one because of worsening of the dermatitis.

Comment

We found no RCTs on the treatment of perioral dermatitis with topical tetracycline.

Topical erythromycin

Quality of evidence: IV

We found no good evidence for the effective treatment of perioral dermatitis with topical erythromycin.

Efficacy

Six patients in a case series were treated with 1·5% erythromycin topical solution twice daily in combination with hydrocortisone valerate cream.[15] Topical 1·5% erythromycin was effective in the treatment of perioral dermatitis, with a mean treatment duration of 4·5 weeks.

Drawbacks

None were reported.

Comment

No RCTs have evaluated the use of topical erythromycin in the treatment of perioral dermatitis.

What are the effects of non-fluorinated corticosteroids?

Hydrocortisone butyrate

Quality of evidence: IV

We found insufficient evidence on the effects of non-fluorinated corticosteroids in patients with perioral dermatitis. We found one study, a split-face randomised trial which, in addition to perioral dermatitis, evaluated rosacea and atopic dermatitis.

Efficacy

We found no systematic review.

Hydrocortisone butyrate versus 1% hydrocortisone alcohol cream

One double-blind, split-face randomised trial with 28 patients (8 patients with perioral dermatitis, 18 patients with rosacea, and 2 patients with atopic dermatitis), randomly treated one side of their face with hydrocortisone alcohol 1% cream and the other side with 0·1% hydrocortisone butyrate.[16] Only patients with severe disease were selected. Participants were instructed to apply the creams twice daily to the appropriate side of the face. Six of 8 patients with perioral dermatitis were also given oxytetracycline, 250 mg twice daily. Patients were re-examined weekly by the same physician until more improvement was noted on one side of the face compared with the opposite side. If no difference was detected, treatment continued for up to 3 months. In addition, patients were re-examined 1 week after treatment was withdrawn to determine whether any rebound occurred. Two patients with perioral dermatitis achieved better results with hydrocortisone alcohol 1% cream (mean duration of therapy 3·5 weeks; range 3–4 weeks), four patients improved with hydrocortisone butyrate (mean duration 3–5 weeks; range 2–5 weeks) and two patients found the two treatments to be equally effective.

Drawbacks

Two patients with perioral dermatitis showed a moderate rebound of the eruption after withdrawal of topical treatment, in each case on the hydroxybutyrate treated side of the face.

Comment

In view of the study design and the small numbers of patients, it is difficult to draw conclusions.

Key points

- Very few RCTs have been conducted to determine appropriate therapies for the treatment of perioral dermatitis.
- It appears that tetracyclines and other oral antibiotics have been used as a standard

treatment with some efficacy, but only one RCT has been reported.
- Topical 1% metronidazole cream has been shown to be effective in one RCT.
- Most of the available evidence for these and other treatments comes from case reports.

References

1. Wilkinson D. What is perioral dermatitis? *Int J Dermatol* 1981;**20**:485–6.
2. Cox NH, Eedy DJ, Morton CA. Guidelines for management of Bowen's disease. *Br J Dermatol* 1999;**141**:633–41.
3. Veien NK, Munkvad JM, Nielsen AO. Topical metronidazole in the treatment of perioral dermatitis. *J Am Acad Dermatol* 1991;**24**:258–60.
4. Manders SM, Lucky AW. Perioral dermatitis in childhood. *J Am Acad Dermatol* 1992;**27**:688–92.
5. Miller SR, Shalita AR. Topical metronidazole gel (0·75%) for the treatment of perioral dermatitis in children. *J Am Acad Dermatol* 1994;**31**:847–8.
6. Macdonald A, Feiwel M. Perioral dermatitis: aetiology and treatment with tetracycline. *Br J Dermatol* 1972;**87**:315–19.
7. Bendl BJ. Perioral dermatitis: etiology and treatment. *Cutis* 1976;**17**:903–8.
8. Coskey RJ. Perioral dermatitis. *Cutis* 1984;**34**:55–7.
9. Cotterill JA. Perioral dermatitis. *Br J Dermatol* 1979;**101**:259–62.
10. Urabe H, Koda H. Perioral dermatitis and rosacea-like dermatitis: clinical features and treatment. *Dermatology* 1976;**152**(Suppl. 1):155–60.
11. Wilkinson DS, Kirton V, Wilkinson JD. Perioral dermatitis: a 12-year review. *Br J Dermatol* 1979;**101**:245–57.
12. Sneddon I. Perioral dermatitis. *Br J Dermatol* 1972;**87**:430–4.
13. Cochran REI, Thomson J. Perioral dermatitis: a reappraisal. *Clin Exp Dermatol* 1979;**4**:75–80.
14. Wilson RG. Topical tetracycline in the treatment of perioral dermatitis. *Arch Dermatol* 1979;**115**:637.
15. Bikowski JB. Topical therapy for perioral dermatitis. *Cutis* 1983;**31**:678–82.
16. Sneddon I. A trial of hydrocortisone butyrate in the treatment of rosacea and perioral dermatitis. *Br J Dermatol* 1973;**89**:505–8.

16
Hand eczema

Pieter-Jan Coenraads, A Marco van Coevorden and Thomas Diepgen

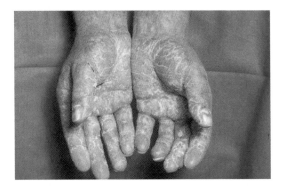

Figure 16.1 One of the several manifestations of chronic hand eczema

Background
Definition

The term "hand eczema" implies an inflammation of the skin (dermatitis) that is confined to the hands. Clinically, the condition is characterised by signs of redness, vesicles (tiny blisters), papules, scaling, cracks and hyperkeratosis (callous-like thickening), all of which may be present at different points in time. Itch, sometimes severe, is a common feature. Microscopically, the disease is characterised by spongiosis with varying degrees of acanthosis, and a superficial perivascular infiltrate of lymphocytes and histiocytes.

Incidence/prevalence

Hand eczema is considered a common condition, with a point prevalence of 1–5% among adults in the general population, and a 1-year prevalence of up to 10%, depending on whether the disease definition includes, more pronounced or mild cases. The prevalence may be higher in some countries. Recently, a decreased prevalence was stipulated, attributed to decreased occupational exposure to irritants. Hand eczema is twice as common in women than in men, with the highest prevalence in young women. Reasons for this sex difference are unknown, although greater exposure of women to wet work is probably contributory. Reliable data on incidence are scarce, and are mainly confined to estimates in particular occupational groups. Estimates vary from 0·5 per 1000 in the general population to 7 per 1000 per year in high-risk occupations such as bakers and hairdressers.

Aetiology

Aetiology is multifactorial. Contact irritants are the commonest external causes. Hand eczema caused by such irritants, or mild toxic agents, is called irritant contact dermatitis. Causal factors that are less common than irritants are contact allergens. Hand eczema caused by skin contact with allergens is called allergic contact dermatitis. Ingested allergens (for example nickel) may also provoke hand eczema. Water is a contact irritant and thereby an external causal or contributing factor. Being atopic (a tendency to develop asthma, hay fever or eczema) is the major predisposing factor responsible for hand eczema. There are several types of hand eczema of which the cause or predisposing factor is unknown. These (partly overlapping) types are not precisely defined and are commonly described as: hyperkeratotic, tylotic, endogenous, dyshidrotic, pompholyx and nummular. In particular, dyshidrotic eczema is the subject of debate: a hallmark is recurrent vesiculation, which may or may not be associated with factors such as nickel allergy, atopy and other factors. In many patients a combination of the aforementioned factors seems to play a role. The relevance of psychosomatic factors remains speculative.

Prognosis

When there is a single, easily avoidable contact allergic factor, the prognosis is good. Several studies, however, have suggested that hand eczema tends to run a long lasting and chronic relapsing course, probably because of the multifactorial origin.

Diagnostic tests

Diagnosis is mainly based on history and clinical signs; there are no standardised diagnostic criteria. Patients are patch-tested to detect or rule out a contact allergy. In addition, prick tests are performed to detect atopy, and skin scrapings are performed to rule out a mycotic infection. In the majority of cases, no relevant contact allergy can be detected. Specific prick tests are of additional value in only very special cases (such as eczematised urticarial reactions).

Aims of treatment

Treatment is aimed at reducing clinical symptoms (including the disabling itch), preventing relapses and improving quality of life by allowing resumption of daily manual tasks.

Relevant outcomes

- Percentage of patients with patient-stated good/excellent response
- Percentage of patients with investigator-stated good/excellent response

- Reduction in severity (patient and doctor rated scoring systems)
- Dose reduction
- Time until relapse

Methods of search

Controlled trials dating back to 1977 were located by searching the *Cochrane Library*, Medline, Embase, Pascal and Jicst-Eplus. In addition, a hand-search was performed on any trial (including uncontrolled trials but excluding single case reports) in major English, German, French, Italian and Dutch dermatology journals.

QUESTIONS

Because of the tendency of hand eczema to develop a chronic or relapsing course, all questions below deal with chronic hand eczema. In the context of this chapter, chronicity can arbitrarily be defined as more than 6 months' duration. Because prescription topical corticosteroids are the most common treatment at present, they are the major comparator in the questions below.

> In adults with chronic hand eczema, do topical corticosteroids lead to better patient- and doctor-rated reduction in symptom scores than topical coal tar preparations?

No systematic review was found, and no trial (controlled or uncontrolled) could be identified. Trials may be detected in older (pre-1977) literature.

> In adults with chronic hand eczema, do short bursts of potent topical corticosteroids (class 3 or 4) lead to better patient- and doctor-rated scores than continuous mild (class 1 or 2) topical steroids?

We found no studies comparing the effect of short bursts of strong (class 3 or 4) topical steroids (for example twice weekly, or weekends only) with continuous application of milder (class

1 or 2) topical steroids. One randomised controlled trial (RCT) compared three-times-weekly application versus weekend application of the same steroid, with limited evidence that the three-times-weekly application was better.

Efficacy

No systematic reviews were found.

Three-times-weekly versus weekend application

There is limited evidence of a preferential effect of three-times-weekly application of mometasone in an RCT of a 30-week maintenance phase (i.e. after induction of remission).[1] The primary outcome variable was the number of recurrences of hand eczema.

Once-daily versus twice-daily application

Three studies compared once- versus twice-daily application. One RCT found no difference between the two application schedules for the same corticosteroid used for 3 weeks.[2] The other two studies were left–right comparisons of two different corticosteroids.[3,4]

Two different concentrations

One left–right RCT of 2 weeks' duration comparing different concentrations of the same corticosteroid applied twice daily detected no difference.[5]

Drawbacks

Mild skin atrophy was reported in one study.[1]

Comment

Except for the study on three-times-weekly versus weekend application, all studies were of short duration. Of the two studies comparing different steroids, it was not clear how many patients with hand eczema were enrolled. No study had tachyphylaxis or atrophy as outcome parameters. No uncontrolled trials were detected. Older (pre-1977) literature may give some insight into this issue.

Implications for clinical practice

The choice for an optimal topical steroid treatment schedule cannot be derived from the current literature on hand eczema trials. Evidence from studies on other eczematous diseases may have to be considered.

> In adults with chronic hand eczema, are oral immunosuppressive agents (ciclosporin, methotrexate, mycophenolate mofetil) better in maintaining a long-term (more than 6 months) reduction of patient- and doctor-rated scores than topical corticosteroids?

Two RCTs were identified, one of which showed that ciclosporin was effective, but not better than topical corticosteroids in terms of clinical signs.[6] The other RCT, studying the same patients, also showed no comparative advantage of ciclosporin over topical steroids in terms of quality of life.[7]

Efficacy

No systematic review was found.

Ciclosporin versus topical betamethasone

One RCT compared ciclosporin with betamethasone dipropionate 0·05% twice daily. The study had three phases, none of which showed a comparative advantage in terms of clinical signs, global assessment or cumulative relapse rate.[6] The first treatment phase was 6 weeks; the second and third amounted to 30 weeks. Quality of life was the outcome parameter in another study of the same design and of the same patients;[7] this parameter showed no comparative advantage.

Methotrexate

We identified no controlled trials. One uncontrolled study indicated an effect in pompholyx-type eczema.[8]

Drawbacks

Paraesthesia, dizziness, insomnia and increase in serum creatinine were reported. An uncontrolled long-term follow up study on ciclosporin did not explicitly evaluate side-effects.[9]

Comment

The comparator in the ciclosporin studies was a relatively strong corticosteroid. Two uncontrolled studies on ciclosporin were found[9,10]: one had enrolled patients who had participated in the aforementioned trial.[7] One uncontrolled study on oral methotrexate was identified, which was description of a case series of five patients.[8] Several single case reports were identified, only one of which was on mycophenolate mofetil.

Implications for clinical practice

Ciclosporin may be useful to obtain short-term control, but cannot be recommended for maintenance therapy.

In adults with chronic hand eczema, does treatment with ionising radiation (x rays) lengthen the time to relapse compared with topical corticosteroids?

We identified six RCTs, all of which had a left–right design (i.e. the contralateral hand of each patient served as control). Two RCTs found no evidence that x rays were superior to conventional topical medication. None of the trials had a follow up time longer than 6 months; therefore there was no evidence that ionising radiation induced a longer remission period than conventional topical medication.

Efficacy

No systematic reviews were found.

Versus topical medication

One 18-week study of Grenz rays using a grading system as outcome parameter[11] and one study of superficial radiotherapy, using (nearly) clearing as an outcome parameter,[12] found no beneficial effect. One 10-week RCT of Grenz rays[13] and one 18-week RCT of superficial x rays[14] found a beneficial effect.

Versus topical PUVA

One trial found a superior effect of radiotherapy at 6 weeks, but after 18 weeks follow up there was no difference in reduction of severity scores.[15]

Superficial x rays versus Grenz rays

One study of 18 weeks' duration found a superior effect of conventional x rays from the doctor's point of view but the patients' rating showed no difference.[16]

Drawbacks

Three trials mentioned the absence of adverse reactions during treatment.[13,14,16] No study could assess the possible long-term harmful effects of the radiotherapy.

Comment

No trial used time to relapse as the outcome variable. No study gave a rationale for the sample size, which was between 15 and 30 patients. None of the trials stated explicitly which conventional topical therapy was the comparator; at best it was described as steroids and/or tar. Overall, the studies did not explicitly describe the types of hand eczema of the patients: four studies specified the type of eczema as constitutional[11,14–16]; the other two gave only very partial results among some types of hand eczema.[12,13] Older literature may give an indication about possible long-term harm.

Implications for clinical practice

Given the uncertainties about the long-term effects of this treatment modality, and the very limited evidence of a short-term effect, radiotherapy cannot be recommended.

Does the daily application of a bland emollient lead to dose and/or frequency reduction of topical corticosteroids in adults with chronic hand eczema?

No RCTs addressing this issue could be identified. Only one controlled study compared an emollient with two different topical steroids.

Efficacy
No systematic review was found.

Emollient versus topical corticosteroids
One controlled trial indicated a beneficial effect of a chamomile-extract-containing cream over a cream with 0·25% hydrocortisone, but not in comparison with 0·75% fluocortin butylester cream.[17] Uncontrolled studies noted a reduction in steroid use in patients treated with a moisturising cream and in patients treated with a protective foam.[18,19]

Versus each other
In one left–right RCT, using patient preference as outcome parameter, there was limited evidence in favour of Aquacare HP over Calmurid, both of which contained 10% urea.[20] One controlled clinical trial (CCT) with a left–right design did not detect an advantage of a urea cream over an aqueous cream.[22]

Drawbacks
No major side-effects were reported. Burning and worsening of the pre-existing hand eczema were reported.[20] Patients were concerned with greasiness of their hands, and with staining of objects they handled.

Comments
Several poor-quality uncontrolled studies were identified, none of which had steroid dose reduction as the outcome parameter.

Implications for clinical practice
Despite their widespread use, there is insufficient documented evidence of any steroid-sparing or additive effect in the treatment of hand eczema. In general, there seems to be no harm either, apart from the occasional contact allergy to an ingredient.

Is treatment of chronic hand eczema with local PUVA or UVB irradiation better in reducing patient- and doctor-rated severity scores than topical corticosteroids?

We identified no trial explicitly comparing PUVA or UVB therapy with topical steroids; only one RCT had ordinary topical treatment (not specified) as comparator. A further four controlled trials, one of which was an RCT, were identified that compared the efficacy of PUVA or UVB therapy with a control group or using a right–left design. Numerous case series without a control group reported the efficacy of different modalities of photo(chemo)therapy. There is insufficient evidence that PUVA/UVB therapy is more effective than conventional topical steroid therapy.

Efficacy
No systematic reviews were found.

PUVA versus UVA
In a double-blind randomised within-patient trial of 15 patients with chronically relapsing vesicular hand eczema, topical PUVA and UVA treatment showed improvement of the severity score over the 8-week treatment period but no statistical difference between the treated hands at any stage.[22]

UVB versus topical treatment
Eighteen patients with chronic hand eczema resistant to conventional topical therapy with potent corticosteroids were randomly divided into three treatment groups: UVB of the hands only, placebo irradiation, and whole-body UVB irradiation.[23] Local UVB irradiation of the hands was significantly better than placebo; whole-body UVB irradiation with additional irradiation of the

hands was significantly better than the continuing local treatment alone (not specified) according to a simple clinical grading (cleared, improved, unchanged/worse). A 3-month follow up demonstrated the fast relapse of hand eczema.

Topical PUVA treatment

In a left–right design, there was little difference between topical 8-methoxypsoralen (8-MOP) bath PUVA and topical 8-MOP lotion PUVA therapy in 24 patients with chronic hand or foot eczema; there was greater than 80% clearing with both modalities.[24] After 1 month the most successful treatment was continued on both sides until lesions cleared; there was no difference in the length of the relapse-free period. A small controlled pilot trial comparing topical PUVA, systemic PUVA and topical corticosteroids was inconclusive.[25]

Systemic PUVA therapy versus no therapy

This was compared in a right–left (within-patient) study of seven patients with dyshidrotic hand eczema.[26] All patients responded and remained disease-free on a maintenance schedule for 2–6 months. Out of 20 patients with different conditions, five patients with endogenous eczema were treated in a controlled study of PUVA therapy versus no treatment but it was unclear how many of the treated hands responded.[27]

Drawbacks

PUVA treatment can cause side-effects such as burning episodes, subacute eczema and acute exacerbation of eczema. UV therapy may also induce skin cancer as a long-term effect.

Comment

In most studies patients continued their topical medication or emollients. There is no study comparing UVB/PUVA therapy with the conventional topical steroid therapy. There is also no evidence that UV therapy is the most effective for hand eczema (see the next question).

Implications for clinical practice

PUVA or UVB is effective. The choice for this treatment option is guided by considerations other than proven clinical superiority over other modalities.

> In adults with chronic hand eczema, does treatment with PUVA irradiation (oral or topical psoralen) lead to better reduction in patient- and doctor-rated scores and remission periods than UVB irradiation?

We identified one RCT on oral PUVA and two CCT's on oral/topical PUVA. The controlled trial on topical bath PUVA demonstrated no comparative advantage, whereas the RCT on oral PUVA showed an effect in favour of PUVA.

Efficacy

No systematic review was found.

Topical bath PUVA versus UVB

A 6-week left–right design CCT of 13 patients showed that, though effective, topical bath PUVA was not better than UVB.[28]

Oral PUVA versus UVB

The only RCT we found, a 3-month study of 35 patients, showed an effect in favour of oral PUVA.[29] In this study, only one hand was treated but in most patients the untreated hand also improved. A CCT comparing UVB used at home with PUVA at the clinic showed no comparative advantage.[30]

Drawbacks

Nausea caused by the oral psoralen was reported. Pain, burning, itching and redness was reported with both therapies, but slightly more from PUVA irradiation.

Comment

Long-term adverse effects could not be assessed. Improvement of the untreated hand may be the result of compliance with topical emollients. More than 17 uncontrolled studies were identified, claiming a beneficial effect of UV treatment (PUVA or UVB), but there was no comparator in any of the studies.

Implications for clinical practice

PUVA or UVB is effective in treating hand eczema. The question of which modality is better is unsolved.

> In adults with chronic hand eczema, is oral treatment with retinoids better in terms of patient- and doctor-rated sign scores than topical corticosteroids?

Two uncontrolled open studies demonstrated limited evidence that oral 9-*cis*-retinoic acid and etretinate are effective in chronic hand eczema. We identified only one CCT comparing topical retinoic acid plus corticosteroids against topical steroids, in 18 patients in a double-blind left–right design. There was no statistically significant difference between the modalities.

Efficacy

No systematic reviews were found.

Topical retinoid versus topical corticosteroids

In a symmetrical double-blind study, the efficacy of triamcinolone acetonide 0·1% cream was compared with the same cream containing, in addition, 0·25% retinoic acid.[31] The study involved 18 subjects with different types of eczema (12 atopic dermatitis, 4 allergic contact dermatitis, 1 nummular eczema, 1 dyshidrosis); the palms and soles were involved in only five patients. The duration of treatment was planned for 2 weeks, with the option to extend treatment to 3 weeks. The same observer scored erythema, oedema, vesicles, crusts, excoriations, scales, lichenifications and pruritus separately on a scale of 0–5. No statistically significant difference between the treatments was observed.

Oral retinoids

In an open uncontrolled study, 15 patients with hyperkeratotic hand eczema were treated with etretinate 25–75 mg daily for 3–20 months.[32] Pronounced improvement was reported but the clinical value was limited because of severe side-effects. Another open study using 9-*cis*-retinoic acid for 1–5 months in 38 patients with refractory therapy-resistant chronic hand eczema showed very good response in 21 patients (55%), a good response in 13 patients (34%), a moderate response in 2 patients (5·5%) and no response in 2 patients (5·5%), as assessed by patient and doctor, and only mild side-effects.[33]

Drawbacks

Topical use of retinoid acid plus steroids is reported to cause significantly more subjective irritation than topical steroids without retinoic acid.[31] Frequent side-effects such as dryness of the mucosae and lips, but also loss of hair and universal pruritus were reported for the treatment with etretinate.[32] Oral 9-*cis*-retinioic acid showed fewer and milder side-effects: cheilitis, 29%; headache, 11%; flush, 11%; conjunctivitis, 3%.[33]

Comment

Oral 9-*cis*-retinioic acid seems to be a promising option but evidence of a comparative advantage is absent. It has to be demonstrated that this new drug with fewer side-effects is more effective than conventional topical steroid or UVB/PUVA therapy.

Implications for clinical practice

Currently there is insufficient evidence to support the prescription of oral retinoids for hand eczema.

> In adults with dyshidrotic hand eczema, does iontophoresis lead to an improvement of patient- and doctor-rated scores compared with topical steroids or UVB/PUVA irradiation?

We identified only one RCT using iontophoresis in patients with dyshidrotic hand eczema. This trial showed a significant improvement of the ionotophoresis-treated side compared with the non-treated side. No trial has compared iontophoresis with topical steroids or UVB/PUVA therapy.

Efficacy

No systematic reviews were found.

Iontophoresis versus no treatment

In a randomised one-sided comparison, the effects of tap-water iontophoresis in addition to steroid-free topical therapy was investigated in 20 patients with dyshidrotic hand eczema.[34] After 3 weeks (20 iontophoresis applications) the parameters "itching" and "vesicle formations" scored significantly better on the iontophoresis-treated side than on the non-iontophoresis-treated side, but redness and desquamation did not differ significantly. In an open study of 54 patients with hyperhidrosis, 20 patients with palmoplantar eczema who continued the iontophoresis treatment at home for at least 6 months were compared with a historical sex- and age-matched control group of eczema

patients without iontophoresis.[35] The relapse-free interval, but not the time needed for clearing, was significantly improved in the iontophoresis-treated group.

Drawbacks

Tap water iontophoresis was always connected with subjective sensations like stinging and discrete paraesthesia ("tingling"). No severe side-effects or possible harmful effects were reported.

Comment

No trial showed sufficient evidence for the benefit of additional iontophoresis therapy compared with conventional topical steroid or UVB/PUVA therapy. The open study that compared the long-term effects of iontophoresis in patients with non-specified hand eczema with historical controls had insufficient evidence to show whether iontophoresis prolongs the relapse-free interval in dyshidrotic hand eczema.[35] Only one study[34] describes the types of dyshidrotic hand eczema of the patients.

Implications for clinical practice

The treatment seems harmless, but is not proven to be effective.

> In adults with hyperkeratotic hand eczema, does dithranol lead to an improvement in patient- and doctor-rated sign scores, and longer remission periods upon clearance, when compared with topical corticosteroids?

No systematic review was found, and no trial (controlled or uncontrolled) of dithranol for any type of hand eczema could be identified. Trials may be detected in older (pre-1977) literature.

> In adults with relapsing vesicular hand eczema based on contact allergy to nickel, does dietary intervention or oral therapy with chelating agents lead to an improvement in patient- and doctor-rated sign scores, when compared with topical corticosteroids?

We identified six trials: two RCTs, one CCT and three open studies. All studies were small, performed in nickel-sensitive patients with hand eczema. Four studies used a nickel-chelating compound and two a low-nickel diet. None of the studies compared the intervention with topical corticosteroids. One multicentre RCT on triethylenetetramine found no significant improvement of hand eczema. The other RCT on disulfiram (tetraethylthiuramdisulphide) found only very limited evidence in favour of this treatment. One controlled trial found no evidence that a low-nickel diet improves dyshidrotic hand eczema.

Efficacy

No systematic reviews were found.

Oral therapy with a nickel-chelating compound

In a multicentre, randomised, double-blind, crossover study, oral treatment with triethylenetetramine, 300 mg daily for a 6-week period, or a lactose-containing placebo was given to 23 nickel-positive patients with chronic hand eczema after a 4-week rest period before crossover.[36] No significant improvement occurred in hand eczema on the basis of either the patients' or the doctor's evaluation. In a double-blind, placebo-controlled RCT, disulfiram with a gradually increased dose was given for at least 6 weeks after having reached the full dosage of 200 mg.[37] Hand eczema was graded according to a semi-quantitative scoring system. During the treatment period, the hand eczema healed in five out of the 11 disulfiram-treated patients, compared with two out of 13 in the placebo group (not significant). Using the semi-quantitative scoring system, results in favour of disulfiram were statistically significant for scaling and frequency of flares but not for the sum of parameters. Two open trials without controls found insufficient evidence on the effect of the nickel-chelating compound disulfiram.[38,39] In one uncontrolled study, two out of 11 patients with

nickel allergy and hand eczema healed and eight improved considerably under the treatment with disulfiram, 200 mg daily for 8 weeks.[38] Mild relapses were observed in all patients within 2–16 weeks after discontinuation of treatment. In the other open study, out of 11 nickel-positive patients with chronic dyshidrotic hand eczema aggrevated by oral challenge with nickel, seven patients cleared, improvement was seen in two patients, and in two the dermatitis remained unchanged during the treatment with disulfiram, 200–400 mg daily for 4–10 weeks.[39]

Low-nickel diet

In a non-randomised trial of 24 patients with dyshidrotic hand eczema caused by nickel, the effects of a low-nickel diet for 3 months (eight patients) were compared with oral disodium cromoglycate for 3 months (nine patients) and with seven patients who did not give consent to the study and who did not receive any treatment.[40] All 24 patients were evaluated blind for itching and number of vesicles. The low-nickel diet did not improve these patients, but those treated with disodium cromoglycate improved significantly and had significantly fewer blisters than the controls and the patients treated by diet. In an open, uncontrolled study, 55 out of 90 nickel-sensitive patients who had had a flare of dermatitis after oral challenge with nickel and adhered to the diet for at least 4 weeks improved or cleared.[41] Forty of these patients reported a long-term improvement when followed up by questionnaire 1–2 years later.

Drawbacks

In one RCT, one patient treated with disulfiram had toxic hepatitis after 8 weeks of treatment and two patients out of 30 patients showed signs of hepatic toxicity.[37] In an open study, treatment with disulfiram, 100 mg, was discontinued in 4 out of 11 patients because of side-effects. Seven out of 11 patients experienced side-effects such as fatigue, headache and dizziness;

in one patient without such side-effects, treatment was stopped when the patient developed viral hepatitis.[39] During the treatment with disulfiram, 200 mg daily over 8 weeks, reversible side-effects of headache, nausea, borborygmus and halitosis were seen in eight out of 11 patients; dizziness was seen in one patient who developed toxic reversible liver damage induced by disulfiram.[38] One RCT mentioned the absence of adverse reactions during the treatment with triethylenetetramine, 300 mg daily for a 6-week period.[36] No study using a low-nickel diet could assess possible harmful effects.

Comment

No trial showed sufficient evidence for the benefit of either a low-nickel diet or a nickel-chelating compound. Only two RCTs with a small number of patients (23 and 11) were performed. On the basis of the harm and the possible side-effects, oral treatment with a nickel-chelating compound cannot be recommended. None of the trials compared treatments with conventional topical medication (for example steroids).

Implications for clinical practice

Given the side-effects and lack of efficacy, oral therapy with a nickel-chelating compound can not be recommended. There is no evidence that a low-nickel diet improves pompholyx-type hand eczema.

In adults with chronic clinically active hand eczema, do protective or occlusive gloves, barrier-creams, avoidance of allergens and irrititants, and other non-pharmacological interventions lead to better patient- and doctor-rated sign scores than topical steroids?

No systematic reviews were found. There is, however, one systematic review being prepared on interventions to prevent occupational hand dermatitis.[42] A number of issues in connection with this question will be dealt with in this review. Information on avoidance of allergens or irritants on a case-by-case basis can be found in the major textbooks on contact dermatitis.[43] The effect of emollients was covered in the fifth question above (p. 136).

No controlled trials on gloves or protective creams were found. We found a few uncontrolled rather descriptive studies indicating some benefit of gloves and/or barrier creams,[19,44] one study having a within-patient left–right design.[45]

Key points

- In general, there is a lack of evidence of comparative advantage for the three most established treatment modalities for hand eczema – topical corticosteroids, topical coal tar and PUVA/UVB.
- Although widely prescribed, there is a lack of evidence of a steroid-sparing effect of emollients.
- There is insufficient clinical evidence for a choice between short bursts of potent topical steroids versus continuous application of mild steroids.
- PUVA and UVB are effective, but there is no evidence of a clinical advantage of one modality over the other.
- There is insufficient evidence for effectiveness of currently marketed retinoids.
- There is insufficient evidence for a comparative advantage of radiotherapy (x rays).
- There is insufficient evidence for oral immunosuppressants as maintenance therapy.
- There is insufficient evidence for low-nickel diet or chelating agents in hand eczema accompanied by nickel allergy.
- Of all the trials that were identified, very few conform to modern quality criteria for an RCT.

References

1. Veien NK, Larsen PØ, Thestrup-Pedersen K, Schou G. Long-term, intermittent treatment of chronic hand eczema with mometasone furoate. Br J Dermatol 1999;**140**:882–6.

2. English JSC, Bunker CB, Ruthven K, Dowd PM, Greaves MW. A double-blind comparison of the efficacy of betamethasone dipropionate cream twice daily versus once daily in the treatment of steroid responsive dermatoses. *Clin Exp Dermatol* 1989;**14**:32–4.

3. Goh CL, Lim JTE, Leow YH, Ang CB, Kohar YM. The therapeutic efficacy of mometasone furoate cream 0·1% applied once daily v clobetasol propionate cream 0·05% applied twice daily in chronic eczema. *Singapore Med J* 1999;**40**:341–4.

4. Levy A. Comparison of 0·1% halcinonide with 0·05% betamethasone dipropionate in the treatment of acute and chronic dermatoses. *Curr Med Res Opin* 1977–78;**5**: 328–32.

5. Uggeldahl PE, Kero M, Ulshagen K, Solberg VM. Comparative effects of desonide cream 0·1% and 0·05% in patients with hand eczema. *Curr Therap Res* 1986;**40**:969–73.

6. Granlund H, Erkko P, Eriksson E, Reitamo S. Comparison of cyclosporine and topical betamethasone 17,21–dipropionate in the treatment of severe chronic hand eczema. *Acta Derm Venereol* (Stockh) 1996;**76**:371–6.

7. Granlund H, Erkko P, Reitamo S. Comparison of the influence of cyclosporin and topical betamethasone-17,21-dipropionate treatment on quality of life in chronic hand eczema. *Acta Derm Venereol* (Stockh) 1997; **77**:54–8.

8. Egan CE, Rallis TM, Meadows KP, Krueger GG. Low-dose oral methotrexate treatment for recalcitrant palmoplantar pompholyx. *J Am Acad Dermatol* 1999;**40**:612–14.

9. Granlund H, Erkko P, Reitamo S. Long-term follow-up of eczema patients treated with cyclosporine. *Acta Derm Venereol* (Stockh) 1998;**78**:40–3.

10. Reitamo S, Granlund H. Cyclosporin A in the treatment of chronic dermatitis of the hands. *Br J Dermatol* 1994;**130**: 75–8.

11. Cartwright PH, Rowell NR. Comparison of Grenz rays versus placebo in the treatment of chronic hand eczema. *Br J Dermatol* 1987;**117**:73–6.

12. King CM, Chalmers RJG. A double-blind study of superficial radiotherapy in chronic palmar eczema. *Br J Dermatol* 1984;**111**:451–5.

13. Lindelöf B, Wrangsjö K, Lidén S. A double-blind study of Grenz ray therapy in chronic eczema of the hands. *Br J Dermatol* 1987;**117**:77–80.

14. Fairris GM, Mack DP, Rowell NR. Superficial X-ray therapy in the treatment of constitutional eczema of the hands. *Br J Dermatol* 1984;**111**:445–9.

15. Sheehan-Dare RA, Goodfield MJ, Rowell NR. Topical psoralen photochemotherapy (PUVA) and superficial radiotherapy in the treatment of chronic hand eczema. *Br J Dermatol* 1989;**121**:65–9.

16. Fairris GM, Jones DH, Mack DP, Rowell NR. Conventional superficial X-ray versus Grenz ray therapy in the treatment of constitutional eczema of the hands. *Br J Dermatol* 1985;**112**:339–41.

17. Aertgeerts P, Albring M, Klaschka F *et al.* Vergleichende Prüfung von Kamillosan Creme gegenüber steroidalen (0·25% Hydrocortisone, 0·75% Fluocortinbutylester) und nichtsteroidalene (5% Bufexamac) Externa in der Erhaltungstherapie von Ekzemerkrankungen. *Z Hautkr* 1985;**60**:270–7.

18. Fowler JF. A skin moisturizing cream containing quaternium-18-bentonite effectively improves chronic hand eczema. *J Cutan Med Surg* 2001;**5**:201–5.

19. Fowler JF. Efficacy of a skin-protective foam in the treatment of chronic hand dermatitis. *Am J Contact Dermatol* 2000;**11**:165–9.

20. Fredriksson T, Gip L. Urea creams in the treatment of dry skin and hand dermatitis. *Int J Dermatol* 1975;**14**:442–4.

21. Anonymous. Carbamide in hyperkeratosis. *Practitioner* 1973;**210**:294–296.

22. Grattan CEH, Carmichael AJ, Shuttleworth GJ, Foulds IS. Comparison of topical PUVA with UVA for chronic vesicular hand eczema. *Acta Derm Venereol* (Stockh) 1991;**71**:118–22.

23. Sjövall P, Christensen OB. Treatment of chronic hand eczema with UV-B Handylux in the clinic and at home. *Contact Dermatitis* 1994;**31**:5–8.

24. Shephard SE, Schregenberger N, Dummer R, Panizzon RG. Comparison of 8-MOP aqueous bath and 8-MOP ethanolic lotion (Meladinine) in local PUVA therapy. *Dermatology* 1998;**197**:25–30.

25. Hogen Esch AJ, Coenraads PJ. Thuisbehandeling van chronisch recidiverend handeczeem met orale PUVA-therapie. *Nederl Tijdschr Dermatol Venereol* 1998;**8**: 267–8.

26. LeVine MJ, Parrish JA, Fitzpatrick TB. Oral methoxsalen photochemotherapy (PUVA) of dyshidrotic eczema. *Acta Derm Venereol* (Stockh) 1981;**61**:570–1.

27. Morison WL, Parrish JA, Fitzpatrick TB. Oral methoxsalen photochemotherapy of recalcitrant dermatoses of the palms and soles. *Br J Dermatol* 1978;**99**:297–302.

28. Simons JR, Bohnen IJWE, Van der Valk PGM. A left–right comparison of UV-B photochemotherapy in bilateral chronic hand dermatitis after 6 weeks' treatment. *Clin Exp Dermatol* 1997;**22**:7–10.

29. Rosén K, Mobacken H, Swanbeck G. Chronic eczematous dermatitis of the hands: a comparison of PUVA and UVB treatment. *Acta Derm Venereol* (Stockh) 1987;**67**:48–54.

30. Sjövall P, Christensen OB. Local and systemic effect of UVB irradiation in patients with chronic hand eczema. *Acta Derm Venereol* (Stockh) 1987;**67**:538–41 [published erratum appears in *Acta Derm Venereol* (Stockh) 1988;**68**:460].

31. Schmied C, Piletta PA, Saurat JH. Treatment of eczema with a mixture of triamcinolone acetonide and retinoic acid: a double blind study. *Dermatology* 1993;**187**:263–7.

32. Reymann F. Two year's experience with Tigason treatment of pustulosis palmo-plantaris and eczema keratoticum manuum. *Dermatologica* 1982;**164**:209–16.

33. Bollag W, Ott F. Successful treatment of chronic hand eczema with oral 9-*cis*-retinoic acid. *Dermatology* 1999;**199**:308–12.

34. Odia S, Vocks E, Rakoski J, Ring J. Successful treatment of dyshidrotic hand eczema using tap water iontopheresis with pulsed direct current. *Acta Derm Venereol* (Stockh) 1996;**76**:472–4.

35. Wollina U, Uhlemann C, Elstermann D, Köber L, Barta U. Therapie der Hyperhidrosis mittels Leitungswasseriontophorese. Positive Effekte auf Abheilungszeit und Rezidivfreiheit bei Hand-Fuß-Ekzemen. *Hautarzt* 1998;**49**:109–13.

36. Burrows D, Rogers S, Beck M *et al.* Treatment of nickel dermatitis with trientine. *Contact Dermatitis* 1986;**15**:55–7.

37. Kaaber K, Menné T, Veien N, Hougaard P. Treatment of nickel dermatitis with Antabuse; a double blind study. *Contact Dermatitis* 1983;**9**:297–9.

38. Christensen OB, Kristensen M. Treatment with disulfiram in chronic nickel hand dermatitis. *Contact Dermatitis* 1982;**8**:59–63.

39. Kaaber K, Menné T, Tjell JC, Veien N. Antabuse treatment of nickel dermatitis. Chelation – a new principle in the treatment of nickel dermatitis. *Contact Dermatitis* 1979;**5**:221–8.

40. Pigatto PD, Gibelli E, Fumagalli M, Bigardi A, Morelli M, Altomare GF. Disodium cromoglycate versus diet in the treatment and prevention of nickel-positive pompholyx. *Contact Dermatitis* 1990;**22**:27–31.

41. Veien NK, Hattel T, Laurberg G. Low nickel diet: an open, prospective trial. *J Am Acad Dermatol* 1993;**29**:1002–7.

42. Cochrane Skin Group Specialist Register. Protocol #28: Interventions to prevent occupational hand dermatitis. www.nottingham.ac.uk/~muzd.

43. Rycroft T, Menne PJ, Frosch PJ, Lepoittevin J-P, eds. *Textbook of Contact Dermatitis, 3rd ed.* Berlin Heidelberg: Springer, 2001.

44. Schleicher SM, Milstein HJ, Ilowite R, Meyer P. Response of hand dermatitis to a new skin barrier protectant cream. *Cutis* 1998;**61**:233–4.

45. Baack BR, Holguin TA, Holmes HS, Prawer SE, Scheman AJ. Use of a semipermeable glove during treatment of hand dermatitis. *Cutis* 1996;**58**:423–4.

Acknowledgement

The authors wish to thank the European Dermato-Epidemiology Network (EDEN) for help with the assembly of the database of trials and for the evaluation of these trials.

17
Atopic eczema

*Hywel Williams, Kim Thomas, Dominic Smethurst,
Jane Ravenscroft and Carolyn Charman*

Since at least 47 groups of interventions have been tried in atopic eczema, coverage of all therapy-related issues for atopic dermatitis is not possible, even in a chapter of this size. Instead, we have opted to introduce the evidence base for treating atopic eczema by means of three common clinical scenarios:

1. a child with moderately severe atopic eczema
2. a person with clinically infected atopic eczema
3. an adult with severe atopic eczema.

Much of the background work and methodology within the sections has been based (with updates) on the results of the UK National Health Service (NHS) systematic review of atopic eczema treatments which was published at the end of 2000. For a more comprehensive and detailed assessment of important areas, such as disease prevention, not covered in this chapter, readers are recommended to read the relevant sections of this report which is available free in the public domain (http://www.ncchta.org). Subsequent editions of this book and the book website will aim to cover these remaining areas. Given the large amount of data described in this chapter, the references are provided at the end of each therapy section, rather than at the end of the chapter.

Hywel Williams was responsible for writing the background section and the evidence summaries of tacrolimus and pimecrolimus, and for editing the other contributions. Jane Ravenscroft and Kim Thomas conducted the updated searches on Medline and Embase. Kim Thomas wrote the sections on emollients and non-pharmacological treatments, and Jane Ravenscroft wrote the section on infected eczema. Carolyn Charman wrote the section on topical steroids and Dominic Smethurst wrote the section on antihistamines and systemic treatments.

Background
Definition and diagnostic criteria
Atopic eczema is a chronic inflammatory skin condition characterised by an itchy red rash that favours the skin creases such as the folds of the elbows, behind the knees and around the neck. The morphology of the eczema lesions themselves varies in appearance from vesicles to gross lichenification on a background of poorly demarcated redness. Other features such as crusting, scaling, cracking and swelling of the skin can occur.[1] Atopic eczema is associated with other atopic diseases such as hay fever and asthma. People with atopic eczema also have a tendency to dry skin, which makes them vulnerable to the drying effects of soaps.

Atopic eczema typically starts in early life, with about 80% of cases starting before 5 years of age.[2] Although the word "atopic" is used when describing atopic eczema, it should be noted that about 20% of people with otherwise typical atopic eczema are not *atopic* as defined by the presence of positive skin-prick test reactions to common environmental allergens or through blood tests that detect specific circulating IgE antibodies.[3] The word *atopic* in the term atopic eczema is simply an indicator of the frequent association with atopy and the need to separate this clinical phenotype from the other forms of "eczema" such as irritant or allergic contact eczema, which have other causes and distinct patterns. The terms *atopic eczema* and *atopic dermatitis* are synonymous. The term atopic eczema or just "eczema" is frequently used in the UK, whereas atopic dermatitis is used more in the US. Much scientific energy has been wasted in debating which term should be used.

Very often, no definition of atopic eczema is given in clinical studies such as clinical trials. This leaves the reader guessing as to what sort of people were studied. Atopic eczema is a difficult disease to define, as the clinical features are highly variable in morphology, body site and time. There is no specific diagnostic test which encompasses all people with typical eczema that can serve as a reference standard. Diagnosis is, therefore, essentially a clinical one.

At least 10 synonyms for atopic eczema were in common usage in the dermatology literature in the 1970s, and it is doubtful if physicians were all referring to the same disease. A major development in describing the main clinical features of atopic eczema was the Hanifin and Rajka diagnostic criteria (1980).[4] These criteria are frequently cited in clinical trial articles, and they at least provide some degree of confidence that researchers are referring to a similar disease when using these features. It should be borne in mind however that these criteria were developed on the basis of consensus, and their validity and repeatability is unknown in relation to physician's diagnosis.[3] Some of the 30 or so minor features have since been shown not to be associated with atopic eczema, and many of the terms, which

> ## Box 17.1 In order to qualify as a case of atopic eczema, the person must have the following[6]:
>
> An itchy skin condition
> Plus three or more of:
>
> - Past involvement of the skin creases such as bends of elbows or behind the knees
> - Personal or immediate family history of asthma or hay fever
> - Tendency towards a generally dry skin
> - Onset under the age of 2 years
> - Visible flexural dermatitis as defined by a photographic protocol

are poorly defined, probably mean something only to dermatologists. Scientifically developed refinements of the Hanifin and Rajka diagnostic criteria, mainly for epidemiological studies, have been developed by a UK working party, and these criteria have been widely used throughout the world.[5] These are shown in Box 17.1.[6]

It is quite possible that there are distinct subsets of atopic eczema, for example those cases associated with atopy and those who have severe disease with recurrent infections. Until the exact genetic and causative agents are known, it is wiser to consider the clinical disease as one condition. Perhaps sensitivity analyses should be done within clinical trials for those who are thought to represent distinct subsets, for example those who are definitely atopic with raised circulating IgE to allergens, and those with severe disease and associated asthma.[3]

Incidence/prevalence

Atopic eczema is a very common problem. European prevalence studies done in the last decade suggest an overall prevalence of 15–20% in children aged 7–18 years.[7] Standardised questionnaire data from 0.5 million children aged

13–14 years in the International Study of Asthma and Allergies in Childhood (ISAAC) suggest that atopic eczema is not just a problem confined to Western Europe, high prevalence being found in many developing cities undergoing rapid demographic change.[8] There is reasonable evidence to suggest that the prevalence of atopic eczema has increased two to threefold over the last 30 years, although the reasons for this are unclear.[9] No reliable estimates of incidence are available for atopic eczema.

Atopic eczema is more frequent in childhood, especially in the first 5 years of life. One study of 2365 patients in Livingston, Scotland who were examined by a dermatologist for atopic eczema suggested that atopic eczema is relatively rare over 40 years of age, with a 1-year period prevalence of 0·2%.[10] Yet, because there are many more adults than children, they may make up over 38% of all atopic eczema cases in that community. Adults also tend to represent a more persistent and severe subset of cases.

Most cases of childhood eczema in any given community are mild. One recent study found that 84% of 1760 children aged 1–5 years from four urban and semi-urban general practices around Nottingham were mild, as defined globally by the examining physician, with 14% of cases in the moderate category and 2% in the severe category,[11] a severity distribution that was very similar to another recent population survey in Norway.[12]

Morbidity and costs

Atopic eczema usually accounts for the worst disturbance in quality of life when compared with other dermatological diseases. Specific aspects of a child's life affected by atopic eczema are[7]:

- itch and its associated sleep loss (which can also cause considerable family disturbance)
- social stigmatisation from other children and parents

- the need for special clothing and bedding
- avoidance of activities such as swimming
- the need for frequent applications of topical treatments and visits to healthcare professionals.

In financial terms, the cost of atopic eczema is potentially very large. One study of an entire community in Scotland in 1995 estimated that the annual personal costs to patients with atopic eczema was £297 million if extrapolated to the entire UK.[13] The cost to the UK NHS was £125 million and the annual cost to society through lost working days was £43 million, making the total expenditure on atopic eczema £465 million per year. This figure is likely to be an underestimate since the prevalence of atopic eczema is lower in Scotland compared with the rest of the UK. Another study from Australia found that the annual personal financial cost of managing mild, moderate and severe eczema was Aus$330, Aus$818 and Aus$1255 respectively, which was greater than the costs associated with asthma in that study.[14]

Aetiology
Genetics
There is good evidence to suggest that genetic factors are important in predisposition to atopic eczema. Twin studies have shown a much higher concordance for monozygotic (85%) than for dizygotic twins (21%),[15] although no single gene has yet emerged as a consistent marker for atopic eczema. There may be several, and it is possible that the tendency to atopic eczema might be inherited independently from atopy.

Environment
There are several general and specific clues that point strongly to a role of the environment in disease expression.[16] It is difficult to explain the large increase in the prevalence of atopic eczema over the past 30 years in terms of genetics.[9] It has been shown that atopic eczema

is more frequent in wealthy families.[17] It is unclear whether this positive social class gradient reflects exposure to indoor allergens or whether it reflects a whole constellation of other factors associated with social "development". Other studies have shown an inverse association between the prevalence of eczema and family size.[18] This observation led to the "hygiene hypothesis" – that children in larger families were "protected" from expressing atopy because of frequent exposure to infections.[19] Some evidence for this "protective" effect of infections on atopic eczema has been shown in relation to measles infection.[20]

Migrant studies also point strongly to the role of environmental factors in atopic eczema. For example, 14·9% of black Caribbean children living in London develop atopic eczema (according to the UK diagnostic criteria) compared with only 5·6% of similar children living in Kingston, Jamaica.[21]

Further work has suggested that the tendency to atopy may be programmed at birth and could be related to factors such as maternal age.[22] The observation that many cases of atopic eczema improve spontaneously around puberty is also difficult to explain in genetic terms alone.[2] Specific environmental risk factors for expression of eczema are still not fully elucidated. Allergic factors such as exposure to house-dust mite may be important, but non-allergic factors such as exposure to irritants, bacteria and hard water may also be important.[23]

Pathophysiology

There appears to be a failure to switch off the natural predominance of TH2 helper lymphocytes that occurs in infancy, which leads to an abnormal response of chemical messengers called cytokines to a variety of stimuli.[1,24] The underlying mechanism of disease may be abnormalities in cyclic nucleotide regulation of marrow-derived cells or allergenic over stimulation that causes secondary abnormalities. Some studies have suggested a defect in lipid composition and barrier function in people with atopic eczema – a defect which is thought to underlie the tendency to dry skin and possibly the enhanced penetration of environmental allergens and irritants, leading to chronic inflammation.

Prognosis

The majority of children with atopic eczema appear to "grow out" of their disease, at least to the point where the condition becomes a problem no longer in need of medical care. A detailed review of prognostic studies reported elsewhere[2] concluded that most large studies of well-defined and representative cases suggest that about 60% of childhood cases are clear or free of disease symptoms in early adolescence. However, many such apparently clear cases are likely to recur in adulthood, often as hand eczema. The most consistent factors that appear to predict persistent atopic eczema are early onset, severe widespread disease in infancy, concomitant asthma or hay fever, and a family history of atopic eczema.

Aims of treatment

Cure is an unrealistic option for the majority of sufferers, the causes of atopic eczema that are amenable to manipulation being poorly understood, and because the effect of conventional treatment on the long-term natural history of the disease is simply not known. Treatment is thus aimed at relieving troublesome symptoms such as itch and soreness and its associated sleep loss, in order to improve the person's quality of life. Improvement in skin appearance may also be important, as is self-esteem, social confidence and the ability to participate freely in recreational activities such as swimming.

Relevant outcomes

Outcome measures used in trials have been reviewed by Finlay.[25] Most outcome measures have incorporated some measure of itch, as assessed by a doctor at periodic reviews or patient self-completed diaries. Other more sophisticated methods of objectively recording itch have been tried. Finlay drew attention to the profusion of composite scales used in evaluating atopic eczema outcomes. These usually incorporate measures of the extent of atopic eczema and several physical signs such as redness, scratch marks, thickening of the skin, scaling and dryness. Such signs are typically mixed with symptoms of sleep loss and itching, and variable weighting systems are used. It has been shown that measuring surface area involvement in atopic eczema is fraught with difficulty,[26] which is not surprising considering that eczema is, by definition, "poorly defined erythema". Charman *et al.* performed a systematic review of named outcome measure scales for atopic eczema and found that of the 13 named scales in current use, only one (SCORAD) had been fully tested for validity, repeatability and responsiveness.[27] Quality-of-life measures specific to dermatology include the Dermatology Quality of Life Index[28] and SKINDEX.[29] The Children's Dermatology Life Quality Index has been used in atopic eczema trials in children.

Most clinical trials of atopic eczema have been very short (i.e. about 6 weeks), which seems inappropriate in a chronic relapsing condition. Few studies have considered measuring number and duration of disease-free periods. In the absence of such long-term studies it is impossible to say whether modern treatments have increased chronicity at the expense of short-term control.

Methods of search

Searching involved updating the trials located in the *Health Technology Assessment (HTA)*[30] using identical optimally sensitive search strings described in Appendix 1 of that report. Both Medline and Embase were searched using these terms up to the end of January 2001 supplemented by additional searches of Pubmed for more recent articles using drug-specific names and synonyms.

Further reading

The epidemiology of atopic eczema has been described in:

The epidemiology, causes and prevention of atopic eczema. In: Williams HC, ed. *Atopic Dermatitis*. Cambridge: Camridge University Press, 2000.

References

1. Archer CB. The pathophysiology and clinical features of atopic dermatitis. Williams HC, ed. *Atopic Dermatitis*. Cambridge: Cambridge University Press, 2000:25–40.

2. Williams HC, Wüthrich B. The natural history of atopic dermatitis. In: Williams HC, ed. *Atopic Dermatitis*. Cambridge: Cambridge University Press, 2000:41–59.

3. Williams HC. What is atopic dermatitis and how should it be defined in epidemiological studies? Williams HC, ed. *Atopic Dermatitis*. Cambridge: Cambridge University Press, 2000:3–24.

4. Hanifin JM, Rajka G. Diagnostic features of atopic eczema. *Acta Derm Venereol* (Stockh) 1980;**92**:44–7.

5. Williams HC. The future research agenda. In: Williams HC, ed. *Atopic Dermatitis*. Cambridge: Cambridge University Press, 2000:247–61.

6. Williams HC, Forsdyke H, Boodoo G, Hay RJ, Burney PGF. A protocol for recording the sign of visible flexural dermatitis. *Br J Dermatol* 1995;**133**:941–9.

7. Herd RM. The morbidity and cost of atopic dermatitis. Williams HC, ed. *Atopic Dermatitis*. Cambridge: Cambridge University Press, 2000:85–95.

8. Williams HC, Robertson CF, Stewart AW, on behalf of the ISAAC Steering Committee. Worldwide variations in the prevalence of atopic eczema symptoms. *J Allergy Clin Immunol* 1999;**103**:125–38.

9. Williams HC. Is the prevalence of atopic dermatitis increasing? *Clin Exp Dermatol* 1992;**17**:385–91.

10. Herd RM, Tidman MJ, Prescott RJ, Hunter JAA. Prevalence of atopic eczema in the community: the Lothian atopic dermatitis study. *Br J Dermatol* 1996;**135**:18–19.

11. Emerson RM, Williams HC, Allen BR. Severity distribution of atopic dermatitis in the community and its relationship to secondary referral. *Br J Dermatol* 1998;**139**:73–6.

12. Dotterud LK, Kvammen B, Lund E, Falk ES. Prevalence and some clinical aspects of atopic dermatitis in the community of Sør-Varanger. *Acta Derm Venereol* 1995;**75**:50–3.

13. Herd RM, Tidman MJ, Prescott RJ, Hunter JAA. The cost of atopic eczema. *Br J Dermatol* 1996;**135**:20–3.

14. Su JC, Kemp AS, Varigos GA, Nolan TM. Atopic eczema: its impact on the family and financial cost. *Arch Dis Child* 1997;**76**:159–62.

15. Schultz-Larsen F, Holm NV, Henningsen K. Atopic dermatitis. A genetic-epidemiological study in a population-based twin sample. *J Am Acad Dermatol* 1986;**15**:487–94.

16. Williams HC. Atopic eczema – why we should look to the environment. *BMJ* 1995;**311**:1241–2.

17. Williams HC, Strachan DP, Hay RJ. Childhood eczema: disease of the advantaged? *BMJ* 1994;**308**:1132–5.

18. McNally N, Phillips D. Social factors and atopic dermatitis. In: Williams HC, ed. *Atopic Dermatitis*. Cambridge: Cambridge University Press, 2000:139–47.

19. Strachan DP. Hayfever, hygiene, and household size. *BMJ* 1989;**299**.1259–60.

20. Shaheen S. Discovering the causes of atopy. *BMJ* 1997;**314**:987–8.

21. Burrell-Morris C, Williams HC. Atopic dermatitis in migrant populations. In: Williams HC, ed. *Atopic Dermatitis*. Cambridge: Cambridge University Press, 2000:169–82.

22. Olesen AB, Ellingsen AR, Olesen H, Juul S, Thestrup-Pedersen K. Atopic dermatitis and birth factors: historical follow up by record linkage. *BMJ* 1997;**314**:1003–8.

23. Hanifin JM. Atopic eczema. In: Marks RM, ed. *Eczema*. London: Martin Dunitz, 1992:77–101.

24. Hanifin JM, Chan S. Biochemical and immunologic mechanisms in atopic dermatitis: new targets for emerging therapies. *J Am Acad Dermatol* 1999;**41**:72–7.

25. Finlay AY. Measurement of disease activity and outcome in atopic dermatitis. *Br J Dermatol* 1996;**135**:509–15.

26. Charman CR, Venn AJ, Williams HC. Measurement of body surface involvement in atopic eczema: an impossible task? *Br J Dermatol* 1999;**140**:109–11.

27. Charman CR, Williams HC. Outcome measures of disease severity in atopic eczema. *Arch Dermatol* 2000; **136**:763–9.

28. Finlay AY, Khan GK. Dermatology Life Quality Index (DLQI): a simple practical measure for routine clinical use. *Clin Exp Dermatol* 1994;**19**:210–16.

29. Chren MM, Lasek RT, Flocke SA, Zyzanski SJ. Improved discriminative and evaluative capability of a refined version of SKINDEX, a quality-of-life instrument for patients with skin diseases. *Arch Dermatol* 1997;**133**:1433–40.

30. Hoare C, Li Wan Po A, Williams H. Systematic review of treatments for atopic eczema. *Health Technol Assess* 2000;**4**(37) (see also http://www.ncchta.org).

Case scenario 1: A child with atopic eczema of moderate severity

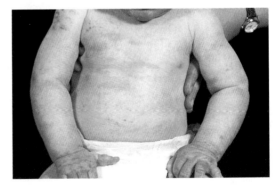

Figure 17.1 A child with flexural atopic eczema

QUESTIONS

What is the role of emollients?

Efficacy

We found no systematic review for emollients in atopic eczema. Five randomised controlled trials (RCTs) are reported here.[1-5] Other studies were excluded because we could not ascertain if they were properly randomised; they included conditions other than atopic eczema (for example Newbold[6]); or they presented only biometric data, the clinical relevance of which was difficult to ascertain (for example Pigatto et al.[7], Hagstromer et al.[8]).

Kantor et al.[1] compared the use of an oil-in-water emollient (Moisturel) versus a water-in-oil emollient (Eucerin) using a left–right comparison design in 50 patients with symmetrical atopic eczema treated for 3 weeks. Test limbs affected by atopic eczema were treated once daily with the emollients and once daily with 2·5% hydrocortisone cream. Global severity showed a statistically significant reduction with both emollients compared with baseline.

The 1998 study by Hanifin et al.[3] compared the effects of adding an emollient called Cetaphil (manufactured by the study sponsor), applied three times daily, to twice-daily application of 0·05% desonide lotion (a topical steroid) versus twice-daily topical desonide alone. Eighty patients with atopic eczema were enrolled for a 3-week period. Outcomes were recorded by an investigator who was blinded to treatment allocation. At the end of 3 weeks the relative reduction in disease severity was 70% for desonide alone, compared with 80% for the desonide/emollient side ($P<0·01$).

The studies by Wilhelm et al.[4] and Andersson et al.[2] both evaluated the benefit of emollients containing urea preparations – a substance intended to improve the water-binding capacity of the outer layer of skin. In the study of Wilhelm et al.,[4] 80 patients were randomised to apply a topical formulation containing 10% urea (manufactured by the study sponsors) versus the vehicle base as "placebo" for 4 weeks in a right–left forearm comparison. Skin redness was improved at 70% of the sites on which 10% urea was applied compared with 30% for the sites where the vehicle was applied.

The study by Andersson et al.[2] compared a "new" cream containing 5% urea as the active substance against an established licensed cream containing 4% urea and 4% sodium chloride. Forty-eight adults with atopic eczema were enrolled in a parallel-group double-blind study. Patients were asked to apply the creams at least once daily for 30 days. Clinical disease severity showed a significant benefit for both creams and there were no statistically significant differences between the preparations.

Larregue and colleagues[5] compared 6% ammonium lactate (another substance designed to improve water-binding capacity of the skin) against its cream base in 46 children aged 6 months to 12 years with atopic dermatitis. The study was a within-person comparison of two symmetrical sites. Lichenification, hyperkeratosis and dryness were reduced in both groups but slightly more so in the ammonium lactate group. This was reported to be statistically significant at day 15 for lichenification and for erythema at day 30 (the final evaluation point of the study). Tolerability, as evaluated by the patients, was very similar in both groups.

Drawbacks

None were reported in the first two studies, with the exception of one patient who experienced a burning sensation when the oil-in-water emollient was applied.[1] In the study by Hanifin et al.,[3] 14% of the patients reported stinging or burning on the side treated with desonide compared with 12% on the side treated with the combination at week 1. Most patients (96% versus 4%) preferred the combination treatment. Transient burning was noticed in four patients treated with urea and in five patients treated with vehicle creams in the study by Wilhelm et al.[4] No adverse effects were described by Andersson et al.[2] Other possible side-effects of emollients include occlusion folliculitis on hair-bearing skin and accidents from slipping whilst climbing into the bath when using emollient bath additives.

Comment

The first two studies were of very short duration, and the quality of reporting was generally poor, with little description of randomisation method, limited blinding and no intention-to-treat (ITT) analysis. The Kantor et al. study[1] failed to show any benefit of one emollient preparation over another (in the presence of a moderate-potency topical steroid), and the Hanifin et al. study[3] suggested that regular use of an emollient with a topical steroid may result in a small increase in treatment response compared with a topical steroid alone. Neither study showed a steroid-sparing effect for emollients.

The first of the two studies on urea preparations[4] showed a possible benefit of a urea-containing preparation compared with vehicle. Comparison of two preparations containing urea in different concentrations failed to show any additional benefit of higher concentrations of urea. Quality of reporting on randomisation, blinding and ITT analysis was poor in both studies. Similar findings were found in the Larregue et al. study.[5]

It is extremely disappointing to see a virtual absence of clinically useful RCT data on the use of emollients in atopic eczema. In addition to measuring efficacy of emollients in treating mild atopic eczema, it is important that future RCTs of emollients measure long-term tolerability, patient preferences and cosmetic acceptability since these are probably key determinants for successful long-term use. There is an urgent need to answer several basic questions, preferably through industry-independent randomised controlled trials. Possible questions that require an answer are as follows.

1. Do emollients have a useful therapeutic effect (with or without wet wraps) for treating minor flares of atopic eczema compared with mild topical steroids?

2. Do emollients have a topical-steroid-sparing effect without loss of efficacy in the long-term management of atopic eczema?

3. Does the regular use of emollients between eczema flares treated by topical steroids help to reduce relapse rates?

4. For children with atopic eczema, do expensive bath emollients provide any additional benefit over application of a cheap emollient directly to the skin after a bath?

5. Does the regular use of emollients reduce the incidence and severity of secondary infection in atopic eczema?

6. Do educational interventions designed to teach the appropriate use of emollients improve the symptoms of atopic eczema?

7. How common is clinically relevant contact sensitisation to emollient constituents such as lanolin?

Implications for clinical practice

There is currently no evidence to doubt the belief that regular emollient use is beneficial for the treatment of atopic eczema. Equally, there is no clear RCT evidence of their benefit. Whether bath additives provide additional benefits to topically applied emollients is particularly unclear.

Key points

- Five RCTs have been summarised. Two examined the possible steroid-sparing effects of emollients, two assessed the benefits of using emollients containing urea and one assessed the benefits of emollients containing ammonium lactate.
- The paucity of good clinical trial evidence does not reflect the importance of emollient therapy for the treatment of atopic eczema and some suggestions for possible future trials have been included.

References

1. Kantor I, Milbauer J, Posner M, Weinstock IM, Simon A, Thormahlen S. Efficacy and safety of emollients as

adjunctive agents in topical corticosteroid therapy for atopic dermatitis. *Today Ther Trends* 1993;**11**:157–66.

2. Andersson AC, Lindberg M, Loden M. The effect of two urea-containing creams on dry, eczematous skin in atopic patients. I. Expert, patient and instrumental evaluation. *J Dermatol Treat* 1999;**10**:165–9.

3. Hanifin JM, Hebert AA, Mays SR *et al.* Effects of a low-potency corticosteroid lotion plus a moisturizing regimen in the treatment of atopic dermatitis. *Curr Ther Res Clin Exp* 1998;**59**:227–33.

4. Wilhelm KP. Scholermann A. Efficacy and tolerability of a topical preparation containing 10% urea in patients with atopic dermatitis. *Aktuelle Dermatol* 1998;**24**:26–30.

5. Larregue M, Devaux J, Audebert C, Gelmetti DR. A double-blind controlled study on the efficacy and tolerability of 6% ammonium lactate cream in children with atopic dermatitis. *Nouv Dermatol* 1996;**15**:720–1.

6. Newbold PC. Comparison of four emollients in the treatment of various skin conditions. *Practitioner* 1980;**224**:205–6.

7. Pigatto PD, Bigardi AS, Cannistraci C, Picardo M. 10% urea cream (Laceran) for atopic dermatitis: a clinical and laboratory evaluation. *J Dermatol Treat* 1996;**7**:171–5.

8. Hagstromer L, Nyren M, Emtestam L. Do urea and sodium chloride together increase the efficacy of moisturisers for atopic dermatitis skin? A comparative, double-blind and randomised study. *Skin Pharmacol Appl Skin Physiol* 2001;**14**:27–33.

Do topical steroids help?

Efficacy
Versus placebo

The effectiveness of topical corticosteroids versus placebo has been demonstrated in one systematic review (search date 1999,13 RCTs)[1] and two further RCTs[2,3] comparing topical steroids with placebo (vehicle) applied for up to 6 weeks in patients with atopic eczema (Table 17.1). Twelve studies found significant improvement with topical steroid compared with placebo.[3–13] Reference 11 includes 2 RCTs – see Table 17.1. The three remaining studies were unable to demonstrate a significant difference between steroid and placebo.[2,14,15] No long-term studies were identified.

Versus each other

One systematic review (40 RCTs) was identified comparing a variety of topical steroids with each other.[1] The review found significant improvements in 13–100% of people after 1–6 weeks of treatment.

Prevention of relapse

One RCT in adults has examined the effectiveness of topical steroids in preventing a relapse of atopic eczema.[16] The study included 54 adults with atopic eczema that had completely healed with a 4-week course of a potent topical steroid (0·005% fluticasone propionate). The study showed that subsequent application of fluticasone propionate 0·005% ointment on two consecutive days a week for 16 weeks was significantly more effective in maintaining an improvement compared with placebo. In a further open uncontrolled study, 90 patients (aged 17–63 years) were treated once daily with mometasone furoate 0·1% cream for 3 weeks. The 78% of patients who had cleared or almost cleared after this time were treated prophylactically with the same preparation twice weekly for 6 months, after which time 90% remained relapse-free.[17]

Application under wet wraps

One RCT (40 children aged 1–15 years) has examined the use of wet-wrap bandaging (wet cotton tubular dressings) applied over diluted topical steroids to improve penetration of topical steroid and control of symptoms.[18] In this study children were treated once daily with either one-tenth strength mometasone furoate 0·005% ointment or one-tenth strength fluticasone

Table 17.1 Topical steroids versus placebo in atopic eczema: results of RCTs[2-15]

Intervention and duration	Number of participants (age in years)	Outcome
Triamcinolone acetonide 0·05% twice daily for 2 weeks[2]	100	Clear or marked improvement: 38% active treatment, 22% controls
Prednicarbate 0·25% ointment twice daily for 4 weeks[3]	51 (18–60)	Excellent, good or fair: 79% active treatment, 37% controls. Significantly reduced pruritus on active treatment
Betamethasone dipropionate 0·05% ointment twice daily for 3 weeks[4]	36 (2–63)	Good or excellent: 94% active treatment, 13% controls
Hydrocortisone valerate 0·2% cream three times daily for 2 weeks[5]	20 (2–75)	Excellent or better: 75% active treatment, 20% controls
Halcinonide 0·1% cream twice daily for 3 weeks[6]	58 (0·8–86)	57% of people achieved a better response with active treatment than control ("better response" not defined)
Halcinonide 0·1% ointment three times daily for 2 weeks[7]	233 (2–67)	Good or excellent: 85% active treatment, 44% controls
Hydrocortisone valerate 0·2% ointment twice daily for 2 weeks[8]	64 (>12)	Disease severity score: 70% reduction with active treatment, 15% with control
Betamethasone dipropionate cream 0·05% twice daily for 4 days[9]	30 (19–57)	Itch-free on days 3–4: 36% active treatment, 22% controls
Desonide cream once daily for 1 week[10]	40 (0·4–15)	Improvement or resolution: 67% active treatment, 16% controls
Fluticasone propionate 0·005% twice daily for 4 weeks[11]	203 (12–82)	Cleared, excellent or good: 80% active treatment, 38% controls
Fluticasone propionate 0.005% twice daily for 4 weeks[11]	169 (12–84)	Cleared, excellent or good: 80% active treatment, 34% controls
Hydrocortisone buteprate 0·1% cream once daily for 2 weeks[12]	194 (17–76)	Excellent or good: 69% active treatment, 26% controls
Clobetasol propionate 0·05% cream twice daily for 4 weeks[13]	81 (>12)	Good, excellent or clear: 82% active, 29% controls
Triamcinolone acetonide 0·5% once daily[14]	40 (2 with atopic dermatitis)	One cleared in actively treated area, the other showed no improvement in either area
Hydrocortisone acetate 1% twice daily for 1 week then emollient only for 1 week versus 2 weeks of emollient only[15]	69 (>16)	Global assessment of parameters showed marked improvement in both groups. Trend towards greater improvement in the steroid group but not statistically significant

propionate 0·005% ointment unoccluded for 2 weeks, and then randomised to receive the same treatment with or without wet-wrap bandaging for a further 2 weeks. Patients treated with wet wraps finished the study with significantly less extensive and less severe disease, and a significant improvement in subjective scores. However, improvement in patients not receiving wet wraps plateaued after week 2 and no statistically significant improvement in disease extent, severity or subjective scores was seen at week 4.

Three further uncontrolled studies have shown improvement in eczema severity with wet wraps over one-tenth strength betamethasone valerate 0·01% cream or various dilutions of fluticasone propionate 0·05% cream, applied for 2–14 days continuously or twice weekly for 3 months.[19–21]

Frequency of application

One systematic review (three RCTs, n = 569) has addressed this issue.[1] The review found no clear evidence to support twice daily over once daily administration of topical corticosteroid, suggesting once daily treatment as a first step in all patients with atopic eczema.

Pulsed or continuous treatment: One RCT (207 children with mild-to-moderate atopic dermatitis, aged 1–15 years) has compared 3-day bursts of a potent topical steroid (betamethasone valerate 0·1% ointment) followed by a 4-day rest period versus continuous use of a mild preparation (hydrocortisone 1% ointment) for 7 days. Participants used the preparations as required over an 18-week trial period. No significant difference in patient symptoms or clinical disease severity was demonstrated between the two treatment groups.[22] Another RCT study of 40 children (published in abstract form) concluded that pulsed clobetasone butyrate 0·05% is more effective than continuous treatment.[23]

Drawbacks

No serious systemic effects or cases of skin atrophy were reported in the short-term RCTs described above. Minor adverse effects such as burning, stinging, irritation, folliculitis, hypertrichosis, contact dermatitis and pigmentary disturbances occurred in less than 10% of patients. No cases of skin atrophy were seen in two longer RCTs (20 and 18 weeks duration) using histological examination and pulsed ultrasound respectively,[16,22] and no serious systemic effects or cases of skin atrophy were reported with regular mild-to-moderate potency topical steroids in a longer cohort study in 14 pre-pubertal children (median treatment 6.5 years).[24] No further RCTs looking at skin atrophy in people with atopic eczema were identified. Enhanced topical steroid absorption and temporary suppression of the hypothalamic–pituitary–adrenal axis have been demonstrated with wet-wrap dressings in uncontrolled studies in patients with severe widespread eczema.[18,20]

Four very small RCTs in healthy volunteers (12 adults) have used ultrasound to evaluate skin thickness after topical steroid application.[25–28] Significant skin thinning occurred after 1 week with twice-daily 0·05% clobetasol 17-propionate and after 3 weeks with twice-daily 0·1% triamcinolone acetate and 0·1% betamethasone 17-valerate. All preparations were used for up to 6 weeks, and skin thinning reversed within 4 weeks of stopping treatment. No significant thinning was reported with twice-daily hydrocortisone prednicarbate or once-daily mometasone furoate after 6 weeks.

Comment

The majority of trials of topical steroids for atopic eczema have been of short duration even though atopic eczema is a chronic relapsing disease in which topical steroids may be required for months or years. Trials have used a wide variety of clinical scoring systems, making it difficult to compare results, and many trials have studied adults only. It is not possible to recommend a "best" topical steroid as most trials have only compared one against another but seldom against the same one and never all together. In the only trial comparing short bursts of potent steroid versus longer duration of mild topical steroids, the majority of patients were recruited from primary care and had mild eczema only. Further trials involving patients with more severe disease are needed to define the most effective method of using topical steroids in the long-term management of the disease and prevention of relapse. The majority of RCTs have not specifically addressed skin atrophy and have been of too short a duration to adequately assess risk with long-term use of topical steroids. The clinical significance of skin thinning as detected by statistically significant changes in total skin thickness when measured by ultrasound is unclear. Only one RCT has addressed the risks of skin atrophy in children,[22] and further trials using a range of topical steroids of different strengths are needed to guide safe prescribing.

Implications for practice

Although topical steroids have been used for the treatment of atopic eczema for over 40 years, surprisingly little work has been done to understand how best to use them for the long-term control of atopic eczema. Most RCTs have compared "me-too" products in studies lasting only a few weeks instead of addressing important questions such as optimum duration of application and whether one should use short bursts of potent steroids followed by milder preparations, or vice versa. The short-term studies have failed to evaluate speed of onset of one type of steroid when compared with another – an important consideration when trying to control the symptoms quickly in the child depicted in the case scenario. Despite widespread concern

about skin thinning with topical steroids, which has arisen from occasional horror stories of people using very potent preparations continuously at sensitive sites such as the face or groin area for inappropriate periods, RCT evidence does not suggest that clinically significant skin thinning is a problem.

In relation to the child portrayed in the case scenario, a possible evidence-based treatment approach could involve the use of a potent topical steroid (for example an inexpensive preparation such as betamethasone valerate once daily) for 2–3 weeks to gain remission, followed by emollient-only "steroid holidays" to allow any skin thinning to recover. Future flares could then be treated with 3-day bursts of the same potent preparation. If this should fail to achieve sufficient overall control in terms of frequency and duration of remission, another approach would be to use the same preparation every weekend on active and previously healed sites.

Key points

- RCTs of topical steroids versus placebo suggest a large treatment effect in atopic eczema.
- It is not possible to make recommendations about the "best" topical steroid as no RCT has compared all available preparations of similar potency.
- There is no clear RCT evidence to support the use of twice daily over once daily topical steroid administration.
- There is no RCT evidence that skin thinning is a problem with correct use of topical steroids, although most RCTs have been of short duration and other non-RCT evidence should be considered before coming to firm conclusions.

References

1. Hoare C, Li Wan Po A, Williams H. Systematic review of treatments of atopic eczema. *Health Technol Assess* 2000;**4**(37).

2. Cato A, Swinehart JM, Griffin EI, Sutton L, Kaplan AS. Azone® enhances clinical effectiveness of an optimized formulation of triamcinolone acetonide in atopic dermatitis. *Int J Dermatol* 2001;**40**:232–6.

3. Lawlor F, Black AK, Greaves M. Prednicarbate 0·25% ointment in the treatment of atopic dermatitis: a vehicle-controlled double-blind study. *J Dermatol Treat* 1995; **6**:233–5.

4. Vanderploeg DE. Betamethasone dipropionate ointment in the treatment of psoriasis and atopic dermatitis: a double-blind study. *South Med J* 1976;**69**:862–3.

5. Roth HL, Brown EP. Hydrocortisone valerate. Double-blind comparison with two other topical steroids. *Cutis* 1978;**21**:695–8.

6. Sudilovsky A, Muir JG, Bocobo FC. A comparison of single and multiple applications of halcinonide cream. *Int J Dermatol* 1981;**20**:609–13.

7. Lupton ES, Abbrecht MM, Brandon ML. Short-term topical corticosteroid therapy (halcinonide ointment) in the management of atopic dermatitis. *Cutis* 1982; **30**:671–5.

8. Sefton J, Loder JS, Kyriakopoulos AA. Clinical evaluation of hydrocortisone valerate 0·2% ointment. *Clin Ther* 1984;**6**:282–93.

9. Wahlgren CF, Hagermark O, Bergstrom R, Hedin B. Evaluation of a new method of assessing pruritus and antipruritic drugs. *Skin Pharmacol* 1988;**1**:3–13.

10. Stalder JF, Fleury M, Sourisse M, Rostin M, Pheline F, Litoux P. Local steroid therapy and bacterial skin flora in atopic dermatitis. *Br J Dermatol* 1994;**131**:536–40.

11. Lebwohl M. Efficacy and safety of fluticasone propionate ointment 0·005% in the treatment of eczema. *Cutis* 1996;**57**(Suppl 2):62–8.

12. Sears HW, Bailer JW, Yeadon A. Efficacy and safety of hydrocortisone buteprate 0·1% cream in patients with atopic dermatitis. *Clin Ther* 1997;**19**:710–19.

13. Maloney JM, Morman MR, Stewart DM, Tharp MD, Brown JJ, Rajagopalan R. Clobetasol propionate emollient 0·05% in the treatment of atopic dermatitis. *Int J Dermatol* 1998;**37**:142–4.

14. Brock W, Cullen SI. Triamcinolone acetonide in flexible collodion for dermatologic therapy. *Arch Dermatol* 1967;**96**:193–4.

15. Gehring W, Gloor M. Treatment of atopic dermatitis with a water-in-oil emulsion with or without the addition of hydrocortisone – results of a controlled double-blind randomized study using clinical evaluation and bioengineering methods. *Zeitschrift Fur Hautkrankheiten* 1996;**71**:554–60.

16. Van der Meer JB, Glazenburg EJ, Mulder PGH *et al.* The management of moderate to severe atopic dermatitis in adults with topical fluticasone propionate. *Br J Dermatol* 1999;**140**:1114–21.

17. Faergemann J, Christensen O, Sjövall P *et al.* An open study of efficacy and safety of long-term treatment with mometasone furoate fatty cream in the treatment of adult patients with atopic dermatitis. *J Eur Acad Dermatol Venereol* 2000;**14**:393–6.

18. Pei AYS, Chan HHL, Ho KM. The effectiveness of wet wrap dressings using 0·1% mometasone furoate and 0·005% fluticasone propionate ointments in the treatment of moderate to severe atopic dermatitis in children. *Pediatr Dermatol* 2001;**18**:343–8.

19. Goodyear HM, Spowart K, Harper JI. "Wet wrap" dressings for the treatment of atopic eczema in children. *Br J Dermatol* 1991;**125**:604.

20. Mallon E, Powell S, Bridgman A. "Wet-wrap" dressings for the treatment of atopic eczema in the community. *J Dermatol Treat* 1994;**5**:97–8.

21. Wolkerstorfer A, Visser RL, De Waard FB *et al.* Efficacy and safety of wet-wrap dressings in children with severe atopic dermatitis: influence of corticosteroid dilution. *Br J Dermatol* 2000;**143**:999–1004.

22. Thomas K, Williams HC, Avery A *et al.* Topical steroids in mild to moderate eczema – short bursts of strong preparations or continuous use of mild ones. *BMJ* 2002; **324**:768–75.

23. Smitt S, Spuls Ph, Van Leent EJM *et al.* Randomized double blind comparison of continuous versus pulsed topical treatment with clobetasone butyrate in 40 children with atopic dermatitis. In: *Proceedings of the International Symposium on Atopic Dermatitis*. National Eczema Association: Portland, Oregon, 2001:24.

24. Patel L, Clayton PE, Addison GM, Price DA, David TJ. Adrenal function following topical steroid treatment in children with atopic dermatitis. *Br J Dermatol* 1995; **132**:950–5.

25. Kerscher MJ, Hart H, Korting HC *et al.* In vivo assessment of the atrophogenic potency of mometasone furoate, a newly developed chlorinated potent topical

glucocorticoid as compared to other topical glucocorticoids old and new. *Int J Clin Pharmacol Ther* 1995;**33**:187–9.

26. Kerscher MJ, Korting HC. Comparative atrophogenicity potential of medium and highly potent topical glucocorticoids in cream and ointment according to ultrasound analysis. *Skin Pharmacol* 1992;**5**:77–80.

27. Korting HC, Vieluf D, Kerscher M. 0·25% Prednicarbate cream and the corresponding vehicle induce less skin atrophy than 0·1% betamethasone-17-valerate cream and 0·05% clobetasol-17-propionate cream. *Clin Pharmacol* 1992;**42**:159–61.

28. Kerscher MJ, Korting HC. Topical glucocorticoids of the non-fluorinated double-ester type. *Acta Derm Venereol* 1992;**72**:214–6.

Do oral antihistamines help?

Only oral antihistamine agents are considered here. For the purposes of answering the question we have included studies whose outcome measures were global indices such as quality of life (which may actually be enhanced in the context of a sedative drug used nocturnally, but is normally decreased in conventional studies where daytime sedation is a side-effect). We also considered trials where specific indices such as disease severity scores or itch assessments were assessed irrespective of the systemic side-effect profile. No new trial results were found subsequent to the NHS *HTA* systematic review of 2000.

Efficacy

The HTA systematic review identified 21 RCTs involving oral antihistamines in the treatment of atopic eczema, summarised in Table 17.2.[1–21] Tabulation and systematic analysis of these trials revealed no clear or powerful effect of administering antihistamines to children or adults. Six of the trials used physician-assessed global severity and five used patient-assessed global severity. The most commonly reported outcome was patient-assessed itch.

Comment

The lack of emergent clarity in these trials reflects the way many dermatology studies are powered: low patient numbers in trials intrinsically demand large treatment effects to be statistically significant. It is therefore likely, from an intuitive point of view, that no large effects will be derived from the use of antihistamines, as the everyday experience of dermatologists will already attest. The individual merits of antihistamine treatments cannot be covered by such a review, and in particular, the patient-specificity of drug effects is necessarily lost when considering aggregated cohorts and statistical means, this is not to mention those differences in "utility" that occur for the same drug in differing contexts. The impact of a specific context of drug administration is nowhere better seen than when comparing the sedative and non-sedative antihistamines across daytime and night-time administrations. It is therefore reasonable to expect that some patients may derive benefits from such interventions, irrespective of the lack of demonstrable effect at a group level. Given the likelihood that further work will return only a mild or non-existent effect and that work is therefore unlikely to inform change, it is debatable whether further large trials are required in this area.

Implications for practice

Collectively, RCTs done to date fail to show convincing evidence of a clear benefit for oral antihistamines, regardless of whether sedative or non-sedating treatments are used. An ongoing systematic review of these trials conducted by individuals within the Cochrane Skin Group may reveal more precise conclusions if data from similar studies can be combined. In relation to the child described in the case scenario, we would not recommend the use of oral antihistamines except for very occasional use as a sedative (in which case other sedatives might be just as good) and the aggregated systematic

Table 17.2 Summary of RCTs of oral antihistamines for atopic eczema

Authors	Main reported results	Authors' conclusions	Comment and quality
Berth-Jones et al. 1989[1]	No evidence of any difference between terfenadine and placebo. Mean scores for itch over the last 4 days of treatment (± SEM): 23·95 (± 4·9) for the terfenadine phase and 25.13 (± 5·1) for the placebo phase. No evidence of carry over or period effect when pruritus scores were assessed	There was no benefit from terfenadine	Method and concealment of randomisation unclear, study described as double blind. Four withdrawals for failure to comply, but not clear at which point and in which initial arm. No ITT analysis. Low power to detect carry-over effect in only 20 patients. No data in graphical form. First and last period data not presented separately. Terfenadine double normal dose
Doherty et al. 1989[2]	Acrivastine significantly reduced itching compared with placebo according to the doctor's assessment ($P = 0·021$). Both acrivastine ($P = 0·026$) and terfenadine ($P = 0·037$) improved the patient's condition significantly more than placebo according to the patient's assessment of the degree of benefit obtained. No significant differences were found between the two active treatments	Acrivastine and terfenadine can partially relieve itching in atopic eczema	Method and concealment of randomisation unclear, study described as double blind. VAS data only given for day 7. Five dropouts (4 active, 1 placebo), no ITT analysis. Unclear what was being assessed and what was meant by "careful examination of the skin"
Foulds and MacKie 1981[3]*†	Although there was a significant difference between individual patients for patient-assessed day pruritus ($P<0·001$) and night pruritus ($0·01<P<0·025$), there was no difference between the treatment periods	Adding an H2 antagonist to the H1 antagonist commonly used in young adults with severe chronic atopic eczema is of no significant advantage.	Method and concealment of randomisation unclear, study described as double blind. Only one loss to follow up, no ITT analysis. No actual data given for clinical outcomes; only P values for statistical comparisons
Frosch et al. 1984[4]*†	No significant difference between cimetidine plus chlorpheniramine and placebo plus chlorpheniramine for day- and night-time patient-assessed itch at weeks 2, 3 and 4	The combination of H1 and H2 antagonists is of no benefit in the treatment of atopic eczema.	Randomisation conducted according to a Latin square, study described as double blind. Baseline itch not given so change cannot be calculated. No standard errors given. Missing baseline data. Two dropouts. No ITT analysis
Hamada et al. 1996*[5]	Itching score and scratch marks improved significantly. Physician's "improved" and "markedly improved" 89.3% in antihistamine-plus-steroid group compared with 50% in topical-steroid-only group	The combination of terfenadine ingestion and topical alclometasone application is more effective than betamethasone alone.	Different topical steroids used in each intervention; no oral placebo. No ITT analysis

(Continued)

Table 17.2 (*Continued*)

Authors	Main reported results	Authors' conclusions	Comment and quality
Hannuksela *et al.* 1993[6*†]	Non-significant difference between groups in intensity of patient-assessed pruritus at baseline. All groups improved significantly ($P = 0.005$). Improvement significantly more pronounced for cetirizine 40 mg than placebo	The sedation observed was probably partly responsible for relief of pruritus. The authors suggest that cetirizine has other properties responsible for skin lesion healing	Method and concealment of randomisation unclear. Dropout rate high: 51–20 for side-effects (mainly sedation) and 19 non-compliers (drug group not specified). No ITT analysis. Possible benefit of cetirizine when used at four times normal dose, but at the expense of sedation
Henz *et al.* 1998[7†]	Mean overall % response rates based on physician's global score were 36·4%, 25·0% and 27·3% in the azelastine, cetirizine and placebo groups, respectively. Baseline data and exact numbers of atopic eczema patients in each group were not stated. Mean itching score decreased from 2·2 to 1·4 in the cetirizine group and from 2·2 to 1·2 in both azelastine and placebo groups (estimated from graphs)	Data underline the low efficacy of antihistamines in atopic eczema	Neither drug reduced itching significantly more than placebo. Statistics not given for atopic eczema patients. No description of what constituted a response. Placebo looks very impressive, clearly no difference in atopic eczema patients. High dropout rate of 37. No ITT analysis
Hjorth 1988[8]	Terfenadine reduced severity of itch in approximately 52% of patients, 34% reported no change and 14% reported increased severity of itch. No data given for placebo	Terfenadine is of value in some patients with atopic eczema and a history of contact urticaria	No outcome data given and no information on placebo response. Method and concealment of randomisation unclear, study described as double blind. Unclear if any dropouts or withdrawals. Author now deceased
Ishibashi *et al.* 1989[9] (Japanese translation)	No significant difference in general improvement rating, overall severity rating and general usefulness rating among the three dose groups of azelastine. A significant difference in improvement ratio was found in three dose groups for the signs of itch, papules, erythema and lichenification	No translated data available	No translated data available
Ishibashi *et al.* 1989[10] (Japanese translation)	No difference in final general improvement rating or general usefulness rating between the three dose groups of azelastine. Effectiveness and usefulness in the treatment of atopic eczema was considered similar for the	No translated data available	No translated data available

(*Continued*)

Table 17.2 (*Continued*)

Authors	Main reported results	Authors' conclusions	Comment and quality
	three groups. Overall safety rating was significantly higher in the 4 mg/day group than in the 2 mg/day group. Overall safety rating similar between the 4 mg/day and ketotifen groups and the 2 mg/day and ketotifen groups		
Klein and Galant 1980[11†]	Hydroxyzine group had a daytime percentage improvement of 32·14 ± 4·98 (mean ± SEM) over baseline pruritus for the entire week, which is significantly greater (P<0·001) than the percentage improvement for the cyproheptadine group (6·21 ± 4·90)	Hydroxyzine may be more effective than cyproheptadine for the management of pruritus associated with atopic eczema in children	Unstable data shown on a graph with inflationary percentage scale but no actual data given. Method and concealment of randomisation unclear, study described as double blind. Not clear if any dropouts or withdrawals
Langeland et al. 1994[12]	Significant effect of loratadine versus placebo on patient-assessed pruritus during the day and night, and on severity of rash	Loratadine may be tried as an adjuvant therapy in the management of severe and moderate atopic eczema, in patients complaining of pruritus	Complex design – six consecutive crossovers. Changes in pruritus on VAS all small. No data for period or carryover effects shown. Method and concealment of randomisation unclear, study described as double blind (block randomised)
LaRosa 1994[13]	Patient diary card scores showed a statistically significant decrease in erythema and other cutaneous symptoms such as lichenification in the cetirizine group. Baseline total mean global score reduced from 230 at baseline to 155 after 8 weeks' treatment with cetirizine, and from 205 at baseline to 180 after 8 weeks' treatment with placebo (estimated from graph)	The results of this preliminary study suggest that cetirizine can effectively control pruritus and other cutaneous symptoms in children suffering from atopic eczema, without noticeable side-effects	Method and concealment of randomisation unclear, study described as double blind. Only one dropout (voluntary withdrawal). Higher baseline scores in those on active treatments suggests that regression to means could partly amount for results
Monroe 1992[14]	Daily pruritus score decreased by 57% in the 14 patients treated with loratadine, 38% in the 14 patients treated with hydroxyzine, and 33% in the 13 placebo patients	Loratadine demonstrates a significant antipruritic effect in atopic eczema.	Patients excluded if unresponsive to antihistamines. No baseline values given. Method and concealment of randomisation unclear, study described as double blind. Very short study (1 week)
Patel et al. 1997[15†]	Loratadine reduced patient-perceived severity of overall condition by 20·8% at endpoint. Incidence of somnolence 9% with cetirizine and 3% with loratadine	In the management of symptoms of atopic eczema, loratadine is as effective as	Study excluded non-responders before study started: number not reported. Report suggests ITT but failed to

(*Continued*)

Table 17.2 (*Continued*)

Authors	Main reported results	Authors' conclusions	Comment and quality
		carry it out. Unc ear if either drug is of benefit in absence of placebo group. Method and concealment of randomisation unclear, study described as double blind	
Savin *et al.* 1979[16]	Neither drug altered likelihood of scratching bouts beginning in wakefulness or in any stage of sleep. However, sleep was less broken with both drugs, but particularly trimeprazine, and the reduced time spent in stage-1 sleep accounted for a modest reduction in the overall amount of scratching during the night	Both trimeprazine and trimipramine resulted in less broken sleep, with a lessening of time awake and in stage-1 sleep. These actions, which may be helpful to some patients, were associated with a modest reduction in the number and length of scratching bouts	Unclear if parallel or crossover study. Length of study unclear. Method and concealment of randomisation unclear, study described as double blind. Withdrawals or dropouts not mentioned. Unclear if changes in sleep patterr helped the patient's eczema
Savin *et al.* 1986[17]	No significant difference between limb movement (measured by limb movement meters) on placebo and on active treatment with LN2974. Difference between the mean scores of the VAS assessment of itching cn placebo and on LN2974 were not significant but favoured LN2974	No significant suppression of scratching or itching was demonstrated	No actual data given. Method and concealment of randomisation unclear, study described as double blind. Unclear if any withdrawals or dropouts
Simons *et al.* 1984[18]	Scores for atopic eczema severity and distribution were significantly reduced at the end of treatment for both doses of hydroxyzine ($P \le 0.05$)	Hydroxyzine 0·7 mg/kg three times daily was as effective as hydroxyzine 1·4 mg/kg three times daily in relieving pruritus and promoting resolution of skin lesions	This trial was buried in the middle of a case series. Only presented mean score at end of treatment rather than mean change in score. Itch data and baseline scores not given. Sample size unclear. Point of randomisation was after the single-cose study. Method and concealment of randomisation unclear, study described as double blind. Unclear if any withdrawals or dropouts. Far too small a study to establish equivalence effects
Simons and Estelle 1999[19]	During the 18-month long study, or ly 48 children treated with cetirizine and 51 treated with placebo dropped out	The safety of cetirizine has been confirmed in this	Well reported study. Good description of randomisation and blinding. Ninety-nine dropouts. No ITT analysis

(Continued)

Table 17.2 (*Continued*)

Authors	Main reported results	Authors' conclusions	Comment and quality
	"for any reason" ($P = 0.737$), only 11 and 15 children, respectively, dropped because of symptoms or events ($P = 0.421$). Serious events were reported in 37 children (9.3%) receiving cetirizine and in 54 children (13.6%) receiving placebo. Hospitalisations were reported in 36 children receiving cetirizine and 47 receiving placebo ($P = 0.189$). Fatigue and insomnia were slightly raised in the cetirizine group. There was no difference in somnolence between cetirizine and placebo. No efficacy data were given	prospective study, the largest and longest randomised, double blind, placebo-controlled safety investigation of any H1 antagonist ever conducted in children and the longest prospective safety study of any H1-antagonist conducted in any age group	Efficacy outcome data eagerly awaited.
Wahlgren *et al.* 1990[20]	No significant changes in difference in itch intensity between the three treatment periods were detected with Pain-Track, and there was no difference in time awake without pruritus. No significant changes in itch magnitude appeared during each period (days 0–3)	The antipruritus effect of 3 days' treatment with terfenadine (non-sedative) and clemastine (sedative) did not differ from that found with placebo	Very short trial (3 days). Method and concealment of randomisation unclear, study described as double blind. No withdrawals or dropouts. Underpowered
Zuluaga de Cadena *et al.* 1989[21] (Colombia, translated)	At the end of the 4-week evaluation period, 8 out of 15 patients on terfenadine compared with 8 out of 17 patients on astemizole and 6 out of 8 patients on hydroxyzine had improvement in itch. Global improvement was noticed in 14 out of 15, 15 out of 17 and 7 out 8 cases, respectively. Improvements in other outcome measures were similar in groups. Other laboratory measures were also recorded	Antihistamines may be beneficial in atopic eczema, with astemizole conferring a prolonged benefit	Outcome measures and their combinations quite complex. Method and concealment of randomisation unclear. Study described as single (investigative) blind. No ITT analysis. Small numbers and no placebo group

*used physician-assessed global severity

†used patient-assessed global severity

ITT, intention to treat; VAS, visual analogue scale

review is unlikely to be specific enough to inform this particular process.

Key points

- Oral antihistamines have been extensively studied.
- Scholarly approaches to this treatment modality have resulted in few assertions.
- Antihistamines are not demographically effective and classical interpretations of RCTs have discouraged their use.
- The individuality of effect of an antihistamine on any one person or given situation is variable enough to allow us to ignore pooled studies and to go on to recommend antihistamines in those contexts, or for those patients, where a potential benefit is obvious or already noted by either the patient, physician or carer.

References

1. Berth-Jones J, Graham-Brown RA. Failure of terfenadine in relieving the pruritus of atopic dermatitis [see comments]. Br J Dermatol 1989;121:635–7.

2. Doherty V, Sylvester DG, Kennedy CT, Harvey SG, Calthrop JG, Gibson JR. Treatment of itching in atopic eczema with antihistamines with a low sedative profile. BMJ 1989;298:96.

3. Foulds IS, MacKie RM. A double-blind trial of the h2 receptor antagonist cimetidine, and the h1 receptor antagonist promethazine hydrochloride in the treatment of atopic dermatitis. Clin Allergy 1981;11:319–23.

4. Frosch PJ, Schwanitz HJ, Macher E. A double blind trial of h1 and h2 receptor antagonists in the treatment of atopic dermatitis. Arch Dermatol Res 1984;276:36–40.

5. Hamada T, Ishii M, Nakagawa K et al. Evaluation of the clinical effect of terfenadine in patients with atopic dermatitis. A comparison of strong corticosteroid therapy to mild topical corticosteroid combined with terfenadine administration therapy. Skin Res 1996;38:97–103.

6. Hannuksela M, Kalimo K, Lammintausta K et al. Dose ranging study: cetirizine in the treatment of atopic dermatitis in adults. Ann Allergy 1993;70:127–33.

7. Henz BM, Metzenauer P, O'Keefe E, Zuberbier T. Differential effects of new-generation h1-receptor antagonists in pruritic dermatoses. Allergy 1998;53:180–3.

8. Hjorth N. Terfenadine in the treatment of chronic idiopathic urticaria and atopic dermatitis. Cutis 1988;42:29–30.

9. Ishibashi Y, Ueda H, Niimura M et al. Clinical evaluation of E-0659 in atopic dermatitis in infants and children. Dose-finding multicenter study by the double-blind method. Skin Res 1989;31:458–71.

10. Ishibashi Y, Tamaki K, Yoshida H et al. Clinical evaluation of E-0659 on atopic dermatitis. Multicenter double-blind study in comparison with ketotifen. Rinsho Hyoka (Clinical Evaluation) 1989;17:77–115.

11. Klein GL, Galant SP. A comparison of the antipruritic efficacy of hydroxyzine and cyproheptadine in children with atopic dermatitis. Ann Allergy 1980;44:142–5.

12. Langeland T, Fagertun HE, Larsen S. Therapeutic effect of loratadine on pruritus in patients with atopic dermatitis. A multi-crossover-designed study. Allergy 1994;49:22–6.

13. La Rosa M, Ranno C, Musarra I, Guglielmo F, Corrias A, Bellanti JA. Double-blind study of cetirizine in atopic eczema in children. Ann Allergy 1994;73:117–22.

14. Monroe EW. Relative efficacy and safety of loratadine, hydroxyzine, and placebo in chronic idiopathic urticaria and atopic dermatitis. Clin Ther 1992;14:17–21.

15. Patel P, Gratton D, Eckstein G et al. A double-blind study of loratadine and cetirizine in atopic dermatitis. J Dermatol Treat 1997;8:249–53.

16. Savin JA, Paterson WD, Adam K, Oswald I. Effects of trimeprazine and trimipramine on nocturnal scratching in patients with atopic eczema. Arch Dermatol 1979;115:313–15.

17. Savin JA, Dow R, Harlow BJ, Massey H, Yee KF. The effect of new non-sedative h1-receptor antagonist (In 2974) on the itching and scratching of patients with ectopic eczema. Clin Exp Dermatol 1986;11:600–2.

18. Simons R, Estelle F, Simons KJ, Becker AB, Haydey RP. Pharmacokinetics and antipruritic effects of hydroxyzine in children with atopic dermatitis. J Pediatr 1984;104:123–7.

19. Simons R, Estelle F. Prospective long term safety evaluation of the H1-receptor antagonist cetirizine in very young children with atopic dermatitis. J Allergy Clin Immunol 1999;104(2 pt 1):433–40.

20. Wahlgren CF, Hagermark O, Bergstrom R. The antipruritic effect of a sedative and a non-sedative antihistamine in atopic dermatitis. *Br J Dermatol* 1990;**122**:545–51.

21. Zuluaga de Cadena A, Ochoa de V A, Donado JH, Mejia JI, Chamah HM, Montoya de Restrepo F. Estudio comparativo del efecto de la hidroxicina la terfenadina y el astemizol en ninos con dermatitis atopica: Hospital General de Medellin-Centro de Especialistas C.E.S. 1986–1988 / Comparative study of the effect of the hidroxicina the terfenadina and the astemizol in children with atopic dermatitis: Hospital General de Medellin-Centro de Especialistas C.E.S. 1986–1988. *CES Med* 1989;**3**:7–13.

What about topical tacrolimus?

Tacrolimus is a powerful immunosuppresant drug used to prevent the rejection of organ transplants. Chemically, it is a macrolide lactone isolated from the bacterium *Streptomyces tsukabaensis*. A topical form of tacrolimus (FK506) has been developed to treat atopic eczema. It is thought to act in atopic eczema by inhibiting phosphatase activity of calcineurin and thereby the dephosphorylation of the nuclear factor for activated T-cell protein, which is necessary for the expression of inflammatory cytokines. Downregulation of the high-affinity IgE receptor on Langerhans cells and inhibition of release of inflammatory mediators from mast cells and basophils may also partly explain the effect of tacrolimus in atopic eczema.[1,2]

Efficacy

One systematic review published in 2000[3] was found, which described four RCTs (three in adults[4,5] and one in children[6]). Since then, a further three RCTs have been published in full.[7–9] All seven RCTs are described in detail in Table 17.3. We also discovered another RCT published in Japanese in 1997[10] (not listed on Medline or Pubmed) which was identified when searching citations of one of the most recently published RCTs.[9] This has been kindly translated by a Japanese colleague (Dr Yukihiro Ohya) who also came across another RCT published in Japanese[11] and also not listed on Medline or Pubmed. We suspect that there are other unpublished or published RCTs that are concealed in less accessible journals, in addition to ongoing studies sponsored by the manufacturer.

Table 17.3 shows that topical tacrolimus is clearly more effective than vehicle alone. There appear to be slight gains in efficacy for 0·1% compared with 0·03% topical tacrolimus preparations. About a third of study participants with moderate-to-severe atopic eczema achieve excellent results, defined as at least 90% improvement in physicians' global assessment.

When tested against a very mild topical steroid (hydrocortisone 1% ointment) in a short-term study, both 0·1% and 0·03% concentrations of tacrolimus ointment were more effective than 1% hydrocortisone.[8] These finding were similar to that of an early study which tested 0·1% tacrolimus against aclometasone dipropionate for atopic eczema of the head and neck.[11] When tested against hydrocortisone butyrate (potent), efficacy of the topical steroid and 0·1% tacrolimus was similar, and both were significantly better (statistically and clinically) than the 0·03% tacrolimus group.[9] Similar equivalence between 0·1% tacrolimus and a standard potent topical steroid (betamethasone valerate) was found in an earlier study published in Japanese only.[10]

All the studies were sponsored by the manufacturer, and none was specifically conducted on people in whom topical steroids had failed.

Table 17.3 Chronological summary of nine randomised controlled trials identified up to April 2002 comparing various strengths of topical tacrolimus to vehicle or various topical corticosteroids

Authors, date (country)	Interventions, comparator (co-treatments)	Study participants	Trial design and follow up	Outcome measures	Main reported results	Quality of reporting	Comment
FK506 Study group 1997 (Japan)[11]	Twice-daily tacrolimus 0·1% ointment v 0·1% aclometasone dipropionate	Multicentre Japanese study of 151 people (tacrolimus: n = 75; aclometasone: n = 76) over 15 years of age with moderate-to-severe atopic dermatitis of face and neck	Two parallel groups evaluated for 1 week	Improvement in physician-assessed global improvement (6 categories) for head and neck dermatitis. Safety in physician-assessed adverse events and patient-assessed irritation	86.3% v 35.7% were reported as showing "remarkable improvement" according to the physician in the tacrolimus group and aclometasone groups respectively ($P<0.001$); irritation reported in 80% of tacrolimus group vs of the 6.6% aclometasone group ($P<0.001$)	Good concealment of allocation and ITT analysis. Method of randomisation generation unclear. Good description of dropouts and adverse events. High frequency of irritation in tacrolimus group suggested that blinding was not successful	A manufacturer sponsored short-term study which shows that a 1-week blast of tacrolimus is more effective than 0·1% aclometasone dipropionate in moderate to severe atopic dermatitis of the face and neck, albeit at the cost of topical irritation. Used non-validated scales. Some concerns regarding increased acne in tacrolimus groups (3 in FK506 group versus 1 in AP group)
FK506 Study group 1997 (Japan)[10]	Twice-daily tacrolimus 0·1% ointment vs 0·12% betamethasone valerate	Multicentre Japanese study of 181 people (tacrolimus: n = 89; betamethasone: n = 92) over 15 years of age, with moderate-to-severe atopic dermatitis of	Two parallel groups evaluated for 3 weeks; trunk and limbs only	Improvement in physician-assessed global rating (six categories); Safety in physician-assessed adverse events and patient-assessed irritation	Moderate or greater improvement as judged by the investigator seen in 93.6% of the tacrolimus group and 90.5% in the betamethasone group; test of equality verified as being within 10%;	Good concealment of allocation and ITT analysis Method of randomisation generation unclear. Good description of dropouts and adverse events.	A manufacturer sponsored short-term study which shows that a 3-week blast of tacrolimus is as effective a 0·12% betamethasone valerate in moderate to severe atopic dermatitis affecting the

(Continued)

Table 17.3 (Continued)

Authors, date (country)	Interventions, comparator (co-treatments)	Study participants	Trial design and follow up	Outcome measures	Main reported results	Quality of reporting	Comment
		the trunk and extremities			Irritation occurred 59·1% of tacrolimus group and 8·9% of betamethasone groups (P<0·001).		trunk and limbs. Used non-validated scales
Ruzicka et al. 1997 (Germany)[5]	Twice-daily tacrolimus ointment 0·03%, 0·1% and 0·3% v vehicle alone (emollients and bath oils only)	Multicentre European study of 215 people aged 13–60 years with moderate-to-severe atopic dermatitis	Parallel study of 4 groups evaluated for 3 weeks	Overall disease score based on 6 signs and 2 symptoms and improvement in an area selected at baseline; investigator and patient global measures	For trunk and limbs, median % decrease in composite severity score 66·7%, 83·3%, 75·0% and 22·5% in the 0·03%, 0·1%, 0·3% tacrolimus and vehicle groups, respectively; differences between active and placebo significant (P<0·001) but not between the tacrolimus concentrations	Method of randomisation and subsequent concealment unclear. No participant flow diagram. Blinding suspect given that many in the tacrolimus group noticed a burning sensation. ITT analysis done.	Short-term study sponsored by manufacturers showing clear effect of tacrolimus compared with vehicle. Patient's assessment data not shown. Used a non-validated and complex measurement scale.
Boguniewicz et al. 1998 (USA)[6]	Twice-daily tacrolimus ointment 0·03%, 0·1% and 0·3% v vehicle alone (emollients only)	Multicentre US study of 180 children aged 7–16 years, with moderate-to-severe atopic dermatitis	Parallel study of 4 groups of up to 22 days' treatment followed up for 2 weeks	Primary: physician global score Others: modified EASI, head and neck score, patients' global and duration of remission	Primary outcome: 69%, 67%, 70% and 38% improved in the 0·03%, 0·1%, 0·3% tacrolimus and vehicle groups, respectively; other	Excellent description of randomisation and subsequent concealment. Clear flow diagram of participants.	Very well reported short-term study which shows that a 3-week blast of tacrolimus is more effective than vehicle only in moderate-to-severe atopic

(Continued)

Table 17.3 (*Continued*)

Authors, date (country)	Interventions, comparator (co-treatments)	Study participants	Trial design and follow up	Outcome measures	Main reported results	Quality of reporting	Comment
					outcomes similar	All those receiving at least 3 days treatment were analysed – not quite the same as ITT	dermatitis in children. Used a variety of non-validated new and composite scales. Interestingly, 52% of patients in the vehicle-only group felt "much better" at study end
Paller et al. 2001 (US)[7]	Twice-daily tacrolimus ointment 0·03% and 0·1% v vehicle only (emollients)	Three US centres; 351 children aged 2–15 years with moderate-to-severe atopic dermatitis	Parallel study of 3 groups of 12 weeks duration; tacrolimus applied until lesions cleared plus 1 week after clearing	Primary: % of patients achieving at least "excellent" improvement compared with baseline according to global physicians' assessment on a 7-category scale Others: extent, EASI, and patients' assessments	35·9%, 40·7% and 6·9% of children in the 0·03%, 0·1% and vehicle groups respectively, achieved investigator-rated excellent improvement (differences between active and vehicle statistically significant); other outcomes consistent	Unclear method of randomisation generation and subsequent concealment. ITT analysis and good description of dropouts and adverse events	Topical tacrolimus clearly more effective than vehicle when given in a prolonged blast of up to 12 weeks. No clinically important difference between the two concentrations. Patient-assessment data not shown. Safety data on systematic absorption quite reassuring. Some concerns regarding increased incidence of herpes simplex in tacrolimus groups

(*Continued*)

Table 17.3 (*Continued*)

Authors, date (country)	Interventions, comparator (co-treatments)	Study participants	Trial design and follow up	Outcome measures	Main reported results	Quality of reporting	Comment
Hanifin et al. 2001 (US)[4]	Twice-daily tacrolimus ointment 0·03% and 0·1% v vehicle only (emollients)	Two RCTs from 41 US centres; 633 adults aged 15–79 years; moderate-to-severe atopic dermatitis; quarter African–American. n = 304 for ths study (Study 1)	Parallel-group study of 12 weeks duration; tacrolimus applied until lesions cleared plus 1 week after clearing	Primary: % of patients achieving excellent or clear skin defined as at least 90% improvement in the physician-assessed global rating. Others: EASI, surface area involved, individual signs and patient-assessed itching	Of the 304 persons analysed in Study 1, 7·8%, 29·1% and 35·4% in the vehicle, 0·03% and 0·1% tacrolimus groups respectively achieved at least 90% improvement; secondary outcomes consistent. When both studies combined, 0·1% tacrolimus was slightly more effective than 0·03% (37% versus 28% "success", P = 0·04), especially in those with severe disease, extensive disease and African–Americans (post hoc).	Method of generating and subsequent concealment of the randomisation sequence unclear. Described as "double-blind" but success of blinding and its execution not described. No ITT, although 632/633 randomised received at least one application of study drug and were analysed.	Unclear why two identical RCTs were done separately then combined, with only some results published separately. Published in an industry-sponsored supplement. Given that this was a dose-finding study, this may have increased the power of showing a significant difference between 0·1% and 0·3% tacrolimus. Clear benefits of both concentrations of tacrolimus when compared with vehicle, but even so, treatment "failed" in about 70% according to the stringent primary outcome measures
Hanifin et al. 2001 (US)[4]	Twice-daily tacrolimus ointment 0·03% and 0·1% v vehicle only (emollients)	Same US multicentre study as above; n = 328 in this study (Study 2)	Parallel-group dose-finding study of 12 weeks' duration; tacrolimus applied	Primary: % patients achieving excellent or clear skin defined as at least 90% improvement in the	5·5%, 25·9% and 38·2% in the vehicle, 0·03% and 0·1% tacrolimus groups, respectively achieved at least 90%	Same concerns as above regarding lack of reporting of randomisation generation and	Same as above. Added benefit of continuing with treatment for 1 week after lesion clearance difficult to evaluate in both of these

(*Continued*)

Table 17.3 (*Continued*)

Authors, date (country)	Interventions, comparator (co-treatments)	Study participants	Trial design and follow up	Outcome measures	Main reported results	Quality of reporting	Comment
			twice daily until lesions cleared plus 1 week after clearing	physician-assessed global rating. Others: EASI, surface area involved, individual signs and patient-assessed itching	improvement; other secondary outcomes consistent, but these were not given for each study separately.	concealment, blinding and ITT analysis.	studies. Safety results were reported in an adjoining article in the same industry-sponsored supplement.
Reitamo et al. 2002[8] (Europe and Canada)	Twice-daily 0·03% and 0·1% tacrolimus ointment v 1% hydrocortisone ointment (emollients and bath oils)	560 children aged 2–15 years with moderate to severe atopic dermatitis recruited from 27 centres in 6 European countries and Canada. Children had to have at least 5% but less that 60% body surface area involvement	Parallel group study of 3 weeks duration; preparations applied for 1 week after clearing	Primary: sensitive area-under-the-curve method assessing improvement in a composite score (mEASI) over the entire 3-week period. Other: outcomes included physician-global rating, adverse events and laboratory markers	Both tacrolimus concentrations were superior to 1% hydrocortisone – with mEASI area-under-the-curve change as a % of baseline of 64·0%, 44·8% and 39·8% for the 1% hydrocortisone, 0·03% and 0·1% tacrolimus groups respectively (lower scores signify greater benefit). Similar trends seen for those with head and neck eczema and for children aged 2–6 years v 7–15	Very well reported study in terms of randomisation generation, concealment, ITT analysis and balanced style of writing. Some doubt regarding success of blinding given that more children in the tacrolimus group experienced transient burning and itching	Although topical tacrolimus is clearly superior to 1% hydrocortisone in this industry study, this is hardly a fair comparison given that it is very weak steroid preparation. It is surprising that ethical permission was granted for allocating children with severe disease to 1% hydrocortisone for 3 weeks. Trial was of very short duration making it difficult to assess long-term control. Validity of modifying the EASI scale not established, and

(*Continued*)

Table 17.3 (*Continued*)

Authors, date (country)	Interventions, comparator (co-treatments)	Study participants	Trial design and follow up	Outcome measures	Main reported results	Quality of reporting	Comment
					years (data not shown). Hydrocortisone effects seem to plateau at 1 week. For physicians' global assessment, 15·7%, 35·8% and 48·4% of children in the 1% hydrocortisone, 0·03% and 0·1% tacrolimus groups, respectively had at least 90% improvement. Skin burning and itching more common in tacrolimus groups		difficult to understand the magnitude of changes in relation to clinical practice
Reitamo et al. 2002[3] (Europe) (virtually same study team as above minus Canadian collaborators)	Twice-daily 0·03% and 0·1% tacrolimus ointment v hydrocortisone butyrate ointment (emollients and bath oils)	570 adults aged 16–70 years with moderate-to-severe atopic dermatitis recruited from 27 centres in 8 European countries. Participants had to have at least 5%	Parallel group study of 3 weeks duration; preparations applied to active lesions for entire 3-week period	Identical to above	Efficacy of hydrocortisone butyrate was very similar to 0·1% tacrolimus; both were superior to 0·03% tacrolimus. The mEASI % change from baseline for area under the curve method was	Well reported study with high follow up rate. Good concealment of allocation, and ITT analysis. Method of randomisation not described. Blinding suspect given that	Virtually identical study to above in terms of design and write-up except that adults were studied and hydrocortisone butyrate (a potent topical steroid) was used as comparator instead of 1% hydrocortisone.

(*Continued*)

Table 17.3 (*Continued*)

Author, date (country)	Interventions, comparator (cotreatments)	Study participants	Trial design and follow up	Outcome measures	Main reported results	Quality of reporting	Comment
		body surface area involvement			36·1%, 36·5% and 47·0%, respectively (lower scores suggest more improvement). Differences were consistent for physicians' global assessment, with 51·4%, 49·2% and 37·6% of participants in the hydrocortisone, 0·1% and 0·03% tacrolimus groups respectively, achieving at least 90% improvement. Skin burning occurred in almost half the tacrolimus group, leading to 8 withdrawals	half in the tacrolimus group experienced burning. The discrepancy between the % experiencing burning in the adults versus children's study above (50% versus 20%) suggests that parents under-reported burning in the children's study.	Hydrocortisone butyrate was found to be equivalent to the strongest preparation of tacrolimus (0·1%) and more effective than the 0·03% preparation

EASI, a composite score of signs plus extent; mEASI is a modification of EASI (based on four signs and extent) with the symptom of itching added in

ITT, intention-to-treat

Drawbacks

The RCTs and various safety studies published to date[12-14] suggest that topical tacrolimus is a safe drug, at least in the short term. Very little of the drug is absorbed systemically. Transient burning at the site of application is a common phenomenon, occurring in about half of adults. Topical irritation increases to 80% for 0·1% tacrolimus when applied to the head and neck area.[11]

Comment

There is little doubt that topical tacrolimus is an effective drug for atopic eczema when compared with vehicle, with some slight gains in efficacy for the stronger 0·1% preparation. The drug appears to be safe in the short term, although it should be borne in mind that tacrolimus is a potent immunosuppressive and more data will be needed on skin infections such as herpes simplex and eczema herpeticum. Longer-term surveillance data will also be needed on subsequent risk of internal malignancies. Given that topical tacrolimus is likely to be applied frequently to facial skin, this being a frequent site for atopic eczema involvement, there is a need to carefully evaluate the risk of excess skin cancer on areas of the skin exposed to the sun.

Topical tacrolimus is a welcome addition to the physician's armamentarium for this troublesome disease. What is less clear for the practising physician is where topical tacrolimus fits in with the other currently available therapies, most notably the topical corticosteroids – an obvious point noted by others.[15]

Topical tacrolimus has been licensed in the US and UK for the treatment of people with moderate-to-severe atopic eczema that is not adequately responsive or who are intolerant of conventional therapies. Rather oddly, however, none of the RCTs has been conducted specifically in people in whom topical steroids have failed. This raises the question of why product licenses were granted for such second-line use, given the lack of relevant evidence to inform such a decision. The percentage of atopic eczema sufferers who are truly "unresponsive" to topical steroids is probably very small (around 10% of *severe* cases seen in secondary care).[16] It is likely, therefore, that the drug will be used in a much wider group of atopic eczema patients as an alternative to topical corticosteroids – a prediction that is likely to be fulfilled given existing widespread and often unjustified public fear of using topical steroids.[16]

The lack of skin thinning with prolonged use of topical tacrolimus is a distinct advantage over topical steroids when the latter have to be used in excessive quantities for sites that are prone to skin thinning, such as the face. Even so, clinically significant skin thinning with intermittent use of topical steroids is exceedingly rare in modern clinical practice. Some case series have suggested good response of facial atopic eczema and atopic blepharitis to topical tacrolimus,[18-20] and these may be two scenarios in which the drug will prove to be particularly useful.

In terms of comparison with topical steroids, the physician is still left with considerable difficulty in deciding when to use topical tacrolimus. The study by Reitamo *et al.*[8] suggested that topical tacrolimus is more effective that 1% hydrocortisone acetate, but this is hardly a fair comparison given that 1% hydrocortisone is very weak and arguably an inappropriate and unethical treatment for people with severe atopic eczema.[8] Three short-term studies have compared 0·1% tacrolimus against potent topical steroids and found it to be equivalent in terms of efficacy.[9-11] It might have been more appropriate to test topical tacrolimus against short bursts of a modern once-daily potent topical steroid such as mometasone or fluticasone over a long period so that the effects of disease chronicity and clinically important skin thinning could be evaluated.

Tacrolimus has not been compared head to head with ascomycin (syn. pimecrolimus), a closely related topical preparation, which is manufactured by another company. This lack of head-to-head comparison seems odd for two such similar drugs competing for the same market. This may be because tacrolimus is aimed at the more severe end of the spectrum in secondary care, with pimecrolimus targeting the much bigger market of primary care.

No data on cost-effectiveness is available, and topical tacrolimus is at least ten times more expensive at present than topical steroids. None of the efficacy studies has been sufficiently long to evaluate effects on disease chronicity.

In view of the above concerns, two key studies are needed:

- a comparison of topical tacrolimus, ascomycin and continued use of topical steroids (with or without bandaging) in people with severe atopic eczema inadequately responsive to topical steroids
- a long-term pragmatic RCT of topical tacrolimus versus topical ascomycin versus standard practice of intermittent use of a potent topical steroid such as fluticasone propionate. Such a study should capture disease chronicity and cost-effectiveness and employ simple categorical patient-derived outcome measures.

None of the studies has been conducted independently of the manufacturers, and it is not clear how many unpublished or ongoing studies exist.

Implications for clinical practice

Given the lack of crucial comparisons surrounding the introduction of topical tacrolimus, physicians and patients are left guessing as to how and when it should be used. The lack of skin thinning effect may point to it being particularly useful when patients with moderate-to-severe disease are "stuck" on their topical steroid preparations and have to use such preparations almost continuously. Topical tacrolimus may be particularly useful for resistant facial atopic eczema, for similar reasons. Physicians should resist using such a preparation as a "steroid alternative" until more relevant RCT and safety data becomes available.

Key points

- It is heartening to see the advent of a new effective topical treatment for people with moderate-to-severe atopic eczema.
- Topical tacrolimus (0·03% and 0·1%) has been shown to be effective when compared with vehicle only in five RCTs.
- Topical tacrolimus has been shown to be superior to a very weak topical corticosteroid (1% hydrocortisone) in children with moderate-to-severe atopic eczema.
- 0·1% topical tacrolimus appears to be equivalent in efficacy to a potent topical steroid (hydrocortisone butyrate), although the 0·03% preparation is inferior to both these preparations.
- 0·1% topical tacrolimus is of similar potency to betamethasone valerate but it is at least ten times more expensive.
- Topical tacrolimus appears to be safe in the short term.
- Transient burning occurs in about half of adults, but is rarely severe enough to warrant stopping the preparation.
- Long-term data are needed on local and systemic infection, and internal and skin cancer rates.
- All of the studies released to date into the public domain have been sponsored by the manufacturer.
- There is a need to test topical tacrolimus as a second-line treatment for atopic eczema in an RCT setting.
- There is a need for a head-to-head comparison of the cost-effectiveness of topical tacrolimus against topical pimecrolimus and intermittent use of potent modern topical steroids.

In relation to the child described in the case scenario, we would use topical tacrolimus only when standard therapy with short bursts of once daily potent topical steroids (or very mild preparations for the face), emollients and educational support had failed.

Acknowledgements

We thank Dr Yukihiro Ohya of the National Children's Hospital, Tokyo, Japan for identifying and translating Japanese studies and Professor Masutaka Furue of Kyushu University, Fukuoka, Japan for data on topical steroid responsiveness.

References

1. Reitamo S. Tacrolimus: a new topical immunomodulatory therapy for atopic dermatitis. *J Allergy Clin Immunol* 2001;**107**:445–8.

2. Nghiem P, Pearson G, Langley RG. Tacrolimus and pimecrolimus: from clever prokaryotes to inhibiting calcineurin and treating atopic dermatitis. *J Am Acad Dermatol* 2002;**46**:228–41.

3. Hoare C, Li Wan Po A, Williams H. Systematic review of treatments for atopic eczema. *Health Technol Assess* 2000;**4**(37).

4. Hanifin JM, Ling MR, Langley R, Breneman D, Rafal E. Tacrolimus ointment for the treatment of atopic dermatitis in adult patients: part I, efficacy. *J Am Acad Dermatol* 2001;**44**:S28–38.

5. Ruzicka T, Bieber T, Schopf E *et al*. A short-term trial of tacrolimus ointment for atopic dermatitis. European Tacrolimus Multicenter Atopic Dermatitis Study Group. *N Engl J Med* 1997;**337**:816–21.

6. Boguniewicz M, Fiedler VC, Raimer S, Lawrence ID, Leung DY, Hanifin J. A randomized, vehicle-controlled trial of tacrolimus ointment for treatment of atopic dermatitis in children. Pediatric Tacrolimus Study Group. *J Allergy Clin Immunol* 1998;**102**:637–44.

7. Paller A, Eichenfield LF, Leung DY, Stewart D, Appell M. A 12-week study of tacrolimus ointment for the treatment of atopic dermatitis in pediatric patients. *J Am Acad Dermatol* 2001;**44**:S47–57.

8. Reitamo S, Van Leent EJM, Ho V *et al*. Efficacy and safety of tacrolimus ointment compared with that of hydrocortisone acetate ointment in children with atopic dermatitis. *J Allergy Clin Immunol* 2002;**109**:539–46.

9. Reitamo S, Rustin M, Ruzicka T *et al*. Efficacy and safety of tacrolimus ointment compared with that of hydrocortisone butyrate ointment in adult patients with atopic dermatitis. *J Allergy Clin Immunol* 2002;**109**:547–55.

10. FK506 Ointment Study Group. Phase III comparative study of FK506 ointment versus betamethasone valerate ointment in atopic dermatitis (trunk/extremities) (in Japanese). *Nishinihon J Derm* 1997;**59**:870–9.

11. FK506 Ointment Study Group. Phase III comparative study of FK506 ointment versus aclometasone dipropionate ointment in atopic dermatitis (face/neck) (in Japanese). *Hihuka Kiyo (Dermatol Bull)* 1997;**92**:277–82.

12. Kang S, Lucky AW, Pariser D, Lawrence I, Hanifin JM. Long-term safety and efficacy of tacrolimus ointment for the treatment of atopic dermatitis in children. *J Am Acad Dermatol* 2001;**44**:S58–64.

13. Soter NA, Fleischer AB Jr, Webster GF, Monroe E, Lawrence I. Tacrolimus ointment for the treatment of atopic dermatitis in adult patients: part II, safety. *J Am Acad Dermatol* 2001;**44**:S39–46.

14. Reitamo S, Wollenberg A, Schopf E *et al*. Safety and efficacy of 1 year of tacrolimus ointment monotherapy in adults with atopic dermatitis. The European Tacrolimus Ointment Study Group. *Arch Dermatol* 2000;**136**:999–1006.

15. Boucher M. Tacrolimus ointment for the treatment of atopic dermatitis. *Issues Emerg Health Technol* 2001;**19**:1–4.

16. Furue M, Terao H, Rikihisa W et al. Clinical dose and adverse effects of topical steroids in daily management of atopic dermatitis. *Br J Dermatol* 2002 (in press).

17. Charman CR, Morris AD, Williams HC. Topical corticosteroid phobia in patients with atopic eczema. *Br J Dermatol* 2000;**142**:931–6.

18. Sugiura H, Uehara M, Hoshino N, Yamaji A. Long-term efficacy of tacrolimus ointment for recalcitrant facial

erythema resistant to topical corticosteroids in adult patients with atopic dermatitis. *Arch Dermatol* 2000;**136**: 1062–3.

19. Kawakami T, Soma Y, Morita E *et al.* Safe and effective treatment of refractory facial lesions in atopic dermatitis using topical tacrolimus following corticosteroid discontinuation. *Dermatology* 2001;**203**:32–7.

20. Mayer K, Reinhard T, Reis A, Bohringer D, Sundmacher R. [FK 506 ointment 0·1 % – A new therapeutic option for atopic blepharitis. Clinical trial with 14 patients]. *Klin Monatsbl Augenheilkd* 2001;**218**:733–6.

How might topical pimecrolimus be used?

Like tacrolimus, pimecrolimus is a macrolide immunosupressive drug. It is currently available in the US and is due to be launched in the EU for the treatment for atopic eczema.[1] The US approved indication for pimecrolimus is for "short-term intermittent long-term therapy in the treatment of *mild-to-moderate* atopic dermatitis in non-immunocompromised patients 2 years of age and older, in whom the use of alternative, conventional therapies is deemed inadvisable because of potential risks, or in the treatment of patients who are not adequately responsive to or are intolerant to conventional therapies".[2] The indications for use in the EU and elsewhere are likely to be similar, although a case is being made to use pimecrolimus for intermittent long-term treatment to prevent progression of flares in patients aged 3 months and older. The primary indication of use is almost identical to that described for topical tacrolimus, the only difference being that pimecrolimus is aimed at mild-to-moderate atopic dermatitis and tacrolimus for moderate-to-severe atopic dermatitis. Given that mild atopic eczema is about ten times more frequent than moderate-to-severe disease,[3] the market could be a lot larger for pimecrolimus.

The mode of action of pimecrolimus is thought to be similar to tacrolimus and ciclosporin in preventing the release of calcineurin-mediated cytokine and pro-inflammatory mediators from mast cells and T cells.[4] Preliminary animal studies published in abstract form have suggested that pimecrolimus has little effect on systemic immune responses.[5]

Efficacy

Only four RCTs have been published in full in three papers at the time of this summary (two trials in adults, n = 34 and n = 260, and two trials in children combined into one, n = 403).[6–8] It is likely that there are many more unpublished and ongoing studies.

In the first study, 34 patients with moderate atopic eczema were randomised within a right–left body comparison study.[6] Topical 1% pimecrolimus (syn. with ascomycin) was applied twice daily (n = 16) or once daily (n = 18) and compared with the corresponding vehicle cream for symmetrical lesions on one or other side of the body. The trial was very short (3 weeks) and all participants were adults. At the end of 21 days, those in the twice-daily pimecrolimus group showed a 71·9% decrease in baseline severity scores compared with 10·3% in the placebo group ($P<0·001$). The magnitude of benefit was less impressive in the once-daily pimecrolimus group, with a 37·7% reduction in the severity index in the active-treatment group, compared with a 6·2% reduction in the vehicle group ($P = 0·002$). None of the patients in the once-daily group (neither active nor placebo) showed total clearance of their lesions. This compared with 3 out of 15 patients showing total clearance in the twice-daily pimecrolimus group.

The large dose-finding RCT[7] enrolled 260 adults who were randomised to 0·05% (n = 42), 0·2% (n = 46), 0·6% (n = 42) or 1% (n = 45) pimecrolimus, matching vehicle cream (n = 43) or betamethasone 17-valerate cream (n = 42) twice daily for 3 weeks.[7] The results were analysed on an ITT basis and 23·5% discontinued from the trial (mainly because of treatment failure in the vehicle and low-strength pimecrolimus groups). Outcomes as assessed by a modified EASI score (a composite scale of the four signs of erythema, papulation/induration, excoriation and lichenification combined with extent, taking into account omission of head and neck) suggested dose-related improvements in all parameters in the 0·2%, 0·6% and 1% pimecrolimus groups but little or no benefit in those using the 0·05% strength. The greatest improvement was seen in the betamethasone group. At 12 weeks, the median percentage changes from baseline were −2·7, −14·8, −17·3, −27·6, −37·9 and −64·1 in the vehicle, 0·05%, 0·2%, 0·6%, 1% pimecrolimus and betamethasone valerate groups, respectively. Pruritus and patient-derived scores were similar, 88·1% of patients in the betamethasone group showed greater than 50% improvement compared with 53·3% in the 1% pimecrolimus group.

The third report[8] evaluated twice-daily 1% pimecrolimus cream versus vehicle cream (randomised 2:1 respectively) for 6 weeks in 403 people aged 1–17 years with predominantly moderate atopic eczema affecting at least 5% of body surface area. This report represented combined data from two almost identical industry-sponsored multicentre studies in the US. At the end of the 6-week treatment period, those in the active group demonstrated clear gains in efficacy when compared with the vehicle group. For the primary outcome measure, 35% of those using 1% pimecrolimus, compared with 18% using vehicle were clear or almost clear according to the investigator, using an ITT analysis ($P = 0·05$). Similar differences in favour of pimecrolimus were shown for other outcome measures such as EASI, and patient-reported itch.

Drawbacks

Data from RCTs do not suggest any serious adverse effects to date. Application reactions of burning, warmth, stinging and soreness have been consistently reported in the RCTs and are dose related. Systemic absorption does occur with pimecrolimus, but this is very small in the majority of people.[9,10] No skin atrophy has been observed in a detailed study comparing topical pimecrolimus with 0·1% betamethasone valerate cream when applied to the forearms of healthy volunteers continuously for 4 weeks.[11] Such a study is difficult to interpret however because potent topical steroids are not used in this way, and the effects of disease on skin thickness cannot be assessed.

As pimecrolimus is an immunosuppresive agent, theoretical long-term risk of cancer needs to be monitored, given that the drug is likely to be prescribed in large quantities to millions of children with mild forms of this common disease. In the Food and Drug Administration letter approving use of pimecrolimus in the US, reference is made to preclinical rodent studies that found an increased risk of lymphomas and follicular cell thyroid cancer in the studies evaluating oral formulations.[2] Reference is also made to preclinical mouse photocarcinogenicity studies showing accelerated rates of skin cancers in such mice. Licensing was granted with requirement for further specific studies to assess such possible long-term risks.[2]

Comment

The quality of reporting of the pimecrolimus studies was generally good. In the third study of pimecrolimus versus vehicle in children, it is unclear why separate but identical multicentre studies were initially set up by the sponsoring company and then combined in a final analysis.[8] The study was reasonably reported, except that the method of randomisation and subsequent concealment and the success of blinding were unclear. It was also unclear whether participants were allowed to use any concomitant treatments such as emollients or rescue therapy for uncontrolled flares (which would have been likely given that 65% "failed" to achieve "success" in the pimecrolimus group).

Topical pimecrolimus has not been compared head to head with topical tacrolimus. However, there is a hint from the second RCT that pimecrolimus is not as effective as potent topical corticosteroids that are of similar strength to tacrolimus.[7,12] This may explain why pimecrolimus has been targeted for mild-to-moderate atopic eczema.

So far, all we are able to say is that 1% pimecrolimus cream is more effective than placebo and that it is much less effective than a potent topical steroid. It appears safe in the RCTs that have been conducted to date, although these are not suitable for excluding long-term rare and more serious risks such as internal and skin malignancies, however unlikely they may seem due to current known mechanisms.

As with tacrolimus, the manufacturers have not performed a long-term study comparing pimecrolimus against typical current best treatment of bursts of potent or even mild topical steroids, and no cost-effectiveness data are available for such head-to-head comparisons. Pimecrolimus has not been evaluated in patients in whom topical corticosteroid have failed, making it difficult to say whether it will be useful as a second-line agent.

As with tacrolimus, it is good to see new and effective topical treatments for atopic eczema that appear to be safe in the short term. What is more difficult for the prescribing physician or patient at the moment is to be clear about the indications for use of the drug in the absence of some key studies. The wording of the indications in the opening paragraph of this section are vague and unhelpful and could include every person with a concern about using topical corticosteroids, however unjustified that may seem.

It is also unclear from the studies whether pimecrolimus should be used continuously or intermittently for flares. The RCTs that have been conducted to date have used treatment regimens that involve applying the cream continuously for several weeks. A recently completed study (published in abstract form only at the time of writing) hints at another way in which the manufacturers may like to see pimecrolimus being used. This was a 6-month study involving 250 infants aged 3–23 months, in whom pimecrolimus was used as soon as the signs of eczema or itching occurred and was compared against a vehicle ointment to see how many flare ups requiring topical corticosteroids could be prevented.[13] Only 32% of those in the control group were free from flare ups compared with 70% of those in the active group. Another similar study of 713 patients aged 2–17 years showed that 51% of those in the pimecrolimus group did not have flare ups requiring potent topical corticosteroids, compared with 28% using emollients only.[14] At face value, both these studies appear convincing until one realises that they are effectively placebo-controlled studies. It could have been the case that early treatment with 1% hydrocortisone ointment would have averted the development of flares equally well. Again, the physician and patient is left guessing how pimecrolimus compares with best standard therapy.

Implications for practice

In relation to the child described in the case scenario, the lack of crucial comparisons makes it impossible for to decide with the child's parents when and how to use topical pimecrolimus. On the basis of the current data, I would only use pimecrolimus in the rare situation of a child with mild-to-moderate atopic eczema who needs to use potent topical steroids almost continuously in order to gain reasonable quality of life, or perhaps in a child whose parents allow their child to suffer terrible symptoms of disease because of an irrational fear of using any form of topical steroids. I might be persuaded to use topical pimecrolimus to prevent flares in childern with brittle disease if early use of 1% hydrocortisone was ineffective.

Key points

- 1% pimecrolimus cream is more effective than vehicle cream in children and adults with mild-to-moderate atopic eczema.
- 1% pimecrolimus does not cause skin thinning.
- 1% pimecrolimus cream is much less effective than topical betamethasone valerate in atopic eczema. It has not been compared against 1% hydrocortisone.
- It is not known how pimecrolimus compares against topical tacrolimus in people with atopic eczema.
- It is not known whether pimecrolimus is effective in people with atopic eczema not well controlled with topical steroids.
- The cost-effectiveness of pimecrolimus versus standard therapy is not known.
- It is not known whether early treatment with topical tacrolimus is any better than early treatment with a weak topical steroid such as 1% hydrocortisone in preventing more severe flares that require potent steroids.
- Independent studies are needed to compare the cost-effectiveness of pimecrolimus versus standard bursts of topical steroids in the short-term control of mild atopic eczema in children and to see whether early use of either treatment approach improves disease control over a longer period.
- Until such crucial comparisons become available, the role of topical pimecrolimus

in the management of atopic eczema will remain unclear.
- Despite these limitations, pimecrolimus is likely to secure a large market for a host of indications because there is so much public fear of using topical steroids.

References

1. Wellington K, Jarvis B. Topical pimecrolimus: a review of its clinical potential in the management of atopic dermatitis. *Drugs* 2002;**62**:817–40.

2. Anon. FDA licensing review of pimecrolimus. www.fda.gov/cder/foi/nda/2001/21-302_Elidel.htm. (accessed 27 Aug, 2002)

3. Emerson RM, Williams HC, Allen BR. Severity distribution of atopic dermatitis in the community and its relationship to secondary referral. *Br J Dermatol* 1998;**139**:73–6.

4. Nghiem P, Pearson G, Langley RG. Tacrolimus and pimecrolimus: from clever prokaryotes to inhibiting calcineurin and treating atopic dermatitis. *J Am Acad Dermatol.* 2002;**46**:228–41.

5. Meingassner JG, Hiestand P, Bigout M *et al.* SDZ ASM 981 is highly effective in animal models of skin inflammation, but has only low activity in models indicating immunosuppresive potential (abstract). *J Invest Dermatol* 2001;**117**:532.

6. Van Leent EJ, Graber M, Thurston M, Wagenaar A, Spuls PI, Bos JD. Effectiveness of the ascomycin macrolactam SDZ ASM 981 in the topical treatment of atopic dermatitis. *Arch Dermatol* 1998;**134**:805–9.

7. Luger T, Van Leent EJ, Graeber M *et al.* SDZ ASM 981: an emerging safe and effective treatment for atopic dermatitis. *Br J Dermatol* 2001;**144**:788–94.

8. Eichenfield LF, Lucky AW, Boguniewicz M *et al.* Safety and efficacy of pimecrolimus (ASM 981) cream 1% in the treatment of mild and moderate atopic dermatitis in children and adolescents. *J Am Acad Dermatol* 2002;**46**:495–504.

9. Van Leent EJ, Ebelin ME, Burtin P, Dorobek B, Spuls PI, Bos JD. Low systemic exposure after repeated topical application of pimecrolimus (Elidel), SDZ ASM 981, in patients with atopic dermatitis. *Dermatology* 2002;**204**:63–8.

10. Robinson N, Singri P, Gordon KB. Safety of the new macrolide immunomodulators. *Semin Cutan Med Surg* 2001;**20**:242–9.

11. Queille-Roussel C, Paul C, Duteil L *et al*. The new topical ascomycin derivative SDZ ASM 981 does not induce skin atrophy when applied to normal skin for 4 weeks: a randomized, double-blind controlled study. *Br J Dermatol* 2001;**144**:507–13.

12. FK506 Ointment Study Group. Phase III comparative study of FK506 ointment versus betamethasone valerate ointment in atopic dermatitis (trunk/extremities) (in Japanese). *Nishinhon J Derm* 1997;**59**:870–9.

13. Abstract presented at the 10th Congress of the European Academy of Dermato-Venereology, Munich 2001.

14. Luger T, Molloy S, Graeber M *et al*. SDZ ASM 981 cream 1%: a new approach to long-term management of atopic dermatitis. Abstract presented at the International Symposium on atopic dermatitis. National Eczema Association: Portland, Oregon, 2001.

Will interventions to reduce house dust mite improve this child's eczema?

Efficacy

This section deals with house dust mite eradication for cases of established atopic eczema. No systematic review was found for house dust mite reduction. Six RCTs[1-6] evaluating the role of house dust mite reduction in the treatment of *established* atopic eczema were identified and are summarised in Table 17.4. In general, the evidence to support the efficacy of house dust mite eradication for the treatment of atopic eczema is of poor quality. Interventions such as vacuuming and the use of synthetic mattress covers appear to be most effective in reducing the house dust mite load, but how this impacts on disease severity is still unclear.

Drawbacks

None of the studies reported any adverse events of the house dust mite removal treatments. This does not necessarily imply that none occurred. The imposition of daily vacuuming for a long period has a cost in terms of time for parents and sufferers, as does the purchase of a high-filtration vacuum cleaner, impermeable mattress covers and mite sprays.

Comment

Given the strong circumstantial evidence to suggest that house dust mite allergens may play a part in atopic eczema, it is a pity that so few studies on house dust mite avoidance have been performed. Those that have been done tend to be small and it is difficult to generalise in the absence of more pragmatic studies. In none of the studies was the method of randomisation and concealment reported, and no ITT analyses were performed (although dropouts were quite low).

Further studies that separate the different interventions for reducing house dust mite are needed. It is important that such trials are as pragmatic as possible to determine which groups respond best, which interventions are the most cost-effective, and whether the laborious interventions are sustainable in less motivated people.

Implications for clinical practice

In the absence of strong clinical trial data to support the use of house dust mite avoidance measures, the decision as to whether the cost and effort of implementing such procedures is warranted probably lies with the individual families.

Key points

- Six randomised, controlled trials have been reported, although methodological difficulties and small sample sizes limit the interpretation of the results.
- Future, large-scale pragmatic trials are needed if this issue is to be resolved.
- In the meantime, the use of allergen-impermeable mattress and pillow covers, coupled with regular vacuuming of the room seem to be the best way of reducing house dust mite if such changes are truly beneficial.

Will an exclusion diet (such as a milk- or egg-free diet) help to reduce the symptoms of this child's atopic eczema?

Table 17.4 RCTs of dust mite reduction for the treatment of established atopic eczema

Study	Intervention	Population and sample size	Design and period of follow up	Main outcome measures	Main results	Quality of reporting	Comment
Colloff et al. 1989[1] (UK)	Daily natamycin (spray to kill house dust mites) v placebo spray, with and without vacuum cleaning of the mattress (i.e. four treatment groups)	20 young adults with atopic eczema and a positive RAST for house dust mite IgE. Active spray + vacuuming (n = 6), active spray, no vacuuming (n = 4), placebo spray + vacuuming (n = 5), placebo spray, no vacuuming (n = 5)	Parallel-group, double-blind, factorial RCT; follow up: 4 months	House dust mite load; disease severity (six features at 16 sites – not a validated scale)	Vacuum cleaning (not natamycin spray) had a significant impact on reducing house dust mite numbers. Reduction in house dust mite was not associated with improvements in clinical severity	Method of randomisation and concealment not reported; no ITT analysis; very small sample size	This trial was too small to provide generalisable results. Nevertheless, the effectiveness of vacuuming compared with sprays may be useful in informing future study design
Tan et al. 1996[3] (UK)	Active intervention: Goretex bedcovers, benzyltannate spray and daily high-filtration vacuuming. Placebo intervention: cotton covers, water and ethanol spray and daily vacuum cleaning with a normal machine	30 adults and 30 children (aged >7 years) with atopic dermatitis; 48 completed the study – active group (n = 28), placebo group (n = 20)	Parallel-group, double-blind, placebo-controlled trial; follow up: 6 months.	House dust mite load; house dust mite allergen Der p1; disease severity (SASSAD)	Although the weight of dust removed was significantly lower for the active versus the placebo group, the level of the major dust allergen Der p1 in bedroom carpets was dramatically reduced in both groups. Disease severity reduced by a small amount in both groups, but more	Method of randomisation and concealment not reported; no ITT analysis; small sample size	This was a small but important study. Blinding may not have been successful, given the very different vacuum cleaners used. This study suggests that vacuuming with an ordinary household cleaner achieves similar reductions in house dust mite antigen levels in bedroom carpets to those achieved by the

(Continued)

Table 17.4 (*Continued*)

Study	Intervention	Population and sample size	Design and period of follow up	Main outcome measures	Main results	Quality of reporting	Comment
					so in the active group (12·6 v 4·2 units). Subgroup analysis suggested that only children had a statistically significant improvement and that there was no correlation between clinical improvement and positive skin prick tests at study outset		more expensive high-filtration vacuum cleaners
Endo *et al.* 1997[2] (Japan)	Intensive vacuum cleaning of carpets, mattresses and quilts by researchers every 3 weeks *v* the same cleaning with the vacuum cleaner on 50% power	30 children with atopic eczema	Parallel-group, randomised controlled trial; follow up: 1 year	Physician-assessed severity; house dust mite load	A statistically significant decrease in mite numbers in favour of the intensive cleaning group was only noted for the room floors. Clinical scores were significantly improved in the active group compared with baseline but not in the control group	Method of randomisation and concealment not reported; no ITT analysis; clinical scores were given in graphical form only and the appropriate statistical test of mean difference between the two treatments was not reported	Patients were probably not blinded adequately, although clinical scores were assessed by a physician blind to treatment allocation. Comparison with normal vacuuming would have been helpful

(*Continued*)

Table 17.4 (Continued)

Study	Intervention	Population and sample size	Design and period of follow up	Main outcome measures	Main results	Quality of reporting	Comment
Ricci et al. 2000[6] (Italy)	Active intervention: encasing mattresses and pillows, hot weekly wash of bedding, living room and bedroom vacuumed twice a week, soft toys washed weekly and removed from the bedroom. Control intervention: normal cleaning	41 children aged ≥ 2 years with atopic dermatitis	Two-part study. Part 1: single-blind randomised controlled trial of 2 months duration. Part 2: all patients allocated to active intervention and followed up from 2 months to 1 year	Disease severity (SCORAD). House dust mite load; house dust mite allergens Dep p1 and Der f1	Severity scores in the active group improved from 33 to 26 (21%) at 2 months. In the control group, scores reduced from 27 to 24 (11%). Dust mite load and allergens were reduced in both groups. Follow up study: after 12 months, both groups showed improvements in clinical severity and dust load, but there was no longer a control group	Randomisation method not clear and probably inappropriate; no ITT analysis; the appropriate statistical test of mean difference between the two groups was not reported	This study had an unusual design and it is not entirely clear why they abandoned the initial randomised groupings after 2 months. The active intervention was very intensive and probably not appropriate for wide-scale implementation
Gutgesell et al. 2001[5] (Germany)	Active intervention: allergen-impermeable mattress cover, plus acaricide spray (tannic acid and benzylbenzoate). Placebo intervention: cotton bed covers, plus water and ethanol spray)	20 adults with moderate to severe atopic dermatitis with sensitisation to the house dust mite	Double-blind, placebo-controlled randomised controlled trial. Follow up: 1 year	Disease severity (SCORAD); dust mite allergen (Der p); topical steroid usage; patient-assessed pruritus and pruritus-induced sleep loss	A significant reduction in dust mite allergen was found, but this did not translate into significant improvements in clinical severity, topical steroid use or patient-assessed pruritus.	Randomisation method was not clear but otherwise the methods were reasonably robust. The most limiting factor of the study was its small sample size, although all 20 patients did complete the study	This is again a very small study. Nevertheless, Gutgesell et al. should be commended for the inclusion of patient-specific outcome measures in this study, as the clinical relevance of small improvements on disease severity scales is often difficult to assess

(Continued)

Table 17.4 (Continued)

Study	Intervention	Population and sample size	Design and period of follow up	Main outcome measures	Main results	Quality of reporting	Comment
Holm et al. 2001[4] (Sweden)	Active intervention: mattress and pillow covers, duvets washed monthly at >60°, carpets and mattress vacuumed weekly. Placebo intervention: cotton covers only	43 adults with atopic dermatitis. Exclusion criteria included the use of potent topical steroids	Follow up: 1 year. Double-blind, placebo-controlled trial. Follow up: 1 year	Disease severity (SCORAD); house dust mite load; total IgE and IgE to house dust mite in blood serum; weekly diary of itch intensity (not mentioned in results)	Disease severity was reduced in both groups (45% in the active group, 39% in the control group). Compared with baseline, house dust mite exposure was significantly reduced in the active group, as was house dust mite specific IgE. Patients not sensitised to house dust mite allergens benefited from the bedcovers as much as sensitised patients	Randomisation method and concealment were unclear; no ITT analysis was performed and the appropriate statistical test of mean difference between the two groups was not reported	This was a small and relatively inconclusive study. The active intervention was very intensive

ITT, intention-to-treat; SASSAD Six Area Six Sign Atopic Dermatitis, SCORAD, severity scoring of atopic dermatitis

Efficacy

This section deals with exclusion diets for cases of established atopic eczema. No systematic reviews of dietary manipulation in established atopic eczema could be identified, although some of the published studies have been reviewed by Charman.[7] The nine RCTs examining the role of elimination diets in established atopic eczema are summarised in Table 17.5.[8-16]

The key benefits to emerge from this review are:

- There is little evidence to support an egg-and-milk-free diet in unselected patients with atopic eczema.
- There is no evidence to support the use of an elemental or few-foods diet in atopic eczema.
- There is some evidence that the addition of a probiotic such as *Lactobacillus* may be beneficial for atopic eczema in those already on a cows'-milk-whey-hydrolysate diet, although in the absence of a control group on no special diet it is hard to say if this is a real benefit.
- There is some evidence to support the use of an egg-free diet in infants with suspected egg allergy who have positive specific IgE to eggs.

Drawbacks

Calcium, protein and calorie deficiency are risks of dairy-free diets in children. Such diets should only be used under medical supervision.

Comment

Methodological difficulties mean that interpretation of these trials is difficult. RCTs that employ a parallel design with an unblinded normal control diet may introduce bias in favour of the active group. In addition, those trials that place all participants on exclusion diets and then re-introduce the suspected offending food compared with a control, risk introducing another allergen (for example soya) or introducing the suspected allergen (for example cows' milk) in a way that does not mimic real life. Poor concealment of randomisation allocation, lack of blinding and high dropout rates without an ITT analysis all mean that the above studies should be interpreted with great caution. Future studies should ideally be longer term, more pragmatic and ensure that randomisation is concealed.

Uncontrolled elimination diets followed by double-blind, placebo-controlled challenges with foods suspected to aggravate symptoms have also been tried in atopic eczema.[17-21] These studies are not the same as RCTs of food elimination. Instead they try to answer the question: "Does food X make a particular child's atopic eczema worse?". The precise relationship between such food challenge studies and long-term benefits of exclusion of the suspected foods to atopic eczema sufferers is not clear. Blood and skin prick tests are usually only helpful in predicting clinical response if they are negative.[22,23] It should also be borne in mind that this high negative predictive value has only been shown in relation to provocation of symptoms after double-blind challenge, and not clinical response following food elimination, which are not necessarily the same thing. The relationship between atopic eczema and food sensitivity is a complex one and readers are referred to a clear evidence-based work by David for further information.[24]

Implications for clinical practice

Elimination diets are difficult for families and patients to follow, even in the highly motivated environment of a clinical trial. In the absence of clear evidence of the involvement of a particular food substance, the possible harms may outweigh the benefits. For cases where exclusion diets are indicated, appropriate dietary advice and support should be made available.

Table 17.5 Studies of elimination diets in the treatment of those with established atopic eczema

Study	Interventions [co-treatments]	Study population and sample size	Design and period of follow up	Main outcome measures	Main results	Quality of reporting	Comment
Atherton 1978[8] (England)	Egg and cows' milk exclusion diet (with soya milk substitution) v control diet with eggs and cows' milk [hydrocortisone, emollients and antihistamines]	36 children aged 2–8 years with clinically typical atopic eczema attending a dermatology clinic	Crossover design with three 4-week periods. During two of the 4-week periods patients were placed on an egg and milk elimination diet. For the other 4-week period children ate their normal diet. The ordering of these three periods was randomly allocated	Eczema area and activity using an unpublished composite score; degree of adherence to diet; skin prick tests	Of 20 children who completed the trial, 13 showed an improvement during the trial diet period, 6 showed no change and 1 showed deterioration. On control diet period, 3 showed improvement, 11 no change and 6 deteriorated. Itch was not statistically significant between the two groups	Method of randomisation and concealment unclear; study described as double blind although some unblinding of parents cannot be excluded; no ITT analysis; high dropout rate (44%)	Marked order effect i.e. improvements greater at end of first versus second period whatever the diet; soya milk (which itself can be allergenic in atopic eczema) used as "control" food
Munkvad 1984[9] (Denmark)	Elemental diet (amino acids, essential fatty acids, glucose, trace elements, sorbic acid and vitamins) v a blended diluted diet of foodstuffs consumed by hospital inpatients	33 adults with atopic eczema covering more than 10% of the body, 13 of whom had a history of intolerance to one or more food elements	Parallel-group RCT of hospitalised patients on diets for 3 weeks	Various unpublished extent and intensity signs scored between −3 and +3; photographs before and after; patient itch and sleep; various serum markers of inflammation; A	Of 25 evaluable patients, 5 of 16 improved on the elemental diet compared with 4 of 9 on the placebo diet. Itch, sleeplessness, antihistamine use and immunological tests were no different between the two groups	Method of randomisation and concealment unclear; unclear if the reported "double blinding" was successful in view of the different composition of the two diets; no ITT analysis; 24% dropout rate	History of food intolerance in patients not confirmed during study; small study of an intervention which is unpalatable, impractical and requires hospitalisation and dietetic input

(Continued)

Table 17.5 (*Continued*)

Study	Interventions, [co-treatments]	Study population and sample size	Design and period of follow up	Main outcome measures	Main results	Quality of reporting	Comment
	[emollients, a topical steroid and antihistamines]			"major activity score of >100" was defined as the criterion for a positive response to treatment			
Cant 1986[10] (England)	Exclusion of egg and cows' milk (with soya substitute) in mothers of infants with atopic eczema who were exclusively breastfeeding versus inclusion of egg and milk [topical steroids and emollients]	19 mothers and babies with established atopic eczema	12-week crossover study divided into three 4-week periods. During the first two periods mothers excluded cows' milk, egg and other foods from their diet and were randomised in the first or second period for milk substitutes containing cows' milk and egg or soya. Normal diet in the third period	Combined area/intensity score (unpublished) with a maximum score of 60	Of 17 mothers completing the study, the activity scores decreased by 20% in four babies on soya and in 1 on egg and milk; no statistically different mean scores between the two groups; marked period effect in that children of mothers on normal diet in third period continued to improve	Method of randomisation described; concealment of allocation unclear; study described as double-blind although almost half of the mothers correctly identified substitutes; ITT analysis was attempted	Well reported although very small study conducted alongside a before-and-after study; soya used as control diet

(*Continued*)

Table 17.5 (*Continued*)

Study	Interventions, [co-treatments]	Study population and sample size	Design and period of follow up	Main outcome measures	Main results	Quality of reporting	Comment
Nield 1986[11] (England)	Egg- and cows'-milk-free diet (using soya as substitute) v normal diet [topical steroids and antihistamines]	53 unselected atopic eczema outpatients aged 1–23 years	Crossover trial with three 6-week periods. During first and third periods, patients were randomised to either receive an egg and cows' milk exclusion diet (a soya-based milk substitute) or an egg and cows' milk preparation as the control intervention	Patient-reported itch and sleep loss; use of co-treatments; composite score of area and intensity; skin prick tests	Of 40 evaluable patients, there was little difference for change in score (area, itch, co-treatment use) between the treatment periods and none were statistically significant	Method of randomisation and concealment of allocation unclear; study reported as double-blind although test substances might have tasted different; no ITT analysis; high dropout rate (25%)	High dropout rate because diet too difficult to adhere to; unclear if there was a period or carry-over effect; confidence intervals suggested that if anything, patients did worse on the exclusion diet than on the normal diet
Mabin 1995[12] (England)	Children allocated to three groups: i) few-foods diet (eliminating all but 5–8 foods) plus whey hydrolysate; ii) few-foods diet plus casein hydrolysate; iii) remain on usual diet [antihistamines and topical steroids]	85 children (median age 2·3 years) with atopic eczema which persisted despite conventional treatment and involving more than 12% of body; breastfed children were excluded	Parallel single-blind RCT with follow up until 6 weeks	Skin severity score incorporating extent and severity; parental record of itch, sleep loss and global improvement	Of 46 evaluable patients, 16 (73%) of the 22 controls and 15 (58%) of the 24 who received the diet showed >20% improvement in skin severity score; improvement in skin severity score in controls, and daytime itch score in the whey hydrolysate group was statistically significant	Method of randomisation clearly described; concealment of allocation unclear; study described as investigator blind; no ITT analysis; very high dropout rate (46%)	Good description of patient flow and interventions; 35 of 39 dropouts were in the diet group, illustrating the difficulty of adopting the few-foods diet even in a motivated hospital group; no evidence to support benefit from diet and some evidence suggesting that control diet was better

(*Continued*)

Table 17.5 (Continued)

Study	Interventions, [co-treatments]	Study population and sample size	Design and period of follow up	Main outcome measures	Main results	Quality of reporting	Comment
Isolauri 1995[3] (Finland)	Children with atopic eczema allocated to whey hydrolysate v an amino-acid-derived formula containing no peptides	45 children who were not being breastfed, who had been fed substitute cows' milk for at least 6 months and who showed a positive reaction to a masked challenge with cows' milk	Parallel prospective randomised study drawing patients from an initial study to determine cows' milk allergy. Children were followed up for 8 months	Atopic eczema severity (extent, intensity of signs and symptoms) measured by the SCORAD system; infants' growth also measured	Weight gain and infant length statistically less in the whey hydrolysate group; eczema severity decreased from a SCORAD of 17 (baseline) to 5 in 22 children on whey hydrolysate compared with 21 (baseline) to 4 at 8 months in the amino acid group	Method and concealment of randomisation allocation unclear; randomised part of the study probably not blinded; no dropouts	Highly selected population; study mainly concerned comparison of growth in amino-acid v hydrolysate formulae; main statistical comparison of change in eczema severity between the two groups not reported in results although children in amino acid group had higher baseline score in the 12 statistical outcome comparisons made
Majamaa 1997[14] (Finland)	Cows' milk elimination (extensively hydrolysed whey formula) with and without a probiotic (*Lactobacillus* GG)	27 infants with clinical history suggestive of cows'-milk allergy who were confirmed as being sensitive to cows' milk by double-blind placebo-controlled	Parallel randomised prospective study monitored for 1 month	Atopic eczema severity measured by SCORAD; no *a priori* statement of minimum clinically significant benefit	Of 27 evaluable children, the median SCORAD at baseline was 21 and 26 in the whey alone versus whey plus probiotic groups respectively. These decreased to 19 and 15 respectively at the end of 1 month	Method and concealment of randomisation allocation unclear; no blinding reported; no dropouts	Authors reported statistical significance for the change in score from baseline to the end of the study separately for each intervention, but did not test the difference between the two treatments. Regression to *(Continued)*

Table 17.5 (*Continued*)

Study	Interventions, [co-treatments]	Study population and sample size	Design and period of follow up	Main outcome measures	Main results	Quality of reporting	Comment
		challenge; 19% of the children also had gastrointestinal symptoms					the mean could have accounted for the greater improvement in the probiotic group
Lever 1998[15] (Scotland)	Egg exclusion diet for young children as advised by a dietitian v general advice from a dietitian only [mild-to-moderate topical steroids and emollients]	62 children all with positive IgE blood antibodies to egg, only 7 of which had a history suggestive of egg allergy	Parallel randomised prospective study of 4 weeks duration	Eczema severity as assessed by extent as a percentage and as a composite severity score in 16 body sites	Of 55 evaluable children, the area involved by eczema reduced from 19·6% to 10·9% in the egg-free group compared with 21·9% to 18·9% in the control group (P = 0·02). Severity score reduced from 33·9 to 24·0 in the egg-free group compared with 36·7 to 33·5 in the control group (P = 0·04)	Method of randomisation unclear; randomisation performed by same dietitian who was giving the intervention; parents unblinded; assessor reported as blinded; no ITT analysis; co-treatment use not reported	Study suggested that egg-free diet in those with a positive RAST test to egg may be useful. Methodological concerns such as lack of randomisation concealment and increased motivation and ancillary care in intervention group could have resulted in bias.
Niggemann 2001[16] (Germany, Finland, France)	Extensively hydrolysed cows' milk formulae v amino acid based formulae [mild-or-moderate topical steroids]	73 infants aged 1–10 months, with atopic dermatitis and cow's milk allergy/intolerance (proven by double-blind, placebo-controlled food challenge)	Multicentre, parallel-group, RCT of 6 months duration.	Disease severity (SCORAD); growth (length and weight-for-length)	Both groups showed significant improvements in disease severity compared with baseline (P<0·001); no significant differences between the two groups at 6 months; mean scores for each group reported in graphical form only	Method of randomisation unclear; no mention of blinding, or standardisation of methods between centres; unclear if all patients completed	Study suggested extensively hydrolysed milk formulae and amino-acid based formulae helpful in reducing disease severity in children with proven cow's milk intolerance. However, in absence of control group, interpretation difficult

ITT, intention to treat; RAST, radio-allergosorbent test; SCORAD, severity scoring of atopic dermatitis,

Key points

- There is insufficient evidence relating to exclusion diets for patients with atopic eczema.
- The most common diets used are milk- or egg-free diets.
- The possible risks of impaired growth and development in children should be recognised.

Do Chinese herbal medicines improve the symptoms of atopic eczema?

Efficacy

We located one systematic review of Chinese herbal medicines for atopic eczema.[25] This review reported two randomised trials of atopic eczema, one on adults[26] and one on children.[27] The authors concluded "At present it is unclear whether Chinese herbal treatments of eczema do more good than harm".

A further two trials have now been identified.[28,29] All four trials evaluated an oral Chinese herbal decoction comprising *Ledebouriella seseloides, Potentilla chinensis, Clematis armandii, Rehmannia glutinosa, Paenia lactiflora, Lophatherum gracile, Dictamnus dasycarpus, Tribulus terrestris, Glycyrrhiza glabra* and *Schizonepeta tenuifolia*, except Sheehan *et al.*[26] who used *Anebia clematidis* instead of *Clematis armandii*.

Sheehan *et al.*[26] compared Chinese herbs (as above) in a decoction and a placebo comprising of a mixture of "inert" plant materials, once daily for 8 weeks in 47 children with atopic eczema. Median percentage changes in the clinical scores for erythema compared with baseline were 51% for Chinese herbs and 6·1% for placebo. Change in surface damage was 63·1% and 6·2% in the Chinese herb and

placebo groups, respectively. A 1-year follow up study of the children concluded that Chinese herbal medicine, in the medium term, was helpful for approximately half the children who originally took part in the RCT.[30]

Sheehan *et al.*[27] also compared the Chinese herbs (as above) in a decoction and an "inert plant" placebo, once daily, in 40 adult patients with atopic dermatitis. Significant improvements were reported for erythema ($P<0·001$) and surface damage ($P<0·001$) with the herbs compared with the placebo.

The study by Latchman *et al.*[29] evaluated the same combination of Chinese herbs finely ground and in a more palatable form of freeze-dried granules over an 8-week period in 18 patients with atopic eczema. There was a significant reduction in erythema and surface damage compared with baseline ($P<0·001$). There were no difference in clinical outcome between formulations.

The study by Fung *et al.*[28] evaluated the same combination of Chinese herbs compared with "inert plant" placebo over an 8-week period in 40 patients with atopic eczema. There was a general trend of clinical improvement for both Chinese herbs and placebo.

Drawbacks

Both active and placebo herbs were reported to be unpalatable and caused 10[26] and 8[27] dropouts in the two studies by Sheehan *et al.* Other adverse effects included abdominal distension, headaches, transient dizziness, gastrointestinal upsets, one case of lichenoid eruption and one case of facial herpes. The potential for hepatotoxicity is a concern with Chinese herbs. However, the three studies that carried out pre- and post-treatment liver function tests found no abnormalities.[26–28]

Comments

All studies were randomised but method and concealment of allocation were not described. All were described as double-blind, except Latchman et al.,[29] where no blinding was mentioned. No ITT analysis was carried out. It is also questionable whether the placebo plants were truly inert. The study by Sheehan et al.[26] reported large effects in children, highlighting a promising treatment of atopic eczema. This has not been replicated in the other studies, although they are all quite similar. Clearly larger scale RCTs of longer duration are needed.

Implications for clinical practice

There is currently little convincing evidence to support the use of Chinese herbal medicines for the treatment of atopic eczema, although some studies have reported large effects. Further work is needed to address the long-term safety implications.

Key points

- Four randomised controlled trials are reported, all of which used the same herbs for the active intervention group.
- Results are conflicting and further large-scale studies are needed.
- A number of side-effects were identified, the true implications of which cannot be addressed without long-term studies.

Do washing powders exacerbate the symptoms of atopic eczema?

Efficacy

Detergent enzymes may cause skin irritation, leading some physicians to advise patients with atopic eczema to avoid the use of such detergents in favour of alternative "non-biological" detergents.[31] We located one RCT testing the hypothesis that enzyme-containing detergents are more likely to aggravate atopic eczema than a non-biological detergent,[32] and one that looked at the impact of using fabric softeners in adults with atopic dermatitis.[33]

In the first study,[32] 26 adults with mild-to-moderate atopic eczema (mean age 25 years) were randomised in a double-blind crossover study to use either a trial detergent containing enzymes or a visually identical detergent without enzymes for one month. There was a 1-month wash-out period before randomisation, when participants used their usual washing powder. Topical steroids were permitted during the study and were weighed. In the 25 patients who completed the trial there was no difference between the two groups in terms of disease severity (SCORAD scores of 29 in each group, 95% CI for mean difference −4 to +5). Similar results were found for the use of topical steroids, patient-reported itch and eczema activity.

The study looking at fabric softeners[33] was a single-blind randomised trial using a left–right comparison design for a period of 12 days. Twenty volunteers with a history of atopic dermatitis were enrolled in the study (none had active lesions at the time of enrolment). In order to simulate realistic conditions of skin damage, sodium lauryl sulphate was applied to each volar forearm under occlusion 3 days before the start of the study. A control patch using water was also applied to each arm. Repetitive wash tests were performed three times a day using softened or unsoftened fabric in random order to each arm. The investigator was blinded to the fabric used at each site. Both for the control and pre-irritated skin, all measured parameters indicated that "softened" fabric was less aggressive to the skin than "unsoftened" fabric.

Drawbacks

No patients had contact dermatitis to enzymes when patch tested at the end of the study, and there was no evidence of specific blood IgE against any of the enzymes.[32]

Comment

Although the study by Andersen et al.[32] was small, the virtual absence of any differences between the enzyme and non-enzyme detergents and the corresponding narrow confidence intervals provide convincing evidence of a lack of harmful effect. The study was not sponsored by industry. Further long-term studies using a pragmatic design may be helpful in determining any potential benefit from using fabric softeners for patients with atopic eczema.

Implications for clinical practice

There is currently no evidence to suggest that parents should switch from a biological to non-biological washing powder.

Key points

- Although parents of children with atopic eczema commonly avoid washing powders that contain enzymes (biological powders), evidence from a small RCT did not support the belief that washing detergents containing enzymes have a provoking effect on eczema severity compared with washing detergents without enzymes.
- There is limited evidence to suggest that softened fabrics may be less likely to exacerbate the symptoms of eczema than unsoftened fabrics, although further pragmatic studies are needed.
- We found no studies looking at the effect of avoiding all contact with washing detergents.

Can specialised clothing help to reduce the symptoms of atopic eczema?

Efficacy

We found no systematic review, but found three RCTs evaluating clothing material in atopic eczema.[34–36] Diepgen et al. in 1990[31] and 1995,[32] evaluated the irritative capacity of shirts made of four different materials (cotton and synthetics of different fibre structure). The other RCT by Seymour et al.[36] evaluated the clinical effects of different types of nappies on the skin of normal infants and infants with atopic eczema.

In the 1990 study by Diepgen et al.,[34] 55 patients with atopic eczema were compared with 31 control patients without atopic eczema and were randomised to wear shirts of one of four different types of fibre. At the end of week 2 of the study those wearing cotton shirts reported better comfort compared with the other textile shirts in increasing order of weight and fibre roughness.

The 1995 study by Diepgen et al.[35] (published in a German textile journal) evaluated seven different garments on 20 patients with mild-to-moderate atopic eczema. The garments were either cotton or polyester, with different fibre roughness, yarn roughness and fabric weaves. The study was a randomised crossover study (Diepgen T, personal communication, January 2000), with each garment worn under standardised conditions on four consecutive days. Comfort was statistically significantly higher for warp-knit shirts compared with jersey-knit shirts, but was no different for cotton and polyester of fine fibre construction (assessed by scanning electron microscopy).

In the Seymour et al. study,[36] cloth nappies were compared with cellulose-core nappies and cellulose-core nappies containing absorbent gelling material. Eighty-five babies with atopic eczema who were less than 20 months of age were recruited. Eczema severity and degree of nappy rash were scored by an independent dermatologist. At the end of the 26-week period, there was no clinical or statistical difference between the different nappy types for overall grade of atopic eczema. However, nappy rash was significantly less in the group using cellulose nappies with absorbent gelling material compared with the others at 26 weeks and throughout the trial ($P < 0.05$).

Drawbacks

None were reported, although specialised cotton clothing for atopic eczema sufferers is more expensive than other synthetic fibres. No adverse events were reported in the trial of different nappies.

Comment

The success of blinding in both of the trials conducted by Diepgen and colleagues[34,35] is questionable because of the different roughness of the various shirt fibres. The magnitude of effects was not stated in the 1995 paper, and it is possible that small differences in comfort between cotton and polyester fabrics were missed. Both RCTs suggest that the smoothness of the fabric is more important than the type of fabric used. Synthetic fibres that are just as comfortable for people with atopic eczema can be manufactured with smooth fibres using yarns and fabric construction.

From the Seymour et al.[36] study it was unclear if the group with atopic eczema who wore cloth nappies were randomised in the same way as the other two groups and whether statistical comparisons were made with the control population who were not part of the same randomised group. The study, nevertheless, suggests that nappy rash is less severe in atopic infants who wear nappies with absorbent gelling material. There was no evidence to support any benefit of conventional disposable nappies over cloth nappies, although the study may have lacked power to demonstrate small differences. The environmental implications of the different types of nappies were not discussed.

Implications for clinical practice

There is no need for parents of children to buy expensive cotton clothes if their child finds that other fine-weave synthetics are just as comfortable. The type of nappy used is unlikely to affect the severity of atopic eczema.

Key points

- Two small randomised controlled trials found that, in people with atopic eczema, the roughness of clothing textiles is a more important factor for skin irritation than the type of textile fibre (synthetic or natural).
- Polyester and cotton of similar textile fineness seem to be equally well tolerated.
- We found no evidence on the long-term effect of different textiles on the severity of atopic eczema.
- It is possible that nappy rash may be less severe in babies using nappies with an absorbent gel.

What is the role of psychological interventions for the treatment of atopic eczema?

Efficacy

It has been postulated that scratching becomes a habit in atopic eczema, and that it is detrimental because it damages the skin further. Habit-reversal is a modified behavioural technique which teaches patients to recognise the habit and then to progressively train them to develop a "competing response practice" such as simply touching, squeezing or tapping the itching area or to develop other ways of moving their hands away from the itching area.[37] The technique has been described in two RCTs[38,39] conducted by the same team from Sweden and compared against topical cortiscosteroids. A further RCT evaluated the potential benefit of three psychological approaches versus dermatological education in the prevention of relapse in atopic eczema.[40]

In the first habit-reversal study,[38] 17 patients with atopic eczema aged 19–41 years were randomised into two groups. The interventions consisted of hydrocortisone cream plus two sessions of habit-reversal treatment, received during week 1, (active-treatment group) or hydrocortisone cream alone (comparator group). The study was unblinded and of 28 days duration. At the end of the assessment period the mean reduction in global eczema score was 67% in the active-treatment group compared with 37% in the comparator group ($P<0.05$). Total score of self-assessed annoyance was also markedly reduced in the active versus comparator groups. Mean percentage reduction of scratching episodes per day was 79% in the active-treatment group compared with 49% in the comparator group ($P<0.01$).

In the later study conducted by the same team[39] 45 patients were randomised to four groups for a period of 5 weeks. One group applied hydrocortisone cream for the entire 5-week period, another group applied betamethasone valerate (a strong topical steroid) for 3 weeks followed by hydrocortisone for the remaining 2 weeks. Another group applied hydrocortisone plus habit-reversal for the 5-week period and another group, betamethasone plus habit-reversal for the first 3 weeks followed by hydrocortisone plus habit-reversal for the remaining 2 weeks. The study was unblinded. Significant differences were reported between the behavioural-therapy groups and those taking steroids alone for total skin status. Scratching was reduced by 65% in the hydrocortisone-only group, 74% in the betamethasone followed by hydrocortisone group, 88% in the hydrocortisone plus habit-reversal group, and 90% in the betamethasone plus hydrocortisone plus habit-reversal group.

The study by Ehlers and colleagues in 1995[40] evaluated the use of an autogenic training programme (ATP) as a form of relaxation therapy versus a cognitive-behavioural treatment (BT), versus a standard dermatological educational programme (DE) versus combined DE and BT

(DEBT). A total of 113 secondary-care patients were randomised to these four groups and were also compared with an additional standard medical treatment group who were not part of the random assignment. Investigators were blinded to the group allocation. The intervention was for 3 months and patients were followed up for 1 year. At the end of 1 year, mean skin severity lesion score dropped from 29·5 to 28·8 in the DE group, from 33·7 to 19·8 in the ATP group, from 31·0 to 20·7 in the BT group and from 35·4 to 25·8 in the DEBT group. There were no significant differences in mean severity of itching between the four groups. The DEBT treatment led to significantly greater improvement in global skin severity than intensive education (DE) alone and this was also accompanied by significant reductions in topical steroid use.

Drawbacks
In the study by Ehlers and colleagues,[40] the behavioural approaches required 12 weekly group sessions of 1·5–2 hours, each with 5–7 patients. No adverse events were reported in any of the trials, although some of the dropouts could possibly be related to the fact that extra visits were needed for the behavioural technique.

Comment
The Ehlers *et al.* study[40] was clearly reported and although no ITT analysis was performed, dropouts were low (9 out of 113 at 3 months). However, over 14 outcome measures were reported, which introduces the possibility of multiple hypothesis testing. The authors also performed statistical comparisons against a non-randomised control group, which may not be justified. Nevertheless, the magnitude of improvement for those receiving behavioural techniques in addition to their standard dermatological care (which included topical corticosteroids) was moderately large, and carried more weight than the other two studies[38,39]

because assessments were made by an investigator blinded to the treatment allocation.

Implications for clinical practice

The combination of habit-reversal plus judicious use of topical corticosteroids seems an attractive one, and evidence from two RCTs supports its use. However, the lack of suitably qualified personnel may limit the ability to deliver this intervention in many settings.

Key points

- Three RCTs suggested that psychological interventions such as habit-reversal techniques are a useful adjunct to dermatological treatment in atopic eczema.
- Further studies are required to assess how these findings can be generalised to other settings and patient groups.

References

1. Colloff MJ, Lever RS, McSharry C. A controlled trial of house dust mite eradication using natamycin in homes of patients with atopic dermatitis: effect on clinical status and mite populations [see comments]. *Br J Dermatol* 1989;**121**:199–208.

2. Endo K, Fukuzumi T, Adachi J *et al.* Effect of vacuum cleaning of room floors and bed clothes of patients on house dust mites counts and clinical scores of atopic dermatitis. A double blind control trial. *Arerugi (Jpn J Allergology)* 1997;**46**:1013–24.

3. Tan BB, Weald D, Strickland I, Friedmann PS. Double-blind controlled trial of effect of housedust-mite allergen avoidance on atopic dermatitis. *Lancet* 1996;**347**:15–18.

4. Holm L, Ohman S, Bengtsson A, van Hage-Hamsten M, Scheynius A. Effectiveness of occlusive bedding in the treatment of atopic dermatitis – a placebo-controlled trial of 12 months duration. *Allergy* 2001;**56**:152–8.

5. Gutgesell C, Heise S, Seubert S *et al.* Double-blind placebo-controlled house dust mite control measures in adult patients with atopic dermatitis. *Br J Dermatol* 2001;**145**:70–4.

6. Ricci G, Patrizi A, Specchia F *et al.* Effect of house dust mite avoidance measures in children with atopic dermatitis. *Br J Dermatol* 2000;**143**:379–84.

7. Charman C. Atopic eczema. In: Godlee F, ed. *Clinical Evidence.* London: BMJ Publishing Group, 2001.

8. Atherton DJ, Sewell M, Soothill JF, Wells RS, Chilvers CE. A double-blind controlled crossover trial of an antigen-avoidance diet in atopic eczema. *Lancet* 1978; **1**:401–3.

9. Munkvad M, Danielsen L, Hoj L *et al.* Antigen-free diet in adult patients with atopic dermatitis. A double-blind controlled study. *Acta Derm Venereol* 1984;**64**:524–8.

10. Cant AJ, Bailes JA, Marsden RA, Hewitt D. Effect of maternal dietary exclusion on breast fed infants with eczema: two controlled studies. *BMJ (Clin Res Ed)* 1986;**293**:231–3.

11. Neild VS, Marsden RA, Bailes JA, Bland JM. Egg and milk exclusion diets in atopic eczema. *Br J Dermatol* 1986;**114**:117–23.

12. Mabin DC, Sykes AE, David TJ. Controlled trial of a few foods diet in severe atopic dermatitis. *Arch Dis Child* 1995;**73**:202–7.

13. Isolauri EMD, Sutas YMD, Makinen-Kiljunen SMSc, Oja Simo S MD, Isosomppi RMSc, Turjanmaa KMD. Efficacy and safety of hydrolyzed cow milk and amino acid-derived formulas in infants with cow milk allergy. *J Pediatr* 1995;**127**:550–7.

14. Majama H, Isolauri E. Probiotics: a novel approach in the management of food allergy. *J Allergy Clin Immunol* 1997;**99**:179–85.

15. Lever R, MacDonald C, Waugh P, Aitchison T. Randomised controlled trial of advice on an egg exclusion diet in young children with atopic eczema and sensitivity to eggs. *Pediatr Allergy Immunol* 1998;**9**:13–19.

16. Niggemann B, Binder C, Dupont C, Hadji S, Arvola T, Isolauri E. Prospective, controlled, multi-center study on the effect of an amino-acid-based formula in infants with cow's milk allergy/intolerance and atopic dermatitis. *Pediatr Allergy Immunol* 2001;**12**:78–82.

17. Sloper KS, Wadsworth J, Brostoff J. Children with atopic eczema I: clinical response to food elimination and subsequent double-blind food challenge. *Q J Med* 1991;**80**:677–93.

18. Devlin J, David TJ. Tartrazine in atopic eczema. *Arch Dis Child* 1992;**67**:709–11.

19. James JM, Bernhisel-Broadbent J, Sampson HA. Respiratory reactions provoked by double-blind food challenges in children. *Am J Respir Crit Care Med* 1994;**149**:59–64.

20. Fuglsang G, Madsen G, Halken S, Jorgensen S, Ostergaard PA, Osterballe O. Adverse reactions to food additives in children with atopic symptoms. *Allergy* 1994;**49**:31–7.

21. Kanny G, Hatahet R, Moneret-Vautrin DA, Kohler C, Bellut A. Allergy and intolerance to flavouring agents in atopic dermatitis in young children. *Allerg Immunol* (Paris) 1994;**26**:204–6.

22. Sampson HA. Comparative study of commercial food antigen extracts for the diagnosis of food hypersensitivity. *J Allergy Clin Immunol* 1988;**82**:718–26.

23. Sampson HA, Ho DG. Relationship between food-specific IgE concentrations and the risk of positive food challenges in children and adolescents. *J Allergy Clin Immunol* 1997;**100**:444–51.

24. David TJ. *Food and Food Additive Intolerance in Childhood*. Oxford: Blackwell Scientific Publications, 1993.

25. Armstrong NC, Ernst E. The treatment of eczema with Chinese herbs: a systematic review of randomised clinical trials. *Br J Clin Pharmacol* 1999;**48**:262–4.

26. Sheehan MP, Atherton DJ. A controlled trial of traditional chinese medicinal plants in widespread non-exudative atopic eczema. *Br J Dermatol* 1992;**126**:179–84.

27. Sheehan MP, Rustin MH, Atherton DJ *et al*. Efficacy of traditional Chinese herbal therapy in adult atopic dermatitis. *Lancet* 1992;**340**:13–17.

28. Fung AY, Look PC, Chong LY, But PP, Wong E. A controlled trial of traditional Chinese herbal medicine in Chinese patients with recalcitrant atopic dermatitis. *Int J Dermatol* 1999;**38**:387–92.

29. Latchman Y, Banerjee P, Poulter LW, Rustin M, Brostoff J. Association of immunological changes with clinical efficacy in atopic eczema patients treated with traditional Chinese herbal therapy (zemaphyte). *Int Arch Allergy Immunol* 1996;**109**:243–9.

30. Sheehan MP, Atherton DJ. One year follow-up of children treated with Chinese medicinal herbs for atopic eczema. *Br J Dermatol* 1994;**130**:488–93.

31. Rothe MJ, Grant-Kels JM. Diagnostic criteria for atopic dermatitis. *Lancet* 1996;**348**:1391–2.

32. Andersen PH, Bindslev-Jensen C, Mosbech H, Zachariae H, Andersen KE. Skin symptoms in patients with atopic dermatitis using enzyme-containing detergents. A placebo-controlled study. *Acta Derm Venereol* 1998;**78**:60–2.

33. Hermanns J, Goffin V, Arrese J, Rodriguez C. Beneficial effects of softened fabrics on atopic skin. *Dermatology* 2001;**202**:167–70.

34. Diepgen TL, Stabler A, Hornstein OP. Irritation from textiles in atopic eczema and controls. Textile intolerance in atopic eczema: a controlled clinical study. *Z Hautkr* 1990;**65**:907–10.

35. Diepgen TL, Salzer B, Tepe A, Hornstein OP. A study of skin irritations by textiles under standardized sweating conditions in patients with atopic eczema. *Melliand English* 1995;**12**:268.

36. Seymour JL, Keswick BH, Hanifin JM, Jordan WP, Milligan MC. Clinical effects of diaper types on the skin of normal infants and infants with atopic dermatitis. *J Am Acad Dermatol* 1987;**17**:988–97.

37. Noren P. Habit reversal: a turning point in the treatment of atopic dermatitis. *Clin Exp Dermatol* 1995;**20**:2–5.

38. Melin L, Frederiksen T, Noren P, Swebilius BG. Behavioural treatment of scratching in patients with atopic dermatitis. *Br J Dermatol* 1986;**115**:467–774.

39. Noren P, Melin L. The effect of combined topical steroids and habit-reversal treatment in patients with atopic dermatitis. *Br J Dermatol* 1989;**121**:359–66.

40. Ehlers A, Stangier U, Gieler U. Treatment of atopic dermatitis: a comparison of psychological and dermatological approaches to relapse prevention. *J Consult Clin Psychol* 1995;**63**:624–35.

Case scenario 2: How should infected atopic eczema be treated?

The relationship between *Staphylococcus aureus* and atopic eczema disease activity has been debated for many years. Most physicians recognise clinically infected eczema as recent onset of weeping, oozing and serous crusting or overt pus overlying the eczematous lesions. In this situation *S. aureus* is isolated in 90–100% of cases, usually in high numbers.[1,2] In around 30% of cases, beta haemolytic streptococci are also isolated.[1] Clinical infection is undoubtedly a

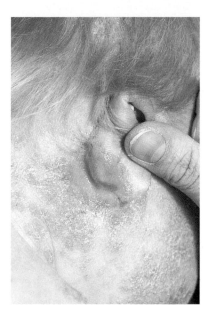

Figure 17.2   Infected atopic eczema

major problem for some atopic eczema sufferers.[3]

S. aureus is also isolated from the lesions of atopic eczema in 50–90% of patients without overt signs of infection.[4,5] Here, the role that S. aureus plays is much less clear. The idea that it may contribute to disease activity has led to the development of many antimicrobial compounds and their widespread use in the management of clincally non-infected atopic eczema. This section evaluates the possible benefit of these agents, primarily for clinically infected atopic eczema. Their use in clinically non-infected (colonised) eczema will also be commented on.

One systematic review was located,[6] which has been the source of much of the data in this section. A total of eight RCTs evaluating the possible benefit of oral or topical antimicrobials in clinically infected eczema were located and are summarised in Table 17.6. Additional RCTs evaluating the possible benefit of antiseptics in atopic eczema are presented in Table 17.7.

QUESTIONS

How useful are systemic antibiotics?

Effectiveness
Only two RCTs evaluating systemic antibiotics for clinically infected eczema were located.[2,7]

Versus placebo
Oral cefadroxil showed significant benefit over placebo for all clinical and microbiological outcomes.[2]

Versus each other
Erythromycin acistrate and erythromycin stearate both improved clinical and microbiological outcomes. There was no significant difference between the preparations.[7]

For non-infected eczema
Two further important RCTs have compared systemic antibiotics with placebo in the treatment of non-clinically infected atopic eczema. In the first,[8] oral flucloxacillin 250 mg four times daily for 4 weeks showed no benefit over placebo in terms of clinical efficacy, despite significantly reducing S. aureus counts. The second study[9] showed a similar absence of benefit for 2 weeks oral cefuroxime. Rapid recolonisation occurred in both groups after cessation of treatment.

Possible drawbacks
Gastrointestinal side-effects occurred in 50% of patients in each group taking erythromycin, and in one patient on cefuroxime. Emergence of methicillin-resistant S. aureus was noted in the flucloxacillin study, which persisted for 2 weeks after completion of treatment.

Comment and clinical implications
The quality of reporting in studies was generally poor, with small numbers of patients. It is

Table 17.6 Randomised controlled trials that have evaluated treatments for clinically infected atopic eczema

Study	Interventions and comparator	Study population and sample size	Trial design, description and follow up	Outcome measures	Main reported results	Quality of reporting	Comment
Oral antimicrobials							
Salo et al. 1988[7] (Finland)	Oral erythromycin acistrate (EA) 400 mg three times daily v oral erythromycin stearate (ES) 500 mg three times daily for 5–12 days (topical steroids and emollients)	42 adults admitted with clinically infected atopic eczema. Most had bacteriological isolates of S. aureus and four had combined staphylococcal/ streptococcal infection	Parallel-group, randomised, double-blind study; 5–12 days	Investigator and patient assessment of treatment efficacy on a 5-point scale	At the end of treatment, 75% and 83% of those in the EA and ES groups respectively showed "good" or "very effective" improvement; similar results according to patients; gastrointestinal side-effects similar in both groups	Method of randomisation and concealment unclear; no ITT analysis	Difficult to evaluate since two "actives" were being compared in the presence of inpatient care and potent co-treatment; that 7 patients with clinically infected eczema did not have positive bacteriology underscores the difficulty understanding the link between disease and bacteria
Weinberg et al. 1992[2] (South Africa)	Oral cefadroxil 50 mg/kg/day in two equal doses v placebo for 2 weeks (no mention of co-treatments)	33 children with bacteriologically confirmed infected atopic eczema caused by either S. aureus or mixed staphylococcal/ streptococcal infection	Parallel-group, randomised, double-blind study; 2 weeks	Clinical clearance of infection; eczema severity; number of patients with positive cultures; global improvement	Of 30 evaluable patients, all 13 in the cefadroxil group no longer had clinical evidence of superinfection at the end of the study, compared with 6 of 15 in the placebo group. Positive isolates fell from 13 to 4 and from 17 to 9 in the cefadroxil and placebo groups, respectively	Method of randomisation and concealment unclear; no description of blinding; no ITT analysis	Results clearly in favour of cefadroxil for these children with infected atopic eczema; poor quality of reporting

(Continued)

Table 17.6 (Continued)

Study	Interventions and comparator	Study population and sample size	Trial design, description and follow up	Outcome measures	Main reported results	Quality of reporting	Comment
Topical treatments							
Wachs and Maibach, 1976[13] (USA)	Betamethasone valerate cream v gentamicin/ betamethasone valerate versus gentamicin cream three times daily	83 pateints with infected moderate-to-severe atopic dermatitis	Prospective, randomised, parallel study; 22 days	Global assessment and overall severity; degree of inflammation; degree of infection, erythema, pruritus, pustules, crusting, exudation, vesiculation, lichenification	Improvement over baseline on a scale of 0–10: betamethasone/ gentamicin group baseline score of 6·1 reduced to 1·0; betamethasone 6·1 reduced to 1·8; gentamicin group 6·6 reduced to 4·2	Method and concealment of randomisation unclear; study described as double blind; 4 dropouts; no ITT analysis	Treatment responses were slightly larger for steroid/antibiotic combination but none were statistically significant; bacterial growth similar in all three groups
Hjorth et al. 1985[16] (Denmark)	0·1% betamethasone 17-valerate v betamethasone 17-valerate plus 2% fusidic acid	60 atopic dermatitis patients with "potentially infected" atopic eczema	Prospective, randomised, left–right, parallel study; 7 days duration	Bacteriological swabs; clinical symptoms: vesicles, oedema, erythema, excoriation, crusting, lichenification, itching	Data for mean atopic dermatitis score not given; only result is investigator preference: 29 no preference, 22 preferred betamethasone plus fusidic acid, 9 preferred betamethasone alone	Method and concealment of randomisation unclear; study described as double blind; no dropouts or withdrawals	More data requested from author but is sadly deceased. Study provides no evidence of improved efficacy of betamethasone/ fusidic acid combination above betamethasone alone in infected atopic eczema
Wilkinson and Leigh 1985[17] (UK)	0·1% betamethasone plus 2% fusidic acid cream v 0·1% betamethasone plus 0·5% neomycin cream two or three times daily	43 infected or potentially infected atopic eczema patients	Prospective, randomised, parallel study; 2 weeks duration	Severity of lesions assessed by patient and doctor as either very severe, severe, moderate, mild, minimal, or absent; swabs taken for infection	95% patients (91% doctors) felt lesions improved after betamethasone plus fusidic acid after 2 weeks versus 100% patients (100% doctors) with betamethasone plus	Method and concealment of randomisation unclear; study described as double blind, 9 withdrawals and dropouts but unclear which type	Impossible to assess the additional benefit of antibiotics in the absence of a steroid-only group

(Continued)

Table 17.6 (Continued)

Study	Interventions and comparator	Study population and sample size	Trial design, description and follow up	Outcome measures	Main reported results	Quality of reporting	Comment
					of eczema these patients had (7 types of dermatoses reported)	neomycin; no separate data for bacteriological efficacy for atopic dermatitis	
Thaci et al. 1999[15] (Germany)	2% fusidic acid plus 0·1% betamethasone cream v 2% fusidic acid plus 0·1% betamethasone ointment vs ointment vehicle twice daily	59 patients with potentially infected atopic dermatitis	Prospective, randomised, parallel study; 10 days duration	Bacteriological tests; signs and symptoms on a four-point scale; investigator-assessed overall clinical response	Overall clinical response assessed by investigator as "clearance" or "marked improvement" in 92% of fusidic acid/betamethasone cream group, in 84% of fusidic acid/beta- methasone ointment group, and 25% of ointment vehicle group; no statistically significant difference between the two formulations	Method and concealment of randomisation unclear; study described as double-blind; no withdrawals or dropouts mentioned	Abstract only; only results reported in text given
Meenan[18] 1988 (Eire)	0·1% hydrocortisone 17-butyrate plus 3% chlorquinaldol (Locoid C) v 0·1% triamcinolone aceton-ide plus 0·25% neo-mycin plus 0·025% gramicidin plus nystatin (Triadcorty®)	40 children with eczema for 3 months to 14 years with secondary infection	Prospective, randomised, parallel study; 14 days duration	Pruritus, erythema, lichenification, oozing/crusting, scaling; skin swabs for infection; patient and physician global scores	"Both treatments produced a highly significant (P<0·001) linear reduction in the scores for all para-meters, no significant difference between treat-ments"; "highly significant reduction in infection for both treatments (P<0·001)	Method and concealment of randomisation unclear; study described as double-blind; no data on withdrawals or dropouts given	Another uninformative study because both agents contain an antimicrobial/antiseptic, and no steroid-only comparator

(Continued)

Table 17.6 *(Continued)*

Study	Interventions and comparator	Study population and sample size	Trial design, description and follow up	Outcome measures	Main reported results	Quality of reporting	Comment
Zienicke 1993[19]	Prednicarbate 0·25% cream v prednicarbate 0·25% cream plus didecyldimethylamm-oniumchloride 0·25%	180 patients with superinfected atopic eczema	Prospective, randomised, parallel study; 34 days duration	Redness, swelling, papulovesicles, vesicles, pustules, bullae, papules, oozing, crusting and scaling on a score of 1–5	Clinical score at baseline of over 25 for both drugs reduced to 13·5 for prednicarbate and 13 for prednicarbate plus didecyldimethyl-ammoniumchloride; 30% of patients still had S. aureus at day 34 compared with 100% at start	Method and concealment of randomisation unclear; study described as double-blind; 44 withdrawals/dropouts; no ITT analysis	Duplicate publication[28], no clinical or statistical difference between groups

Table 17.7 Randomised controlled trials that have evaluated antiseptics for atopic eczema

Study	Interventions and comparator	Study population and sample size	Trial design, description and follow up	Outcome measures	Main reported results	Quality of reporting	Comment
Stalder et al. 1992[10] (France)	Proprietary brand of chlorhexidine solution compared against 1:20 000 dilution of potassium permanganate solution for 7 days in addition to topical desonide (topical steroid)	20 children aged 5 months to 9 years; no details of whether they were clinically infected	Parallel-group, double-blind, randomised study; 1 week duration	Bacterial counts; composite clinical severity score; patient-reported tolerance	Total severity score fell from 8·8 at day 0 to 5·7 at the end of the 7 days for chlorexidine and from 11·1 to 8·8 for the permanganate group ($P = 0.63$). Intensity and number of affected sites also showed very little difference between the two groups. Bacterial counts fell substantially in both groups but they were not statistically significant ($P = 0.37$) and baseline scores in the two groups were quite different. Clinical tolerance was "good" in both groups	Poor quality of reporting with very few methodological details	Difficult to interpret such a small study which compares two active treatments; clinical tolerance data were useful
Harper 1995[22] (England)	Standard proprietary bath emollient (Oilatum) v the same with added	30 children aged 1-9 years with recurrent infections and/or frequent	Randomised crossover study of two 4-week treatment periods	Composite sign and symptom score (max. 100), patient recorded global	On the basis of 26 evaluable patients, the change from baseline score (baselines scores	Method of randomisation described, but no ITT analysis; statistical	Study published in a "round table" discussion document sponsored by the manufacturer.

(Continued)

Table 17.7 (Continued)

Study	Interventions and comparator	Study population and sample size	Trial design, description and follow up	Outcome measures	Main reported results	Quality of reporting	Comment
	antiseptic 6% w/w benzalkonium chloride and 2% triclosan (Oilatum plus)	exacerbation	with a 2-week wash-out period in between	overall impression, and global change scales	not given) was 9·0 for those using the antiseptic emollient compared with 2·7 for those with regular emollient at 4 weeks. Patient-rated scores were not significantly different between the two treatments (data not shown)	tests of change in scores from baseline for each treatment separately rather than the appropriate test of the difference in score changes between the two treatments	Difficult to interpret in view of the wrong statistical tests used and missing patient-reported data
Holland et al. 1995[23] (England)	Comparison of a standard proprietary bath emollient (Oilatum) v same emollient with 6% w/w benzalkonium chloride and 2% triclosan (Oilatum plus)	15 patients aged 4–34 years with moderate-to-severe atopic eczema with S. aureus on their skin	Parallel-group, randomised, double-blind study; 4 weeks duration	Clinical scores of signs, symptoms and extent and bacterial counts	At the end of 4 weeks' treatments, clinical scores in the emollient/antiseptic group had fallen more than those in the emollient-only group, but these were not statistically significant. There was no statistically significant difference in S. aureus counts between the two groups at the end of the treatment period. Five dropouts in the emollient-only group	No description of randomisation process or ITT analysis; although described as a parallel study, patients were paired for matching pre-treatment S. aureus population densities	Difficult to interpret the lack of efficacy in such a small study with high dropout rate

(Continued)

Table 17.7 *(Continued)*

Study	Interventions, and comparator	Study population and sample size	Trial design, description and follow up	Outcome measures	Main reported results	Quality of reporting	Comment
Sasai-Takedatsu et al. 1997[26] (Japan)	Comparison of spraying infants with water twice a day for 1 week or an acid electrolytic water (pH<2.7) using a spray gun (no co-treatment allowed in this period)	22 children aged 2–56 months with mild-to-moderate atopic eczema	Parallel-group, randomised, double-blind study; 1 week duration	Colony counts of *S. aureus*; composite grading score; scores for itching and sleep disturbance	Colony counts decreased by around 50% in the active but not in the water group (though baseline scores were quite different). Global severity scores fell from 9 to 5 in the active group compared with a rise from 7 to 8 in the water group; scores for itching and sleep also decreased in the active group but not in the water group. Although the authors found a statistically significant change in all of these measures for the active group compared with baseline, they did not do the appropriate test of difference between the two groups	Although described as randomised, this is suspect because authors state that the 22 patients were "arbitrarily divided by a referee physician into two groups of 11"; blinding also seems unlikely because of the taste and sensation of the acid	Difficult to interpret because the correct statistical comparison was not done and because of the short duration of the study. Some serious concerns about the study quality. The ethics of spraying an acid onto young infants is also questionable
Hizawa et al. 1998[25]	Daily povidone-iodine solution to one	16 volunteers with atopic eczema aged	Right–left, investigator-blinded	Physician-assessed before and after	Of 15 evaluable patients, physicians reported an	Unclear method and concealment of	Inconclusive study in view of threat of unblinding,

(Continued)

Table 17.7 (*Continued*)

Study	Interventions and comparator	Study population and sample size	Trial design, description and follow up	Outcome measures	Main reported results	Quality of reporting	Comment
(Japan)	arm versus nothing else on opposite side (emollients only)	12–29 years with similar eczema lesions in each elbow fold	comparison study; 1 week duration	photographs; colony counts of after of *S. aureus*	improvement in the povidone-treated sites (*P*<0·01), but not on the control sites. Bacterial colonisation was significantly reduced on the treated but not the untreated sites. No summary data of differences between treatments reported	randomisation; investigator masking suspect as iodine stains the skin	short duration and failure to perform the appropriate statistical tests. Worth pursuing in a larger double-blind study as povidone iodine is a cheap antiseptic with good anti-staphylococcal properties.
Breneman et al. 2001[24] (USA)	1·5% triclocarban bar v placebo soap	50 patients with moderately severe atopic eczema	Prospective, randomised, double-blind study; 14-day standardisation period followed by 42-day treatment period and 21-day regression period	Rating scale of extent and severity of disease including itch; investigators global evaluation of change from day 0 to days 14, 28 and 42 on a scale of −5–5; bacterial counts and topical steroid usage were also recorded	Mean global improvement scores from start of treatment through to end of regression period shown on graph only. Comment that global improvement was significantly greater in antibacterial than placebo (no *P* value or CI given) group. Microbiology results shown on graph – selected only patients with *S. aureus* at start.	Method of randomisation and concealment not given; blinding difficult to assess; one dropout because of adverse event mentioned; not clear how many dropouts altogether and not clear if ITT; lack of actual data for most results	Although the authors claim a statistically significant improvement in the group using the antibacterial soap throughout, no actual data are given. The data shown in graphical form show a marked difference in baseline scores, followed by a parallel degree of improvement in each group

CI, confidence interval; ITT, intention-to-treat

common practice to prescribe a short course of oral antibiotics in acute infected eczema. There is some evidence to support this, and no evidence of a detrimental effect. In contrast, there is no evidence to support the use of longer-term antibiotics in people with atopic eczema whose skin is colonised with *S. aureus*, and there is some evidence that use of such antibiotics may promote antibiotic resistance.

Do topical steroids help in clinically infected atopic eczema?

Efficacy
Versus vehicle
We found no RCTs that addressed this question in clinically infected atopic eczema.

Non-infected eczema
We located three RCTs that have demonstrated the effectiveness of topical steroids in reducing *S. aureus* in clinically non-infected atopic eczema. In the study by Stalder *et al.*[10] topical desonide was significantly better than its excipient alone at reducing *S. aureus* and global clinical score. In the second study,[11] Group A compared a moderate-strength steroid with an alternative similar steroid in propylene glycol (antiseptic) base; Group B compared a potent steroid with potent steroid plus neomycin (antibiotic). In both groups, the addition of the antimicrobial did not improve clinical outcome. In the third study[12] 1% hydrocortisone was as effective as 1% hydrocortisone/2% fusidic acid in terms of overall clinical outcome, although the combination treatment was more effective at reducing *S. aureus*.[12]

Possible drawbacks
Minor skin irritation or flare of eczema occurred in 1–3% of patients across the study groups.

Comment and implications
There is evidence that topical steroids alone are effective in reducing bacterial counts in clinically non-infected eczema. No studies have evaluated the efficacy of topical steroids alone for clinically infected atopic eczema.

How effective are topical antibiotics in clinically infected atopic eczema?

Effectiveness
One RCT evaluated topical antibiotics in the treatment of clinically infected atopic eczema (Table 17.6). Gentamicin cream was significantly less effective at reducing dermatitis activity than betamethasone valerate/gentamicin or betamethasone alone.[13]

Non-infected eczema
Two RCTs have looked at topical antibiotics in people with clinically non-infected atopic eczema. In the first, which compared mupirocin ointment with placebo ointment (both with steroid), mupirocin (but not placebo) significantly reduced *S. aureus* compared with baseline, and clinical scores were significantly better in the mupirocin group than placebo. However, recolonisation occurred in the 4-week follow up period.[14] Ramsay *et al.*[12] showed that fusidic acid 2% cream resulted in more treatment failures than hydrocortisone/fusidic acid.

Possible drawbacks
Minor skin irritation or eczema flare occurred in 18% of patients in the fusidic acid group, compared with only 3% in the steroid/fusidic acid group.[12]

Comment and implications
These studies are in keeping with current clinical practice, which recognises the need for topical

steroids in the treatment of clinically infected eczema. There is concern about emergence of resistant organisms resulting from the use of topical antibiotics.

Is the addition of antibiotics to topical steroids beneficial?

Effectiveness
We found four RCTs evaluating steroid/antibiotic combinations for clinically infected atopic eczema[13,15-17] (Table 17.6).

Versus vehicle
The study by Thaci et al.[15] showed superior benefit of both betamethasone/fusidic acid ointment and cream over vehicle alone, with no significant difference between cream and ointment.

Versus topical steroid
Two RCTs found no significant difference in clinical signs or symptoms when betamethasone valerate/fusidic acid[16] or betamethasone/gentamicin[13] were compared with topical steroid alone.

Versus each other
There was no significant difference between 0·1% betamethasone/2% fusidic acid and 0·1% betamethasone/0·5% neomycin in terms of clinical efficacy or ability to eradicate S. aureus.[17]

Non-infected eczema
One further RCT was located that has evaluated topical steroid/antibiotic treatment for non-clinically infected atopic eczema. In this study, 2% fusidic acid/1% hydrocortisone showed no clear benefit over 1% hydrocortisone alone in reducing atopic eczema activity, but it was significantly better at reducing S. aureus.[12]

Possible drawbacks
Minor skin irritation, flare of dermatitis and possible hypersensitivity reactions occurred in 1–3% of patients across the groups. Despite the concern about emergence of resistant organisms resulting from the use of topical antibiotics, this was not recorded in any of the studies.

Comment and implications
There is a conspicuous lack of evidence that topical steroid/antibiotic combinations are more effective than topical steroids alone in improving the clinical signs and symptoms of clinically infected atopic eczema despite their widespread use. The same applies to non-clinically infected eczema.

How useful are topical steroid/antiseptic combinations?

Effectiveness
We found 2 RCTs that evaluated topical steroid/antiseptic combinations in the treatment of clinically infected atopic eczema[18,19] (Table 17.6). The first study, by Meenan, showed no difference in efficacy between Triadcortyl cream and Locoid C.[18] In the second study by Zienicke,[19] a topical steroid/antiseptic was compared with topical steroid alone; 0·25% prednicarbate/didecyldimethylammoniumchloride cream and 0·25% prednicarbate cream were both effective at reducing clinical scores and bacterial counts, with no significant difference between them.[19]

Possible drawbacks
Minor skin irritation was reported in one patient in one study.

Comment and implications

There is no evidence to support a benefit from topical steroid/antiseptic combinations over topical steroid alone.

How effective are topical antifungals?

Effectiveness

One RCT evaluated a combination of topical steroid/antibiotic/antifungal versus topical steroid/antiseptic in clinically infected atopic eczema (Table 17.6).[18] Both combinations produced a highly significant reduction in clinical scores and bacterial counts, with no significant difference between treatments.[18]

Non-infected eczema

We located two further RCTs evaluating topical antifungals in non-clinically infected atopic eczema.[20,21] The first small study compared topical steroid/antibiotic/antifungal against topical steroid/antibiotic, and showed a significant improvement in the four patients treated with 0·1% triamcinolone acetonide/0·35% neomycin/ undecylenic acid compared with the six receiving the same steroid/antibiotic combination but without undecylenic acid.[20] In the second study, Broberg et al.[21] attempted to evaluate the role of antifungals in atopic eczema of the head and neck area. All patients received oral antibiotics, followed by randomisation to either miconazole-hydrocortisone cream plus ketoconazole shampoo or hydrocortisone cream plus placebo shampoo. There was no significant difference between the groups in clinical outcome.[21]

Possible drawbacks

Where side-effects were documented, minor skin irritation and possible hypersensitivity reactions were seen in up to 5% of patients across the groups.

Comment and implications

It is difficult to draw conclusions about the role of antifungals from these small and disparate studies. There is no current evidence to support their routine use in the treatment of clinically infected atopic eczema.

How useful are antiseptics agents in clinically infected atopic eczema?

This section includes antiseptic emollients, bath additives and other antiseptic treatments.

Efficacy

There are no RCTs of antiseptics in clinically infected atopic eczema.

Non-infected eczema

We located six RCTs of antiseptics in non-clinically infected eczema,[22–27] summarised in Table 17.7.

Antiseptic versus standard bath emollient:

Two RCTs have compared a standard bath emollient, Oilatum (acetylated wool alcohols 5%, liquid paraffin 63·4%) with an emollient plus antiseptic, Oilatum Plus (benzalkonium chloride 6%, triclosan 2%, light liquid paraffin 52·5%). No significant difference was demonstrated in terms of clinical or microbiological outcomes.[22,23]

Antiseptic soap versus placebo soap

This study compared a soap containing 1·5% triclocarban with an identical placebo soap. The authors state that the global change in atopic eczema severity was significantly greater in the treatment than the placebo group, but the actual data are missing. Graphical data suggest a similar degree of improvement in both groups.[24]

Topical antiseptic versus no topical antiseptic

Two RCTs were identified. The first study reported improvement on the arm treated with daily povidine iodine solution but not on the untreated side, compared with baseline.[25] In the second study, acid electrolytic water sprayed onto infants significantly reduced clinical scores and *S. aureus* counts compared with baseline. Neither study reported a comparison of treatments.[26]

Comparison of two topical antiseptics

This study compared a proprietary brand of chlorhexidine with a 1:20 000 dilution of potassium permanganate, in addition to topical steroid in both groups, and found no significant difference in clinical or bacteriological outcomes.[10]

Drawbacks

Skin irritation, pruritus and worsening of dermatitis were the main side-effects reported in the studies where adverse events were documented. These were reported more frequently overall in the antiseptic-treated groups.

Comment and clinical implications

Antiseptic-containing preparations are in common use in the management of atopic eczema. There are no RCTs of many of the commonly used preparations. The current evidence base for the use of such preparations in infected or clinically non-infected atopic eczema does not provide any clear support for their use. Further large studies with appropriate comparators are required.

References

1. Hauser C, Wuethrich B, Matter L *et al. Staphylococcus aureus* skin colonisation in atopic dermatitis patients. *Dermatologica* 1985;**170**:35–9.

2. Weinberg E, Fourie B, Allmann B, Toerien A. The use of cefadroxil in superinfected atopic dermatitis. *Curr Ther Res Clin Exp* 1992;**52**:671–6.

3. David TJ, Cambridge GC. Bacterial infection and atopic eczema. *Arch Dis Child* 1986;**61**:20–3.

4. Leyden JE, Marples RR, Kligman AM. *Staphylococcal aureus* in the lesions of atopic dermatitis. *Br J Dermatol* 1974;**90**:525–30.

5. Goh CL, Wong JS, Yoke CG. Skin colonisation of *Staphylococcus aureus* in atopic dermatitis patients seen at the National Skin Centre, Singapore. *Int J Derm* 1997;**36**:653–7.

6. Hoare C, Li Wan Po A, Williams H. Systematic review of treatments for atopic eczema. *Health Technol Assess* 2000;**4**(37).

7. Salo OP, Gordin A, Brandt H, Antikainen R. Efficacy and tolerability of erythromycin acistrate and erythromycin stearate in acute skin infections of patients with atopic eczema. J Antimicrob Chemother 1988;**21**(Suppl. D):D 101–6.

8. Ewing CI, Ashcroft C, Gibbs AC, Jones GA, Connor PJ, David TJ. Flucloxacillin in the treatment of atopic dermatitis. *Br J Dermatol* 1998;**138**:1022–9.

9. Boguniewicz M, Sampson H, Leung S, Harbeck R, Leung DYM. Effects of cefuroxime axetil on *Staphylococcus aureus* colonisation and superantigen production in atopic dermatitis. *J All Clin Immunol* 2001;**108**:651–2.

10. Stalder JF, Fleury M, Sourisse M *et al.* Local steroid therapy and bacterial skin flora in atopic dermatitis. *Br J Dermatol* 1994;**131**:536–40.

11. Nilsson EJ, Henning CG, Magnusson J. Topical corticosteroids and *Staphylococcus aureus* in atopic dermatitis. *J Am Acad Derm* 1992;**27**:29–34.

12. Ramsay CA, Savoie JM, Gilbert M, Gidon M, Kidson P. The treatment of atopic dermatitis with topical fusidic acid and hydrocortisone acetate. *J Eur Acad Dermatol Venereol* 1996;**7**(Suppl. I):S15–22.

13. Wachs GN, Maibach HI. Co-operative double-blind trial of an antibiotic/corticoid combination in impetiginized atopic dermatitis. *Br J Dermatol* 1976;**95**:323–8.

14. Lever R, Hadley K, Downey D, Mackie R. Staphylococcal colonization in atopic dermatitis and the effect of topical mupirocin therapy. *Br J Dermatol* 1988;**119**:189–98.

15. Thaci D, Kokorsch J, Kaufmann R. Fusidic acid/betamethasone 17-valerate in potentially infected

atopic dermatitis. *J Eur Acad Dermatol Venereol* 1999;**12**(Suppl. 2):S163.

16. Hjorth N, Schmidt H, Thomsen K. Fusidic acid plus betamethasone in infected or potentially infected eczema. *Pharmatherapeutica* 1985;**4**:126–31.

17. Wilkinson RD, Leigh DA. Comparative efficacy of betamethasone and either fusidic acid or neomycin in infected or potentially infected eczema. *Curr Ther Res* 1985;**38**:177–82.

18. Meenan FO. A double-blind comparative study to compare the efficacy of locoid c with tri-adcortyl in children with infected eczema. *Br J Clin Pract* 1988;**42**:200–2.

19. Zienicke H. Topical glucocorticoids and anti-infectives: a rational combination? *Curr Probl Dermatol* 1993;**21**:186–91.

20. Anonymous. Treatment of eczemas and infected eczemas. *Br J Clin Pract* 1967;**21**:505–7.

21. Broberg A, Faergemann J. Topical antimycotic treatment of atopic dermatitis in the head/neck area. A double-blind randomised study. *Acta Derm Venereol* 1995;**75**:46–9.

22. Harper J. Double-blind comparison of an antiseptic oil-based bath additive (Oilatum Plus) with regular Oilatum (Oilatum Emollient) for the treatment of atopic eczema. In: Lever R, Levy J, eds. *The Bacteriology of Eczema*. London: The Royal Society of Medicine Press, 1995.

23. Holland KT, Bojar RA, Cunliffe WJ. A comparison of the effect of treatment of atopic eczema with and without antimicrobial compounds. In: Lever R, Levy J, eds. *The Bacteriology of Eczema*. London: The Royal Society of Medicine Press, 1995.

24. Breneman DL, Hanifin JM, Berge CA, Keswick BH, Neumann PB. The effect of antibacterial soap with 1·5% triclocarban on *Staphylococcus aureus* in patients with atopic dermatitis. *Cutis* 2000;**66**:296–300.

25. Hizawa T, Sano H, Endo K, Fukuzumi T, Kataoka Y, Aoki T. Is povidone-iodine effective to the lesions of atopic dermatitis? *Skin Res* 1998;**40**(Suppl. 20):134–9.

26. Sasai-Takedatsu M, Kojima T, Yamamoto A *et al.* Reduction of *Staphylococcus aureus* in atopic skin lesions with acid electrolytic water – a new therapeutic strategy for atopic dermatitis. *Allergy* 1997;**52**:1012–16.

27. Stalder JF, Fleury M, Sourisse M *et al.* Comparitive effects of two topical antiseptics (chlorhexadine *v* KMnO$_4$) on bacterial skin flora in atopic dermatitis. *Acta Dermato Venereol* 1992;**Suppl 176**:132–4.

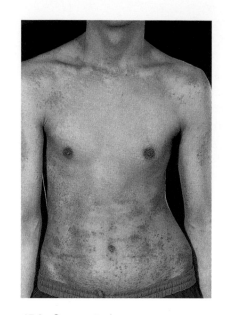

Figure 17.3 Severe atopic eczema

28. Korting HC, Zienicke H, Braun-Falco O, Bork K, *et al.* Modern topical glucocorticoids and anti-infectives for superinfected atopic eczema: do predicarbate and didecyldimethylammoniumchloride form a rational combination? *Infection* 1994;**6**:390–4.

Case scenario 3: an adult with severe atopic eczema
QUESTIONS

What is the role of systemic immunosuppressive therapy?

Immunosuppressive therapy is generally of proven benefit in the short- and intermediate-term (few months) management of atopic dermatitis. Immunomodulatory therapy (platelet activating factor, immunoglobulins, levamisole, etc.), however, is rarely used. We found immunomodulatory therapy to be poorly reported. We decided that the use of less concrete therapies such as anthelmintics and injections of antibodies/antigen complexes should not be considered here. Instead, we have concentrated on commonly used systemic immunosuppressive agents such as photochemotherapy, ciclosporin, azathioprine and systemic steroids. We examined global indices of well-being and also disease-specific indices such as patient-assessed itch. The long-term morbidity associated with such potentially highly toxic treatments is unclear. Here we concentrate on short-term treatments of the crisis-intervention type, this being the most common use of immunosuppressive treatments in dermatology. Much of the information is based on the NHS systematic review of treatments for atopic eczema highlighted in the opening section of this chapter.

Effectiveness
Azathioprine
No systematic review and no RCTs inform us about the use of azathioprine. Its use is confined to certain specialists and, anecdotally, it appears to have limited efficacy. An ongoing RCT has been identified on the Cochrane Skin Group's ongoing clinical trials register (see http://www.nottingham.ac.uk/~muzd) which is due to report in late 2002.

Systemic steroids
Systemic prednisolone is commonly used in short bursts (a few weeks) for severe atopic eczema. The systematic review concluded that the potency of this approach beyond that of placebo was large (Table 17.8).[2,4,10] There are no trials that properly evaluate the treatment according to Helsinki protocols (i.e. against another validated form of immunosupression such as ciclosporin). The trials also did not report long-term relapse rates or follow up disease severity.

Ciclosporin
The systematic review found ciclosporin to be effective, although of unknown efficacy compared with systemic steroids. Of the 10 available trails,[1,3,11,14–18,20,21] three studies[11,15,18] were systematically pooled with respect to itch scores. The pooled mean difference in itch scores was 15 (95% CI 9 to 23) points lower for ciclosporin, as assessed by a self-reported visual analogue scale (up to 100 mm).

The degree of stress, brought upon physician and patient alike by the use of this drug with potentially serious side-effects,[19] is almost certainly significant and might reasonably be expected to impact upon quality-of-life scores. This omission in the studies and lack of comparison with the "best of the rest" of the immunosuppressive agents makes it difficult to know if ciclosporin can be recommended in preference to systemic steroids.

Phototherapy and photochemotherapy
Broadly speaking, light therapy appears to improve responses in patients, and these responses are extremely significant if the placebo effect is included (tanning makes placebo effect dissociations near impossible). The extent to which the disease is improved by the physiological response of tanning compared to the psychological effect of being tanned is a fundamental problem. The systematic review identified six RCTs[5–9,12] and we identified a further one[13] (Table 17.9). The seven trials differed in methodology, with randomisation, blinding and controls proving difficult. Most of the trials suggest positive results.

Drawbacks
All of the immunosuppressants currently available carry potentially serious side-effects such as kidney damage (ciclosporin), bone marrow suppression (azathioprine), osteoporosis (systemic steroids) and skin cancer (photochemotherapy). These are described in more detail in the systematic review. It is difficult to make any statements about how useful these drugs are in comparison with one another because the impact of these adverse effects (for example azathioprine-induced bone marrow

Table 17.8 Randomised controlled trials of systemic corticosteroids in atopic dermatitis

Study	Interventions and comparator	Study population and sample size	Trial design, description and follow up	Outcome measures	Main reported results	Quality of reporting	Comment
Dickey 1976[2‡‡] (USA)	Betamethasone sodium phosphate 4·0 mg/ml injection v dexamethasone sodium phosphate 4·0 mg/ml injection once daily	22 patients with moderate-to-severe atopic dermatitis	Prospective, randomised, parallel study; 24 hours duration	Inflammation, vesiculation, pruritus, exudation, excoriations, overall evaluation	Overall evaluation on a four-point rating scale: with betamethasone, 3·44 (baseline) reduced to 2·89; with dexametha-sone 3·62 (baseline) reduced to 2·69	Method and concealment of randomisation unclear; study described as double-blind; withdrawals and dropouts not mentioned	Although a placebo group might have been ethically difficult, patient-based views on treatment response would have been useful
Heddle et al. 1984[‡‡] (UK)	Oral plus nasal beclomethasone dipropionate three times daily v placebo	27 children with moderate-to-severe atopic eczema	Prospective, randomised, crossover study; 4 weeks duration	Patient-assessed itch and sleep loss (VAS); physician-assessed redness, vesiculation, crusting, excoriation, lichenification	Only parental score for itch and antihistamine use were significantly lower on beclomethasone than on placebo; use of topical steroids and sleep loss did not show any significant change; other significant changes, particularly surface damage	Method and concealment of randomisation unclear; study described as double-blind; 1 withdrawal, no ITT	Crossover study with significant treatment order interactions; large treatment effects
La Rosa et al. 1995[‡*10] (Italy)	Systemic flunisolide 640–1200 micrograms twice daily v placebo	20 children with severe atopic dermatitis	Prospective, randomised, crossover study; 2 weeks duration	Pruritus, erythema/oedema, excoriation, papulation/erosion/ scaling, lichenification	Improvement over baseline for total clinical severity score: group A, 75 reduced to 34; group B, 74 reduced to 29	Method and conceal-ment of randomisation unclear; study descri-bed as double-blind; withdrawals/dropouts not mentioned	Big treatment effects

*used physician-assessed global severity

‡used patient-assessed global severity

Table 17.9 Randomised controlled trials of phototherapy and photochemotherapy in atopic dermatitis

Study	Interventions and comparator (co-treatments)	Study population and sample size	Trial design, description and follow up	Outcome measures	Main reported results	Quality of reporting	Comment
Reynolds et al. 2001[13] (UK)	Twice-weekly TLO-1 NBUVB (150 mJ/cm²) v UVA 15 J/cm² for 12 weeks or visible fluorescent light	73 patients; 16–65 years old	Prospective, controlled randomised study with follow up 3 months after last dose	Patient-assessed itch scales, area scores and physician assessed 6-site score summation for disease activity	UVB reduced disease score by 6·7 points (95% CI 2 to 12) over visible light. UVA reduced the same by 1 points (95% CI –5 to 3).	Structured ITT analysis and adequately attempted blinding	13 dropouts had to be included; advantage of UVA over UVB; not significant despite conclusion
Jekler and Larko, 1988[6] Study 1 (Swe)	Three-times-weekly UVB (20–153 mJ/cm² up to 63–816 mJ/cm²) v placebo (visible light), three times per week (emollients and hydrocortisone)	17 patients over 15 years of age, most of whom had skin type III (tans easily, seldom burns)	Prospective, randomised, controlled left–right parallel study of 8 weeks duration	Patients assessed for pruritus, lichenification, scaling, xerosis, vesiculation, excoriations, erythema; variables assessed on a scale of 0–3, plus a global assessment	Improvement from baseline of 1·5 (mean) to 0·7 for UVB and 1·4 for placebo for overall clinical response (P<0·001) Thus the total score was significantly lower for the UVB-treated side	Described as randomised but method unclear; blinding unlikely because of mild burning on UVB-treated side; no ITT analysis	Unclear if randomisation referred to side of active/placebo treatment or to type of MED: large treatment effect for all parameters; many dropouts (11/17) because of "intercurrent disease" and lack of time for treatments
Jekler & Larko, 1988[6] Study 2 (Swe)	Three-times-weekly UVB given at 80% MED versus UVB at 40% of MED (emollients and hydrocortisone)	25 patients, mean age 25·9 years, most with skin type III	Randomised right/left side parallel study for 8 weeks	As for Study 1 above	Clearing or considerable improvement in 15/25 on high-dose UVB v 16/25 with low-dose (not statistically significant)	Methods very scanty; randomisation unclear; probably unblinded; no ITT analysis	Further details of study found in Jeckler 1992 thesis. This study of high-v low-dose UVB suggested very little difference between the two, but power of study is very limited
Jekler and Larko, 1991[7]	UVA (average 8·1 mW/cm²) v UVB (0·85 mW/cm²)	33 patients, mean age 23·3 years; mean disease	Prospective, randomised left right parallel study	Patients assessed for pruritus, lichenification, scaling,	Improvement from mean baseline of 10·3 (range 6–18) for clinical sign	Described as single blind and randomised but methods unclear;	Both treatments induced large improvements compared with baseline,

(*Continued*)

Table 17.9 (*Continued*)

Study	Interventions and comparator (co-treatments)	Study population and sample size	Trial design, description and follow up	Outcome measures	Main reported results	Quality of reporting	Comment
(Swe)	Three-times-weekly (emollients and hydrocortisone)	duration of 19·6 years; most with skin type III	of 8 weeks duration	xerosis, vesiculation, excoriations, erythema and an overall evaluation on a score of 0-3 (none to severe); healing evaluated on a scale of 3 to −1 (3 = healed, −1 = worse)	(total score) decreased to 5·5 for UVA and 6·4 for UVB. Pruritus scored separately with baseline of 2·2, improving to 1·1 after UVA and 1·3 after UVB.	differential tan on side of the body likely to have unblinded study; 12 withdrawals and dropouts, no description given; no ITT analysis	with some small statistically significant change in favour of UVA. Most patients preferred UVA
Jekler 1992[5] (Swe)	Mixed UVA (74%) and UVB (26%) v UVB Three-times per week	30 patients, mean age 24·8 years; mean disease duration 20·5 years	Prospective, randomised left-right parallel study of 8 weeks duration	Patients assessed for pruritus, lichenification, scaling, xerosis, vesiculation, excoriations, erythema and an overall evaluation on a score of 0-3 (none to severe); healing evaluated on a scale of 3 to −1 (3 = healed, −1 = worse)	A decrease from baseline score of 10·8 to 5·2 for UVA/B and 6·1 for UVB (P = 0·002 for difference in scores between treatments); 21/24 patients reported mild burning with UVB (severe in 6 patients) compared with 3 episodes of mild burning with UVA/B (none severe)	Described as randomised but method unclear; no blinding; no withdrawals or dropouts	This thesis also presents the two studies reported in Jekler and Larko, 1988[6] in more detail; a further three small left-right comparison studies are also described comparing UVA v UVB, low-dose UVB v UVA/B, and UVA v UVA/B, but it is unclear if these were RCTs
Krutmann et al. 1992[8] (Ger)	High-dose UVA1 (0–130 J/cm² once daily) v UVA/B therapy (up to 30 J/cm² UVB and 7.5	25 young adults with atopic eczema and definite atopy	Prospective, randomised, parallel study of 15 days duration	Costa scoring system: erythema, oedema, vesicles, exudation, crusts, excoriations, scales,	A decrease from baseline of 53 (overall score) to 14 after UVA1 (P<0·001 against comparator change); comparative	Described as "randomly selected patients" but method unclear; (personal communication)	Unclear if patients randomised but confirmed by authors; large treatment effects, all in favour of high-dose UVA

(*Continued*)

Table 17.9 (*Continued*)

Study	Interventions and comparator (co-treatments)	Study population and sample size	Trial design description and follow up	Outcome measures	Main reported results	Quality of reporting	Comment
	J/cm² UVA daily (emollients)			lichenification, pruritus, loss of sleep on a seven-point scale (0 = no lesion, 6 = extremely severe)	data for UVA/B not given but shown in graphical form only; baseline score of 52 decreased to 38 with UVA/B (estimated from graph)	"treatments randomly allocated"; no blinding; no dropouts or withdrawals	over UVA/B
Krutmann et al. 1998[9] (Ger)	High-dose UVA 130 J/cm² once daily v once-daily fluocortolone 0·5% cream or ointment v UVA/B MED once daily	53 patients with acute severe exacerbation of atopic eczema	Prospective, randomised, parallel study of 10 days duration	Costa scoring system: erythema, oedema, vesicles, exudation, crusts, excoriations, scales, lichenification, pruritus, loss of sleep on a seven-point scale (0 = no lesion, 6 = extremely severe)	Improvement over baseline for total clinical score: high-dose UVA1 baseline of 56 reduced to 26; fluocortolone baseline of 60 reduced to 35; UVA/B baseline of 60 reduced to 42 (all after 10 days' treatment) P<0·0001.	"A randomisation sequence generated by random numbers"; no blinding; no withdrawals or dropouts	Very short duration; results had to be estimated from graphs; useful to have a comparison with topical steroids; study suggests superiority of high-dose UVA over a topical steroid
Reynolds et al. 1999[12] (UK)	NBUVB (up to 1·2 J/cm²) v UVA (up to 15 J/cm²) or placebo	73 adult patients with moderate-to-severe atopic eczema	Prospective, randomised, double-blind	Five clinical features at 6 separate body sites plus itch and	Mean reduction in total disease activity was 9·7 for 21 evaluable patients on NBUVB, 4·8 on UVA and 0·4 on placebo, the change significant at the 5% level (P<0·05) for NBUVB v placebo only	Study described as randomised (in balanced blocks),	Published in abstract form only at time of report; only 47 out of 73 patients

(*Continued*)

Table 17.9 (*Continued*)

Study	Interventions, co-treatments	Study population and sample size	Trial design description and follow up	Outcome measures	Main reported results	Quality of reporting	Comment
	(visible light) all twice weekly (mild-to-moderate topical steroids plus emollients)		parallel study of 12 weeks duration	sleep loss (VAS), and extent of disease recorded by one observer	90% (P=0·02) for NBUVB, 63% for UVA and 53% for placebo (P=0·02 compared with placebo); changes for sleep loss failed to reach statistical significance	controlled, and double blind; no ITT analysis	completed the study; study possibly partly unblinded because of lack of pigmentary changes on one side and burning on other
Der-Petrossian et al. 2000[22] (Austria)	NBUVB v bath PUVA 1 mg/l as 8-MOP three times per week	12 patients with severe/chronic atopic dermatitis, age 27 ± 11·3 years (mean ± SD)	Prospective, randomised, single-blind half-side comparison; 6 weeks duration	Patient-rated itch and sleep loss (VAS 0–10 cm) as part of SCORAD, doctor-rated global severity and global changes of modified SCORAD for eight signs and symptoms	Baseline scores of 100% SCORAD for bath-PUVA and UVB reduced by 65·7% for bath-PUVA treated side and 64·1% for UVB treated side (P=0·48)	Study described as randomised, and investigator blinded; no ITT analysis; two withdrawals, one due to exacerbation of atopic dermatitis, one because of fewer erythema reactions to the bath-PUVA side	A small study which took care to ensure that both treatments were given in equal doses; big falls in SCORAD scores for both treatments with little difference between the two

CI, confidence intervals; NBUVB, narrow-band UVB; MED, minimal erythema dose (i.e. minimal dose to produce redness); 8-MOP, 8-methoxypsoralen; SCORAD, severity scoring of atopic dermatitis VAS, visual analogue scale toxicity) can be predicted by tests beforehand and others (for example kidney damage with ciclosporine) can be identified at an early stage before any permanent damage has occurred. The relative efficacies of systemic immunosuppressants are therefore contingent upon the way they are used.

Clinical implications

Both ultraviolet light and systemic treatments such as short courses of oral steroids and ciclosporin are probably useful and safe to use in the person depicted in the case scenario. Safety is a factor limiting the long-term use of all of these agents. Planned short-term use (2–3 months) to try and gain a remission or give the person a "holiday" from severe symptoms seems a reasonable option, resorting to topical treatments such as intermittent use of potent topical steroids or tacrolimus once control is achieved.

Key points

- There is reasonable RCT evidence to support the use of systemic immunosuppressive therapies such as oral corticosteroids and ciclosporin.
- Both of these therapies are associated with significant side-effects which limit their short-to-medium-term use for major disease flares, with return to conventional topical treatment inbetween such flares.
- Photochemotherapy has consistently been shown to benefit atopic dermatitis, but is limited by the long-term risk of skin cancer after many treatments.
- The use of other common treatments such as azathioprine are not currently supported by RCT evidence.
- There is need for longer term studies of systemic immunosuppressive treatment for atopic dermatitis to evaluate long-term safety and whether use of these agents alters the natural history of the disease.

References

1. Cordero Miranda MA, Flores Sandoval G, Orea Solano M, Estrada Parra S, Serrano Miranda E. Safety and efficacy of treatment for severe atopic dermatitis with cyclosporin A and transfer factor. *Revista Alergia Mexico* 1999;**46**:49–57.

2. Dickey RF. Parenteral short-term corticosteroid therapy in moderate to severe dermatoses. A comparative multiclinic study. *Cutis* 1976;**17**:179–83.

3. Harper JI, Ahmed I, Barclay G *et al.* Cyclosporin for severe childhood atopic dermatitis: Short course versus continuous therapy. *Br J Dermatol* 2000;**142**:52–8.

4. Heddle RJ, Soothill JF, Bulpitt CJ, Atherton DJ. Combined oral and nasal beclomethasone diprorionate in children with atopic eczema: a randomised controlled trial. *BMJ Clin Res Ed* 1984;**289**:651–4.

5. Jekler J. Phototherapy of atopic dermatitis with ultraviolet radiation. *Acta Derm Venereol Suppl* 1992;**171**:1 37.

6. Jekler J, Larko O. UVB phototherapy of atopic dermatitis. *Br J Dermatol* 1988;**119**:697–705.

7. Jekler J, Larko O. UVA solarium versus UVB phototherapy of atopic dermatitis: a paired-comparison study. *Br J Dermatol* 1991;**125**:569–72.

8. Krutmann J, Czech W, Diepgen T, Niedner R, Kapp A, Schopf E. High-dose UVA1 therapy in the treatment of patients with atopic dermatitis. *J Am Acad Dermatol* 1992;**26**:225–30.

9. Krutmann J, Diepgen TL, Luger TA, Grabbe S, Meffert H, Sonnichsen N *et al.* High-dose UVA1 therapy for atopic dermatitis: results of a multicenter trial. *J Am Acad Dermatol* 1998;**38**:589–93.

10. La Rosa M, Musarra I, Ranno C *et al.* A randomized, double-blind, placebo-controlled crossover trial of systemic flunisolide in the treatment of children with severe atopic dermatitis. *Curr Ther Res Clin Exp* 1995;**56**:720–6.

11. Munro CS, Levell NJ, Shuster S, Friedmann PS. Maintenance treatment with cyclosporin in atopic eczema. *Br J Dermatol* 1994;**130**:376–80.

12. Reynolds NJ, Franklin V, Gray JC, Diffey BL, Farr PM. Effectiveness of narrow-band UVB (TL01) compared to UVA in adult atopic eczema: a randomised controlled trial. *Br J Dermatol* 1999;**141**(Suppl. 55):20.

13. Reynolds NJ, Franklin V, Gray JC, Diffey BL, Farr PM. Narrow-band ultraviolet B and broad band ultraviolet A phototherapy in adult atopic eczema: a randomised controlled trial. *Lancet* 2001;**357**(9273):2012–16.

14. Salek MS, Finlay AY, Luscombe DK *et al.* Cyclosporin greatly improves the quality of life of adults with severe atopic dermatitis. A randomized, double-blind, placebo-controlled trial. *Br J Dermatol* 1993;**129**:422–30.

15. Sowden JM, Berth-Jones J, Ross JS *et al.* Double-blind, controlled, crossover study of cyclosporin in adults with severe refractory atopic dermatitis [see comments]. *Lancet* 1991;**338**:137–40.

16. van Joost T, Heule F, Korstanje M, van den Broek MJ, Stenveld HJ, van Vloten WA. Cyclosporin in atopic dermatitis: a multicentre placebo-controlled study. *Br J Dermatol* 1994;**130**:634–40.

17. Wahlgren CF. Itch and atopic dermatitis: clinical and experimental studies. *Acta Derm Venereol Suppl* 1991;**165**:4–53.

18. Wahlgren CF, Scheynius A, Hagermark O. Antipruritic effect of oral cyclosporin a in atopic dermatitis. *Acta Derm Venereol* 1990;**70**:323–9.

19. Zaki I, Emerson R, Allen BR. Treatment of severe atopic dermatitis in childhood with cyclosporin. *Br J Dermatol* 1996;**135**:21–4.

20. Zonneveld IM, De Rie MA, Beljaards RC *et al.* The long-term safety and efficacy of cyclosporin in severe refractory atopic dermatitis: a comparison of two dosage regimens. *Br J Dermatol* 1996;**135**(Suppl. 48):15–20.

21. Zurbriggen B, Wuthrich B, Cachelin AB, Wili PB, Kagi MK. Comparison of two formulations of cyclosporin A in the treatment of severe atopic dermatitis. A double-blind, single-centre, cross-over pilot study. *Dermatology* 1999;**198**:56–60.

22. Der-Petrossian M, Seeber A, Honigsmann H, Tanew A. Half-side comparison study on the efficacy of 8-methoxypsoralen bath-PUVA versus narrow-band ultraviolet B phototherapy in patients with severe chronic atopic dermatitis.*Br J Dermatol* 2000;**142**:39–43.

Summary of the evidence base for atopic eczema

- Although around 300 RCTs have been conducted for atopic dermatitis, they have a limited ability to inform us about everyday management of patients. This is partly due to a generally poor quality of study reporting. All dermatology journals have a role to play here by insisting on basic standard of clinical trial reporting, as outlined in the CONSORT statement (http://www.consort-statement.org).

- Most of the trials of people with atopic dermatitis have reflected the agenda of the drug industry. This has meant introducing more "me-too" drugs on to the market and cleverly introducing them in a way that makes comparison with existing treatments impossible.

- Independent trials are needed to make head-to-head comparisons.

- Cost-effectiveness studies of topical steroids compared with the newer topical immunomodulatory agents are needed.

- Cheap and well-tried systemic agents such as oral steroids and azathioprine need to be compared against each other and against the more expensive agents such as ciclosporin that have found their way on to the market through mainly placebo-controlled studies.

- Some interventions (for example topical steroids and ultraviolet light therapy) are well supported by RCT evidence.

- For other interventions (such as Chinese herbs and house dust mite reduction) there is simply insufficient evidence to decide whether they are effective – better research is needed.

- In some areas (for example topical steroid/antibiotic combinations or bath antiseptics) the RCT evidence did not support a clinically useful effect, providing dermatologists and patients with an opportunity to disinvest in such treatment rituals.

- Some treatments currently in use (for example oral azathrioprine) have not been tested within RCTs at all, making primary research in these areas an urgent research priority.

18
Seborrhoeic dermatitis

Mauro Picardo and Norma Cameli

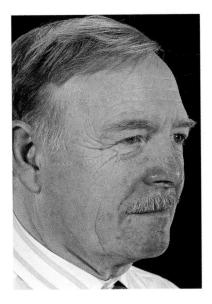

Figure 18.1 Patient with seborrhoeic dermatitis

Background
Definition

Seborrhoeic dermatitis is a chronic inflammatory skin disease characterised by erythematous and scaling plaques, with a distinctive distribution in areas rich in sebaceous glands, such as the scalp, eyebrows, nasolabial folds, retroauricular regions, sternum and between the shoulder blades.[1] Pruritus and dandruff of the scalp are often associated with the condition.

Incidence/prevalence

The prevalence of seborrhoeic dermatitis is 1–3% in the general population and 3–5% in young adults. In patients with acquired immunodeficiency syndrome (AIDS), the incidence is increased (30–80%), probably related to CD4 levels (altered immune surveillance).[2]

Aetiology/risk factors

The aetiology of seborrhoeic dermatitis is not clear. Several factors, such as sebaceous output, androgenic hormones, mycological infection and neurological disturbances can have a major effect on the development of the condition. In particular, qualitative and quantitative abnormalities in the composition of sebum have been suggested but not clearly defined. The non-pathogenic fungus *Malassezia furfur (Pityrosporum ovale* and *P. orbiculare)* may play a role[3] but the mechanism has not been established.[4] Increased keratinocyte and sebocyte turnover has been reported in association with altered keratinisation. Systemic lipid metabolism and antioxidants may play a role in modulation of the disease onset and the inflammatory reaction. A few studies have linked the onset or relapses with psychological situations, alcohol intake, psychotropic drugs and a deficiency of micronutrients (lithium, zinc, magnesium, biotin).

Prognosis

Although there are many treatments for seborrhoeic dermatitis, recurrences are very common, with the disease typically relapsing for years. Even if the prognostic studies that we found were not long term, preventive regimens have been developed and can help to reduce the severity of the disease. They include improvement of lifestyle, intake of nutrients and sun exposure.

Aims of treatment

The aims of treatment are reduction of symptoms and relapses, and cosmetic improvement of the disease with a short-term treatment.

Outcomes

We found no standard scales for the assessment of the severity of seborrhoeic dermatitis. Outcomes used include severity of symptoms (erythema, desquamation, itching), rate of recurrence, number of *P. oribculare* colonies, patient satisfaction and cosmetic acceptability.

Search methods

We found few RCTs that met clinical evidence criteria, so we included observational studies (Medline 1981–October 2001).

QUESTIONS

What are the effects of topical treatment?

Antifungals

Topical antifungals are well established in the treatment of seborrhoeic dermatitis. We found several clinical trials showing that different topical antifungals improve seborrhoeic dermatitis.

Efficacy

We found no systematic review.

Ketoconazole

We found six double-blind placebo-controlled trials using cream or shampoo.[5-10] The largest trial using 2% ketoconazole shampoo (n = 565) reported an excellent response in 88% of the patients treated and effectiveness in preventing relapses when used prophylactically once a week.[5] A randomised controlled trial (RCT) comparing 2% ketoconazole shampoo with 2·5% selenium sulphide shampoo found both treatments to be better than placebo; ketoconazole was statistically superior to selenium sulphide ($P = 0·0026$) and better tolerated.[6] In a double-blind crossover study the change in clinical score with ketoconazole shampoo was significant ($P<0·01$).[7] Two RCTs demonstrated the clinical efficacy of 2% cream compared with placebo in 37[8] and 20[9] patients, respectively. One open randomised parallel study showed that the 2% formulation was significantly more effective than a 1% formulation ($P<0·001$) and that intermittent application of 2% ketoconazole shampoo can successfully prevent relapse.

A long-term prophylactic treatment has to meet a high standard with regard to patient safety.[11] The safety of 2% ketoconazole shampoo is supported by absorption studies and by local irritancy and contact sensitivity studies. Ketoconazole shampoo does not influence sebum production but improves its delivery onto the skin surface.[12]

Bifonazole

We found three double-blind controlled trials and two open studies.[13-15] The largest, involving 100 patients, reported that bifonazole 1% cream was significantly better than placebo ($P<0·05$).[13]

Ciclopirox olamine

One placebo-controlled double-blind study of ciclopirox olamine 1% cream in facial seborrhoeic dermatitis (57 patients in the ciclopirox olamine group and 72 in the vehicle group) found a statistically significant ($P<0·01$) difference between the two treatment groups at the end of the initial phase (twice daily for

28 days) and the maintenance phases (once daily for 28 days).[16]

Other antifungals

We found one RCT,[17] in which the lesions cleared in 11 of 18 eligible patients after treatment with terbinafine 1% solution once daily for 4 weeks. Beneficial effects have been reported in open studies with fluconazole[18] and fenticonazole.[19]

Drawbacks

The few adverse effects reported include erythema, dryness and pruritus.

Comment

The various antifungal drugs have not been compared. The possible mechanisms of action of these compounds include antifungal and anti-inflammatory effects.

Corticosteroids

Over the past years we have found little information about use of topical steroids.[20–25] The drugs, applied for 1–4 weeks, improve seborrhoeic dermatitis and do not cause systemic effects, but relapses were more frequent than with topical antifungals.

Efficacy

No systematic reviews were found. In one RCT, 1% hydrocortisone solution was compared with miconazole and a combination of miconazole and hydrocortisone in 70 patients[20]; the combination was most effective. The largest number of patients with recurrence was seen in the hydrocortisone group. We found one randomised double-blind controlled trial of 2% ketoconazole cream versus 0·05% clobetasol 17-butyrate cream,[21] and one trial comparing topical application of 0·02% flumethasone

pivalate with 2% eosin in 30 infants with seborrhoeic dermatitis; the two treatments had comparable effects.[22]

Drawbacks

Long-term corticosteroid therapy may induce adverse effects such as skin atrophy and telangectasia.[25]

Comment

No recent RCTs demonstrate the efficacy of corticosteroids, although they are used as comparative drugs.

Lithium succinate

RCTs have found that lithium succinate improves seborrhoeic dermatitis compared with placebo.

Efficacy

We found two randomised, double-blind, placebo-controlled trials and one open trial with 8% lithium succinate ointment.[26–28] One crossover trial in nine centres (200 patients) and a parallel-group study in two centres (27 patients) showed that symptom score improved significantly in the lithium group ($P<0·0001$).[26] The other double-blind trial, conducted in twelve patients with AIDS-associated seborrhoeic dermatitis, showed a rapid (2–5 days) and significant ($P<0·01$) clinical improvement in patients treated with lithium succinate.[27]

Drawbacks

Adverse effects were skin and eyelid irritation in a few patients.

Comment

Lithium inhibits growth in small colony strains of *Pityrosporum* and blocks the release of free fatty acids from tissue. Lithium also has potentially anti-inflammatory actions.

Antibacterials

We found only a few studies of metronidazole.

Efficacy

We found no systematic review. A double-blind study (n = 44) showed a significant improvement after using 1% metronidazole gel compared with placebo for 8 weeks. Fourteen patients in the metronidazole group and two in the placebo group had complete improvement.[29]

Drawbacks

Metronidazole gel was well tolerated and did not produce adverse effects.

Comment

The mechanism of action of metronidazole is not known.

Benzoyl peroxide

Two controlled studies have reported the efficacy of benzoyl peroxide.

Efficacy

We found two studies. One open trial found improvement in 28 of 30 patients treated for several months with 2·5% benzoyl peroxide.[30] The second, a double-blind RCT in 59 people, comparing 5% benzoyl peroxide with placebo for 4 weeks, reported a significant improvement in erythema, pruritus and scaling in the group treated with benzoyl peroxide ($P<0·05$).[31]

Drawbacks

Skin irritation was reported as a side-effect.

Propylene glycol

We found one double-blind controlled study in which 39 patients with seborrhoeic dermatitis of the scalp were treated with a solution containing 15% propylene glycol.[32] The lesions improved in 89% of patients treated with propylene glycol, compared with 32% in the placebo group. *In vitro*, the *P. orbiculare* and *P. ovale* counts were reduced significantly after treatment with propylene glycol, but not in the placebo group.

Miscellaneous

Several treatments have been claimed to be effective in uncontrolled studies. A blind, randomised, parallel-group study in 80 patients found 1% ichthyol to be superior to 4% coal tar in seborrhoeic dermatitis of the scalp.[33]

Tacalcitol (1a-24-R-dihydroxycholecalciferol) was used in four patients with good results,[34] crude honey (30 patients),[35] borage oil, 40% urea ointment,[36] dithranol (18 patients),[37] pyridoxine and cystine[38] have been reported as beneficial in uncontrolled studies.

Ultraviolet light

RCTs have found that phototherapy improves seborrhoeic dermatitis.

Efficacy

No systematic reviews were found. Limited evidence suggests that natural sunlight has a significant effect on seborrhoeic dermatitis.[39,40] One RCT (n = 48) found improvement in 85% of patients receiving selective ultraviolet phototherapy, and in 76% of the PUVA-treated patients after a mean of 26 treatments.[41] In an open prospective study, 18 patients with severe seborrhoeic dermatitis were treated in an open study with narrow-band UVB (TL-01) phototherapy, three times weekly, starting with

70% of the minimum erythema dose, up to maximum of 8 weeks. All patients responded to narrow-band UVB; 12 completed the study, six had complete remission and six had marked improvement.[42]

Drawbacks

No side-effects were reported except rare episodes of moderate erythema.

Comment

The trials of phototherapy were too few to evaluate its effectiveness.

What are the effects of systemic treatments?

Antifungal drugs

We found limited evidence that oral antifungals are beneficial.

Efficacy

We found no systematic reviews.

Ketoconazole

One double-blind placebo-controlled crossover study in 19 patients compared ketoconazole, 200 mg/day for 4 weeks, with placebo. Seventy per cent of subjects showed a significantly greater improvement, particularly on the scalp, with ketoconazole compared with 10% of subjects receiving placebo ($P<0.01$).[43]

Terbinafine

In one placebo-controlled trial (n = 60), oral terbinafine 250 mg once daily for 4 weeks significantly reduced scores ($P<0.0001$) compared with baseline and control groups.[44]

Drawbacks

Ketoconazole damages the liver and interferes with testosterone metabolism. No side-effects were reported during the terbinafine study.

Comment

Seborrhoeic dermatitis relapses when the drugs are stopped so that prolonged treatment is often needed. Systemic antifungal drugs are not suitable for this.[45]

What are the effects of nutrients?

We found no controlled studies of the effects of nutrients, vitamins and trace elements on seborrhoeic dermatitis. On the basis of limited observational evidence, seborrhoeic dermatitis is said to have improved after administration of vitamins A, E, D, B1, B2, B6 and C, niacin, biotin, selenium, zinc or iron.[46,47]

Do treatments that reduce sebaceous secretions improve the symptoms?

Retinoids and antiandrogens

We found that few drugs interfere with sebum secretion and insufficient evidence that controlling sebum production leads to improvement of seborrhoeic dermatitis.

Efficacy

Oral retinoids reduce sebaceous gland size, suppress sebum production and inhibit sebocyte differentiation; they also have anti-inflammatory activity.[48] Antiandrogen and 5-alpha-reductase inhibitors reduce the size of the sebaceous glandular lobules and ducts.[49]

We found no evidence to support the hypothesis that reducing sebum production decreases the probability of developing seborrhoeic dermatitis.

Key points

- RCTs show that topical antifungal treatment and metronidazole are effective.
- Limited evidence suggests that systemic antifungal therapy can be useful in controlling the disease.
- Few RCTs have examined the efficacy of topical steroids.
- We found limited or no evidence on the effect of natural sunlight or systemic nutrients.

References

1. Plewig G, Jansen T. Seborrheic dermatitis. In: Freedberg IM, Eisen AZ, Wolff K *et al.*, eds. *Fitzpatrick's Dermatology in General Medicine, 5th ed.* Volume 1. New York: McGraw Hill, 1999:1482–9.

2. Schaub NA, Drewe J, Sponagel L *et al.* Is there a relation between risk groups or initial CD4T cell counts and prevalence of seborrheic dermatitis in HIV-infected patients? *Dermatology* 1999;**198**:126–9.

3. Schmidt A. *Malassezia furfur*: a fungus belonging to the physiological skin flora and its relevance in skin disorders. *Cutis* 1997;**59**:21–4.

4. Faergemann J, Bergbrant I-M, Dohsé *et al.* Seborrhoeic dermatitis and *Pityrosporum (Malassezia) folliculitis* characterization of inflammatory cells and mediators in the skin by immunohistochemistry. *Br J Dermatol* 2001;**144**:549–56.

5. Peter RU, Richarz-Barthauer U. Successful treatment and prophylaxis of scalp seborrhoeic dermatitis and dandruff with 2% ketoconazole shampoo: results of a multicentre, double blind, placebo-controlled trial. *Br J Dermatol* 1995;**132**:441–5.

6. Danby FW, Maddin WS, Margesson LJ *et al.* A randomised, double blind, placebo-contolled trial of ketoconazole 2% shampoo versus selenium sulfide 2·5% shampoo in the treatment of moderate to severe dandruff. *J Am Acad Dermatol* 1993;**29**:1008–2.

7. Carr MM, Pryce DM, Ive FA. Treatment of seborrhoeic dermatitis with ketoconazole: I. response of the scalp to topical ketoconazole. *Br J Dermatol* 1987;**116**:213–16.

8. Skinner RB, Noah PW, Taylor RM *et al.* Double-blind treatment of seborrheic dermatitis with 2% ketoconazole cream. *J Am Acad Dermatol* 1985;**12**:852–6.

9. Green CA, Farr PM, Shuster S. Treatment of seborrhoeic dermatitis with ketoconazole: II Response of seborrhoeic dermatitis of the face, scalp and trunk to topical ketoconazole. *Br J Dermatol* 1987;**116**:217–21.

10. Faergemann J. Treatment of seborrhoeic dermatitis of the scalp with ketoconazole shampoo. *Acta Derm Venereol* 1990;**70**:171–2.

11. Pierard-Franchimont C, Pierard GE, Arrese JE *et al.* Effect of ketoconazole 1% and 2% shampoos on severe dandruff and seborrhoeic dermatitis: clinical, squamometric and mycological assessments. *Dermatology* 2001;**202**: 171–6.

12. Dobrev H, Zissova L. Effect of ketoconazole 2% shampoo on scalp sebum level in patients with seborrhoeic dermatitis. *Acta Derm Venereol* 1997;**77**:132–4.

13. Zienicke H, Korting HC, Braun-Falco O *et al.* Comparative efficacy and safety of bifonazole 1% cream and the corresponding base preparation in the treatment of seborrhoeic dermatitis. *Mycoses* 1993;**36**:325–31.

14. Segal R, David M, Ingber A *et al.* Treatment with bifonazole shampoo for seborrhoea and seborrhoeic dermatitis randomised, double-blind study. *Acta Derm Venereol* 1992;**72**:454–5.

15. Massone L, Borghi S, Pestarono A *et al.* Seborrhoeic dermatitis in otherwise healthy patients and in patients with lymphadenopathy syndrome/AIDS-related complex: treatment with 1% bifonazole cream. *Int J Mediterranean Soc Chemother* 1988;**7**:109–12.

16. Dupuy P, Maurette C, Amoric JC, Chosidow O. Randomized, placebo-controlled, double-blind study on clinical efficacy of ciclopiroxolamine 1% cream in facial seborrhoeic dermatitis. *Br J Dermatol* 2001;**144**:1033–7.

17. Faergemann J, Jones TC, Hettler O *et al.* Pityrosporum ovale *(Malassezia furfur)* as the causative agent of seborrhoeic dermatitis: new treatments. *Br J Dermatol* 1996;**134**(Suppl 46):12–5.

18. Rigopoulos D, Katsambas A, Antoniou C *et al.* Facial seborrhoeic dermatitis treated with fluconazole 2% shampoo. *Int J Dermatol* 1994;**33**:136–7.

19. Merlino A, Malvano L, Cervetti O *et al.* Role of *Malassezia furfur* in seborrhoeic dermatitis in adults and therapeutic efficacy of fenticonazole. *Giorn It Derm Vener* 1988;**123**: 37–49.

20. Faergemann J. Seborrhoeic dermatitis and *Pityrosporum orbiculare*: treatment of seborrhoeic dermatitis of the scalp with miconazole-hydrocortisone (Daktacort), miconazole and hydrocortisone. *Br J Dermatol* 1986; **114**:695–700.

21. Pari T, Pulimood S, Jacob M *et al.* Randomised double blind controlled trial of 2% ketoconazole cream versus 0·05% clobetasol 17–butyrate cream in seborrhoeic dermatitis. *J Eur Acad Dermatol Venereol* 1998;**10**:89–90.

22. Shohat M, Mimouni M, Varsano I. Efficacy of topical application of glucorticosteroids compared with eosin in infant with seborrheic dermatitis. *Cutis* 1987;**40**:67–8.

23. Prakash A, Benfield P. Topical mometasone. A revew of its pharmacological properties and therapeutic use in

the treatment of dermatological disorders. *Drugs* 1998;**55**:145–63.

24. Pierard-Franchimont C, Willemaers V, Fraiture AL *et al.* Squamometry in seborrheic dermatitis. *Int J Dermatol* 1999;**38**:712–5.

25. Pierard-Franchimont C, Hermanns JF, Degreef H *et al.* From axioms to new insights into dandruff. *Dermatology* 2000;**200**:93–8.

26. Efalith Multicenter Trial Group. A double-blind, placebo-controlled, multicenter trial of lithium succinate ointment in the treatment of seborrheic dermatitis. *J Am Acad Dermatol* 1992;**26**:452–7.

27. Langtry JA, Rowland Payne CM, Staughton RC *et al.* Topical lithium succinate ointment (Efalith) in the treatment of AIDS-related seborrhoeic dermatitis. *Clin Exp Dermatol* 1997;**22**:216–9.

28. Cuelenaere C, De Bersaques J, Kint A. Use of topical lithium succinate ointment in the treatment of seborrhoeic dermatitis. *Dermatology* 1992;**184**:194–7.

29. Parsad D, Pandhi R, Negri KS *et al.* Topical metronidazole in seborrhoeic dermatitis – a double-blind study. *Dermatology* 2001;**202**:35–7.

30. Bonnetblanc JM, Bernard P. Benzoyl peroxide in seborrheic dermatitis. *Arch Dermatol* 1986;**122**:752.

31. Bonnetblanc JM, De Prost Y, Bazex J *et al.* Treatment of seborrheic dermatitis with benzoyl peroxide. *Ann Dermatol Venereol* 1990;**117**:123–5.

32. Faergemann J. Propylene glycol in the treatment of seborrhoeic dermatitis of the scalp: a double-blind study. *Cutis* 1988;**42**:69–71.

33. Michel V, Reygagne P, Dupuy P. Results of a clinical study comparing 1% icthiol with 4% coaltar in seborrhoeic dermatitis of the scalp. *J Eur Acad Dermatol Venereol* 1997;**9**:186.

34. Nakayama J. Four cases of sebopsoriasis or seborrhoeic dermatitis of the face and scalp successfully treated with 1a-24-R-dihydroxycholecalciferol (tacalcitol) cream. *Eur J Dermatol* 2000;**10**:528–32.

35. Al Waili NS. Therapeutic and prophylactic effects of crude honey on chronic seborrhoeic dermatitis and dundruff. *Eur J Med Res* 2001;**6**:306–8.

36. Shemer A, Nathansohn N, Kaplan B *et al.* Treatment of scalp seborrheic dermatitis and psoriasis with an ointment of 40% urea and 1% bifonazole. *Int J Dermatol* 2000;**39**:532–4.

37. Wolbling RH, Scofer H, Milbradt R. Treatment of seborrhoeic dermatitis with low-dosage dithranol. *Hautzart* 1985;**36**:529–30.

38. Melli MC, Giorgini S. Clinical evaluation of the efficacy of a topical preparation containing pyridoxine and cystine in seborrhoeic dermatitis an in seborrhoeic condition of the face. *Giorn It Derm Vener* 1986;**121**:LI–LIII.

39. Berg M. Epidemiological studies of the influence of sunlight on the skin. *Photodermatology* 1989;**6**:80–4.

40. Maietta G, Rongioletti F, Rebora A. Seborrheic dermatitis and daylight. Acta Derm Venereol 1991;**71**:538–9.

41. Salo O, Lassus A, Juvakoski T. Treatment of atopic dermatitis and seborrheic dermatitis with selective UV-phototherapy and PUVA. A comparative study. *Dermatol Monatsschr* 1983;**169**:371–5.

42. Pirkhammer D, Seeber A, Honigsmann H *et al.* Narrow-band ultraviolet B (TL-01) phototherapy is an effective and safe treatment for patients with severe seborrhoeic dermatitis. *Br J Dermatol* 2000;**143**:964–8.

43. Ford GP, Farr PM, Ive FA *et al.* The response of seborrhoeic dermatitis to ketoconazole. *Br J Dermatol* 1984;**111**:603–7.

44. Scaparro E, Quadri G, Virno G *et al.* Evaluation of the efficacy and tolerability of oral terbinafine (Daskil) in patients with seborrheic dermatitis. A multicentre, randomised, investigator-blinded, placebo-controlled trial. *Br J Dermatol* 2001;**144**:854–7.

45. Faergemann J. Treatment of seborrhoeic dermatitis with oral terbinafine? *Lancet* 2001;**358**:170.

46. Brenner S, Horwitz C. Possible nutrient mediators in psoriasis and seborrheic dermatitis. *World Rev Nutr Diet* 1988;**55**:165–82.

47. Passi S, Morrone A, De Luca C *et al.* Blood levels of vitamin E, polyunsaturated fatty acids of phospholipids, lipoperoxides and glutathione peroxidase in patients affected with seborrheic dermatitis. *J Dermatol Sci* 1991;**2**:171–8.

48. Orfanos CE, Zouboulis ChC. Oral retinoids in the treatment of seborrhoea and acne. *Dermatology* 1998;**196**:140–7.

49. Ye F, Imamura K, Imanishi N *et al.* Effects of topical antiandrogen and 5–alpha-reductase inhibitors on sebaceous glands in male fuzzy rats. *Skin Pharmacol* 1997;**10**:288–97.

19
Psoriasis

Robert JG Chalmers

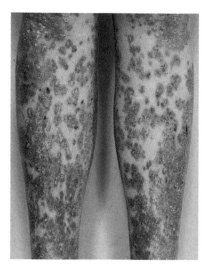

Figure 19.1 Chronic plague psoriasis

Background
Definition

Psoriasis is an inflammatory disease of the skin characterised by an accelerated rate of epidermal turnover, with hyperproliferation and defective maturation of epidermal keratinocytes. In the majority of cases psoriasis is a chronic disease which, in its most common form – chronic plaque psoriasis – manifests itself as well-demarcated, often symmetrically distributed, thickened, red, scaly plaques. These may vary considerably both in size and in number and may involve any part of the skin, although they are found most typically on the extensor surfaces of the knees and elbows, in the sacral area and on the scalp. Appearances may be modified by the site of involvement, with flexural areas showing beef-red shiny plaques without scale (flexural or inverse psoriasis), palms and soles showing marked hyperkeratosis and fissuring, and nails becoming distorted by thimble-pits, thickening and nail-plate detachment. Up to 8% of people with psoriasis may have an associated inflammatory arthropathy,[1] which in severe cases may be the dominant cause of morbidity.

Acute inflammatory forms of psoriasis may develop *de novo* or may complicate existing chronic plaque psoriasis. Acute guttate psoriasis characteristically affects children and young adults following streptococcal infection.[2] Typically, showers of tiny red papules (likened to raindrops or guttae) erupt over large areas of the skin surface 1–2 weeks after an episode of acute streptococcal pharyngitis or tonsillitis. Erythrodermic and generalised pustular psoriasis are uncommon but severe and potentially life-threatening forms of psoriasis; they may be complicated by high-output cardiac failure, temperature dysregulation and septicaemia, particularly in the elderly.

Localised pustular forms of psoriasis, which may cause long-lasting disability, include chronic palmoplantar pustular psoriasis (palmoplantar pustulosis) and acropustulosis (acrodermatitis continua of Hallopeau). Only a minority of patients with these relatively uncommon variants have evidence of psoriasis at other sites[3] and their relationship to ordinary psoriasis remains poorly understood.

Prevalence

Psoriasis first manifests itself most commonly in the second and third decades of life but can present at any age.[4] Its prevalence varies from 0·3% or less in Mongoloid and Amerindian ethnic groups to more than 2% in parts of Scandinavia.[4,5] In both North America and Europe the prevalence has been estimated to be between 1% and 2% as, for instance, in a recent community-based study from the UK where a point prevalence of 1·48% was found.[5,6]

Aetiology

Epidermal turnover is greatly accelerated in psoriasis such that keratinocytes within active psoriatic plaques may travel from the basal layer of the epidermis to the stratum corneum in as little as 4 days rather than the normal 28 days. Exactly what drives this process is incompletely understood but it is agreed that it is mediated by activated T lymphocytes and that there is a strong genetic component.[7] Stress, heavy alcohol consumption, smoking, infection and local trauma (Koebner phenomenon) are all thought to influence the severity of psoriasis.[2,4,7,8]

Prognosis

Chronic plaque psoriasis, as its name implies, tends to last years or decades but is subject to periods of remission and relapse. At the time of the UK study referred to above,[5,6] in which the mean duration of psoriasis was about 20 years, 9% of patients were in remission but only 7% estimated that their psoriasis had been in remission for more than a quarter of the time since its original onset. The prognosis following a first attack of guttate psoriasis has not been properly quantified but only a third of a small group of such patients reviewed at 10 years had had further psoriasis.[9]

Aims of treatment

Until there is a safe and effective cure for psoriasis, a balance must be struck between patients' individual perceptions of disability from psoriasis, their willingness to devote time and effort to managing the disease and their preparedness to accept risks from treatment. Successful management may therefore range from reassurance and provision of simple emollients to the use of powerful and potentially hazardous systemic agents.

Relevant outcomes

Outcomes should reflect the above aims and will therefore most importantly address patient satisfaction with treatment and changes in disease-related quality of life. Outcomes should thus include proportions of patients reporting good or excellent response to treatment and reporting that treatment is "worthwhile". Similarly, proportions of patients achieving clearance or near clearance of disease are more robust outcomes than are absolute or relative changes in disease severity scoring systems such as the psoriasis area and severity index (PASI). Adverse effects and their frequency are equally important because they may limit the utility of otherwise effective interventions.

Methods of search

The search strategy [Psoria* or "Acrodermatitis continua of Hallopeau" or (Impetigo and herpetiformis) or ((Palm* or Plant* or Sole* or Bacterid) and (Pustul* or Psoria*)) or Acropustulosis] was used to search the Cochrane Central Register of Controlled Trials (Issue 3, 2001) and the European Dermato-Epidemiology Network (EDEN) database of psoriasis trials, and filtered using the Cochrane optimal search strategy for randomised controlled trials (RCTs),[10] Medline and Embase (both to August 2001). The results were crosschecked against the Salford Database of Psoriasis Trials developed for the systematic review published in 2000.[11]

Presentation of the evidence

There is a large amount of RCT evidence on the effects of treatments for psoriasis. This review does not aim to be comprehensive in its coverage of all areas of psoriasis management but concentrates on presenting data on systemic therapies and on evidence from systematic reviews and meta-analyses

QUESTIONS

How effective are treatments for limited stable chronic plaque psoriasis?

Emollients and occlusive dressings

Psoriatic plaques are dry, scaly and frequently itchy. Emollients may help to soften psoriatic scale by increasing its water content, either by forming an occlusive layer on the skin surface (for example white soft paraffin) or by an osmotic effect (for example urea containing creams). Most topically applied therapies for psoriasis are formulated in emollient bases but emollients on their own are frequently advocated for psoriasis. They are claimed to reduce dryness, scaling and itch. There is little published evidence documenting the efficacy of emollient therapy alone in the management of psoriasis, although many studies have compared the effects of emollient bases with the same bases containing "active" ingredients. Some evidence suggests that emollients may have a steroid-sparing effect in psoriasis managed with topical corticosteroids.

Occlusive dressings have also been used for treating psoriatic plaques, often to enhance penetration of active drugs such as topical corticosteroids, but they have also been examined on their own. Hydrocolloid gel dressings may be useful on their own for selected recalcitrant psoriatic plaques and may enhance the response to topical corticosteroids and calcipotriol.

Efficacy
Emollients

Many studies have shown an improvement over baseline after regular application of emollient creams or ointments. In one open-label study in which within patient comparisons were made in two separate cohorts of 48 patients with chronic plaque psoriasis, the combination of a once-daily application of a water-in-oil cream or lotion with once-daily betamethasone dipropionate cream was found to be more effective than once-daily and of equal efficacy to twice-daily betamethasone dipropionate cream.[12] In another within patient study (n = 43) the application of an oil-in-water emollient cream before UVB exposure significantly enhanced the rate of psoriasis improvement with UVB phototherapy. The authors suggest that the emollient may have altered the optical properties of the epidermis. Another small within patient study compared a 10% urea ointment with its base or with no therapy (n = 10). Two weeks' therapy with the urea ointment produced a >50% reduction in clinical score compared with the untreated side; however, the ointment base alone also produced a significant improvement in clinical score.[13] In another RCT (n = 40), a 12% urea and 12% sodium chloride cream was shown to be superior to the cream base and to have comparable efficacy to salicylic acid ointment at removing scale from psoriatic plaque.[14]

Hydrocolloid dressings

In a small open prospective bilateral comparison study involving 26 patients with stable symmetrical plaque psoriasis, 47% of treated plaques resolved after weekly applications of an adhesive hydrocolloid occlusive dressing for 10 weeks. Furthermore, the dressing was found to be more effective than twice-daily applications of a potent corticosteroid cream (fluocinolone acetonide) for 10 weeks (12% resolution rate) although less effective than erythemogenic UVB phototherapy given five times weekly for the same duration (67% resolution rate).[15] The results from another small RCT suggest that 3 weeks' therapy with a hydrocolloid dressing or with a potent corticosteroid cream (0·1% triamcinolone acetonide) is insufficient to induce resolution but that a combination of the two is significantly more effective.[16] Hydrocolloid dressings have also been used with the topical vitamin D analogue, calcipotriol. In a small single-blind controlled trial in 15 patients, symmetrical chronic plaques were treated with either calcipotriol ointment or a superpotent corticosteroid ointment (0·05% clobetasol propionate) under hydrocolloid occlusion; dressings were changed every 4 days. Two patients were withdrawn because of irritation by calcipotriol; in the remaining 13 patients all treated plaques had cleared by day 12.[17]

Drawbacks

Local irritation and, rarely, allergic contact dermatitis may result from use of emollients or occlusive dressings.

Comment

Patients with mild psoriasis may choose to use emollients alone because of their convenience and lack of adverse effects. Usually, however, emollients are used as adjuncts to other therapies. Hydrocolloid gel dressings may be useful on their own for selected recalcitrant psoriatic plaques and may enhance the response to topical corticosteroids and calcipotriol.

Keratolytics

Salicylic acid is the most commonly used keratolytic agent and is often advocated for removing psoriatic scale. It is considered beneficial not only because it reduces scaling and skin shedding but also because it thereby removes a barrier to the penetration of more active compounds into the skin. Concentrations between 2% and 10% in an ointment base are usually dispensed. Salicylic acid is often used in combination with coal tar or corticosteroids. There is little information from RCTs on the efficacy of salicylic acid monotherapy as a descaling agent.

Efficacy

There is RCT evidence (n = 408) that the addition of salicylic acid to a topical corticosteroid preparation enhances efficacy in psoriasis.[18]

Drawbacks

Topical salicylic acid may be absorbed through the skin and could thus cause systemic toxicity (salicylism),[19] but this seems to be rare in practice.[19,20] It may irritate and inflame the skin. Salicylic acid has been shown to interfere with UVB absorption into the skin and, in one RCT, the addition of salicylic acid to an emollient applied before UVB phototherapy decreased the rate of clearance of psoriasis.[21]

Comment

Topical salicylic acid is widely accepted as an effective keratolytic and rarely causes significant side-effects.

Vitamin D analogues

The vitamin D analogue calcipotriol was introduced in the early 1990s as a topical treatment for mild-to-moderate plaque psoriasis. Since then other vitamin D derivatives have been studied. One systematic review of calcipotriol found that it was at least as effective as potent topical corticosteroids, calcitriol, short-contact anthralin (dithranol) therapy and coal tar. Its main drawback is that it may cause skin irritation. Much less evidence is available for other vitamin D analogues, including tacalcitol and maxacalcitol.

Efficacy

One systematic review of calcipotriol (search date 1999, 37 RCTs, 6038 people)[22] has been published. The authors concluded that calcipotriol is an effective treatment for mild-to-moderate chronic plaque psoriasis, more so than calcitriol, tacalcitol, coal tar or short contact anthralin and that, amongst topical therapies with which it has been compared, only potent topical corticosteroids seem to have comparable efficacy at 8 weeks. Although calcipotriol causes more skin irritation than topical corticosteroids, this has to be balanced against the potential long-term effects of corticosteroids. Skin irritation rarely led to withdrawal of calcipotriol treatment. The combination of calcipotriol cream applied in the morning with a moderately potent to potent topical corticosteroid at night has been shown to be at least as effective as twice-daily calcipotriol cream but to cause significantly less irritation.[23] More recently, a compound ointment containing calcipotriol, 50 microgram/g and betamethasone dipropionate, 0·5 mg/g, has been evaluated in a RCT involving 1106 people with chronic psoriasis. Participants were randomised to receive 4 weeks' twice-daily treatment with the combination ointment or with marketed formulations of one or other of its two active constituents, followed by twice-daily calcipotriol, 50 microgram/g ointment for a further 4 weeks.[24] The mean percentage decrease in psoriasis severity score at 4 weeks was 74·4% in the combination group (n = 372), 55·3% in the calcipotriol group (n = 369) and 61·3% in the betamethasone group (n = 365). These differences were highly significant. At the end of 8 weeks, however, the severity scores did not differ.

Drawbacks

Calcipotriol monotherapy causes more irritation than potent topical corticosteroids (number needed to harm (NNH) 10, 95% confidence intervals (CI) 6 to 34).[22] Perilesional irritation from calcipotriol has been reported in as many as 25% of people, the face and flexures being most susceptible. Hypercalciuria is a dose-related side-effect of therapy, and application of large amounts of calcipotriol can cause hypercalcaemia. To avoid these problems it is recommended that patients should not use more than 100 g 0·05% calcipotriol cream or ointment per week.

Comment

Calcipotriol has been extensively studied and shown to be of value in suppressing mild-to-moderate psoriasis. Psoriasis may improve more rapidly when calcipotriol is initially combined with a potent corticosteroid for 4 weeks but by 8 weeks response rates are no different.

> How effective are treatments for severe chronic plaque psoriasis?

Phototherapy and photochemotherapy

Many different schedules for delivery of phototherapy to people with psoriasis are in current use. One systematic review of treatments for severe psoriasis[25] concluded that:

- photochemotherapy (PUVA) using a combination of either oral or topical psoralen with UVA was effective in clearing psoriasis
- oral and topical PUVA were of comparable efficacy
- UVA alone did not clear psoriasis
- broad-band 290–320 nm ultraviolet B (BBUVB) was effective in clearing psoriasis
- narrow-band 311 nm UVB (NBUVB) offered the possibility of clearance with fewer episodes of erythema and may require a lower cumulative dose of UVB to achieve this
- PUVA or UVB in combination with systemic retinoids appeared to be more effective than either therapy alone

- it was not possible to reach a conclusion on the effects of combining topical tar or anthralin with phototherapy
- PUVA is of similar efficacy to daily anthralin dressings in clearing psoriasis
- combinations of either UVB or PUVA either with vitamin D3 analogues or with topical corticosteroids all appeared to be superior to each agent used alone.

More recent evidence suggests that NBUVB phototherapy used three times weekly is of similar efficacy to twice-weekly PUVA.[26]

There is little evidence to support the use of balneophototherapy in which phototherapy is combined with bathing in various mineral or salt waters.[27] Heliotherapy using natural sunlight is effective at clearing psoriasis[28] but is associated with an increased risk of skin cancer.[29] The main risks of PUVA therapy are photoageing (premature skin ageing) and skin cancer, notably squamous cell carcinoma[30] and, to a lesser extent, malignant melanoma.[31] It is therefore advisable to limit the number of treatments to 200 or the cumulative UVA dose to 1500 J/cm.[2,32] Therapeutic BBUVB irradiation does not appear to be associated with development of skin cancer. There are no long-term studies to assess whether NBUVB carries a risk of skin cancer.

Efficacy

One systematic review of phototherapy and photochemotherapy for psoriasis (search date 1999, 51 RCTs, 2864 people),[25] one meta-analysis of squamous cell carcinoma risk from PUVA (search date 1998, nine studies, 12 142 people)[30] and one meta-analysis of balneophototherapy (search date 2000, three RCTs, 119 people)[33] have been published. A further 12 RCTs were identified by the current search.

Clearance with BBUVB

BBUVB has not been compared directly with placebo. In one case series (n = 87), clearance

(defined as >80% reduction in psoriasis severity score) was obtained in 81% of people with psoriasis given BBUVB four times weekly in a mean of 24 treatment sessions.[34] The investigators noted however that clearance was significantly less likely in people with >50% body surface area involvement. In another series (n = 165) clearance (defined as complete resolution of at least 90% of psoriasis present before treatment) was achieved in a mean of 27 treatment sessions in 81% of the 128 people who had BBUVB at least three times weekly.[35] The optimal frequency of therapy is unknown but an uncontrolled study found no difference in response rate between three- and five-times-weekly regimens (n = 46).[36] A recent small RCT (n = 20) has highlighted the importance of optimising UVB dosimetry for each patient in order to achieve optimal response rates with BBUVB.[37]

Maintenance of remission with BBUVB

One RCT (n = 94) examined the value of maintenance therapy with BBUVB after initial clearance followed by consolidation with up to six treatments in the 3 weeks after clearance. Patients randomised to receive weekly maintenance therapy thereafter were calculated to have a 75% chance of remaining clear (no more than 3% increase in body surface area involved) for a further 16 weeks and >50% chance of still being clear at 23 weeks. By contrast, a quarter of patients who discontinued therapy had relapsed by 8 weeks and only 28% were still clear at 23 weeks.[35]

Clearance with NBUVB

The efficacy of NBUVB has been compared with BBUVB in four small RCTs which, with one exception, failed to show clear superiority of one over the other.[25,38] In the case of the exception, nine of ten patients cleared more rapidly on the half of the body randomised to receive NBUVB.

In the remaining patient NBUVB and BBUVB were equally effective.[38] In two of the studies, however, clearance could be achieved with a 6–10-fold reduction in UV irradiance. (In the third study, greater irradiances were given to the patients receiving NBUVB than to those receiving BBUVB because of a high rate of interruption of therapy in the latter group as a result of episodes of burning.) One RCT (n = 21) has compared three- versus five-times-weekly NBUVB therapy and concluded that, although clearance could be achieved more quickly with five-times-weekly treatments (median 35 versus 40 days), this was at the expense of a greater number of treatment sessions (median 23·5 versus 17), a greater overall UVB irradiance (median 94 versus 64 × minimal erythema dose) and greater inconvenience to the patients. The authors therefore recommended the three-times-weekly regimen.[39]

Maintenance of remission with NBUVB

Longer term maintenance studies with this newer form of treatment have not been reported.

Clearance with heliotherapy (natural sunlight)

Many people with psoriasis report that their skin improves greatly after exposure to natural sunlight. In one RCT with an open crossover design, 95 Finns with psoriasis were randomised to receive a 4-week heliotherapy course in the Canary Islands during the Finnish winter either immediately or after a delay of 12 months. Exposure was gradually increased over the 4 weeks from 0·5–1·0 hour of midday sunshine to a maximum of 6 hours daily sunshine. All patients were kept under review for 24 months. All conventional antipsoriatic therapy was allowed in the observation period before and after heliotherapy. Over 90% of patients achieved clearance of psoriasis following 4 weeks' heliotherapy. In the 12 months following treatment the mean cumulative period for which

patients required active therapy was 25 weeks in both groups; this was much less than the 38 weeks in the group observed for 12 months before heliotherapy (P<0·001). The reduction was mainly due to a reduction in the use of topical corticosteroids and systemic retinoids. Nevertheless, 54% of patients had relapsed to pretreatment severity levels by 6 months and only 15% had not reached 50% of their pretreatment score by this time.[40]

Clearance with balneophototherapy

Balneophototherapy is popular in some countries, particularly in Europe, for the treatment of severe psoriasis. It involves bathing in spa waters containing a variety of concentrations of minerals and salt before artificial UVB irradiation. A systematic review (search date 2000, n = 119) found no evidence of superiority of spa waters or salt water over tap water.[27] A recent RCT (n = 71) comparing balneophototherapy using high mineral content saline spa water followed by NBUVB phototherapy with NBUVB phototherapy alone found no evidence of benefit from the spa water.[41]

Clearance with UVA sunbed

Thirty-eight people with mild-to-moderate psoriasis (median modified PASI score 4·4) were treated three times weekly for 4 weeks with a modified commercial low-UVB-emission UVA sunbed unit. Patients were randomised to receive UVA-filtered visible light to one half of the body and UVA to the other. In over half the patients (53%), the response of the UVA treated side was the same or worse than the visible light treated side. Despite the apparently minimal improvements seen (median reduction in pretreatment disease severity scores by 11% and 5%, respectively), 64% of patients felt that the response was sufficiently good to warrant using a sunbed again to treat their psoriasis.[42]

Clearance with oral PUVA

PUVA has not been compared directly with placebo but two large prospective studies have been published. The first, in 1308 people with psoriasis with a mean 33% body surface area involvement, achieved clearance with 29 exposures or fewer in 69% people given oral PUVA twice or three times weekly; a further 19% cleared with longer treatment courses.[43] In the second study, where more aggressive dosing was used and where patients were treated four times weekly, clearance was achieved in 65% of 3175 people with severe psoriasis in an average of 20 treatments; a further 24% improved markedly.[44] Comparable results have been obtained in patients treated in the oral PUVA arm of RCTs; for instance, a 74% clearance rate was achieved in a median of 16·5 exposures in 50 patients receiving twice-weekly oral PUVA.[45] A higher and more rapid response rate was seen in another RCT where people had possibly less extensive psoriasis than in the studies quoted above (mean 26–29% body surface area involvement), clearance of psoriasis being achieved in a mean of 14.6 treatments in 91% of 113 patients randomised to receive oral PUVA three times weekly.[46] Several studies have examined the effects of different doses and types of psoralen. One RCT (n = 56) has shown that when 8-methoxypsoralen is given at a dose of 40 mg rather than 10 mg, not only is there a greater success rate (rate difference 0·72, CI 0·54 to 0·90) but success can be achieved with a significantly lower cumulative UVA dose (mean (range): 54 (14·5–115) versus 77 (46–113) J/cm^2). Another RCT (n = 106) has shown that when 5-methoxypsoralen is given at 1·2 mg/kg rather than 0·6 mg/kg, a similar reduction in cumulative UVA dose can be achieved (means ± SD: 53 ± 33 versus 132 ± 87 J/cm^2). The two psoralens have been compared and were found in one study to have comparable efficacy at the higher doses given above. In another, however, 5-methoxypsoralen appeared to be less effective, possibly because peak plasma levels had not been reached at the time UVA was administered. The incidence of side-effects (severe erythema, pruritus and nausea) was much lower with 5- than with 8-methoxypsoralen (6% versus 38%).[25] Different incremental schedules for UVA dosing have been advocated based either on skin type (assessed by recalled susceptibility to sunburn) or on phototesting for minimal phototoxic dose. Two RCTs failed to demonstrate a clear advantage of one method over the other.[25]

Maintenance of remission with oral PUVA

The largest RCT, involving 1005 people whose psoriasis had been cleared by oral PUVA, found that maintenance treatment reduced relapse at 18 months from 62% with no maintenance to 27%, 30% and 34% of patients receiving maintenance treatments once every 1, 2 and 3 weeks, respectively.[43] In view of the concerns over cumulative UVA dose in patients receiving PUVA, long-term maintenance therapy is no longer recommended.[32]

Clearance with bath PUVA

As an alternative to oral ingestion, psoralen may be applied directly to the skin. For people with widespread psoriasis this is achieved by adding psoralen to bath water in which the body is immersed before UVA irradiation. This may be useful particularly where a person cannot tolerate oral psoralen, usually because of nausea. Three RCTs have compared bath PUVA with oral PUVA in a total of 171 people with widespread plaque psoriasis.[47–49] All three studies concluded that bath PUVA was of similar efficacy to oral PUVA. All found that less UVA was required to achieve clearance when bath PUVA was employed (reported reductions in mean UVA dose ranged from 60% to 80%). The biological significance of this is unknown, although some evidence suggests that the risk of squamous cell carcinoma may be lower following bath PUVA (see Drawbacks below).[28]

Clearance with psoralen and natural sunlight

The systematic review identified three RCTs involving psoralen and natural sun.[25] Clearance was achieved in 12 of 20 Indians with psoriasis who were randomised to a regimen of oral 8-methoxypsoralen 40 mg followed 150–180 minutes later by exposure of the skin to direct Indian sunlight for 25–30 minutes; 18 of the 20 (90%) showed a marked improvement or better.[50] No improvement was seen in the 20 people randomised to placebo capsules and sunlight. On the other hand Parrish found that white-skinned people with psoriasis improved with sunlight alone. Although response rates were better with 8-methoxypsoralen, 0·6 mg/kg, and sunlight, some patients had severe phototoxic burns.[51] Psoralen and sunlight therapy may be of value for darker-skinned people in parts of the world where access to alternative treatments is limited.

PUVA versus NBUVB

Five controlled trials were identified, but it was possible to extract a response rate from only three of these. In 100 people with chronic plaque psoriasis randomised to twice-weekly treatment with either NBUVB or PUVA, clearance was achieved in a significantly greater proportion of those treated with PUVA (84%) than in those treated with NBUVB (63%) (odds ratio in favour of PUVA 3·04; CI 1·18 to 7·84) with significantly fewer treatments (median number of treatments for clearance: 16·7 with PUVA versus 25·3 with NBUVB; ratio of medians 1·52; CI 1·24 to 1·86). Only 12% of those treated with NBUVB were clear of psoriasis 6 months after finishing treatment, compared with 35% for PUVA.[52] Others have argued, however, that optimal responses with NBUVB require three-times-weekly administration.[53] In a small randomised left–right comparison of bath PUVA and NBUVB administered three times weekly to 28 people, clearance was achieved in 75% of sides receiving NBUVB compared with 54% of sides receiving bath PUVA (intention-to-treat analysis; 95% CI for difference between treatments 4% to 37%);[53] however, only 18 patients completed the study. In a larger parallel-group RCT in which 54 patients with >10% coverage with psoriasis were randomised to standard regimens of PUVA (twice weekly) or NBUVB (three times weekly), no difference in response was found. Clearance was achieved in medians of 66 days (interquartile range 50·5–116) and 67 days (43–94·75), with medians of 19 (13·5–27·5) and 25·5 (17·2–35·8) treatments, respectively; relapse rates were similar (193 and 191 days to reach 50% of baseline severity score).[26] The authors thought that NBUVB probably had a more favourable adverse effect profile than PUVA, and so recommended that NBUVB should be preferred. Another RCT compared twice-weekly PUVA with twice-weekly psoralen plus NBUVB in 100 people with psoriasis; clearance rates were similar (success rate difference –0·12, 95% CI –0·28–0·04).[45]

PUVA versus retinoids

In one RCT (n = 40) good or excellent responses were seen in 80% of people treated with PUVA and in 55% of those given etretinate at an initial dose of 50–60 mg daily and then reduced according to response and side-effects.[54]

Retinoids + UVB versus UVB alone

See systemic retinoids.

Retinoids + PUVA (RePUVA) versus PUVA alone

See systemic retinoids.

PUVA or UVB versus other systemic therapies

No RCTs comparing phototherapy with other systemic therapies such as ciclosporin or methotrexate were identified.

PUVA or UVB versus topical therapies

In a comparison of a standard regimen using daily anthralin paste with PUVA three times weekly (n = 224), clearance was achieved in 91% of the 113 in the PUVA group but in only 82% of the anthralin group; clearing, however, took longer with PUVA (mean ± SEM 34·4 ± 1·8) than with anthralin (20·4 ± 0·9).[50]

Combinations of PUVA or UVB with topical therapies versus phototherapy alone

The combination of calcipotriol cream twice daily and BBUVB twice weekly was compared with placebo cream and three-times-weekly BBUVB over 12 weeks in 164 patients with extensive psoriasis. Three-quarters of patients in each group achieved an 80% reduction in psoriasis severity score. The calcipotriol group required fewer exposures (12 versus 19) and less cumulative UVB irradiance (median 1570 versus 5430 mJ/cm^2).[55] In another RCT (n = 53) in which all participants received low-dose NBUVB phototherapy, just under half were randomised to receive calcipotriol ointment, 50 microgram/g twice daily, to affected skin. Low-dose NBUVB phototherapy was found to be effective but the addition of calcipotriol ointment did not improve treatment outcome.[56] Some evidence indicates that the addition of topical corticosteroids to either UVB or PUVA therapy is of no benefit.[25] Although the Goeckerman regimen of tar and UVB phototherapy has been widely used since the 1920s, little RCT evidence exists on whether the combination is better than phototherapy alone.[25] Five small RCTs with conflicting results have compared different combinations of anthralin and phototherapy.[25,57] The evidence is insufficient to evaluate whether combination therapy is more effective than either component alone.

Drawbacks

Exposure to natural UV radiation is associated in humans with photoageing and skin cancer. In a 25-year follow up of 1738 Danish patients with psoriasis treated by heliotherapy at the Dead Sea during 1972–73, the risks of basal cell and squamous cell carcinoma of the skin were 4·2 and 10·7 times higher, respectively, than expected in the general population.[29] The authors point out that such patients will have had many other exposures to UV radiation but the risk from exposure to sunlight is clearly increased. There is, however, little evidence to suggest that therapeutic BBUVB irradiation for psoriasis conveys a significantly increased risk of developing skin cancer. There is as yet little evidence as to whether NBUVB is more or less harmful than BBUVB.[33] The main risks of PUVA therapy are photoageing (premature skin ageing) and skin cancer. In addition to the characteristic changes of photoageing (dry skin, wrinkles, elastosis), people who have received large doses of PUVA are prone to developing widespread irregular dark freckling (PUVA lentigines) which may be cosmetically disfiguring and may be difficult to differentiate from early malignant melanoma. Skin cancer is a well-recognised effect of long-term PUVA therapy. In a meta-analysis of nine patient series including data on 12 142 people treated with PUVA followed up for between 5–13 years, a dose-dependent increase in incidence of squamous cell carcinoma was found, with a 14-fold increase in risk in recipients of >200 treatments or >2000 J/cm^2 (CI 8·3 to 24·1); on the other hand there was little evidence that people who had received <100 treatments or <1000 J/cm^2 were at significantly increased risk compared with the normal population.[30] Risk of squamous cell carcinoma was increased in people with fairer skin types (types I and II). A combined analysis of two cohort studies of bath PUVA (n = 944) excluded a threefold excess risk of squamous cell carcinoma after a mean follow up of 14·7 years, suggesting that bath PUVA is possibly safer than oral PUVA.[28] The risks of developing basal cell carcinoma do not appear to be substantially increased except in patients exposed to very high cumulative doses of UVA.[58] A fourfold increase in the incidence of malignant melanoma has been found after long-term (15 years or more) follow up of people exposed to at least 200 PUVA treatments compared with those exposed to fewer (n = 1380, CI 2·0 to 9·2).[31]

Comment

Phototherapy is suitable for inducing remission of psoriasis but not for long-term maintenance of remission. Exposure to both natural sunlight and PUVA increases the risk of developing skin cancer. It is advisable to limit the lifetime number of PUVA treatments given to any one individual to fewer than 200 (or to a cumulative UVA dose of 1500 J/cm²). Patients who have received large doses of oral PUVA require long-term follow up to monitor for the development of skin cancer. NBUVB phototherapy when used three times weekly appears to be of similar efficacy to PUVA and offers a number of advantages over the latter. It may be less likely to increase skin cancer risk, but data to confirm this are not available.

Ciclosporin

The immunosuppressive drug ciclosporin has been used for treating severe psoriasis since the early 1980s. One systematic review concluded that ciclosporin is more effective at inducing remission at 5 mg/kg/day than at 2·5 mg/kg/day.[59] Further increases in the dose produce little extra benefit and are limited by side-effects, particularly on renal function. Continuous therapy is usually required to maintain remission; furthermore, doses below 2·5 mg/kg/day appear to be insufficient to achieve this. Ciclosporin appears to be more effective than etretinate. It appears to achieve more rapid improvement of psoriasis than methotrexate but produces similar benefit by 16 weeks.

Efficacy

One systematic review of ciclosporin for severe psoriasis has been published (search date 1999,

18 RCTs, 2240 people).[59] One additional as yet unpublished RCT was identified.

Versus placebo for induction of remission

Different dosage regimens for induction of remission have been compared with placebo in nine intervention groups in five RCTs (n = 289). A dose of 1·25 mg/kg/day was ineffective whereas 5 mg/kg/day appeared to be more effective than 2·5 mg/kg/day. Higher doses appeared to give little extra benefit.

Comparison of dosage schedules for induction of remission

The superiority of 5 mg/kg/day over 2·5 mg/kg/day was confirmed in two RCTs (n = 432). In the larger of these (n = 251), 92% of people receiving the higher dose were judged to have responded satisfactorily, compared with only 52% on the lower dose.[60]

Versus placebo for maintenance of remission

Two RCTs (n = 202) examined low (1·25 mg/kg/day) and intermediate (3·0 mg/kg/day) dose schedules for maintenance of remission induced by ciclosporin. The higher dose was required to achieve superiority over placebo, although even then only 57% and 58% of people continuing therapy for 16 or 24 weeks, respectively, were considered to have remained in remission. Since the definitions of remission used in these studies allowed for relapse to up to 50% of the pretreatment disease extent, it may be difficult to maintain acceptable levels of control with ciclosporin alone at these relatively low doses.[61,62]

Comparison of drug formulations

In 1995 a new formulation of ciclosporin (Neoral) was introduced to improve reliability of gastrointestinal absorption. Two RCTs (n = 345) found no difference in efficacy at 12 weeks between Neoral and its precursor Sandimmun, although the new formulation may have had a more rapid onset of action.[63]

Versus etretinate

Two RCTs (n = 286) concluded that etretinate was less effective than ciclosporin at inducing remission of psoriasis within 10 to 12 weeks.[64,65]

Versus methotrexate

One RCT (n = 85) compared various dose regimens of methotrexate 15–22·5 mg weekly and ciclosporin 3–5 mg/kg/day for 12 weeks followed by tapered withdrawal to 16 weeks (Spuls P, International Psoriasis Symposium, San Francisco, June 2001, personal communication). There was no significant difference in response at 16 weeks, although ciclosporin appeared to act more rapidly.

Drawbacks

In a retrospective study of 122 consecutive patients given ciclosporin for psoriasis at a dose not exceeding 5 mg/kg/day for between 3 and 76 months, impairment of renal function, as evidenced by an increase in serum creatinine levels to >30% above the baseline value, occurred in 53 (43%) patients after a median treatment time of 23 months.[66] Hypertension developed in 29 (24%) patients after a median treatment time of 53 months. The risk of having to discontinue therapy because of side-effects rose to 41% (± 6·7%) by 48 months. This risk increased with the age of the patient and with pre-existing hypertension or high serum creatinine levels. In a smaller study of 20 patients who had received ciclosporin for an average of 6 years (range 5–8 years), nine (45%) developed persistent increases in serum creatinine of >30% from baseline and five (25%) showed persistent increases of >50%. The renal glomerular filtration

rate showed a persistent decrease of >30% in seven patients and of >50% in two patients.[67]

Comment

Although ciclosporin is highly effective at inducing remission of psoriasis when used at the upper end of the recommended dose range, maintenance of remission requires continued therapy, with a significant risk of eventual hypertension and/or impairment of renal function.

Systemic retinoids

Systemic therapy with retinoic acid derivatives has been used for treating psoriasis since the late 1970s. Most clinical studies have been of etretinate and its hydrolysis product acitretin, which has now replaced it. One systematic review has examined the use of retinoids for psoriasis.[68] It concluded that relatively high doses (approximately 1 mg/kg/day) are needed for monotherapy to show superiority over placebo and that the responses achieved are less than those achieved with low-dose ciclosporin. Combinations of retinoids with PUVA, UVB, topical corticosteroids and topical calcipotriol have been shown to be more efficacious than the individual components of each combination. The use of retinoids is limited by their liability to cause birth defects in women of child-bearing potential and by the high incidence of symptomatic mucocutaneous side-effects. Nevertheless they retain an important place in the management of severe psoriasis.

Efficacy

One systematic review (search date 1999, 32 RCTs, 2530 people) has been published.[69] Two additional RCTs were identified.

Versus placebo

Ten reports involving 395 people were available for analysis: five concerning etretinate and five acitretin. Inclusion criteria varied markedly (from >5% to >20% body surface area affected; "psoriasis of long duration" or not reported). Doses ranged considerably, from 10 mg/day to 75 mg/day; study duration varied from 8 to 52 weeks. Three of the trial protocols permitted the concomitant use of topical corticosteroid. Success criteria were generally an improvement of at least 75% in severity score, but the reporting of three trials did not allow differences in success rates to be calculated. Unsurprisingly, the results were heterogeneous. Nevertheless it appeared that doses of 75 mg/day (or 1 mg/kg/day) were required to show superiority over placebo.

Acitretin versus etretinate

Six patient series (n = 508) could be analysed. Etretinate and acitretin were of equal efficacy in inducing remission of psoriasis.

RePUVA versus PUVA alone

The results from six patient series using retinoid doses of at least 50 mg/day (n = 283) demonstrated a small increase in success rate of RePUVA over PUVA alone (rate difference 0·14, CI 0·04 to 0·23). Five trials for which results were available found a clear trend towards a reduction in the UVA dose required to achieve clearance when PUVA was given with retinoid therapy.

Retinoids + UVB versus UVB alone

Three RCTs (n = 149) showed a benefit of the combination over UVB alone.[69–71]

Versus ciclosporin

Two RCTs (n = 286) concluded that etretinate was less effective than ciclosporin at inducing remission of psoriasis within 10–12 weeks.[64,65]

Retinoids + topical corticosteroids versus retinoids alone

The results from two patient series (n = 160) showed that the combination of a moderately potent to potent topical corticosteroid with systemic retinoid therapy increased response rates.

Retinoids + topical calcipotriol versus retinoids alone

One study (n = 86) showed a clear benefit over the untreated side from 0·05% calcipotriol cream applied twice daily to one half of the body in patients receiving etretinate 50 mg daily for 9 weeks.[69] In a second study (n = 135) the addition of twice-daily 0·05% calcipotriol cream to low-dose acitretin (20 mg daily) increased success rates (clearance or marked improvement) at 12 weeks from 41% to 67% (rate difference 0·26, CI 0·10 to 0·42).[73]

Retinoids + fish oil versus retinoids alone

A small open RCT (n = 40) has claimed benefit from the addition of eicosapentaenoic acid to low-dose etretinate in the treatment of stable, chronic plaque psoriasis.[74]

Drawbacks

Most people who receive etretinate or acitretin develop reversible, dose-dependent mucocutaneous side-effects, including chapped lips, a tendency to nose bleeds, hair loss and dry or peeling skin. Hyperlipidaemia occurs frequently. In a small open study in 25 psoriasis patients with retinoid-induced hyperlipidaemia, fish oil supplementation (providing 3 g omega-3 fatty acids daily) resulted in a 27% reduction in triglyceride levels and an 11% reduction in the ratio of total to high-density lipoprotein cholesterol after 4 weeks.[75] As fish oil may also have a mild antipsoriatic effect, it was felt that it could prove a useful adjunct in such patients. In a prospective study of 128 adults with chronic, stable psoriasis treated with oral acitretin for 2 years, there was no evidence from serial liver biopsy of cumulative hepatotoxicity.[76] A 5-year prospective study of 956 patients with psoriasis treated with etretinate provided no evidence for an increased risk of cardiovascular disease, cancer, diabetes or inflammatory bowel disease in association with long-term use.[77]

Oral retinoids are teratogenic. Etretinate may be detected in body fat stores for up to 2 years after discontinuation of therapy; acitretin, although normally excreted much more rapidly, may in certain circumstances be converted *in vivo* to etretinate. For these reasons both drugs should normally be avoided in women of child-bearing potential.

Comment

Retinoid therapy is not suitable for every patient with severe psoriasis. It should normally be used in combination with either phototherapy or topical therapy, when lower doses may suffice to achieve satisfactory control. Apart from the risk of teratogenicity, the potential for serious harm from retinoid therapy appears to be less than from other interventions used in severe psoriasis such as methotrexate, PUVA or ciclosporin.

Methotrexate

Methotrexate has been widely used to treat severe psoriasis since the 1960s. It was the first potent systemic antipsoriatic agent to be introduced into practice and has continued to play a vital role in the management of severe psoriasis, despite the advent of newer treatments. It has not been subjected to the same rigorous evaluation as some newer agents and a recent systematic review found no RCT in which standard methods of methotrexate administration for psoriasis were compared with placebo or with any alternative treatment modality in patients with chronic plaque psoriasis.[78] Evidence from case series supports the place of methotrexate as one of the most powerful drugs in common use for severe psoriasis. Only recently has it been formally compared with another systemic agent. No significant difference in response at 16 weeks was found in 85 patients randomised to receive either methotrexate or ciclosporin, although the latter appeared to act more rapidly (Spuls P,

personal communication). Methotrexate is normally well tolerated, although nausea is common and can cause patients to stop therapy. Acute myelosuppression is a more important cause of serious morbidity and mortality than the chronic liver damage for which methotrexate is well recognised.

Efficacy

One systematic review (search date 1999, no RCT) has been published.[78] One as yet unpublished RCT was identified. In addition, a systematic review of treatments for psoriatic arthritis included two RCTs of methotrexate versus placebo, both demonstrating benefit for arthritis.[79]

Versus placebo

No RCTs have compared the effects of methotrexate on the skin of psoriasis patients with placebo. Published studies would suggest that methotrexate can reduce disease severity by at least 50% in at least three-quarters of patients treated.[78] For example, in an uncontrolled series of 113 people with severe psoriasis, treatment with weekly low-dose methotrexate (maximum dose 15 mg) gave satisfactory control in 81% people over a mean treatment duration of 8 years.[80] Of 252 psoriasis patients followed for up to 20 years, Zachariae stated that methotrexate greatly improved 60%, and modestly improved 30%; only 10% were not improved.[81] In another retrospective study of 98 patients with a history of psoriasis which had previously relapsed rapidly following clearance by the Ingram method (inpatient anthralin and UVB phototherapy), maintenance treatment with methotrexate was commenced during a further course of Ingram therapy; relapse rates were compared with historical controls available for 46 patients in the cohort. Without methotrexate maintenance, psoriasis had begun to reappear within 1 month and had relapsed to pretreatment severity by 5 months. Methotrexate at weekly doses averaging 7·5–15 mg lengthened these intervals to about 1 year and to considerably more than 3 years, respectively.[82]

Versus ciclosporin

One RCT (n = 85) compared various dose regimens of methotrexate, 15–22·5 mg weekly, and ciclosporin, 3–5 mg/kg/day, for 12 weeks followed by tapered withdrawal to 16 weeks.[83] There was no significant difference in response at 16 weeks, although ciclosporin appeared to act more rapidly.

Drawbacks

The most frequent symptomatic side-effect of low-dose methotrexate therapy is nausea, which may affect up to one-third of treated people.[80] The most important potential side-effect is acute myelosuppression, which is the cause of most of the rare deaths attributable to methotrexate when used as a therapy for psoriasis.[84] Methotrexate is eliminated largely via the kidneys, and toxic levels may build up rapidly in the presence of renal impairment. Particular care is required in the elderly in whom renal function may deteriorate rapidly in response to acute illness; dietary folate deficiency may add to toxicity. Recent work has shown that circulating homocysteine levels are elevated in psoriasis patients receiving methotrexate but that folate supplementation can reverse this abnormality[85]; since raised homocysteine levels have been associated with atherothrombotic vascular disease, it may be advisable for all patients on methotrexate to receive folate supplements. Certain drugs, particularly non-steroidal anti-inflammatory drugs, aspirin, trimethoprim and sulphonamides, may interfere with methotrexate pharmacokinetics and thus increase the risk of toxicity, particularly when renal function is impaired.[86] Regular monitoring of the full blood count is essential. Long-term methotrexate

treatment carries with it a risk of hepatic fibrosis and cirrhosis, which is related to the dosage regimen employed. The original method of administering methotrexate in small daily doses was shown to be much more hepatotoxic than the same overall amount given as a single weekly dose.[87,88] An alternative regimen in which the weekly dose is divided into three parts taken at 12-hourly intervals is still widely used[89] although the theoretical basis from which it was devised is unlikely to be valid.[90] Liver toxicity is enhanced by alcohol abuse, and patients who cannot restrict alcohol consumption are not suited to methotrexate therapy.[84] On the other hand, if patients are carefully monitored and both methotrexate dose and alcohol consumption are restricted, then many patients may continue therapy safely for prolonged periods. In two case series examining long-term once-weekly low-dose (<20 mg) methotrexate therapy (n = 49 and 55; mean duration of therapy 9·7 and 7·5 years, respectively),[80,91] no correlation between cumulative methotrexate dose or duration of therapy and the risk of liver fibrosis or cirrhosis was found. Unfortunately standard tests of liver function do not reliably detect liver toxicity; they may remain normal in the presence of hepatic cirrhosis. The Psoriasis Task Force of the American Academy of Dermatology recommends that liver biopsy should be performed on psoriasis patients after treatment has been established and thereafter with each cumulative dose of 1·5 g methotrexate – in practice about every 18 months to 2 years for the average patient.[92] Others have argued that the morbidity and potential hazards of performing regular liver biopsy in patients receiving long-term low-dose methotrexate for psoriasis are difficult to justify when measured against the low yield of information resulting in a change of management.[91] A number of workers have recommended that a serological marker of hepatic fibrosis, the aminoterminal peptide of Type III procollagen, may be used to screen for underlying hepatic damage and that liver biopsy may then be reserved for those with consistently abnormal results.[93,94]

Comment

Methotrexate continues to play an important role in the management of severe psoriasis despite the advent of newer therapies. It appears to be particularly valuable for patients with concomitant arthritis. Overall, it is probably safer for long-term use than other therapies such as ciclosporin and PUVA.

Hydroxyurea

Hydroxyurea is a systemic therapy for severe psoriasis which is mainly used as a substitute for more commonly used systemic drugs such as ciclosporin or methotrexate when these are contraindicated. The evidence for its efficacy has been considered in a systematic review.[59] Hydroxyurea has not been directly compared with other systemic therapies. Side-effects include bone-marrow suppression and teratogenicity. There is a need for high-quality RCTs of hydroxyurea both against placebo and against other systemic agents.

Efficacy

One systematic review (search date 1999) identified only one RCT. This compared hydroxyurea, 1 g daily, with matching placebo, each given for 4 weeks in a crossover study involving 10 people. Improvement was noted by the investigators in seven of 10 and by the participants in nine of 10 periods of active therapy as opposed to only one of 10 periods of placebo therapy.[95]

Drawbacks

The doses of hydroxyurea advocated for psoriasis are close to those that may cause bone-marrow suppression. There is little information on long-term toxicity.

Comment

The study referred to allowed for the continuation of hydroxyurea therapy in an open assessment.[95] The authors commented that it took 6 weeks for maximal improvement to be achieved. Hydroxyurea has been used for treating psoriasis for nearly 30 years. The fact that it has not been nearly so widely used as other treatment modalities and that it has been seen necessary to use it in combination with other powerful antipsoriatic drugs suggest that dermatologists have not found it very effective compared with treatments such as methotrexate, ciclosporin or photochemotherapy (PUVA). The available data do not allow a direct comparison with these treatments. Nevertheless there is some evidence that individual patients may respond well. Hydroxyurea has the advantage that it may be possible to use it in circumstances where other treatments are contraindicated.

Fumarates

For some 20 years a mixture of dimethyl and monoethyl esters of fumaric acid has been used widely in Northern Europe, particularly in German-speaking countries, as a systemic treatment for severe psoriasis. The evidence for the efficacy of oral fumaric acid therapy has been considered in a systematic review[59] which concluded that it is an effective systemic treatment for psoriasis. Of the constituents of the standard compound fumaric acid ester therapy in use in Northern Europe (Fumaderm), dimethylfumarate appears to be the principal active component although only the compound mixture has thus far been licensed for clinical use. Formal comparisons with topical or with other systemic therapies have not been performed. The incidence of symptomatic side-effects is high.

Efficacy

One systematic review (search date 1999, 6 RCTs, 258 people)[59] included all the RCTs identified by the present search.

Versus placebo

In the two RCTs comparing the standard compound fumaric acid ester therapy (maximum dose 1290 mg ester mixture daily) with placebo (n = 123), 34 of 61 (56%) people treated for up to 16 weeks achieved at least a 70% reduction in PASI score whereas only 5 of 62 (8%) receiving placebo showed similar improvement (rate difference 0·47, CI 0·33–0·61).[96,97] Two RCTs comparing fumaric esters monotherapy with placebo showed benefit from dimethylfumarate (n = 42) but not monoethylfumarate (n = 38).[98]

Fumaric acid ester regimens compared

In one RCT (n = 45) no difference in efficacy between Fumaderm and dimethylfumarate monotherapy could be demonstrated.[99]

Drawbacks

Symptomatic side-effects (flushing and gastrointestinal disturbance) are frequent but result in discontinuation of therapy in fewer than 10% of patients.[97,100] Eosinophilia and mild lymphocytopenia are common. Serious side-effects appear to be rare.

Comment

Similar response rates have been reported in a prospective open study.[100] In those who completed 4 months' therapy (70 of 101 people enrolled) an average 80% reduction in PASI score was seen. Seven per cent discontinued therapy because of side-effects. Little information is available on the long-term success of treatment with fumarates.

Azathioprine

Oral azathioprine has been used to a limited extent for treating severe psoriasis for many years but there is little evidence to support its use. It may cause catastrophic myelosuppression. Its efficacy has not been compared in RCTs with either placebo or other systemic therapies. The fact that nowadays azathioprine is rarely used in psoriasis suggests that it is not as effective as other systemic therapies such as methotrexate, ciclosporin and PUVA.

Efficacy

One systematic review[59] and the present search both failed to identify any RCTs of azathioprine treatment in psoriasis.

Drawbacks

In people who cannot metabolise the drug normally because of a deficiency in thiopurine methyltransferase, there is a high risk of catastrophic bone marrow suppression. Nausea and vomiting are common. A drug-induced hepatitis may occur.

Comment

One uncontrolled study published in the early 1970s reported benefit in 19 of 29 people treated.[101]

Sulfasalazine

Sulfasalazine is an anti-inflammatory drug which is widely used for the treatment of inflammatory polyarthritides. The findings in one RCT suggest that it is a moderately effective treatment for severe psoriasis although probably less so than acitretin, ciclosporin, PUVA and methotrexate. Further RCTs comparing sulfasalazine with placebo and with other systemic therapies are justified.

Efficacy

One systematic review (search date 1999)[59] identified the single RCT located by the present search. Sulfasalazine, 3–4 g daily for 8 weeks, produced >60% improvement in seven of 23

(30%) patients compared with none of the 27 who received placebo.[102] Altogether 14 (61%) patients receiving sulfasalazine and only one (4%) receiving placebo were judged to have shown >30% reduction in clinical severity score (rate difference 0·57, CI 0·36 to 0·78).

Drawbacks

The most common side-effects are headache, nausea and vomiting. In general these are dose related.

Comment

Larger studies for longer treatment periods would be required to assess the place of this drug in psoriasis therapy.

How effective are treatments for guttate psoriasis?

We found two systematic reviews from the same group of investigators; one examined antistreptococcal interventions for both guttate and chronic plaque psoriasis (search date 2000, one RCT, 20 people)[103] whilst the second examined other interventions for guttate psoriasis (search date 2000, one RCT, 21 people).[104] We found no additional RCTs not considered by these investigators. No published report could be found to support or to challenge current commonly used methods of management of guttate psoriasis, which include tar, topical corticosteroids, vitamin D analogues and UVB phototherapy.

Although it is well known that guttate psoriasis may be precipitated by streptococcal infection, and antibiotics have frequently been advocated for patients with recurrent guttate psoriasis, the authors of the reviews concluded that there was no firm evidence to support the use of antibiotics either in the management of established guttate psoriasis or in preventing the development of guttate psoriasis following streptococcal sore throat.

Tonsillectomy has been advocated for patients with recurrent streptococcal sore throat associated with either recurrent guttate psoriasis or recalcitrant chronic plaque psoriasis; although an uncontrolled prospective study claimed clearance in five of six people with recurrent guttate psoriasis subjected to tonsillectomy,[104] there is no firm evidence to date that such intervention is beneficial.

Efficacy

The reviews did not identify any trials of standard therapies (tar, topical corticosteroids, vitamin D analogues, phototherapy) for guttate psoriasis.

Omega-3 fatty acids

One RCT (n = 21) compared the effects of daily intravenous infusions of lipid-rich emulsions containing either fish-oil-derived omega-3 fatty acids or placebo (omega-6 fatty acids) in hospitalised patients with acute guttate psoriasis. The former produced a rapid beneficial effect (improvement in severity scores of 45–76% over 10 days) not seen in patients receiving omega-6 supplementation (16–25% over 10 days).[106] It is not known whether oral supplementation with omega-3 fatty acids would have similar effects, although they have been shown to have a modest effect in chronic plaque psoriasis.

Antibiotic therapy

Despite recommendations in many standard texts that antibiotics should be given to people with recurrent guttate psoriasis, the only RCT examining their use found no evidence of benefit in any patient receiving either of two antibiotic regimens.[107]

Tonsillectomy

No RCT examining the effects of tonsillectomy on recurrence or persistence of guttate psoriasis was found.

Drawbacks

There is insufficient information. Tonsillectomy carries with it a small risk of serious adverse outcome.

Comment

There is very little information to guide practice, particularly with regard to the place of and optimal regimen for phototherapy in guttate psoriasis.

How effective are treatments for chronic palmoplantar pustular psoriasis?

We found one systematic review examining interventions for chronic palmoplantar pustular psoriasis (search date 2001, 23 RCTs, 724 people).[108] We did not find further RCTs not included in this review.

Topical corticosteroids with and without occlusion

Moderately potent corticosteroids under hydrocolloid occlusion may induce rapid clearance of chronic palmoplantar pustular psoriasis; such therapy is more effective than superpotent corticosteroids without occlusion. Because of side-effects associated with long-term corticosteroid use and the rapid relapse seen after interruption of therapy, it is likely to be helpful mainly as an adjunct to other interventions.

Efficacy

In one RCT (n = 19) identified in the review,[108] 12 of 19 sides receiving medium-strength corticosteroid under hydrocolloid occlusion for 4 weeks cleared compared with 3 of 19 sides receiving highly potent corticosteroid twice daily (success rate difference 0·47 (CI 0·20 to 0·75). Relapse to pretreatment severity occurred within 4 weeks of discontinuing therapy.

Drawbacks

Prolonged use of potent corticosteroids results in skin atrophy.

Comment

This is the only form of topical therapy which has been subjected to rigorous assessment.

Systemic retinoid monotherapy

Systemic retinoids are widely used for treating chronic palmoplantar pustular psoriasis. Most of the available studies were carried out when etretinate was available but this has now been replaced by acitretin. The review[108] found that the two drugs are of comparable efficacy and that about two in five patients achieve a good or excellent response. There is evidence that improvement may be maintained by continuing therapy at a lower dose. Retinoid therapy is more effective than photochemotherapy (PUVA).

Efficacy
High-dose retinoid versus placebo for induction of remission

The review identified four RCTs involving 127 people. Twenty-six of 67 (39%) patients who received etretinate (modal dose 1 mg/kg/day) as compared with 10 of 60 (17%) who received placebo achieved a good or excellent response (intention-to-treat analysis) with a success rate difference of 0·22 favouring retinoids (CI 0·07 to 0·36).

Low-dose retinoid versus placebo for maintenance of remission

The review found two RCTs involving 45 people. Thirteen of 21 (62%) who had responded to initial high dose (1 mg/kg/day) etretinate therapy maintained clinical remission for 3 months with low-dose etretinate (20–30 mg daily) as compared with five of 24 (21%) who received placebo. Success rate difference was 0·42 in favour of etretinate (CI 0·16 to 0·68).

Acitretin versus etretinate
One RCT (n = 60) found no difference in efficacy of the two retinoids as judged by reduction in pustule counts.

Versus PUVA
Two RCTs involving 121 people compared etretinate with PUVA (both topical and systemic). Seventeen of 43 (40%) cleared with retinoid compared with seven of 78 (9%) who received PUVA. The success rate difference was 0·38 in favour of retinoid therapy (CI 0·21 to 0·54).

Drawbacks
Systemic retinoids have well-known mucocutaneous side-effects which limit their acceptability to many patients. Both etretinate and acitretin are unsuitable for use in women at risk of pregnancy.

Comment
Even at high doses, systemic retinoids achieve a good response in under half of people treated.

Photochemotherapy alone
The review[108] found that there is little to support the use of topical psoralen photochemotherapy (topical PUVA) but that oral psoralen photochemotherapy (systemic PUVA) cleared chronic palmoplantar pustular psoriasis in a minority of people.

Efficacy
Versus placebo
Four RCTs involving 90 people compared either topical or systemic PUVA with placebo. Fifteen of 36 (42%) receiving oral PUVA cleared, compared with 0 of 36 (0%) receiving placebo: success rate difference 0·42 (CI 0·25 to 0·58). One of 54 (2%) receiving topical PUVA cleared, compared with none of 54 receiving placebo: success rate difference 0·02 (CI –0·04 to 0·08).

Topical PUVA versus systemic PUVA
In the one RCT identified (n = 64), 4 of 51 (8%) cleared with topical PUVA compared with none of 13 who received systemic PUVA: success rate difference 0·08 (CI –0·05 to 0·21).

Versus retinoids
See above.

Drawbacks
Topical PUVA causes blistering and irritation of the skin in a minority of treated patients. Systemic PUVA has well-known potential side-effects. The risk of carcinogenesis is likely to be considerably less where only the palms and soles are irradiated.

Comment
The failure of palmoplantar pustular psoriasis to clear in any of the 13 patients who received oral PUVA in the study comparing systemic and topical PUVA is at variance with the findings from the two studies comparing oral PUVA with placebo. This may be a chance difference as numbers involved are small.

RePUVA
The review[107] identified three RCTs examining RePUVA. These studies demonstrated that the combination is more effective than either PUVA or retinoids alone and suggest that this modality is the most effective treatment available for achieving remission of palmoplantar pustular psoriasis.

Efficacy

In two RCTs (n = 54) systemic PUVA was used; the other (n = 20) employed topical 8-MOP. Overall, 28 of 41 (68%) cleared with PUVA-etretinate compared with 9 of 33 (27%) receiving PUVA alone: success rate difference 0·44 (CI 0·24 to 0·63). In the two studies where an analysis could be made, the clearance rate in sites treated with retinoids alone was 15%, compared with 61% for the combination with PUVA: success rate difference 0·45 (CI 0·25 to 0·66).

Drawbacks

Although patients are exposed to the risks of both retinoids and PUVA, some evidence suggests that lower doses of UVA are required than when PUVA monotherapy is used.

Comment

The clearance rates achieved here are higher than with any other reported intervention.

Ciclosporin

Although measurable improvement has been demonstrated with ciclosporin, there is no good RCT evidence to date that it can induce clearance of chronic palmoplantar pustular psoriasis. This may be because the published studies have been too short and have used inadequate doses. Uncontrolled studies have reported good to excellent results in patients treated for longer periods at higher doses if required (for example more than two-thirds good or excellent response at 1 year in 58 people receiving up to 4 mg/kg/day for a year[109]).

Efficacy

Two RCTs (n = 98) were identified in the review.[108] Both were short (4 weeks) and used low doses of ciclosporin (1 and 2·5 mg/kg/day). Thirty of 47 (64%) people receiving ciclosporin improved, compared with 10 of 51 (20%) receiving placebo: success rate difference 0·44 (CI 0·27 to 0·60). Improvement was defined as a 50% reduction in pustule count; no reports of clearance were given.

Drawbacks

Ciclosporin has well known side-effects including hypertension and renal impairment.

Comment

Further studies are required to establish the place of this drug in the management of chronic palmoplantar pustular psoriasis.

Tetracycline antibiotics

There is good RCT evidence that tetracyclines may induce limited improvement in chronic palmoplantar pustular psoriasis.

Efficacy

Two RCTs of crossover design (240 treatment courses with either tetracycline or clomocycline in 100 patients) were identified in the review.[108] Overall, improvement was seen in 58 of 120 (48%) tetracycline treatment courses compared with 23 of 120 (19%) placebo courses: success rate difference 0·29 (CI 0·19 to 0·40). Few patients achieved clearance.

Drawbacks

Tetracyclines are normally well tolerated but may cause gastrointestinal upset.

Comment

Tetracycline therapy is generally safe and well tolerated but the limited degree of benefit seen may not justify routine use for chronic palmoplantar pustular psoriasis.

Other therapies

The review[108] identified limited benefit from Grenz ray therapy and little to support the use of tar, anthralin, colchicine or methotrexate.

Efficacy

In one RCT of Grenz ray therapy, 13 of 17 sides receiving Grenz ray showed greater improvement than the contralateral side; by comparison an advantage was seen in only one of 17 sides receiving placebo. The author commented that the degree of improvement was modest. One of two RCTs comparing colchicine with placebo claimed benefit from the former but at the expense of troublesome side-effects. There is no good evidence from RCTs to support the use of tar or anthralin. There are no RCTs of methotrexate therapy for chronic palmoplantar pustular psoriasis. In an uncontrolled prospective study eight of 25 people given methotrexate, 25 mg weekly for 2 months, achieved a good or excellent response. The response rate appeared greater in those with evidence of psoriasis elsewhere (six of 12) than in those without (two of 13).[110]

Drawbacks

Colchicine commonly causes gastrointestinal disturbances. Methotrexate can cause myelosuppression and liver damage and is now usually used at a lower dose than in this study.

Comments

A comparison of methotrexate with retinoid therapy might help to establish whether there is a place for the former in this disease, the ideal therapy for which remains elusive.

How effective are treatments for acrodermatitis continua of Hallopeau?

We found no RCT of treatments for this uncommon but disabling pustular form of psoriasis, which can cause marked destruction of fingernails, toenails and surrounding tissues. The greatest number of published case reports in which successful response to treatment is claimed is for ciclosporin, although acitretin, methotrexate and dapsone have been reported in individual case reports to produce resolution.

Key points

- The current review does not claim to be comprehensive and in particular has not considered commonly used topical agents including anthralin (dithranol), tar and topical corticosteroids, nor all variants of psoriasis (for example nail psoriasis, scalp psoriasis, generalised pustular psoriasis).
- Many psoriasis trials are too small and of too short a duration to be able to draw robust conclusions. Few trials record patients' own evaluations of treatment efficacy and tolerability. There is, however, a considerable amount of information to help guide practice.

Chronic plaque psoriasis

- There is firm RCT evidence of effectiveness of a range of treatments for chronic plaque psoriasis, specifically:

  - calcipotriol
  - ciclosporin
  - systemic retinoids (acitretin and etretinate), especially in combination with phototherapy
  - phototherapy including broadband ultraviolet B (UVB), narrowband UVB and psoralen photochemotherapy (PUVA)
  - combinations of topical vitamin D_3 analogues and topical corticosteroids with either UVB or PUVA
  - heliotherapy (natural sunlight)
  - fumaric acid esters

- methotrexate, although effectiveness of this widely accepted drug has been examined specifically in chronic plaque psoriasis in only one RCT.

- There is evidence of lack of efficacy of UVA sunbed (with low UVB emission) and balneotherapy (spa water).
- There is a lack of firm RCT evidence of effectiveness of other therapies for chronic plaque psoriasis, including tacalcitol, azathioprine, hydroxyurea and sulfasalazine (although one small RCT has shown moderate efficacy from sulfasalazine).
- It is clear that there is a paucity of studies addressing long-term management of severe chronic plaque psoriasis. There is, however, good evidence of risk of serious harm from the major treatment modalities used for treating severe psoriasis, including skin cancer from PUVA and heliotherapy, hypertension and renal impairment from ciclosporin, myelosuppression and hepatic fibrosis from methotrexate, and teratogenicity from systemic retinoids.

Gutatte psoriasis

- There is virtually no guidance from controlled trials on how to manage guttate psoriasis.

Palmoplantar pustular psoriasis

- There is no ideal treatment for chronic palmoplantar pustular psoriasis but there is RCT evidence to support the use of topical corticosteroid under hydrocolloid occlusion, systemic retinoids, systemic PUVA, and systemic retinoids in combination with systemic PUVA. Of these, the last appears to give the greatest chance of disease control.
- There is some evidence that modest improvements may be attained with low-dose ciclosporin, tetracycline antibiotics, and Grenz ray therapy.
- There is little evidence to support the use of colchicine, topical PUVA, hydroxyurea or methotrexate.

References

1. Franssen MJAM, van den Hoogen FHJ, van de Putte LBA. Psoriatic Arthropathy. In: van de Kerkhof PCM, ed. *Textbook of Psoriasis*. Oxford: Blackwell Science, 1999:30–42.

2. Telfer NR, Chalmers RJ, Whale K, Colman G. The role of streptococcal infection in the initiation of guttate psoriasis. *Arch Dermatol* 1992;**128**:39–42.

3. van de Kerkhof PCM. Clinical features. In: van de Kerkhof PCM, ed. *Textbook of Psoriasis*. Oxford: Blackwell Science, 1999:3–29.

4. Farber EM, Nall L. Epidemiology: natural history and genetics. In: Roenigk HH, Maibach HI, eds. *Psoriasis, 3rd ed*. New York: Marcel Dekker, 1998:107–57.

5. Camp RDR. Psoriasis. In: Champion RH, Burton JL, Burns DA, Breathnach SM, eds. *Textbook of Dermatology, 6th edn*. Oxford: Blackwell Science, 1998:1589–1649.

6. Nevitt GJ, Hutchinson PE. Psoriasis in the community: prevalence, severity and patients' beliefs and attitudes towards the disease. *Br J Dermatol* 1996;**135**:533–7.

7. van de Kerkhof PCM. Pathogenesis. In: van de Kerkhof PCM, ed. *Textbook of Psoriasis*. Oxford: Blackwell Science, 1999:79–105.

8. Savin JA. Psychosocial Aspects. In: van de Kerkhof PCM, ed. *Textbook of Psoriasis*. Oxford: Blackwell Science, 1999:43–53.

9. Martin BA, Chalmers RJ, Telfer NR. How great is the risk of further psoriasis following a single episode of acute guttate psoriasis? *Arch Dermatol* 1996;**132**:717–18.

10. Optimal search strategy for RCTs. From Dickersin K, Larson K. Establishing and maintaining an international register of RCTs. In: Cochrane Collaboration. *Cochrane Library*. Oxford: Update Software, 1996.

11. Griffiths CEM, Clark CM, Chalmers RJG, Li Wan Po A, Williams HC. A systematic review of treatments for severe psoriasis. *Health Technol Assess* 2000;**4**(40):1–115.

12. Watsky KL, Freije L, Leneveu MC, Wenck HA, Leffell DJ. Water-in-oil emollients as steroid-sparing adjunctive therapy in the treatment of psoriasis. *Cutis* 1992;**50**:383–6.

13. Hagemann I, Proksch E. Topical treatment by urea reduces epidermal hyperproliferation and induces differentiation in psoriasis. *Acta Derm Venereol* 1996;**76**:353–6.

14. Fredriksson TLM. A blind controlled comparison between a new cream ("12 + 12"), its vehicle, and salicylic acid in

petrolatum on psoriatic plaques. *Curr Ther Res* 1985;**37**:805–9.

15. Friedman SJ. Management of psoriasis vulgaris with a hydrocolloid occlusive dressing. *Arch Dermatol* 1987;**123**:1046–52.

16. David M, Lowe NJ. Psoriasis therapy: comparative studies with a hydrocolloid dressing, plastic film occlusion, and triamcinolone acetonide cream. *J Am Acad Dermatol* 1989;**21**:511–14.

17. Nielsen PG. Calcipotriol or clobetasol propionate occluded with a hydrocolloid dressing for treatment of nummular psoriasis. *Acta Derm Venereol* 1993;**73**:394.

18. Koo J, Cuffie CA, Tanner DJ *et al.* Mometasone furoate 0·1%-salicylic acid 5% ointment versus mometasone furoate 0·1% ointment in the treatment of moderate-to-severe psoriasis: a multicenter study. *Clin Ther* 1998;**20**:283–91.

19. Zgrzyblowski A, Paradecki W, Przybyla L. Serum levels of salicylic acid in patients with psoriasis treated with 10% salicylic acid ointment. *Przeglad Dermatol* 1990;**77**:20–4.

20. Maune S, Frese KA, Mrowietz U, Reker U. Toxic inner ear damage in topical treatment of psoriasis with salicylates. *Laryngorhinootologie* 1997;**76**:368–70.

21. Kristensen B, Kristensen O. Topical salicylic acid interferes with UVB therapy for psoriasis. *Acta Derm Venereol* 1991;**71**:37–40.

22. Ashcroft DM, Li Wan Po A, Williams HC, Griffiths CE. Systematic review of comparative efficacy and tolerability of calcipotriol in treating chronic plaque psoriasis. *BMJ* 2000;**320**:963–7.

23. Kragballe K, Barnes L, Hamberg KJ *et al.* Calcipotriol cream with or without concurrent topical corticosteroid in psoriasis: tolerability and efficacy. *Br J Dermatol* 1998;**139**:649–54.

24. Douglas WS, Bibby AJ. A new calcipotriol/betamethasone formulation with rapid onset of action is superior to betamethasone dipropionate ointment and calcipotriol ointment in psoriasis. In: *Congress abstracts from European Academy of Dermatology and Venereology 10th Congress.* Munich: EADV, 2001:620.

25. Griffiths CEM, Clark CM, Chalmers RJG, Li Wan Po A, Williams HC. Phototherapy and photochemotherapy. In: *A systematic review of treatments for severe psoriasis.* Health Technol Assess 2000;**4**(40):55–74.

26. Gambichler T, Kreuter JA, Altmeyer P, Hoffmann K. Meta-analysis of the efficacy of balneophototherapy. *Aktuelle Dermatol* 2000;**26**:402–6.

27. Markham T, Rogers S, Collins P. A comparison of oral 8-methoxypsoralen PUVA and narrowband UVB (TL-01) phototherapy in the management of chronic plaque psoriasis. *Br J Dermatol* 2001;**145**(Suppl. 59):12–26.

28. Hannuksela-Svahn A, Sigurgeirsson B, Pukkala E *et al.* Trioxsalen bath PUVA did not increase the risk of squamous cell skin carcinoma and cutaneous malignant melanoma in a joint analysis of 944 Swedish and Finnish patients with psoriasis. *Br J Dermatol* 1999;**141**: 497–501.

29. Frentz G, Olsen JH, Avrach WW. Malignant tumours and psoriasis: climatotherapy at the Dead Sea. *Br J Dermatol* 1999;**141**:1088–91.

30. Stern RS, Lunder EJ. Risk of squamous cell carcinoma and methoxsalen (psoralen) and UV-A radiation (PUVA). A meta-analysis. *Arch Dermatol* 1998;**134**:1582–5.

31. Stern RS. The risk of melanoma in association with long-term exposure to PUVA. *J Am Acad Dermatol* 2001;**44**: 755–61.

32. British Photodermatology Group . British Photodermatology Group guidelines for PUVA. *Br J Dermatol* 1994;**130**: 246–55.

33. British Photodermatology Group. An appraisal of narrowband (TL-01) UVB phototherapy. British Photodermatology Group Workshop report (April 1996). *Br J Dermatol* 1997;**137**:327–30·

34. Boer J, Hermans J, Schothorst AA, Suurmond D. Comparison of phototherapy (UV-B) and photochemo-therapy (PUVA) for clearing and maintenance therapy of psoriasis. *Arch Dermatol* 1984;**120**:52–7.

35. Stern RS, Armstrong RB, Anderson TF *et al.* Effect of continued ultraviolet B phototherapy on the duration of remission of psoriasis: a randomized study. *J Am Acad Dermatol* 1986;**15**:546–52.

36. Adrian RM, Parrish JA, Khosrow M, Karlin MJ. Outpatient phototherapy for psoriasis. *Arch Dermatol* 1981;**117**:623–6.

37. Selvaag E, Caspersen L, Bech-Thomsen N, de Fine Olivarius F, Wulf HC. Optimized UVB treatment of psoriasis: a controlled, left-right comparison trial. *J Eur Acad Dermatol Venereol* 2000;**14**:19–21.

38. van Weelden H, Baaart de la Faille H, Young E, van der Leun JC. A new development in UVB phototherapy of psoriasis. *Br J Dermatol* 1988;**119**:11–19.

39. Dawe RS, Wainwright NJ, Cameron H, Ferguson J. Narrow-band (TL-01) ultraviolet B phototherapy for

chronic plaque psoriasis: three times or five times weekly treatment? Br J Dermatol 1998;**138**:833–839.

40. Snellman E, Aromaa A, Jansen CT *et al.* Supervised four-week heliotherapy alleviates the long-term course of psoriasis. *Acta Derm Venereol* 1993;**73**:388–92.

41. Léauté-Labràze C, Saillour F, Châne G *et al.* Saline spa water or combined water and UVB for psoriasis versus conventional UVB. Lessons from the Salies de Béarn randomized study. *Arch Dermatol* 2001;**137**:1035–9.

42. Turner RJ, Walshaw D, Diffey BL, Farr PM. A controlled study of ultraviolet A sunbed treatment of psoriasis. *Br J Dermatol* 2000;**143**:957–63.

43. Melski JW, Tanenbaum L, Parrish JA *et al.* Oral methoxsalen photochemotherapy for the treatment of psoriasis: a cooperative clinical trial. *J Invest Dermatol* 1977;**68**:328–35.

44. Henseler T, Wolff K, Honigsmann H, Christophers E. Oral 8-methoxypsoralen photochemotherapy of psoriasis. The European PUVA study: a cooperative study among 18 European centres. *Lancet* 1981;**1**:853–7.

45. de Berker DA, Sakuntabhai A, Diffey BL, Matthews JN, Farr PM. Comparison of psoralen-UVB and psoralen-UVA photochemotherapy in the treatment of psoriasis. *J Am Acad Dermatol* 1997;**36**:577–81.

46. Rogers S, Marks J, Shuster S, Briffa DV, Warin A, Greaves M. Comparison of photochemotherapy and dithranol in the treatment of chronic plaque psoriasis. *Lancet* 1979;**1**:455–8.

47. Collins P, Rogers S. Bath-water compared with oral delivery of 8-methoxypsoralen PUVA therapy for chronic plaque psoriasis. *Br J Dermatol* 1992;**127**:392–5.

48. Turjanmaa K, Salo H, Reunala T. Comparison of trioxsalen bath and oral methoxsalen PUVA in psoriasis. *Acta Derm Venereol* 1985;**65**:86–8.

49. Cooper EJ, Herd RM, Priestley GC, Hunter JA. A comparison of bathwater and oral delivery of 8-methoxypsoralen in PUVA therapy for plaque psoriasis. *Clin Exp Dermatol* 2000;**25**:111–14.

50. Sadananda Naik PV, Paily PP, Gopinatha Pillai KG, Asokan PU. Photochemotherapy for psoriasis with psoralen and sunlight. *Indian J Dermatol Venereol Lepr* 1981;**47**:9–16.

51. Parrish JA, White AD, Kingsbury T, Zahar M, Fitzpatrick TB. Photochemotherapy of psoriasis using methoxsalen and sunlight. A controlled study. *Arch Dermatol* 1977;**113**: 1529–32.

52. Gordon PM, Diffey BL, Matthews JN, Farr PM. A randomized comparison of narrow-band TL-01 phototherapy and PUVA photochemotherapy for psoriasis. *J Am Acad Dermatol* 1999;**41**:728–32.

53. Dawe RS, Cameron H, Yule S *et al.* A comparison of TL-01 UVB phototherapy and bath-PUVA for chronic plaque psoriasis. *Br J Dermatol* 2000;**143**(Suppl. 57):15.

54. Lauharanta J, Juvakoski T, Lassus A. A clinical evaluation of the effects of an aromatic retinoid (Tigason), combination of retinoid and PUVA, and PUVA alone in severe psoriasis. *Br J Dermatol* 1981;**104**:325–32.

55. Ramsay CA, Schwartz BE, Lowson D, Papp K, Bolduc A, Gilbert M. Calcipotriol cream combined with twice weekly broad-band UVB phototherapy: a safe, effective and UVB-sparing antipsoriatric combination treatment. The Canadian Calcipotriol and UVB Study Group. *Dermatology* 2000;**200**:17–24.

56. Brands S, Brakman M, Bos JD, de Rie MA. No additional effect of calcipotriol ointment on low-dose narrow-band UVB phototherapy in psoriasis. *J Am Acad Dermatol* 1999;**41**:991–5.

57. Gerritsen MJ, Boezeman JB, Elbers ME, van de Kerkhof PC. Dithranol embedded in crystalline monoglycerides combined with phototherapy (UVB): a new approach in the treatment of psoriasis. *Skin Pharmacol Appl Skin Physiol* 1998;**11**:133–9.

58. Stern RS, Liebman EJ, Vakeva L. Oral psoralen and ultraviolet-A light (PUVA) treatment of psoriasis and persistent risk of nonmelanoma skin cancer. PUVA Follow-up Study. *J Natl Cancer Inst* 1998;**90**:1278–84.

59. Griffiths CEM, Clark CM, Chalmers RJG, Li Wan Po A, Williams HC. Cyclosporin. In: A systematic review of treatments for severe psoriasis. *Health Technol Assess* 2000;**4**(40):13–23.

60. Laburte C, Grossman R, Abi-Rached J, Abeywickrama KH, Dubertret L. Efficacy and safety of oral cyclosporin A (CyA;Sandimmun) for long-term treatment of chronic severe plaque psoriasis. *Br J Dermatol* 1994;**130**:366–75.

61. Ellis CN, Fradin MS, Hamilton TA, Voorhees JJ. Duration of remission during maintenance cyclosporine therapy for psoriasis: Relationship to maintenance dose and degree of improvement during initial therapy. *Arch Dermatol* 1995;**131**:791–5.

62. Shupack J, Abel E, Bauer E *et al.* Cyclosporine as maintenance therapy in patients with severe psoriasis. *J Am Acad Dermatol* 1997;**36**:423–32.

63. Zachariae H, Abrams B, Bleehen SS et al. Conversion of psoriasis patients from the conventional formulation of cyclosporin A to a new microemulsion formulation: a randomized, open, multicentre assessment of safety and tolerability. Dermatology 1998;**196**:231–6.

64. Finzi AF, Mozzanica N, Pigatto PD et al. Cyclosporin versus etretinate: Italian multicenter comparative trial in severe plaque-form psoriasis. Dermatology 1993;**187**:8–18.

65. Mahrle G, Schulze HJ, Farber L, Weidinger G, Steigleder GK. Low-dose short-term cyclosporine versus etretinate in psoriasis: improvement of skin, nail, and joint involvement. J Am Acad Dermatol 1995;**32**:78–88.

66. Grossman RM, Chevret S, Abi-Rached J, Blanchet F, Dubertret L. Long-term safety of cyclosporine in the treatment of psoriasis. Arch Dermatol 1996;**132**:623–9.

67. Powles AV, Hardman CM, Porter WM, Cook T, Hulme B, Fry L. Renal function after 10 years' treatment with cyclosporin for psoriasis. Br J Dermatol 1998;**138**:443–9.

68. Griffiths CEM, Clark CM, Chalmers RJG, Li Wan Po A, Williams HC. Oral retinoids. In: A systematic review of treatments for severe psoriasis. Health Technol Assess 2000;**4**(40):25–49.

69. Ruzicka T, Sommerburg C, Braun-Falco O et al. Efficiency of acitretin in combination with UV-B in the treatment of severe psoriasis. Arch Dermatol 1990;**126**:482–6.

70. Lowe NJ, Prystowsky JH, Bourget T, Edelstein J, Nychay S, Armstrong R. Acitretin plus UVB therapy for psoriasis. Comparisons with placebo plus UVB and acitretin alone. J Am Acad Dermatol 1991;**24**:591–4.

71. Green C, Lakshmipathi T, Johnson BE, Ferguson J. A comparison of the efficacy and relapse rates of narrowband UVB (TL-01) monotherapy v. etretinate (re-TL-01) v. etretinate-PUVA (re-PUVA) in the treatment of psoriasis patients. Br J Dermatol 1992;**127**:5–9.

72. Giannetti A, Coppini M, Bertazzoni MG et al. Clinical trial of the efficacy and safety of oral etretinate with calcipotriol cream compared with etretinate alone in moderate-severe psoriasis. J Eur Acad Dermatol Venereol 1999;**13**:91–5.

73. van de Kerkhof PC, Cambazard F, Hutchinson PE et al. The effect of addition of calcipotriol ointment (50 micrograms/g) to acitretin therapy in psoriasis. Br J Dermatol 1998;**138**:84–9.

74. Danno K, Sugie N. Combination therapy with low-dose etretinate and eicosapentaenoic acid for psoriasis vulgaris. J Dermatol 1998;**25**:703–5.

75. Ashley JM, Lowe NJ, Borok ME, Alfin-Slater RB. Fish oil supplementation results in decreased hypertriglyceridemia in patients with psoriasis undergoing etretinate or acitretin therapy. J Am Acad Dermatol 1988;**19**:76–82.

76. Roenigk HH Jr, Callen JP, Guzzo CA et al. Effects of acitretin on the liver. J Am Acad Dermatol 1999;**41**:584–8.

77. Stern RS, Fitzgerald E, Ellis CN, Lowe N, Goldfarb MT, Baughman RD. The safety of etretinate as long-term therapy for psoriasis: results of the etretinate follow-up study. J Am Acad Dermatol 1995;**33**:44–52.

78. Griffiths CEM, Clark CM, Chalmers RJG, Li Wan Po A, Williams HC. Methotrexate. In: A systematic review of treatments for severe psoriasis. Health Technol Assess 2000;**4**(40):51–3.

79. Jones G, Crotty M, Brooks P. Interventions for treating psoriatic arthritis (Cochrane Review). In: Cochrane Collaboration. Cochrane Library. Issue 4. Oxford: Update Software, 2001.

80. Van Dooren-Greebe RJ, Kuijpers ALA, Mulder J, De Boo T, Van de Kerkhof PCM. Methotrexate revisited: effects of long-term treatment in psoriasis. Br J Dermatol 1994;**130**:204–10.

81. Zachariae H. Methotrexate in psoriasis. In: Burgdorf WHC, Katz SI, eds. Proceedings of the 18th World Congress of Dermatology. New York: Parthenon Publishing Group Inc., 1992:685–7.

82. van de Kerkhof PC, Mali JW. Methotrexate maintenance following Ingram therapy in "difficult" psoriasis. Br J Dermatol 1982;**106**:623–7.

83. Heydendael VMR, Spuls PI, Opmeer BC et al. Effectiveness, safety and quality of life of methotrexate versus cyclosporine A in moderate to severe psoriasis: a randomised controlled trial. Br J Dermatol 2002;**147**:1047–8.

84. Boffa MJ, Chalmers RJ. Methotrexate for psoriasis. Clin Exp Dermatol 1996;**21**:399–408.

85. Hanrahan E, Barnes L. Elevated serum homocysteine levels in patients with psoriasis receiving long-term, low-dose methotrexate therapy. Br J Dermatol 2001;**145** (Suppl. 59):43.

86. Rosenthal D, Guenther L, Kelly J. Current thoughts on the use of methotrexate in patients with psoriasis. J Cutan Med Surg 1997;**2**:41–6.

87. Nyfors A, Brodthagen H. Methotrexate for psoriasis in weekly oral doses without any adjunctive therapy. Dermatologica 1970;**140**:345–55.

88. Weinstein GD, Roenigk H, Maibach M, Cosmides J, Halprin K, Millard M. Psoriasis-liver methotrexate interactions. *Arch Dermatol* 1973;**108**:36–42.

89. Weinstein GD, Frost P. Methotrexate for psoriasis – a new therapeutic schedule. *Arch Dermatol* 1971;**103**:33–8.

90. Zanolli MD, Sherertz EF, Hedberg AE. Methotrexate: anti-infammatory or antiproliferative? *J Am Acad Dermatol* 1990;**22**:523–4.

91. Boffa MJ, Chalmers RJG, Haboubi NY, Shomaf M, Mitchell DM. Sequential liver biopsies during long-term methotrexate treatment for psoriasis: a reappraisal. *Br J Dermatol* 1995;**133**:774–8.

92. Roenigk HH, Auerbach R, Maibach HI, Weinstein GD. Methotrexate in psoriasis: Consensus conference. *J Am Acad Dermatol* 1998;**38**:478–85.

93. Boffa MJ, Smith A, Chalmers RJG *et al*. Serum type III procollagen aminopeptide for assessing liver damage in methotrexate-treated psoriatic patients. *Br J Dermatol* 1996;**135**:538–44.

94. Zachariae H, Heickendorff L, Soegaard H. The value of amino-terminal propeptide of type III procollagen in routine screening for methotrexate-induced liver fibrosis: a 10-year follow-up. *Br J Dermatol* 2001;**143**:100–3.

95. Leavell UW, Yarbro JW. Hydroxyurea. A new treatment for psoriasis. *Arch Dermatol* 1970;**102**:144–50.

96. Nugteren-Huying WM, van der Schroeff JG, Hermans J, Suurmond D. Fumaric acid therapy for psoriasis: a randomized, double-blind, placebo-controlled study. *J Am Acad Dermatol* 1990;**22**:311–12.

97. Altmeyer PJ, Matthes U, Pawlak F *et al*. Antipsoriatic effect of fumaric acid derivatives. Results of a multicenter double-blind study in 100 patients [see comments]. *J Am Acad Dermatol* 1994;**30**:977–81.

98. Nieboer C, de Hoop D, van Loenen AC, Langendijk PN, van Dijk E. Systemic therapy with fumaric acid derivates: new possibilities in the treatment of psoriasis. *J Am Acad Dermatol* 1989;**20**:601–8.

99. Nieboer C, de Hoop D, Langendijk PN, van Loenen AC, Gubbels J. Fumaric acid therapy in psoriasis: a double-blind comparison between fumaric acid compound therapy and monotherapy with dimethylfumaric acid ester. *Dermatologica* 1990;**181**:33–7.

100. Mrowietz U, Christophers E, Altmeyer P. Treatment of psoriasis with fumaric acid esters: results of a prospective multicentre study. German Multicentre Study. *Br J Dermatol* 1998;**138**:456–60.

101. du Vivier A, Munro DD, Verbov J. Azathioprine in psoriasis. *BMJ* 1974;**1**:49–51.

102. Gupta AK, Ellis CN, Siegel MT *et al*. Sulfasalazine improves psoriasis. A double-blind analysis. *Arch Dermatol* 1990;**126**:487–93.

103. Owen CM, Chalmers RJ, O'Sullivan T, Griffiths CE. Antistreptococcal interventions for guttate and chronic plaque psoriasis. In: Cochrane Collaboration. *Cochrane Library*. Issue 2.Oxford: Update Software, 2000.

104. Chalmers RJ, O'Sullivan T, Owen CM, Griffiths CE. Interventions for guttate psoriasis. In: Cochrane Collaboration. *Cochrane Library*. Issue 2. Oxford: Update Software, 2000.

105. Hone SW, Donnelly MJ, Powell F, Blayney AW. Clearance of recalcitrant psoriasis after tonsillectomy. *Clin Otolaryngol* 1996;**21**:546–7.

106. Grimminger F, Mayser P, Papavassilis C *et al*. A double-blind, randomized, placebo-controlled trial of n-3 fatty acid based lipid infusion in acute, extended guttate psoriasis. Rapid improvement of clinical manifestations and changes in neutrophil leukotriene profile. *Clin Investigator* 1993;**71**:634–43.

107. Vincent F, Ross JB, Dalton M, Wort AJ. A therapeutic trial of the use of penicillin V or erythromycin with or without rifampin in the treatment of psoriasis. *J Am Acad Dermatol* 1992;**26**:458–61.

108. Marsland AM, Murphy J, O'Sullivan T, Chalmers RJG, Griffiths CEM. Interventions for chronic palmoplantar pustular psoriasis. In: Cochrane Collaboration. *Cochrane Library*. Oxford: Update Software, submitted for publication 2002.

109. Erkko P, Granlund H, Remitz A *et al*. Double-blind placebo-controlled study of long-term low-dose cyclosporin in the treatment of palmoplantar pustulosis. *Br J Dermatol* 1998;**139**:997–1004.

110. Thomsen K. Pustulosis palmaris et plantaris treated with methotrexate. *Acta Derm Venereol* 1971;**51**:397–400.

20
Lichen planus

Laurence Le Cleach, Olivier Chosidow and Bernard Cribier

Background
Definition
Lichen planus (LP) is a chronic inflammatory disease affecting skin, oral or genital mucosae, nails and/or the scalp. Cutaneous LP is typically a pruritic eruption of shiny, violaceous, flat, polygonal papules mainly localised on the front of the wrists, the lumbar region and around the ankles. The most frequent oral presentation is asymptomatic reticular LP, but painful erosive or ulcerative areas may appear.

Incidence/prevalence
No reliable data exist on population incidence or prevalence. The oral mucosa is the most frequently affected site.

Aetiology
The pathogenesis of LP remains unclear. There is some evidence that T lymphocytes infiltrating epidermis and dermis act as effector agents against keratinocytes but the target antigens are unknown.

Prognosis
Spontaneous remission of cutaneous LP after 1 year occurs in two-thirds of cases.[1] Patients mainly complain of pruritus. The spontaneous remission of oral LP is much rarer and may occur in approximately 5% of patients. The reported mean duration of oral LP is about 5 years, but the erosive form does not resolve spontaneously.[2] The erosive form can be extremely painful, leading to major weight loss because of dysphagia. Malignant transformation of oral LP has occasionally been described. Nail or scalp involvement may result in irreversible scars.

Diagnostic tests
Whatever the clinical presentation, histopathological analysis confirms the diagnosis of LP, showing a dermoepidermal papule with hyperkeratosis, hypergranulosis and acanthosis, a basal cell vacuolisation and a band-like inflammatory infiltrate in the superficial dermis.

Aims of treatment
The objective of treatment depends on the clinical form of LP. In the cutaneous form, the aim of treatment is to reduce pruritus and time to resolution, without inducing severe side-effects. The asymptomatic form of oral LP does not usually require treatment. Symptomatic oral LP may need aggressive treatment to stop the pain and to obtain a remission. The aim of the treatment of nail or scalp involvement is to stop the inflammatory process as soon as possible, in order to avoid scars.

Relevant outcomes
Expected relevant outcomes in cutaneous LP are reduction of pruritus, improved quality of life, and time to resolution. In oral LP, relevant outcomes are reduction of erosive lesions, better quality of life and reduction of pain. In oral LP, the rate of recurrence is high after withdrawal of treatment. Recurrence rate and tolerance of

long-term treatment should be considered. These relevant outcomes were mostly not evaluated in the studies reviewed, which used imprecise global evaluation scores.

Methods of search

We searched Medline and Biosis databases to identify articles published before March 1998[3] and Medline and Embase between March 1998 and July 2001. We used the key words "lichen" and "treatment or therapy" and we combined each treatment modality with "lichen". Because of the small number of controlled studies, we also reviewed the open studies and case reports using treatments usually recommended in textbooks. When mucous and cutaneous LP were evaluated together, we reviewed separately the results obtained in cutaneous and oral LP.

Cutaneous lichen planus

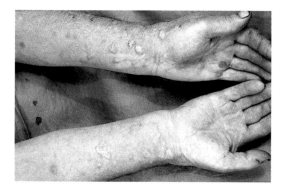

Figure 20.1 Cutaneous lichen planus

QUESTIONS

Do corticosteroids improve cutaneous LP?

Efficacy

One randomised controlled study (RCT) compared the efficacy of prednisolone,

30 mg/day, and placebo administered for 10 days in 38 patients.[4] After follow up for 2 years, results could be evaluated in 28 patients. The median time for LP to clear was 18 weeks in the prednisolone group and 29 weeks in the placebo group ($P = 0.02$); LP did not clear after 2 years in 3 of 14 patients in the placebo group but in none of the corticosteroid group. Five patients in the corticosteroid group relapsed after treatment withdrawal.

We found no clinical trial of topical corticosteroids in cutaneous LP.

Drawbacks

The side-effects were minimal. One patient had mild heartburn and another experienced euphoria.[4]

Comment

Evidence on corticosteroids is scant, although they have been widely used in practice for the past 40 years. In the only available RCT that evaluated systemic corticosteroids, topical corticosteroids were allowed but were not quantified.

Implications for practice

Short courses of systemic corticosteroid therapy and/or topical corticosteroids are usually recommended as first-line treatment for cutaneous LP, although this is not based on relevant clinical trials.

Do retinoids improve cutaneous LP?

Efficacy
Acitretin

We found only one RCT evaluating the efficacy of oral retinoids in cutaneous LP.[5] This double-blind study compared acitretin and placebo in 65 patients with cutaneous LP. Treatment consisted of acitretin, 30 mg/day for 8 weeks. Of the patients on acitretin, 64% (18/28) improved significantly or remitted compared with 13% in the placebo group. One figure showed that papules persisted in the majority of patients on acitretin. Nevertheless, the intensity of pruritus, papulosis and erythema was significantly less in the acitretin group.

Etretinate

We found an open study which evaluated the efficacy of etretinate, 50 mg/day for 2–3 weeks followed by 25 mg/day in 28 patients with cutaneous LP.[6] A "good effect" was reported in 23 patients.

Oral isotretinoin

We found a report of two patients with severe cutaneous and oral LP who were treated successfully with oral isotretinoin, 0·5 mg/kg.[7]

Tretinoin

There is one small series of 13 patients with cutaneous LP treated with oral tretinoin, 10–30 mg/day for 1–10 months.[8] Complete remission occurred in 12 patients.

Drawbacks

Tolerability was considered to be good or very good in 73% of patients in the RCT using acitretin.[5] Side-effects noted in this study were mainly cheilitis and dry mouth. In the study with etretinate,[6] half of the patients experienced side-effects (dryness and swelling of oral mucosae, dermatitis, gastrointestinal disturbances, headache), leading to interruption of the treatment in four patients. Side-effects of systemic retinoids are not exceptional (myalgia, arthralgia, increased blood levels of cholesterol, triglycerides and aminotransferases). The most severe side-effect of retinoids is teratogenicity.

Comment

In the RCT evaluating acitretin in cutaneous LP,[5] neither the duration of the disease before inclusion nor the extent of the lesions were detailed. The criteria for remission and marked improvement were not detailed. The level of evidence of acitretin efficacy is therefore of average quality.

Implications for practice

Because of potential side-effects, acitretin can be recommended only as a second-line treatment for cutaneous LP.

Does photochemotherapy improve cutaneous LP?

Efficacy

We found a small controlled trial in which 10 patients with cutaneous LP were treated with hemicorporeal UV irradiation after ingestion of psoralen.[9] Eight showed partial improvement and three were completely cured. The absence of any observed contralateral effect of the PUVA therapy supports its local efficacy.

A cure rate of 75% after 8 weeks was reported in two open studies conducted in seven[10] and 70 patients.[3]

We found six open studies of bath PUVA therapy.[3] The largest included 75 patients, and found that two cycles of PUVA therapy cured 65% and improved 15% of patients.[11] The relapse rate after 2–5 years' follow up was 25%. The other five studies included smaller groups of patients. One study suggested that exacerbation or relapse of the disease could occur after withdrawal of therapy.[12]

Drawbacks

No adverse effects were described in the PUVA trials. There is probably no major risk of photoageing and/or skin cancer if the treatment is limited to one or two cycles.

Comment

Considering the high rate of spontaneous remission, the evidence for the efficacy of PUVA therapy is weak. Moreover, the possibility of exacerbation of the disease by this treatment has been suggested. The combination of retinoids and PUVA is occasionally recommended, but its efficacy has not been evaluated yet.

Implications for practice

PUVA therapy could be recommended as a second-line treatment in cutaneous LP.

Does ciclosporin improve cutaneous LP?

Efficacy

We found small uncontrolled series and one case report.[13–17] A total of 21 patients with severe cutaneous LP resistant to retinoids or systemic corticosteroid therapy were treated in these series. A complete response occurred in all patients, with doses ranging from 1–6 mg/kg/day, and without relapse during several months of follow up in the majority of patients. Pruritus disappeared after 1–2 weeks of treatment and clearance of the rash was noted in a mean of 6 weeks.

Drawbacks

In these trials, two of the 21 patients had increased triglyceride and/or creatinine levels (both received 3 mg/kg/day). In long-term treatment for psoriasis (more than 6 months) 6–18% of patients interrupted the treatment because of side-effects. The most serious side-effects were high blood pressure, renal toxicity and a potential increase in the risk of cancer.[18] High blood pressure was reported in 5–26% of patients in short-term trials. Renal toxicity from ciclosporin is attributed to a vasoconstrictor effect on kidney arteries.[18] Acute renal side-effects improve after withdrawal of treatment. However, renal impairment from long-term treatment could be irreversible.

Comment

In the absence of controlled study, the level of evidence of ciclosporin efficacy is low. The risk of serious side-effects is high.

Implication for practice

The benefit/harm ratio of ciclosporin is too low in LP. Therefore, its use for cutaneous LP is not recommended.

Does griseofulvin improve cutaneous LP?

Efficacy

We found two trials comparing griseofulvin with placebo in cutaneous LP.[19,20] The first included two groups of 17 patients who received either placebo or griseofulvin, 500 mg/day, for 4–6 weeks.[19] "Complete regression" was observed in 71% of griseofulvin-treated patients compared with 30% of placebo-treated patients. The definition of a cure was based only on flattening of lesions and reduction of itching. In the second study, 44 patients with cutaneous LP were treated with griseofulvin, 500 mg/day, or placebo for 8 weeks.[20] Griseofulvin resulted in "complete improvement" in 82% of patients whereas "partial remission" occurred in 23% of placebo-treated patients.

Drawbacks

Side-effects were not recorded in these studies.

Comments

In the two comparative trials, the methods were incompletely described and the extension and type of lesions were not mentioned. These trials allow no conclusions to be drawn.

Implication for practice

Griseofulvin is not recommended in the treatment of cutaneous LP.

Oral lichen planus

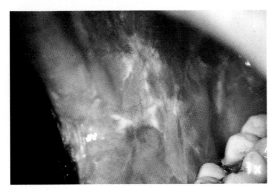

Figure 20.2   Oral lichen planus

QUESTIONS

Do topical corticosteroids improve oral LP?

Efficacy
Fluocinonide

We found one RCT and one open study. The open study was initially conducted as a double-blind trial with crossover, and compared fluocinonide in an adhesive base with placebo in 11 patients.[21] A partial response was observed in five patients and a complete response in six patients in the fluocinonide group, compared with one partial response in the placebo group. Subsequently, 56 other patients were treated openly, 29 obtained a complete response after 2 weeks of therapy. The exact number of relapses is impossible to calculate because various oral diseases were mixed in the follow-up study. In the second RCT,[22] fluocinonide in an adhesive base, applied 6 times per day for 9 weeks, was compared with its vehicle in 40 patients with oral LP. This study included 12 patients with erosive LP, 13 with reticular LP, and 15 with a combination. Thirteen of the 20 treated patients obtained complete remission or had a good response, compared with four good responses in the placebo group.

Betamethasone valerate

We found one open study and one RCT. The RCT[23] compared betamethasone valerate aerosol, four sprays per day for 2 months, with placebo in 23 patients with oral LP, 18 of whom had erosive lesions. After 2 months of therapy, eight of 11 patients had a "good or moderate" response (6 of them having erosive LP) compared with 2 moderate responses in the placebo group.

The open study[24] was conducted in 30 patients with oral LP, treated topically four times daily. Twenty patients showed significant improvement after 1–12 months of treatment.

Drawbacks

In the two RCTs, one with fluocinonide and one with betamethasone valerate, the only adverse effect observed was a case of oral candidiasis.

Comments

The RCT conducted with fluocinonide and with betamethasone valerate included patients with oral LP of varying degrees of severity. The study of fluocinonide gel included only a few patients and used a subjective overall evaluation of responses. Nevertheless, these two RCTs provide an average level of evidence of efficacy of topical corticosteroids in oral LP, with slightly better evidence for fluocinonide gel.

Implication for practice

Topical corticosteroids are the first-line treatment for oral LP.

Which is the most effective topical corticosteroid for oral LP?

Efficacy

One RCT compared 0·1% fluocinolone acetonide with 0·1% triamcinolone acetonide, four applications per day for 4 weeks, to treat oral LP in 40 patients with erosive (18 cases) or atrophic (22 cases) LP.[25] The efficacy was based on the reduction of the surface of lesions. Fluocinolone was found to be more effective, with 13 of 19 patients cured compared with eight of 19 treated with triamcinolone. After a 1 year follow up, only two patients in the fluocinolone group remained completely cured.

Drawbacks

Oral candidiasis was observed in 13 patients, nine of whom were in the fluocinolone group.

Comment

The rate of success according to erosive or atrophic forms of LP was not detailed.

Implications for practice

One per cent fluocinolone acetonide was found to be slightly more effective than 1% triamcinolone acetonide in the treatment of oral LP, with a low level of evidence.

Do systemic corticosteroids improve oral LP?

No controlled studies have evaluated the efficacy of oral corticosteroids in oral LP. However many authors recommend prednisolone, 30–80 mg/day, in erosive oral LP.

Do retinoids improve oral LP?

Efficacy
Topical retinoic acid

We found a few open studies lacking details on dosage and clinical evaluation, and two studies comparing 0·1% retinoic acid with placebo. The first was not randomised.[26] Of 23 patients with atrophic-erosive lesions treated with tretinoin, 71% improved compared with 29% in 15 patients receiving the vehicle. Relapses were common after 3 months.

The second study[27] was randomised and double-blind and included 10 patients in each group, all with plaque-like LP lesions. After 4 months of therapy, nine patients in the tretinoin group had improved or were cured compared with four in the placebo group. The diminution of the lesions was 91% in the tretinoin group and 21% in the placebo group.

Isotretinoin gel

One RCT compared isotretinoin gel with excipient alone for 2 months in 20 patients.[28] The improvement in scores was 90% and 10%, respectively.

Etretinate

We found five open studies and one small RCT.[3] The five open studies included 58 patients. The initial dosage ranged from 0·6 to 1 mg/kg/day, for various durations. A good outcome (without precise criteria) was reportedly obtained in four of the five studies. In one study of 10 patients, efficacy was minimal and was considered to be outweighed by side-effects. The RCT[29] included 28 patients with severe oral LP who were treated with etretinate, 75 mg/day, or placebo for 2 months, followed by crossover to etretinate in nine cases. Improvement (reduction of more than 50% of the erosions and infiltration) was observed in 93% of lesions in the etretinate group compared with 5% of controls. Three months after the end of treatment 66% of the patients had relapsed.

Oral tretinoin and oral isotretinoin

We found only three open studies of different dosages of oral tretinoin and anecdotal reports of oral isotretinoin.[3]

Drawbacks

In the two RCTs on topical retinoic acid and isotretinoin gel, only mild local side-effects (burning, dryness, scaling, redness) were observed. In the etretinate RCT, severe dermatological side-effects and headache led to four withdrawals.

Comments

Both RCTs of topical retinoids were of poor methodological quality, especially because of incomplete clinical data and the small numbers of patients included.

Implications for practice

Topical 0.1% tretinoin gel and 0.1% isotretinoin gel both improve oral LP, but recurrence after withdrawal is frequent. This treatment can be recommended as first-line treatment of oral LP.

> Do topical ciclosporin and tacrolimus improve oral LP?

Efficacy
Topical ciclosporin

We found three RCTs and numerous small open trials, using various doses and methods of application.[3] Most of these uncontrolled trials reported favourable results in severe resistant oral LP but poor efficacy was reported in three small case series.

The three RCTs also used different doses and modalities of application. The first RCT compared efficacy of three washes (1500 mg/day) with placebo in 16 patients with symptomatic oral LP.[30] When compared with the control group, erythema, reticulated lesions, erosions and functional signs were significantly attenuated after 8 weeks' treatment. In the second RCT, 14 patients with erosive oral LP were treated with dosed oral rinses containing either ciclosporin, 500 mg, or placebo.[31] After 4 weeks' treatment, the rate of healing was significantly better with ciclosporin, with reduced pain. In the last RCT, 20 patients with erosive oral LP were treated with a bioadhesive gel containing either ciclosporin or placebo.[32] After 10 weeks' treatment, the rate of complete healing was significantly higher with ciclosporin (50% versus 0%).

Tacrolimus

We found a small series of six cases[33] and one single case[34] reporting efficacy of topical tacrolimus in oral LP. In all cases, tacrolimus 0.1% was applied twice daily for at least 4 weeks. Complete resolution or good improvement was observed but a relapse was noted a few weeks after cessation of therapy.

Drawbacks

The only side-effect reported in the RCT with topical ciclosporin was local burning sensation. No elevated serum ciclosporin levels were observed in any of the 3 studies.

Comments

The three RCTs of topical application of ciclosporin suggested that ciclosporin was more effective than vehicle. However, dosage, treatment duration and modalities of application were different in these studies, thus the level of evidence is low.

Implications for practice

No formulation of local ciclosporin is commercially available. The level of evidence of efficacy is low, with few adverse effects. Local ciclosporin could be a second-line treatment for severe oral LP. No conclusion about topical tacrolimus can be drawn.

Are other topical treatments more effective than topical corticosteroids for treating oral LP?

Efficacy

An RCT compared 0·05% tretinoin with fluocinonide in 33 patients with atrophic and erosive LP.[35] The reduction of severity score was significantly higher with fluocinonide. An RCT compared topical ciclosporin three washes per day (1500 mg/day) with triamcinolone paste in 13 patients.[36] No difference in efficacy was demonstrated. Another controlled trial compared oil-based ciclosporin solution, 50 mg three times daily, with aqueous 1% triamcinolone acetonide solution in 20 patients.[37] No difference was observed.

Comment

In the tretinoin RCT there was only a small decrease in the severity score but the 0·05% concentration may have been too low.

Implication for practice

There is no evidence that topical ciclosporin is more effective than corticosteroids in oral LP.

Does photochemotherapy improve oral LP?

Efficacy
Oral photochemotherapy
We found four open studies and one RCT.[3] The controlled study of oral PUVA therapy was conducted on 18 patients with erosive or ulcerative oral LP, after ingestion of psoralen, 0·6 mg/kg, and randomised unilateral irradiation.[38] The endpoint was comparison of the treated and non-treated sides. After 12 sessions (total dose 16.5 J/cm^2), the treated side showed a marked or slight improvement in 13 patients and the control side improved in six patients.

Extracorporeal photochemotherapy
We found a small series of seven patients with severe resistant erosive oral LP treated with extracorporeal photochemotherapy.[39] Complete remission was obtained in all patients.

Drawbacks

In the RCT of oral photochemotherapy two patients stopped the treatment because of nausea after ingestion of psoralen. In the study of extracorporeal photochemotherapy a progressive decrease in blood lymphocytes was observed in all patients but without significant consequences.

Comments

One small RCT suggested a moderate efficacy of oral photochemotherapy in oral LP.

Implications for practice

In oral photochemotherapy, irradiation is provided by an apparatus designed for light-cured dental fillings, which is not easily available; the level of evidence of efficacy is low. Because of its cost, extracorporeal photochemotherapy has to be reserved for very severe oral LP. No comparative study has yet been performed.

Summary

This review of the literature showed that many drugs or physical treatments have been used in the treatment of LP, but comparative studies are rare. In almost all open studies, the reported efficacy in small groups of patients was based on imprecise global evaluation scores and many studies lack precise inclusion criteria. It is impossible to compare the balance of benefit/harm of these treatments in each clinical form of LP.

Nevertheless, the studies contain enough preliminary data to encourage the planning of larger RCTs. These future RCTs must evaluate cutaneous LP, non-erosive oral and erosive oral LP separately, and use specific objective criteria in each clinical type of LP.

Key points

- Lichen planus is a chronic inflammatory disease mainly affecting skin and oral mucosae. The objectives of the treatment vary according to the clinical forms. There is a lack of large trials comparing the usually recommended treatments with placebo.
- We found no evidence of efficacy of systemic or topical corticosteroids although this treatment is usually recommended as first-line treatment for cutaneous LP.
- We found limited evidence of acitretin efficacy and PUVA therapy efficacy in cutaneous LP.
- We found the benefit/harm ratio of ciclosporin in cutaneous LP to be too low to recommend this treatment.
- We found limited evidence of efficacy of topical corticosteroids, topical 0·1% tretinoin gel and 0·1% isotretinoin gel in oral LP.
- We found no evidence that topical ciclosporin is more effective than topical corticosteroid in oral LP.

References

1. Irvine C, Irvine F, Champion RH. Long-term follow-up of lichen planus. *Acta Derm Venereol* 1991;**71**:242–4.
2. Scully C, El-Kom M. Lichen planus: review and update on pathogenesis. *J Oral Pathol* 1985;**14**:431–58.
3. Cribier B, Frances C, Chosidow O. Treatment of lichen planus. *Arch Dermatol* 1998;**134**:1521–30.
4. Kelett JK, Ead RD. Treament of lichen planus with a short course of oral prednisolone. *Br J Dermatol* 1990;**123**:550–1.
5. Laurberg G, Geiger JM, Hjorth N *et al.* Treatment of lichen planus with acitretine: a double blind, placebo-controlled study in 65 patients. *J Am Acad Dermatol* 1991;**24**:434–7.
6. Schuppli R. The efficacy of a new retinoid (Ro 10-9359) in lichen planus. *Dermatology* 1978;**157**:60–3.
7. Woo TY. Systemic isotretinoin treatment of oral and cutaneous lichen planus. *Cutis* 1985;**23**:385–93.
8. Ott F, Bollag W, Geiger JM. Efficacy of oral low-dose tretinoin (all-trans-retinoic acid) in lichen planus. *Dermatology* 1996;**192**:334–6.
9. Gonzales E, Khosrow MT, Freedman S. Bilateral comparison of generalized lichen planus treated with psoralens and ultraviolet A. *J Am Acad Dermatol* 1984;**10**:958–61.
10. Ortonne JP, Thivolet J, Sannwald C. Oral photochemotherapy in the treatment of lichen planus. *Br J Dermatol* 1978;**99**:315–18.
11. Karvonen J, Hannuksela M. Long term results of topical trioxsalen PUVA in lichen planus and nodular prurigo. *Acta Derm Venereol Suppl* 1985;**120**:53–5.
12. Helander I, Jansen CT, Meurman L. Long-term efficacy of PUVA treatment in lichen planus: comparison of oral and external methoxsalen regimens. *Photodermatology* 1987;**4**:265–8.
13. Higgins EM, Munro CS, Friedmann PS, Marks JM. Cyclosporine A in the treatment of lichen planus. *Arch Dermatol* 1989;**125**:1436.
14. Ho VC, Gupta AK, Nickoloff BJ, Vorhees JJ. Treatment of severe lichen planus with cyclosporine. *J Am Acad Dermatol* 1990;**22**:64–8.
15. Pigatto PD, Chiapino G, Bigardi A, Mozzanica N, Finzi AF. Cyclosporine A for the treatment of severe lichen planus. *Br J Dermatol* 1990;**122**:121–3.
16. Levell NJ, Munro CS, Marks JM. Severe lichen planus clears with very low-dose cyclosporine. *Br J Dermatol* 1992;**127**:66–7.
17. Reiffers-Mettelock J. Acute lichen planus treated by Sandimmun (ciclosporin). *Dermatology* 1992;**184**:84.
18. Le Cleach L, Bocquet H, Roujeau JC. Reaction and interactions of some commonly used systemic drugs in dermatology. *Dermatol Clin* 1998;**16**:421–9.
19. Sehgal VN, Abraham GJS, Malik GB. Griseofulvin therapy in lichen planus: a double-blind controlled trial. *Br J Dermatol* 1972;**87**:383–5.

20. Sehgal VN, Bikhchandani R, Koranne RV, Nayar M, Saxena HMK. Histopathological evaluation of griseofulvin therapy in lichen planus. *Dermatologica* 1980;**161**:22–7.

21. Lozada F, Silverman S. Topically applied fluocinonide in an adhesive base in the treatment of oral vesiculoerosive diseases. *Arch Dermatol* 1980;**116**:898–901.

22. Voute AB, Schulten EA, Langendijk PNJ, Kostense PJ, van der Waal I. Fluocinonide in an adhesive base for the treatment of oral lichen planus: a double-blind, placebo-controlled clinical study. *Oral Surg Oral Med Oral Pathol* 1993;**75**:181–5.

23. Tyldesley WR, Harding SM. Betamethasone valerate aerosol in the treatment of oral lichen planus. *Br J Dermatol* 1977;**96**:659–662.

24. Cawson RA. Treatment of oral lichen planus with betamethasone. *BMJ* 1968;**1**:86–9.

25. Thongprasom K, Luangjamekorn L, Seratat T, Taweesap W. Relative efficacy of fluocinolone acetonide compared with triamcinolone acetonide in treatment of oral lichen planus. *J Oral Pathol Med* 1992;**21**:456–8.

26. Sloberg K, Hersle K, Mobacken H, Thilander H. Topical tretinoin therapy and oral lichen planus. *Arch Dermatol* 1979;**115**:716–18.

27. Boisnic S, Branchet MC, Pascal F, Ben Slama L, Rostin M, Szpirglas H. Trétinoïne topique dans le traitement des lichens plans et des leucoplasies de la muqueuse buccale. *Ann Dermatol Venereol* 1994;**121**:459–63.

28. Giustina TA, Stewart JCB, Ellis CN *et al.* Topical application of isotretinoin gel improves oral lichen planus. *Arch Dermatol* 1986;**122**:534–6.

29. Hersle K, Mobacken H, Sloberg K, Thilander H. Severe oral lichen planus: treatment with an aromatic retinoid (etretinate). *Br J Dermatol* 1982;**106**:77–80.

30. Eisen D, Ellis CN, Duell EA, Griffiths CEM, Voorhees JJ. Effect of topical cyclosporine rinse on oral lichen planus: a double-blind analysis. *N Engl J Med* 1990;**323**:290–4.

31. Harpenau LA, Plemons JM, Rees TD. Effectiveness of low dose of cyclosporin in the management of patients with oral erosive lichen planus. *Oral Surg Oral Med Oral Pathol Oral Radiol Endod* 1995;**80**:161–7.

32. Gaeta GM, Serpico R, Femiano F, La Rotonda MI, Cappello B, Gombos F. Cyclosporin bioadhesive gel in the topical treatment of erosive oral lichen planus. *Int J Immunopathol Pharmacol* 1994;**7**:125–32.

33. Vente C, Reich K, Rupprecht R, Neumann C. Erosive mucosal lichen planus: response to topical treatment with tacrolimus. *Br J Dermatol* 1999;**140**:338–42.

34. Lener EV, Brieva J, Schachter M, West LE, West DP, El-Azhary RA. Successful treatment of erosive lichen planus with topical tacrolimus. *Arch Dermatol* 2001;**137**: 419–22.

35. Vigliola PA. Therapeutic evaluation of oral retinoid RO 10-9359 in severe nonpsoriatic dermatoses. *Br J Dermatol* 1980;**103**:483–7.

36. Sieg P, Von Domarus H, von Zitzewitz V, Iven H, Färber L. Topical cyclosporin in oral lichen planus: a controlled, randomized, prospective trial. *Br J Dermatol* 1995;**132**: 790–4.

37. Lopez Lopez J, Rosello Llabres XR. Cyclosporine A, an alternative to the oral lichen planus erosive treatment. *Bull Group Int Rech Sci Stomatol Odontol* 1995;**38**:33–8.

38. Lundquist G, Forsgren H, Gajecki M, Emstetam L. Photochemotherapy of oral lichen planus:a controlled study. *Oral Surg Oral Med Oral Pathol Oral Radiol Endod* 1995;**79**:554–8.

39. Bécherel PA, Bussel A, Chosidow O, Rabian C, Piette JC, Francès C. Extracorporeal photochemotherapy in the treatment of multiresistant mucosal lichen planus. *Lancet* 1998;**351**:805.

21

Acute urticaria

Torsten Schäfer

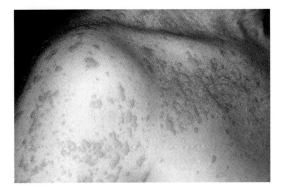

Figure 21.1 Patient with acute urticaria

This chapter deals with the management of a single isolated episode of urticaria (acute urticaria) rather than recurrent episodes observed in chronic urticaria. Discussion is restricted to randomised controlled trials (RCTs). The majority of the RCTs consider the most recently developed drugs. Earlier experimental work with the first antihistamines are not considered because they were not assessed formally in RCTs. It should be noted that many of the reported RCTs have been conducted in emergency departments. It is unclear whether such results also apply to ordinary practice.

Background
Definition
Usual synonyms for urticaria are "hives" or "nettle rash", according to the German term "Nesselsucht", which focuses on the typical reactions following skin contact with the stinging nettle (*Urtica dioica*).

The primary lesions of this monomorphic exanthematous disease are hives or wheals, which are defined as circumscribed white- to pink-coloured compressible skin elevations produced by dermal oedema. Accompanying erythemas in the surrounding area are typical. Pathophysiologically the wheal can be characterised by local vasodilatation and increase of permeability of capillaries and small venules, followed by transudation of plasma constituents into the papillary and upper reticular dermis. Among a large number of substances, such as kinins, leukotrienes, prostaglandins or proteolytic enzymes, histamine is the best known elicitor of typical wheal-and-flare reactions. Eruptions of urticarial lesions are usually associated with intense pruritus.

Although the disease may be easily diagnosed from a clinical point of view, standardised or validated diagnostic criteria for urticaria do not exist. The disease is classified by aetiology or course.

Incidence/prevalence
Valid population-based estimates on the incidence of acute urticaria are lacking. Approximately 20–30% of the general population experience at least one episode of urticaria in their life. There is some consistency in the assumption that acute urticaria is more common in children. Females predominate in acute and chronic forms of the disease.[1]

Aetiology

In principle, the same aetiological considerations as for chronic urticaria apply. In correspondence with the course of the disease, (acute) infections alone or in combination with concomitant drug intake were found to be associated with acute urticaria in 30–50% of cases.[2]

Prognosis

By definition acute urticaria is restricted to an occurrence of no longer than 6 weeks, otherwise it will be classified as chronic urticaria. The disease is therefore considered to be self-limiting.

Diagnostic tests

In principle the same diagnostic considerations as for chronic urticaria apply. However, a full diagnostic workup is rarely indicated in acute cases. A carefully taken history will provide important aetiological hints (infection, drugs).

Aims of treatment

The aims of treatment are to reduce symptoms or to shorten the course of the disease.

Relevant outcomes[1]

- intensity of subjective symptoms (pruritus, sedation)
- disease/wheal intensity
- general physicians' and patients' assessment as assessed by numeric or visual analogue scales (VAS)
- surface area (rule of nine)
- cessation rate

Methods of search[2]

Any RCT (meta-analysis, systematic review or Cochrane review) on "acute" and "urticaria" or "hive" or "wheal" or "nettle and rash" in electronic databases and time periods as indicated in Chapter 6.

QUESTIONS

Which drugs are efficient and safe in the treatment of acute urticaria?

The search of the *Cochrane Library* and the other electronic databases did not reveal a systematic review or meta-analysis on acute urticaria. Recently a consensus report on the management of urticaria appeared as a result of a panel discussion during the clinically oriented European Society for Dermatological Research's symposium *Urticaria 2000*.[3] Besides the elimination of eliciting stimuli, non-sedating H1 antihistamines were recommended as standard and initial treatment, with prednisolone 50 mg/day for 3 days as alternative treatment. A further review, which appeared in 2001, describes the evidence-based evaluation of antihistamines in the treatment of urticaria.[4] The paragraph on acute urticaria discusses two studies, which will also be presented in this chapter.[2,5]

Further search was restricted to RCTs. The *Cochrane Library* listed seven such trials with acute urticaria as primary endpoint of the intervention and not as a reported side-effect. Three further trials were identified in other databases. These trials are summarised in Table 21.1.

Antihistamines (first-generation H1 antagonists and H2 antagonists)

Four studies compared the use of H1 and H2 antagonists or a combination. None of these studies had a placebo arm. Two studies compared diphenhydramine with an H2 antagonist (famotidine or cimetidine).

Moscati *et al.* investigated the efficacy of a single-dose intramuscular cimetidine 300 mg with

Table 21.1 Summary of data from randomised controlled trials of the treatment of acute urticaria

Reference	Intervention	Outcome measures	No. of patients enrolled	Results
Moscati et al.[5]	Single-dose cimetidine 300 mg IM OR diphenhydramine 50 mg IM	Itching, wheal intensity, sedation, wheal extent, overall improvement on a 3–4 point numerical scale; validity and reliability not known	93 No dropouts	No difference for clinical response Diphenhydramine significantly more sedating
Watson et al.[6]	Single-dose H2-receptor antagonist famotidine 20 mg i.m. v H1-receptor antagonist diphenhydramine 50 mg IM in the treatment of acute urticaria Diphenhydramine 50 mg + ranitidine	Pruritus (patient, VAS) Intensity of urticaria (physician, VAS) Surface area (physician, rule of nine) Sedation (patient, VAS)	25 No dropouts	Only within-group comparison (before/after comparison)
Lin et al.[7]	50 mg v diphenhydramine 50 mg + placebo Single-dose diphenhydramine	Presence of urticaria at baseline and after 1 and 2 hours Extent (number of involved areas)	Unclear	Presence of urticaria after 2 hours: 16·2% v 8·3% (+ ranitidine) $P = 0.02$
Runge et al.[8]	50 mg + placebo IV OR cimetidine 300 mg + placebo IV OR diphenhydramine 50 mg + cimetidine 300 mg IV	VAS (110 mm) to assess: Pruritus – throat tightness, and facial swelling (patient) Urticaria – pharyngeal tissue swelling, and facial swelling (physician) Change of 25 mm considered clincally significant Adverse effects	39	More urticaria patients receiving diphenhydramine + cimetidine (11/12) experienced relief compared with those receiving diphenhydramine (5/11, $P = 0.027$) or cimetidine (8/10, ns) alone

(Continued)

Table 21.1 (*Continued*)

Reference	Intervention	Outcome measures	No. of patients enrolled	Results
Simons *et al.*[14]	Oral cetirizine 0·25 mg/kg twice daily v placebo over 18 months in children with atopic eczema	Incidence of diary-reported symptoms typical for acute urticaria	795	Cumulative incidence of urticaria 16·2% v 5·8% during 18-month treatment (*P*<0·001) 4·6% v 3·0% during 6-month follow up (ns)
Pollack and Romano[10]	Single-dose diphenhydramine 50 mg IM. followed by oral hydroxyzine 25 mg every 4–8 hours plus oral prednisone 20 mg twice daily for 4 days or placebo	Pruritus (VAS 10 cm) Adverse effects	43	Significantly more improvement with the addition of steroid
Zuberbier *et al.*[2]	Loratadine 10 mg/day until remission v prednisolone 50 mg/day for 3 days followed by loratadine 10 mg/day until remission	Cessation of whealing	109	Percentage cessation at 5 time points Significant differences only after 3 days (when the intervention arm had received prednisolone only so far) (93·8% v 65·9%)

ns, not significant; IV, intravenous; IM, intramuscular

intramuscular diphenhydramine 50 mg intramuscular in 93 young adults.[5] Both treatments yielded significant reductions in itching, wheal intensity and extent after 30 minutes, with no differences between treatments. A significant increase in sedation was reported by patients in both groups, but was significantly higher in patients treated with diphenhydramine. Absolute changes in the three- and four-point scoring scales appeared to be clinically important. The study is limited by flaws in the process of randomisation and blinding.

Watson *et al.* compared single-dose intramuscular diphen-hydramine 50 mg with intramuscular famotidine 20 mg in 25 adults.[6] After 30 minutes pruritus was reduced significantly by both treatments, with diphenhydramine appearing more effective. Famotidine also significantly reduced the affected body surface area. Physician-rated intensity of urticaria was reduced equally and significantly by both drugs. A non-significant increase in sedation was reported by patients receiving diphenhydramine. The small sample size and unbalanced group size (diphenhydramine n = 10, famotidine n = 15; no block randomisation) does not allow for a meaningful comparison of the groups.

Lin *et al.* compared the efficacy of single-dose intravenous diphenhydramine 50 mg alone or in combination with intravenous ranitidine 50 mg in 91 adults.[7] Significantly more patients receiving the combination therapy (91·7%) were free of symptoms after 2 hours compared with those who received diphenhydramine alone (73·8%). After control for baseline extent, the combination therapy was able to reduce the number of involved areas significantly within 2 hours. Significantly more additional antihistamines were administered in the diphenhydramine group, however, which may have shifted the effect towards the zero-effect level.

Runge *et al.* studied 39 adults with acute allergic reactions, including urticaria.[8] Fourteen patients received a single dose of intravenous diphenhydramine 50 mg, 12 received intravenous cimetidine 300 mg) and 13 received both preparations. After 30 minutes the combination therapy led to significantly higher reduction of urticaria (evaluated using a VAS) compared with diphenhydramine alone. The latter, however, achieved the best results in reduction of pruritus, differences being significant compared with cimetidine. The study is limited by the small sample size and significant differences in mean treatment scores for urticaria between study groups, which were not adjusted for in later analyses.

Pontasch *et al.* compared three oral medication in the treatment of acute urticaria in adults.[9] Seven patients received diphenhydramine, six received famotidine, and another seven received cromolyn sodium. Patient satisfaction was highest with diphenhydramine (6/7), followed by famotidine (3/6) and cromolyn sodium (3/7). Adverse effects were reported in 3/7 treated with diphenhydramine, in 3/6 of the famotidine group and in one patient who received cromolyn sodium.

Corticosteroids

The addition of oral prednisone 20 mg twice daily for 4 days to the standard treatment with H1 antagonists was investigated in 43 adults by Pollack and Romano[10] The intensity of itch, as scored on a VAS, was significantly reduced by both regimens after 2 and 5 days of follow up. However, the addition of prednisone reduced the symptom score significantly more than the standard therapy. Although, standard therapy with antihistamines is generally considered sufficient, in selected cases (severity, need to shorten antihistamines) addition of prednisone seems helpful.

Similar, Zuberbier *et al.* showed that prednisolone 50 mg/day for 3 days led to a significantly higher clearing rate (93·8%) after 3 days than therapy with loratadine 10 mg/day in 109 patients.[2] The study may be limited by aspects of design (open, pseudo-randomisation by consecutive time periods, differential allocation of possibly pregnant women).

Other treatments and non-randomised trials

An early case series of five patients with acute urticaria following insect stings reported good therapeutic effects of intravenous cimetidine 300 mg initially followed by 300 mg orally four times daily) after ineffective administration of epinephrine (adrenaline), H1 antagonists and corti-costeroids.[11]

A further report investigated the effect of flunarizine, a calcium antagonist, in the treatment of acute urticaria. In this uncontrolled trial 20 patients received a single 10 mg sublingual dose of flunarizine. After 3 hours 16 patients had improved, with effects being more pronounced for itching than for reduction of wheals. Four patients remained unresponsive and five other patients reported drowsiness as a major side-effect.[12]

A Chinese publication describes the therapeutic effect of the added ingredient of *Radix angelicae sinesis* in 106 patients with acute urticaria. Unfortunately, the lack of an abstract in English makes it difficult to draw conclusions.[13]

Prevention

The European multicentre study ETAC (Early Treatment of the Atopic Child) investigated the preventive effect of long-term (18 months) administration of cetirizine 0·25 mg/kg twice daily in 1–2-year-old children with atopic eczema and positive family history of allergies.[14] On addition to the primary endpoint (asthma), symptoms typical for acute urticaria were recorded in a diary during the intervention period and a 6-month follow up. During the intervention period significantly fewer episodes of acute urticaria (5·8%) were reported in the intervention group compared with the placebo arm (16·2%). This effect did not persist after medication was stopped (3·0% versus 4·6%).[14]

Harms

On the basis of the available studies on acute urticaria, the major side-effect is sedation associated with the first-generation H1 antagonists. Hauser's chapter on chronic urticaria discusses the newer antihistamines. This chapter has been published on the book website http://www.evidbasedderm.com.

Comment – implications for clinical practice

Generally the available therapeutic evidence for acute urticaria is quantitatively and qualitatively weak. RCTs of the therapeutic efficacy of the second-generation antihistamines are lacking, although one would like to consider these the first choice of therapy based on the studies in chronic urticaria.[3] There is some evidence that the combination of H1 and H2 antagonists has additional beneficial effects. A short-term intervention with corticosteroids seems to be superior to a treatment with antihistamines alone, but should be considered in the context of individual needs.

Key points

- Acute urticaria is a common disease.
- It seems to predominate in children and females.
- The aetiology remains mostly unclear, but there is evidence that (acute) infections and concomitant drugs, as well as (food) hypersensitivity are important elicitors.
- The therapeutic evidence for treatment of acute urticaria is qualitatively and quantitatively poor.

- There is evidence that first- and second-generation antihistamines are effective and that the combination with H2 antagonists may have additional beneficial effects.
- A short-term intervention with corticosteroids seems to be superior to a treatment with antihistamines alone, but should be considered in the context of individual needs.

A chapter by Conrad Hauser on *Chronic Urticaria* has been published on the book website http://www.evidbasedderm.com.

References

1. Schäfer T, Ring J. Epidemiology of urticaria. In: Burr M, ed. *Epidemiology of Clinical Allergy*. Basel: Karger, 1993:49–60. vol 31.

2. Zuberbier T, Ifflander J, Semmler C, Henz B. Acute urticaria: clinical aspects and therapeutic responsiveness. *Acta Derm Venereol* 1996;**76**:296–7.

3. Zuberbier T, Greaves M, Juhlin L, Merk H, Stingl G, Henz B. Management of urticaria: a consensus report. *J Invest Dermatol Symp Proc* 2001;**6**:128–31.

4. Lee E, Maibach H. Treatment of urticaria. An evidence-based evaluation of antihistamines. *Am J Clin Dermatol* 2001;**2**:27–32.

5. Moscati R, Moore G. Comparison of cimetidine and diphenhydramine in the treatment of acute urticaria. *Ann Emerg Med* 1990;**19**:12–15.

6. Watson N, Weiss E, Harter P. Famotidine in the treatment of acute urticaria. *Clin Exp Dermatol* 2000;**25**:186–9.

7. Lin R, Curry A, Pesola G *et al.* Improved outcomes in patients with acute allergic syndromes who are treated with combined H1 and H2 antagonists. *Ann Emerg Med* 2000;**36**:462–8.

8. Runge J, Martinez J, Caravati E, Williamson S, Hartsell S. Histamine antagonists in the treatment of acute allergic reactions. *Ann Emerg Med* 1992;**21**:237–42.

9. Pontasch M, White L, Bradford J. Oral agents in the management of urticaria: patient perception of effectiveness and level of satisfaction with treatment. *Ann Pharmacother* 1993;**27**:730–1.

10. Pollack CJ, Romano T. Outpatient management of acute urticaria: the role of prednisone. *Ann Emerg Med* 1995;**26**:547–51.

11. Rusli M. Cimetidine treatment of recalcitrant acute allergic urticaria. *Ann Emerg Med* 1986;**15**:1363–5.

12. Allegue F, Martin M, Harto A, Ledo A. Treatment of acute urticaria with sublingual flunarizine. *Int J Dermatol* 1988;**27**:265–6.

13. Wang C, Zhang Z, Wang Q. Therapeutic effect of 106 acute urticaria patients with the added ingredient of *Radix angelicae sinesis*. *J Shanxi Coll Trad Chin Med* 1997;**20**:25.

14. Simons F, Group ES. Prevention of acute urticaria in young children with atopic dermatitis. *J Allergy Clin Immunol* 2001;**107**:703–6.

Part 3: The evidence

Section B: Skin cancer

Editor: Hywel Williams

22
Prevention of skin cancer

Ros Weston

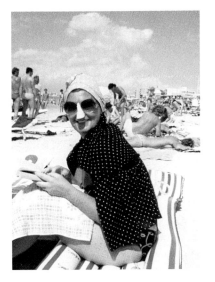

Figure 22.1   The future of skin cancer prevention?

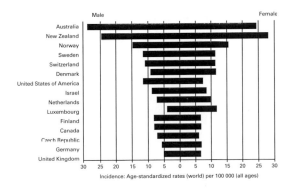

Figure 22.2   Estimated age-standardised rates for cutaneous melanoma of the skin in 1990

Background
Incidence

Skin cancer is more common than any other type of cancer; the estimated age-standardised rates of cutaneous melanoma in several countries are given in Figure 22.2.[1]

Mortality and morbidity

About 106 000 people around the world were diagnosed with cutaneous melanoma in 1990. Since melanoma can be a fatal disease if diagnosed at a late stage, this represents many lost potential life-years, as well as direct costs to health services. It is estimated that at

least 2 750 000 people were diagnosed with non-melanocytic cancers (basal cell carcinoma (BCC) and squamous cell carcinoma (SCC)) of the skin in 1985. These represent more than 30% of newly diagnosed cancers.[2] Mortality from melanoma increased after the 1970s, particularly in white males, possibly as a result of increased recreational exposure to sunlight.[3,4] During the next few years about 51 400 individuals are expected to develop melanoma and almost 7800 to die of the disease.

The incidence increased 126% between 1973 and 1995, at a rate of approximately 6% per year. Non-melanocytic skin cancers are not usually considered life threatening but they represent a huge toll on health service budgets as well as days lost at the workplace and therefore employer and insurance costs. In Australia, and increasingly in the USA, UK and

Europe, rising incidence is causing further increases in direct health costs, as well as in individual morbidity and mortality. The Incidence continues to rise, particularly in males compared with females.[5] Caucasian populations are currently experiencing a reduction in incidence and mortality in some target groups such as young people, with at least one population study showing reduced incidence for BCC but not for SCC. Reduced incidence has also been reported for melanoma in areas where health promotion interventions have encouraged people to reduce their sun exposure.[5,6]

Risk factors

Epidemiological evidence suggests that skin cancers, non-melanocytic skin cancers (NMSCs) and melanoma are caused in the main by exposure to UV radiation (UVR) and repeated episodes of sunburn (erythema) in childhood and adulthood. Genetic susceptibility or phenotype, including the number of naevi on the skin, may have a role in the development of skin cancers for some populations and individuals. Exposure to UVR and susceptibility (phenotype) are risk factors associated with the incidence of sunburn, solar keratoses and precancerous lesions. The type of exposure – intermittent (i.e. lying for long periods in the sun on annual foreign holidays) or continuous (i.e. daily exposure over long periods, as in those working outdoors) – may differ between the three main types of cancer.[7] It is thought that risk increases with increasing intermittency of exposure. Evidence supports this increased risk for melanoma, probably for BCC, but not for SCC. The risk for SCC appears to depend only on the accumulated amount of exposure to the sun.

The incidence of melanoma rises rapidly in Caucasians after 20 years of age. Fair-skinned individuals exposed to the sun are at higher risk. The best risk-reduction strategy is protection from UVR. Individuals with certain types of

pigmented lesions (dysplastic or atypical naevi), several large non-dysplastic naevi, many small naevi, or with moderate freckling have a two- to three-fold risk of developing melanoma. Individuals with familial dysplastic naevus syndrome or with several dysplastic or atypical naevi are at high risk (greater than fivefold) risk of developing melanoma.[8] Evidence for the relationship between total exposure to the sun and melanoma remains to be proved. Further evidence that UVR causes skin cancer has been provided from the observation that people with the rare genetic condition xeroderma pigmentation have a very high risk for skin cancer. Some studies show that individuals who have occupational sun exposure have a lower risk for melanoma than those with less exposure.[9-11]

Mutation of the *p53* gene appears to be an important step in the development of skin cancers. Exposure to sunlight causes a number of chemical changes in DNA. If these changes are not repaired then mutation begins. DNA damage can produce signature mutations in DNA and these are hypothesised as being linked definitively to carcinogenesis. Signature mutations have been found on the tumour suppresser *p53* gene in normal skin cells and their presence has been correlated with extent of exposure. Signature mutations in the *p53* gene have also been found in BCC and SCC of the skin whereas they are rare in this gene in other types of cancer. In the general population there is conflicting evidence about excision repair of DNA and the risk for BCC.[12-14]

Aims for primary prevention

Primary prevention refers to the interventions designed to prevent skin cancer from occurring for the first time. Interventions for primary sun protection aim to change risk behaviour in order to reduce new skin cancers. Studies that evaluate such interventions usually use behaviour change as a surrogate for decrease in melanoma incidence, because of the difficulties in following up very large populations over decades in order to document such incident tumours. Proxy measures such as knowledge and attitudes may also be used. The main sun-protection strategies are the wearing of wide-brimmed hats, staying out of the sun between 11 am and 3 pm, and the use of shade. Sunscreens are a popular prevention strategy; the evidence of their effectiveness in reducing the risk of skin cancers is considered in Chapter 23.

Aims for secondary prevention

Interventions for secondary prevention aim to encourage people to recognise skin changes and to seek early diagnosis and treatment, as well as improving effective diagnosis.

Search strategy

The studies for this review were found by searching PubMed (the original search for these chapters was carried out in 1998 using Medline) combining the following study types as key words: meta-analysis, randomised controlled trials, case-control and direct observation studies with the following cancer terms: melanoma, basal-cell carcinoma, rodent ulcer, squamous cell carcinoma, non-melanoma skin cancers. The Cochrane database and the health-promotion journals *Health Education Research* and *Health Education* were searched for appropriate studies with the additional key words: health promotion interventions. One unpublished meta-analysis done by Girgis *et al.* of the University of Newcastle, New South Wales, Australia in 1998, was included.[15] Very few randomised controlled trials (RCTs) were found for primary prevention although there were more for chemoprevention and secondary prevention. Most studies used direct observation. Randomised population surveys were found for Australia and the US where there has been concerted year-on-year campaigns aimed at changing population behaviour in the sun.

QUESTIONS
Primary prevention

Is there evidence that wearing clothes and hats or that the use of shade reduces the risk of skin cancers?

Few RCTs were found. Those that were found had already been included in an unpublished review of 11 intervention studies, which also included randomised pretest and post-test studies. This review suggested that, where effective interventions have been identified, little work has been undertaken to identify the most effective strategies for disseminating interventions, particularly in schools, the community and workplaces. The analysis indicated a low prevalence of sun-protection behaviours, particularly for the use of hats (randomised observational study) and protective clothing, although the use of shade was increasing in a number of target groups. In a randomised observation study of beach behaviour in Australia, 17% used hats, 15% used shade, and recommended shorts and shirts were used by 15%. Outdoor market traders did not use such clothing.[15–18]

Comment

The review suggests that primary prevention interventions need to be multi-strategic across all health, education and leisure/travel settings. Such interventions should include strategies for motivating individual behaviour change through effective sun-protection policies that include the development of shaded areas, low-cost clothing, and sunscreens. Media dissemination is an important vehicle for reinforcing sun-protection messages through education, public media campaigns and healthcare providers. There is a need for RCTs or controlled studies with multiple outcome measures for prevention aimed at increasing public awareness of reducing exposure to UVR as an effective method of solar protection. Such studies should have specific outcome measures for each component (i.e. hats, clothes and shade). It is imperative that research continues into the relationship between sun exposure and new skin cancers and precancerous lesions such as solar keratoses to establish a dose–response curve for the protective effect of the use of shade, appropriate protective clothing and hats. We have little direct evidence of population knowledge, attitudes and behaviour regarding their use.

Can year-on-year education campaigns reduce the risk of skin cancers?

Hill *et al* (1993) carried out a randomised telephone survey on the prevalence of sunburn and attitudes to sun protection. They collected baseline data for this study in Dec 1987 and Feb 1988. After the SunSmart Campaign in the summers of 1989 and 1990 behavioural and sunburn data were reported for the previous weekend. After adjustment for UVA, temperature, survey month, age, sex and skin type a significant reduction in sunburn was found. Sunburn dropped from 11% to 10% to 7% over the 3-year period. Adjusted odds ratios with 95% CI were:

Year 1–Year 2: 0·75 (CI 0·57–0·99)
Year 1–Year 3: 0·59 (CI 0·43–0·81)

Hat wearing increased significantly each year (19%, 26% and 29% from Year 1 to Year 3) as did sunscreen use (12%, 18% and 21%, respectively).

The main trends in proportion of body surface area covered by clothing were less obvious (0·67, 0·64 and 0·71, respectively Year 1 to Year 3). The authors concluded that a well planned campaign can paly a part in changing sun behaviour.

Comment

The Australian community shows a substantial improvement in sun-protection behaviours over the years, with women showing greater improvement than men and with little or few differences between social class. Further improvements will be harder to achieve as the campaigns move from initiation stage to action and maintenance of change, and researchers will require a longer intervention cycle to bring about health gains for more of the population.[19] Future intervention planners need to continue frequent reminders for protection and argue for structural change (policy development) that makes it easier for people to embrace protective behaviour. There is a need to develop long-term strategies and interventions so that behaviour change becomes habitual, particularly in young people. In primary-care settings there is a need to encourage general practitioners to offer opportunistic advice on sun protection as well as early diagnosis opportunities.

An Australian cohort analysis for melanoma incidence demonstrates a levelling off in younger groups and even slight reduction compared with older cohorts, in whom incidence continues to rise. This could be due to the effect of publicity campaigns. Mortality is also decreasing in younger groups (<18 years of age) as well as in younger women (>18 years of age). This is likely to be the effect of early diagnosis and treatment rather than the single effect of the primary-prevention campaigns, and health promoters and policy makers cannot be complacent. Such campaigns are expensive and it is necessary to have specific outcome objectives for each specific sun-protection strategy.

Can education and information interventions reduce the risk of skin cancer?

Several groups have conducted studies, few randomised, to learn more about the possible intervention strategies for the reduction of exposure to UVR and the development and implementation of sun-protection policies. Many of these studies had knowledge rather than behaviour as their main outcome measure and so have not been included here. The included studies show that education seems to be the most appropriate way to help populations understand the risks associated with sun exposure and sunburn, and sun-protection strategies. Long-term reminders may have some impact on reducing sun exposure in individuals who have been treated for NMSC but it seems to be the educational intervention at the time of treatment that had the greatest impact.[20-22]

Comment

Two studies suggest that educational messages about changes to sun-protection behaviour are more effective when the damage is done. However, in this high-risk group few were able to sustain their sun-protection behaviour in the long term despite their experience. Maintenance of long-term behaviour change continues to be problematic in other lifestyle change behaviours such as smoking, alcohol consumption, healthy eating, weight control and in the recreational use of drugs.[23] Health promoters need to consider designing long-term randomised studies with specific behaviour outcome measures for each element of the intervention. Research on the role of knowledge in behaviour change has shown that knowledge alone does not necessarily lead to behaviour change. The relationship is complex and too many studies rely on a hypothesised link between the two, particularly when knowledge is stated as an outcome measure, thus weakening any evidence accruing from the intervention.

> Does health policy lead to more effective community interventions to reduce the risk of skin cancer?

No randomised studies reported on the effectiveness of sun-protection policies in schools and communities. Only two direct observation studies and one survey were found, even though public health policy is deemed the appropriate context for the promotion of individual behaviour change for sun protection (for example the development of shaded areas in communities, on beaches, in school playgrounds and in other outdoor areas). Schofield et al. reported on the dissemination of sun protection polices in schools and their impact. The schools were randomised but the evidence regarding use of protective clothes, hat wearing and shade was from direct observational studies.[24]

Horsley et al. carried out a survey for the UK Department of Health in 1295 primary schools, 59 middle schools and 216 secondary schools (a 10% sample of schools).[25] In 1995 the Health Education Authority in partnership with the Department of Health and the British Association of Dermatologists introduced Sun Awareness Guidelines to schools. Seven items from the guidelines (education, uniform, shade, outdoor activities, sunscreens, staff awareness and parent and governor alliances) were chosen as outcome measures. The results showed that most schools had taken at least one of the seven actions (mean 2·67, SD 0·88). Of the schools that had addressed sun protection, the majority had done so after the release of the guidelines in 1995. The proportion of schools beginning to take action was greater in the second year of the study than in the first year. Teaching in the curriculum was the most frequent action and was information giving. Brimmed hats and long sleeves were rarely part of summer school wear. Most schools had less than 25% of their outside break in shade but action was being taken to increase this. Sports days were usually scheduled for the afternoon. Sunscreen was allowed in over 80% of schools but its application caused problems for teachers. Few staff manuals included sun awareness issues, few staff attended in-service training on the issue but two-thirds of head teachers would support staff attending such training. The researchers concluded that more support, government guidelines, funding, materials and courses were required if sun awareness is to be improved.[25]

Comment

It is too early to report the effectiveness of such policies. Where such policies have been implemented, reducing skin cancer is only one element of the policy, and other lifestyle issues tend to attract more funding. There is a need to evaluate how the implementation of sun-protection policies influences behaviour in community settings. Such studies need to be long-term randomised population studies that include specific outcome measures for each element of the policy in relation to specific target groups. Research so far shows that they have had a very limited effect in two populations and only for one or two outcome measures. Public health policy was intended to be the driver for more effective interventions and funding but so far it has been difficult to assess how effective this has been. Australia has used policies most effectively to reduce taxes on sun-protection clothing and sunscreens.

Secondary prevention

Can chemoprevention interventions reduce the risk of cancer?

The International Agency for Research on Cancer (IARC: WHO) recently produced three separate meta-analyses – of vitamin A intake,[26] carotenoids,[27] and retinoids[28] – and their effect on cancers, including skin cancer.[28] They concluded that there was no association between the dietary intake of retinol and the risk of skin cancer in a small number of observational studies (one case-control and three cohort studies). These studies were conducted among Caucasian populations with a wide range of disease risk. The risk estimates in the individual studies were generally greater than unity, and in every instance the 95% confidence interval (CI) included 1·0. Two prospective studies of pre-diagnostic levels of retinol and melanoma[28] both reported no significant association on the basis of 30 and 10 cases, respectively. This is consistent with the findings of a case-control study of melanoma and dietary intake of preformed vitamin A.[28]

Evidence suggests that beta-carotene does not prevent cancer when used as a high-dose supplement and there is inadequate evidence with regard to its effect at usual dietary levels. There is inadequate evidence with respect to the possible cancer preventive activity of other individual carotenoids. This is in contrast to some results from animal studies.

A number of randomised studies have evaluated the efficacy of chemoprevention agents such as isotretinoin and beta-carotene for individuals at increased risk of developing NMSC. High-dose isotretinoin was found to prevent new skin cancers in individuals with xeroderma pigmentosum. An RCT of long-term treatment with isotretinoin in individuals previously treated for BCC showed that such treatment did not prevent re-occurrence of new BCC and produced the side-effects characteristic of isotretinoin treatment.[29]

An RCT of the long-term treatment with beta-carotene in individuals treated for NMSC showed no benefit for the occurrence of new NMSCs,[30] concordant with the IARC meta-analysis results. For both these trials it is not known if treatment would benefit individuals at high risk (those who have sun-damaged skin) who have not yet developed skin cancer or if longer follow up would show a long-term effect in the prevention of subsequent skin cancers.

A multicentre double-blind randomised placebo-controlled trial of 1312 patients with a history of BCC or SCC of the skin and a mean follow up of 6·4 years showed that 200 micrograms of selenium (in brewer's yeast tablets) did not have a significant effect on the primary endpoint of the development of BCC or SCC of the skin.[31]

A case-control study found that a significant two-fold increase in the risk of melanoma among current users of the contraceptive pill (relative risk (RR) 2·0, 95% CI 1·2, 3·4) compared with 10 or more years of use (RR 3·4, 95% CI 1·7, 7·0). Risk did not appear elevated among past oral contraceptive users, even among those with longer duration of use, and risk did not decline linearly with time since last use. Risk of premenopausal melanoma may be increased among those with longer duration of use, and further research is needed to determine whether low-dose oestrogen pills in particular are associated with an increase in risk and to describe possible interactions between oral contraceptive use and sun exposure or other risk factors for melanoma.[32]

Comment

The evidence from RCTs suggests that vitamin A and beta-carotene are not effective for the prevention of skin cancers. The evidence for the effect of isotretinoin is equivocal and there is no evidence that brewer's yeast tablets have a preventive effect for NMSCs. There is some evidence from one case-control study that long-term use of oral contraceptives may be associated with increased risk of melanoma.

Can early detection, diagnosis and treatment reduce the risk of skin cancer and melanoma?

Early detection and diagnosis are generally accepted as the most effective secondary prevention intervention likely to reduce the

morbidity and mortality for skin cancer. Melanoma survival rates are linked to early diagnosis and treatment and especially to the thickness of the tumour (Breslow thickness). Patients with thin tumours (less than 1·5 mm) have a 5-year survival rate in excess of 90% compared with a survival rate of 68% for tumours greater than 3 mm in thickness. The major determinant of delay in excising such tumours is delay in seeking advice.[33]

Self-examination for skin pigmentary characteristics associated with melanoma, for example freckling, may be a useful way to identify individuals at increased risk of developing melanoma. Skin type, the propensity to burn after sun exposure, and tanning ability, alone or with other physical characteristics such as hair colour, has been used as a measure of sun sensitivity in epidemiology studies.[34,35]

Other interventions for early detection and diagnosis involve primary-care practitioners and dermatology clinics, and an early study revealed the problems with such a policy. The work overload on dermatology clinics in particular was a major outcome of the Cancer Research Campaign's Mole Watcher seven-centre study.[36] This has implications for policy planners. A recent population cross-sectional study of 1600 participants aged 25–69 years and stratified by a social deprivation score of wards within one general practice in the UK looked at the feasibility of targeted early detection for melanoma using a postal questionnaire and an invitation to screening by a consultant dermatologist. Participants were randomly selected from a population of 8000. A total of 1227 (77%) returned the questionnaire and 896 (56%) attended the screening clinic. Uptake was lower for men ($P<0.001$) and skin types 3 and 4 (men only, $P<0.001$). Twenty per cent of women and 10% of men felt nervous about attending the clinic but only 4% were worried by the questionnaire. The level of agreement between self-assessment and the dermatologist's assessments of risk factors was best for hair colour (κ 0·67; sensitivity 73%; specificity, 98%). People tended to underreport their level of risk. Over 95% knew about at least one major sign of skin cancer, with 54% reporting incorrect signs of melanoma.[37–41]

A recent study in Leicestershire, UK, examined the effect of the introduction of a pigmented lesion clinic on the referral interval for patients with melanoma presenting to their general practitioner.[42] There was a significant initial reduction in the mean referral interval following the introduction of the clinic from 27·9 days (SEM –6·6) in 1984 to 11·3 (2·3) days in1987 ($P<0.01$). This was not maintained over the following 7 years and rose to a mean of 20·4 (4·4) days in 1994. This was not significantly better than the 1985/1986 level. The rise was the result of melanomas being referred directly to other clinics. By 1994 only 48% of melanomas were being referred to the pigmented lesion clinics, compared with 70% in 1987, with more than 50% of melanomas being correctly diagnosed by general practitioners.

Comment

The evidence for the effectiveness of targeted early detection by screening clinics and dermatologists is inconclusive. The limited evidence suggests that targeted screening for melanoma in the UK will be hampered by difficulties in accurately identifying the target population. Strategies to improve skin self-awareness rather than screening should be developed and evaluated.

> **Is dermatoscopic diagnosis more accurate as a diagnostic tool than examination by the naked eye?**

Distinguishing malignant melanoma from benign naevus is often difficult, even for experienced dermatologists. The macroscopic clinical ABCD rule and the Glasgow seven-point checklist are helpful but are often inaccurate, yielding many false-positive and false-negative diagnoses. A Danish meta-analysis of 11 studies reviewed the efficacy of dermatoscopic diagnosis of cutaneous melanoma. Dermatoscopy performed by a trained physician was shown to increase the diagnostic accuracy to a sensitivity of 80%.[43]

A French meta-analysis compared dermoscopy with diagnosis by the naked eye. Eight of the 672 studies retrieved according to specific criteria were included in this meta-analysis. The selected studies represented 328 melanomas (mostly less than 0·76 mm thick) and 1865 mostly melanocytic benign pigmented lesions. For dermoscopic diagnosis of melanoma the sensitivity and specificity ranges were 0·75–0·96 and 0·79–0·98, respectively. Dermoscopy had significantly higher discriminating power than clinical examination, with respective estimated odds ratios of 76 (95% CI 25, 223) and 16 (95% CI 9, –31) ($P=0.88$), and estimated positive likelihood ratios of 9 (95% CI 5·6, 19·0) and 3·7 (95% CI 2·8, 5·3), respectively.[44]

A further study to test the effectiveness of dermatoscopic diagnosis used patients referred to a pigmented lesion clinic by their general practitioner. These patients had melanocytic lesions requiring excision (using dermatological criteria). A set of 74 sequentially observed lesions – 37 melanomas and 37 melanocytic naevi – made up the initial set. A second set of 52 lesions – 32 melanomas and 20 melanocytic naevi – was used to validate conclusions drawn from the original set. The clinical features studied were appearance, history and dermatoscopic features. Following pathological examination, both sets of lesions showed that the most powerful identifying effect of the lesion was the presence of three or more colours on examination by dermatoscopy. In the initial set the age of the patient and the irregular edge and largest diameter of the lesion also contributed to diagnosis, but these were less useful in the second set. The sensitivity and specificity of the three-colour dermatoscopy test for melanoma and naevus were 92% and 51% respectively (the predictive value of a diagnosis of melanoma if three colours are present is 64%, and the predictive value that the lesion will not be melanoma if less than three colours is 85%), with the potential to reduce minor surgical work and patient morbidity.[45]

Comment

The importance of the number of lesions analysed, the percentage of melanoma lesions, the instrument used, and dermoscopic criteria used in each study could not be proved. This limited evidence suggests that, for experienced users, dermoscopy was more accurate than clinical examination for the diagnosis of melanoma pigmented skin lesions. This hypothesis needs further testing in a multicentre study.

Can postgraduate medical training improve accurate diagnosis?

An Australian RCT evaluated the effectiveness of a postgraduate skin cancer training programme for improving doctors' knowledge and clinical practice in skin examinations and diagnosis. Forty-one of 59 family doctors agreed to take part in the training programme. Half were allocated to the intervention group (those that took part in the programme) and others were allocated to the "waiting list status" control group. Data were collected before and after the programme to assess doctors' change in knowledge, perceived confidence and clinical practice. The training programme involved three sessions including information and education, a practical session at the local melanoma clinic and a practical surgical procedure.[46]

Comment

There were significant improvements in accurate diagnosis when lesions were presented on colour slides with accompanying case history, and the correct management was identified. Doctors felt very or extremely confident in their ability to advise patients on screening frequency, to advise on signs of skin cancer and to decide whether changes in lesions were malignant. Significant improvements in clinical practice were found by recording pathology request forms. The study suggested that it was easy to bring about improvement in knowledge through training but more difficult to change clinical practice. This was essentially a pilot study and could be a useful marker for training in general practice.

Implications for practice

The major implication for health promotion practice and research for solar protection interventions resulting from this summary is the need for long-term community-based RCTs using multistrategic primary and secondary interventions across targeted populations within communities. Such trials should use partnership or health alliance models including partners from health, education and workplace settings or use existing partnerships where these are already operational. These trials should include training and education in general practice as well as early detection and diagnosis outcomes. Interventions targeted at high-risk groups could be a discrete element of the trial, and in particular, identification of high-risk patients.

To date there has been a problematic gap between the reporting of initial research studies and the use of the data from these studies to plan and implement long-term randomised trials. Researchers and policy planners have not capitalised on the results from successful early pilot or short-term sun-protection interventions to develop such long-term trials. It is necessary to include behaviour change outcome measures for each specific element of the trial as well as at least one other outcome measure (for example knowledge) for primary prevention interventions. Further research is needed to establish the link between knowledge and behaviour in the process of long-term behaviour change. For secondary prevention, such trials should include behaviour change outcome measures for populations as well as for clinical practice where appropriate. As global warming continues there is an urgent need for more individuals to make long-term behaviour (maintained) changes. Primary-care practitioners need to be convinced that they have a role in both the primary and secondary prevention of skin cancers, and in identifying high-risk individuals. Such improvements and the research required to substantiate them will require considerable funding.

Key points

- There is limited evidence from systematic reviews of population, epidemiological, randomised, observational and case-control studies that primary prevention interventions have had some impact on sun-related behaviour in the short term.
- This is substantially weakened by the design of research studies and the lack of published long-term RCTs. This suggests lack of both funding and commitment to long-term multistrategy outcome measure studies within communities.
- There is no evidence that the development and implementation of public health policy for sun protection has improved intervention design or improved the implementation of long-term trials following effective pilot or short-term studies.
- There is no evidence that funding followed this development either. Australia has used public policy to reduce tax on clothing, hats and sunscreens but there is only very limited evidence that this has changed behaviour (i.e. use of these protectors).
- There is a need for policies to be reviewed and a further consideration of how they can drive intervention development in the long term. There is a need for multi-methodological evaluation of such policy implementation and effect.

- There is some evidence from case-control, observational and epidemiological population studies that primary and secondary prevention programmes may be associated with reduced incidence of skin cancers in specific populations and age groups.
- There is some evidence (weakened by study design and short-term studies) that protective clothing messages are successful in encouraging reduced solar exposure in specific populations and target groups: particularly females and children (by definition of carers' actions and role modelling).
- There is some evidence from surveys that schools have begun to address solar protection education and information giving, but little evidence of behaviour change for solar protection from the sustained use of clothing, especially hats, and shaded areas.
- There is some evidence that information about skin self-examination (signs of change in the skin) is an effective strategy for encouraging specific target groups to seek early diagnosis (more females seek early diagnosis than males).
- There is no evidence that regular screening for skin cancer in general practice settings is a cost-effective prevention strategy for melanoma and NMSCs.
- There is very limited evidence that dermoscopy is a more effective diagnostic tool than the naked eye for diagnosis for melanoma and skin cancers.

References

1. Parkin DM, Pisai P, Farley J. Estimates of the world-wide incidence of 25 major cancers in 1990. *Int J Cancer* 1999;**80**:827–41.
2. Hall HI, Miller DR, Rogers JD *et al.* Update of the incidence and mortality from melanoma in USA. *J Am Acad Dermatol* 1999;**40**:35–42.
3. Wingo PA, Ries LA, Rosenberg HM. Cancer incidence and mortality 1973–1995: *A report card for US cancer* 1998;**82**:1197–207.

4. Hall HI, Miller DR, Rogers JD *et al*. Update on the incidence and mortality for melanoma in USA: *J Am Acad Dermatol* 1998;**40**:35–42.

5. Mathers C, Penm R, Sanson-Fisher R, Campbell E. Health System Costs of Cancer in Australia 1993–94, Canberra: Australian Institute of Health and Welfare, 1998.

6. Baron JA. Prevention of non-melanoma skin cancer: *Arch Dermatol* 2000;**136**:200–45.

7. Armstrong BK. Melanoma: Childhood or lifelong sun exposure. In Grob JJ, Stern RS, MacKie RM, Weinstock WA, eds. *Epidemiology, Causes and Prevention of Skin Diseases*. Oxford: Blackwell Science, 1997.

8. Tucker MA, Halpen A, Holly EA *et al*. Clinically recognized dysplastic nevi: a central risk factor for cutaneous melanoma: *JAMA* 1996;**277**:1439–44.

9. Elwood JM, Jobson J. Melanoma and sun exposure: an overview of published studies: *Int J Cancer* 1997;**73**:198–203.

10. Severi G, Giles GG, Robertson C, Boyle P, Autier P. Mortality from cutaneous melanoma: evidence for contrasting trends between populations. *Br J Cancer* 2000;**82**:1887–91.

11. Whiteman DC, Whiteman CA, Green AC. Childhood sun exposure as a risk factor for melanoma a systematic review of epidemiological studies. *Cancer Causes Control* 2001;**1**:69–82.

12. Zeigler A, Jonason A, Simon J, Leffell D, Brash DE. Tumour suppressor gene mutations and photocarcinogenesis: *Photochem Photobiol* 1996;**63**:432–5.

13. Ibid.

14. Ouhtit A, Ueda M, Nakazawa H *et al*. Quantitative detection of ultra-violet light-specific p53 mutations in normal skin from Japanese patients. *Cancer Epidemiol Biomarkers Prev* 1997;**6**:433–8.

15. Girgis A. Unpublished review of sun protection studies. Faculty of Behavioural Health Science, University of Newcastle, New South Wales, 1998.

16. Girgis A, Sanson-Fisher RW, Tripodi DA, Golding T. Evaluation of interventions to improve solar protection in primary schools. *Health Educ Q* 1993;**20**:275–87.

17. Girgis A, Campbell EM, Redman S, Sanson-Fisher RW. Screening for melanoma: a community survey of prevalence and predictors. *Med J Aust* 1991;**154**:338–43.

18. Girgis A, Sanson-Fisher RW, Watson A. A workplace intervention for increasing outdoor workers' use of solar protection. *Am J Pub Health* 1994;**84**:77–81.

19. Hill D, White V, Marks R, Baland R. Primary prevention of skin cancer: where to now in reducing sunlight exposure? *Eur J Cancer Prev* 1993;**6**:447–56.

20. Robinson JK. Compensation strategies in sun protection behaviours by a population with non-melanoma skin cancer. *Prev Med* 1992;**21**:754–65.

21. Berwick M, Fine JA, Bolognia JL. Sun exposure and sunscreen use following a community skin cancer screening. *Prev Med* 1992;**21**:302–10.

22. Moise AF, Gies HP, Harrison SL. Estimation of the annual solar UVR exposure dose of infants and small children in tropical Queensland, Australia. *Photochem Photobiol* 1999;**69**:457–63.

23. Scott D, Weston R. *Evaluating Health Promotion*. Cheltenham: Nelson Thorne, 1998.

24. Schofield MJ, Edwards K, Pearce R. Effectiveness of two sun protection policy dissemination strategies in New South Wales primary and secondary schools. *Aust N Z J Public Health* 1997;**21**:743–50.

25. Horsley L, Charlton A, Wiggett C. Current action for skin cancer risk reduction in English schools: a report on a survey carried out for the Department of Health. *Health Educ Res* 2000;**15**:249–59.

26. IARC. Handbooks on Cancer Prevention (Vol. 3) Vitamin A. Lyon, France: IARC Press, 1998.

27. IARC. Handbooks on Cancer Prevention (Vol. 2) Carotenoids. Lyon, France: IARC Press, 1998.

28. IARC. Handbooks on Cancer Prevention (Vol. 4) Retinoids (Vol. 4) Lyon, France: IARC Press, 1999.

29. The Isotretinoin-Basal Cell Carcinoma Study Group. Long-term therapy with low dose isotretinoin for prevention of basal cell carcinoma: a multi-centre clinical trial. *J Natl Cancer Inst* 1993;**84**:328–32.

30. The Skin Cancer Prevention Study Group. A clinical trial of beta-carotene to prevent basal cell and squamous cell cancers of the skin. *New Engl J Med* 1990;**323**:789–95.

31. Clark LC, Combs GF, Turnbull BW *et al*. Effects of selenium supplementation for cancer prevention in patients with carcinoma of the skin: a randomized controlled trial. *JAMA* 1996;**276**:1957–63.

32. Feskanich D, Hunter DJ, Willet WC *et al*. Oral contraceptive use and risk of melanoma in premenopausal women. *Br J Cancer* 1999;**81**:918–23.

33. Blois MS, Sagebiel RW, Abarnanel RM *et al*. Malignant melanoma of the skin: the association of tumour depth

and type, and patient sex, age and site with survival. *Cancer* 1983;**52**:1330–41.

34. Friedman RJ, Rigel DS, Kopf AW. Early detection of malignant melanoma: the role of the physician examination and self examination of the skin. *CA Cancer J Clin* 1993;**35**:130–51.

35. MacKie RM, Hole D. Audit of public education campaign to encourage earlier detection of malignant melanoma. *BMJ* 1992;**304**:1012–15.

36. Melia J, Moss S, Graham-Brown R. *et al.* The relation between mortality from maliganant melanoma and early detection in the Cancer research Campaign Mole Watcher Study. *Br J Cancer* 2001;**85**:803–7.

37. Farmer ER, Gonin R, Hanna MP. Discordance in the histopathologic diagnosis of melanoma and melanocytic nevi between expert pathologists. *Hum Pathol* 1996;**27**:528–31.

38. Berwick M, Begg CB, Fine JA. Screening for cutaneous melanoma by skin self-examination. *J Natl Cancer Inst* 1996;**88**:17–23.

39. Ferrini RL, Perlman M, Hill L. Screening for Skin Cancer. American College of Preventive Medicine: Practice Policy Statement, 1998. *Am J Prev Med* 1998;**14**:80–2.

40. Asri GD, Clarke WH Jr, Guerry DV *et al.* (1990) Screening and surveillance of patients at high risk for malignant melanoma result in the detection of earlier disease. *J Am Acad Dermatol* 1990;**22**:1042–8.

41. Melia J, Harland C, Moss S, Eiser JS, Pendry L. Feasibility of targeted early detection for melanoma: a population-based screening study. *Br J Cancer* 2000;**82**: 1605–9.

42. Altman JF, Oliveria SA, Christos PJ, Halpern AC. A survey of skin cancer screening in the primary care setting: a comparison with other cancer screenings. *Arch Fam Med* 2000;**10**:1022–7.

43. Lorentzen HF, Weismann K. Dermatoscopic diagnosis of cutaneous melanoma. Secondary prophylaxis. *Ugeskr Laeger* 1993;**162**:3312–16.

44. Bafounta ML, Beauchet A, Aegerter P, Saiag P. Is dermoscopy useful for the diagnosis of melanoma? Results of a meta-analysis using techniques adapted to the evaluation of diagnostic tests. *Arch Dermatol* 2001;**137**:1343–50.

45. MacKie RM, Fleming C, McMahon AD, Jarrett P. The use of dermatoscope to identify early melanoma using the three colour test. *Br J Dermatol* 2002;**146**:481–4.

46. Girgis A, Sanson-Fisher RW. Skin cancer prevention, early detection, and management: current beliefs and practices of Australian family physicians. *Cancer Detect Prev* 1996;**20**:16–24.

23

Do sunscreens reduce
the incidence of skin cancers?

Ros Weston

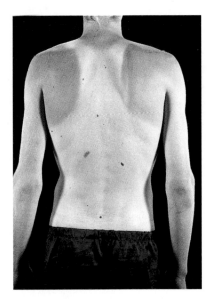

Figure 23.1   Patient with sunburn and dysplastic naevus syndrome

Background
Historical development and SPF

Sunscreens were first used in1928 and became popular with those intentionally trying to gain a suntan. They mainly filter out the wavelengths responsible for sunburn (UVB, 280–315 nm). Following evidence that longer wavelengths of sunlight (UVA, 315–400 nm) are involved in the sunburn reaction and photocarcinogenesis, UVA absorbers have been added to most sunscreens to widen their absorption spectra. There is concordant evidence that sunscreens undoubtedly protect against sunburn, but evidence for a role in the prevention of skin cancers is still somewhat equivocal.[1,2] The concept of a sunscreen effectiveness index (ratio) is attributed to Schulze and Greiter, who proposed the specific term "sun protection factor" (SPF), and the associated method for assessing SPF.[3] SPF activity is the ratio of the least amount of UV energy required to produce erythema (reddening of the skin) on sunscreen-protected skin to the amount of energy to produce the same effect on unprotected skin.

Testing and regulation of sunscreens

Topical sunscreens applied to the skin act by absorbing and/or scattering incident UV radiation (UVR). The shape of the absorption spectrum is the fundamental attribute of a topical sunscreen. It is expressed as the extinction coefficient: the measure of the degree to which the sunscreen absorbs individual wavelengths across the terrestrial UVR spectrum (290–400 nm). Absorption is the product of the extinction coefficient, the concentration of the active ingredient, and the effective thickness of application on exposed parts of the body.

Sunscreens are regulated for specific formulations in most countries. In the EU, Japan, and South Africa they are regulated as cosmetics and in other countries (Australia, Canada and New Zealand) as drugs. Testing for toxic effects is mandatory in each country. Control in Europe is by a directive of the European Commission (2000). This mandates that labelling should include a full list of ingredients in decreasing order of concentration, and that this should be displayed on the containers of all cosmetics that include sunscreen formulations.[4–7] Sunscreens are now readily available in most countries during all seasons. In Australia the availability of sunscreens has been maximised through sales tax exemptions and they are now available in workplaces, schools; their use by children is actively promoted.[8–10]

Paradoxical findings: problems with use of sunscreen as a primary prevention aim

Protecting against sun damage and reducing the risk of sunburn and skin cancers involves behavioural choices. Studies demonstrate that increased use of sunscreens often means a reduction in other photo-protective methods: wearing of hats and protective clothing and the use of shade (see Figure 22.1), thus increasing net sun exposure. Most sunscreens are made to prevent against sunburn and most sunburn, in both children and adults, occurs during intentional exposure to the sun.[11–14] The use of sunscreens, including those with high SPFs, during intentional exposure has been found to have little effect on the occurrence of sunburn.[15–17] This is concordant with the results from surveys of beachgoers which suggest that increased overreliance on sunscreens reduces the use of other protective measures. Individuals seem to balance protective behaviours according to personal motivation and characteristics and the desire for a suntan.[18–24]

Intended and actual sun protection from sunscreens

There is some evidence that the numerical measure of protection indicated on the product pack is generally higher than that achieved in practice. The photoprotection of sunscreens (the SPF) is measured by photo-testing *in vivo* at internationally agreed levels of thickness of application 2 mg/cm². To receive the SPF quoted on sunscreen packaging, an individual would need to use 35 ml of sunscreen for total body surface protection. Studies have demonstrated that individuals are more likely to use 0·5–1·5 mg/cm² and that most users get, in protective terms, the benefit of between one-quarter and one-half of the product.[25] Individuals get sunburnt because they use too little sunscreen, spread it unevenly, miss parts of the body surface exposed to the sun and because sunscreen is rubbed or washed off. Thus, individuals' use of a sunscreen makes a difference in how effective sunscreens are in the prevention of sunburn and explains why sunburn still occurs even with higher SPF sunscreens. If individuals want to be supine in the sun for long periods of time (hours) then it is recommended that SPFs of 20–30 or higher are necessary. Sunscreens need to be applied evenly 30 minutes before going out in the sun. They need to be reapplied at regular intervals as much is washed off by swimming and other water sports and by any abrasive action particularly from sand on the beach.[25]

Possible drawbacks of sunscreens

No published studies have demonstrated toxic effects of sunscreens in humans. Case reports suggest there is an increase in the frequency of photocontact dermatitis among patients who are frequent sunscreen users and who have photodermatoses such as polymorphic light eruption. There is no evidence that sunscreen use affects vitamin D levels.[25] Using sunscreen does not cause adverse effects on reproduction or fetal development, although some effects have been seen with high oral doses of sunscreen ingredients in animal models. In some experimental conditions topically applied sunscreen (in the absence of UVR) affects the immune system but most toxicity studies have shown that the active ingredients in sunscreens are safe when applied topically at recommended concentrations. DNA damage has been reported in one study.[25]

Search strategies

Searches of Medline, PubMed and the *Cochrane Library* was carried out using "sunscreen" as a key word and searching for appropriate meta-analyses and randomised controlled trials (RCTs). Health education and promotion journals were also searched. This search located the International Agency for Research on Cancer (IARC) meta-analysis of sunscreen use.[25]

Outcome measures

Ideally, the main outcome measure of studies addressing sunscreen use and cancer risk would be numbers of incident cancers in those using sunscreens compared with those not using sunscreens. However, this is unrealistic because of the long latency period for a skin cancer to develop and the relative rarity of such events. Surrogate outcome measures such as reported protective behaviour are therefore often used in studies. Intermediate outcomes such as incidence of actinic keratoses or reduction in naevi are also used as short-term surrogates for longer term skin cancer risk. All of these surrogate measures have their problems. There are many confounding factors when assessing sunscreen use. Many studies use behaviour (for example, reported use of suncreen or sun avoidance) as the outcome measure. The data may still be unreliable as recall of use is not necessarily accurate and other protective measures are confounding factors. Lack of

specificity of outcome measures remains problematic.

QUESTIONS

Can the use of sunscreen prevent cutaneous melanoma?

Efficacy

There are no reported RCTs or cohort studies on the use of sunscreens and the risk for cutaneous melanoma. There are a total of 15 case-control studies[26-40] (see Table 23.1). In attempting to assess the evidence from these it is important to note that these studies use very different populations and different cultural groups. This analysis does not compare like with like: each uses a different study design, has different terms of reference and uses different methods for data collection. The term sunscreen is variously described and does not refer to one category. Sun lotion, sun-tanning oil and sun protection factor are used throughout these studies. This makes it particularly difficult to assess the reported results unless these terms were clearly defined to study participants, or confounding factors accounted for, as part of the data analysis process. Overall, however, these studies showed on overall low prevalence of sunscreen use (see Table 23.1)

Klepp and Magnus (1979)[26], Graham *et al.* (1985)[27] and Herzfeld *et al.* (1985)[28] reported an increased risk between sunscreen use and melanoma with Graham *et al.* reporting an increased risk particularly in males. Beitner *et al.* (1990)[29] reported increased risk for those who used sunscreens "often" or "very often". This study controlled for age, sex and hair colouring. Elwood and Gallagher (1999)[30] assessed the relationship between phenotype, history of sun-tanning and sunburn, exposure to sunlight and the risk for melanoma in four western provinces of Canada. Analysis of a subset of cases of

Table 23.1 Case-control studies of sunscreen use and risk for cutaneous melanoma

Population place/date	Type of cases/controls	No. cases/controls	Exposure	RR[a] (95% CI)	Comments	Reference
Norway 1974–75	Hospital cases Other cancer controls	78 cases 131 controls	Sometimes, often or almost always use sun lotion/oil	M 2·8[b] (1·2–6·7) F 1·0[b] (0·42–2·5) T 2·3[b] (1·3–4·1)	Elevated risks among males only. Sunscreens not differentiated from "sun lotions".	Klepp and Magnus (1979)[26]
USA 1974–80	Hospital cases Other cancer controls	404 cases 521 controls	Used sunscreen Used suntan lotion	M 2·2[b] (1·2–4·1) M 1·7 (1·1–2·7) F "no added risk"	Elevated risks among males only	Graham et al. (1985)[27]
USA 1977–79	Population cases and controls	324 male trunk melanoma cases 415 controls	Always used "suntan lotion"	2·6[b] (1·4–4·7) Not significant after control for "tendency to sunburn and water sports"	"Suntan lotions" and "sunscreens" not differentiated in questionnaire	Herzfeld et al.[28] (1993)
Sweden 1978–83	Hospital cases Population controls	523 cases 505 controls	Often used sun protection agents	1·8[b] (1·2–2·7)		Beitner et al.[29] (1990)
Canada 1979–81	Population cases and controls	369 trunk and lower limb melanomas 369 controls	Used sunscreen almost always	1·1 (0·75–1·6)	Highest risk in those using sunscreen "only for first few hours" RR,1·62 (1·04–2·52)	Elwood and Gallagher[30] (1999)
Australia 1980–81	Population cases and controls	507 cases 507 controls	Used sunscreens ≤ 10 years	1·1 (0·71–1·6)		Holman et al.[31] (1986)
USA 1981–86	Population cases and controls	452 cases 930 controls	Always used sunscreens	All cutaneous melanoma 0·62[b] (0·49–0·83) Superficial spreading melanoma (SSM) 0·43 (CI not available)	Study involved only women aged 25–59 at diagnosis. CI estimated. RR for SSM adjusted for host factors and sun exposure	Holly et al.[32] (1995)
Denmark 1982–85	Population cases and controls	474 cases 926 controls	Always used sunscreens	1·1[b] (0·8–1·5)		Osterlind et al. (1997)[33]
Australia 1987–94	Population cases Controls from same	50 cases 156 controls	Always used sunscreens	2·2 (0·4–12) on holidays		Whiteman et al. (1997)[34]

(Continued)

Table 23.1 (*Continued*)

Population place/date	Type of cases/ controls	No. cases/ controls	Exposure	RR[a] (95% CI)	Comments	Reference
	school	All children < 15		0·7 (0·1–6·0) at school		
Sweden 1988–90	Population cases and controls	400 cases 640 controls	Almost always used sunscreens	Trunk 1·4 (0·6–3·2) Other sites 2·0 (1·1–3·7)	No information on duration of use	Westerdahl *et al.* (1995)[35]
Spain 1989–93	Hospital cases Hospital visitors	105 cases 138 controls	Always used sunscreens	0·2 (0·04–0·79)		Rodenas *et al.* (1996)[36]
Spain 1990–94	Hospital cases and controls	116 cases 235 controls	Used sunscreen	0·48 (0·34–0·71)	Inadequate description of measurement of sunscreen use	Espinoza-Arranz *et al.* (1991)[37]
Europe 1991–92	Hospital cases Neighbourhood controls	418 controls 438 controls	Ever use psoralen sunscreens Ever use sunscreen	2·3 (1·3–4·0) 1·5 (1·1–2·1) M 1·8 (1·1–2·7) F 1·3 (0·87–2·0)	Highest risk for sun-sensitive subjects using sunscreens to tan: RR, 3·7 (1·0–7·6)	Autier *et al.* (1995, 1997b)[38]
Austria 1993–94	Hospital cases and controls	193 cases 319 controls	Often used sunscreen	3·5 (1·8–6·6)		Wolf *et al.* (1998)[39]
Sweden 1995–97	Population cases and controls	571 cases 913 controls	Always used sunscreen Used sunscreens to spend more time sunbathing	1·8 (1·1–2·9) 8·7 (1·0–76)		Westerdahl *et al.* (2000)[40]

[a] Relative risk estimates adjusted for phenotype and sun-related factors where possible

[b] Crude relative risk ratio only available

melanoma on intermittently exposed sites (trunk and lower limbs) and controls provided information about the use of sunscreens on these sites during outdoor activity. Risk for those reporting sunscreen "almost always used" was very similar to that of those using sunscreen "sometimes". Those using sunscreen only in first few hours had increased risk after adjustment for hair, eye and skin colouring and propensity to burn.

Holman *et al*, (1986)[31] found that those who had used sunscreens for less than 10 years did not have a reduced risk for cutaneous melanoma: risk was not reduced for those who had used sunscreens for 10–15 years. Frequency of use did not appear to be related to risk. This study did find a positive relationship between the use of sunscreen and the risk for cutaneous melanoma but in the absence of control for pigmentary traits and sun sensitivity. Sunscreens were not available in Australia when the subjects in this study were younger and therefore they were unable to use them at a time when they may have given protection.

Holly *et al.* (1995)[32] found that women who reported "almost always" using sunscreens had a lower risk for cutaneous melanoma than those who reported that they "never" used sunscreens. After controlling for superficial spread of melanoma, sun sensitivity and sunburn history before the age of 12 years the risk for women "almost always" using was lower than for those "never" using. The authors concluded that sunscreen use was strongly protective against melanoma. This study showed that the highest level of risk was for women with the least exposure after controlling for sun sensitivity.

Osterlind *et al.* (1988)[33] found that compared to those who "never" used sunscreens, a small non-significant increase in risk was seen for those who had used them for less than 10 years, or for those using for more than 10 years. Frequency of use was not associated with the risk of melanoma among those "always using" against those who "hardly ever used" or "never used". Effective sunscreens were not available to the study group in their youth.

Whiteman *et al.* (1997)[34] found, after controlling for tanning ability, freckling and number of naevi, those who had "always" used sunscreens while on holiday had a non-significant elevated risk for cutaneous melanoma compared to those not using sunscreens. The use of sunscreens at school was associated with a non-significant reduced risk. The RRs have very wide confidence intervals in this study (only 11 "always" used on holiday and only two reported sunscreen use at school).

Westerdahl *et al.* (1995)[35] found, after controlling for history of sunburn; history of sunbathing; number of raised naevi; freckling and hair colour,

those "almost always" using sunscreen had similar risk estimates to those "never" using in both men and women. Risk for use before age 15, at age 15–19 and at age 19 years reported elevated odds ratios at each stage similar to those of people "always using" sunscreens. Risk for melanomas of the trunk were similar to that found for melanomas of the extremities, and head and neck, after adjustment for sunburns, frequent sunbathing, freckling and naevi.

Rodenas *et al.* (1996)[36] reported that the use of sunscreen appeared to protect against melanoma and that risk was strongly associated to the sensitivity of the skin to the sun (relative risk of 2·0) for those who always burned. This study failed to give a description of how sunscreen use was measured. Espinoza-Arranz *et al.* (1999) found similar results.[37]

Autier *et al.* (1995 and 1997)[38] found that those who had "never" used psoralen-containing sunscreens had an increased risk for cutaneous melanoma after controlling for age, sex, hair colouring, and number of weeks spent in sunny climes each year. An elevated risk was found particularly among those who reported no history of sunburn. Use of psoralen-containing sunscreens, however, was not common. Those "ever" using these sunscreens (psoralen) also had increased risk after adjustment for some factors compared to those "never" using. Increased risk was reported for those using sunscreens and those having light or dark hair. Sensitive and sun-insensitive participants showed an increased risk with the use of sunscreens. The authors concluded that use of sunscreen tended to be associated with higher risk for cutaneous melanoma among sunbathers. Highest risk was for those using sunscreen and who had no history of sunburn after age 14 years. The use of clothing, rather than sunscreen, appeared protective. It was the use of sunscreen, particularly in UVA as well as UVB light, that was found to associated with increased risk.

Wolf et al. (1998)[39] reported "often used" sunscreen had a significant higher risk for melanoma compared to "never used" (study controlled for skin colouring, sunbathing and history of sunburn). The authors concluded that use of sunscreen did not prevent melanoma.

Westerdahl et al. (2000)[40] reported a significantly increased risk for melanoma for regular use (always used) of sunscreen after adjustment for hair colour, history of sunburns, frequency and duration of sunbathing. Risk was significantly increased among those using sunscreens with an SPF less than 10 compared with those who did not use sunscreens and for those with no history of sunburn when they used sunscreens. The risk was even higher for those using sunscreen to increase sunbathing time (deliberate exposure). In an analysis of subsites, risk was significantly increased only for melanoma of the trunk.

The following studies could be assessed as supporting a positive association between sunscreen use and risk of cutaneous melanoma but this tentative conclusion should be viewed cautiously.[26-29,38-40] Confounding factors such as: sunscreen use, sun exposure, sun sensitivity, a history of sun-related neoplasia and sun-protective behaviour such as the use of protective clothing, staying indoors or seeking shade were problematic in these studies. There was idiosyncratic reporting of these confounding factors casting doubt on the significance of the results.

Three studies[30,31,33] reported no increased risk for use of sunscreen and cutaneous melanoma with non-significant increase being reported in one study.[34] Three studies reported sunscreen as protective against cutaneous melanoma.[34,36]

Studies that have assessed naevus count as an indicator of melanoma risk

One study using naevi count as an intermediate endpoint showed that the median number of new naevi in Caucasian children was reduced in the sunscreen users. Sunscreen was more effective in preventing naevi in children who freckled than in those who did not.[41] Difference in exposure time was not a significant variable. One cohort study[42] showed increasing naevi development with sunscreen use. Further analysis showed that this was because children who used sunscreen had longer cumulative exposure time but no data were available to support this conclusion. The cross-sectional study[43] reported that the use of summer sunscreen reduced the number of sunburns but was not associated with annual sun exposure or with naevi number or density. This study was criticised for not reporting all data.

Studies using naevus count as an outcome do not provide any conclusive evidence about the relationship between the use of sunscreen and reduced naevi and thus reduced risk for cutaneous melanoma. In all studies the confounding variables and lack of reported data were problematic. A consistent finding of all these studies was the link between cumulative exposure and risk.

Comment on sunscreen use and melanoma risk

Some studies demonstrate a positive association between sunscreen use and risk for cutaneous melanoma whereas others do not. Many confounding factors prevented any firm conclusions as to the possible protective or harmful effect on the use of sunscreens. The most likely reason for an apparently increased risk is that individuals who use sunscreen stay in the sun longer because they falsely believe that sunscreen protects them. This needs further research, particularly to clarify knowledge and attitudes to suntanning, sunscreen use and knowledge of skin cancer. It would seem that individuals intent on gaining a suntan use sunscreens to give themselves more time in the sun without sunburn. Reducing their risk of cancer is a secondary motive. Risk is also related to phenotype and history of sun exposure and sunburn. There is equivocal evidence about the use of sunscreen and the use of other photo-protective measures. Further research is needed to assess these factors in long-term randomised studies with specific target groups. Such research needs to include a formative stage that seeks to explore knowledge and attitude to sunscreen use and other photo-protective measures. This information will enable specific outcome objectives to be developed for each aspect of the study, thus reducing confounding factors. There is a need for an agreed definition of "sunscreen use" and specific definition and description of such use: how, when and what SPF is used in specific situations.

Can the use of sunscreen reduce the risk of basal cell carcinoma (BCC) and squamous cell carcinoma (SCC)?

The Nambour Skin Cancer Prevention Trial (a randomised study exploring risk of both SCC and BCC) demonstrated that sunscreen use could be significant in reducing the risk of SCC.[44] This was a complex trial including 1850 residents aged 20–69. They were invited to use a daily application of SPF 16 sunscreen and use 30 mg of beta-carotene supplement in the prevention of skin cancer; 1647 attended baseline assessment that included a cancer risk factor assessment and a full skin examination by a dermatologist. Any detected skin cancers were removed at the start of the study. Out of these 1647 residents, 1621 agreed to take part in the study. They were randomised to one of four study groups, sunscreen and beta-carotene; sunscreen and placebo; no sunscreen and beta-carotene; and no sunscreen and placebo. The participants attended a clinic every 3 months to receive new sunscreen and beta-carotene. The weight of the sunscreen returned to these clinics every three months was recorded. A random subgroup of

sunscreen users kept a 7-day diary on three occasions to record their frequency of sunscreen application and sun exposure. Dermatologist examinations were given at these visits and any cancers removed and recorded. No protective effect for prevention of SCC was found in the beta-carotene group. Sunscreen use was analysed for all groups, regardless of beta-carotene use as no interaction was seen between the two interventions (sunscreen and beta-carotene). A total of 28 new SCCs were detected in the group given sunscreen and 46 in those not given sunscreen (RR, 0·61; 95% CI 0·50–1·6) a statistically significant difference. The authors concluded that sunscreen use could be of significant benefit in protecting against SCC. No placebo sunscreen was used and the results need to be interpreted with caution because the comparison group was not ideal, reducing the power of the study to detect an effect of daily sunscreen use. Green et al. (1999)[45] subsequently reported that solar exposure of those given sunscreen did not differ from those not given sunscreen. The prevalence of sunburn was lower for those receiving sunscreen to those not receiving it (tested on a random sample of participants wearing photosensitive badges). The findings suggest that the reduction of incidence of SCC seen in the group using sunscreens was probably due to the attenuation [sic thinning] of the UVR by the sunscreen rather than in behaviour change (reducing time in the sun). Higher factor sunscreen use, especially for older people, may not result in them spending longer time in the sun.

A cohort study by Grodestein et al. (1995)[46] reported that sunscreens used over a 2-year period by women who spent 8 or more hours per week in the sun was not protective by comparison with no use of such agents (RR 1·1; 95% CI 0·83–1·7).

Timing of exposure to UVR was a significant risk factor for SCC in a case-control study by Pogoda and Preston-Martin (1996).[47] There is little evidence that sunscreen use protects against BCC. Some patients may have been advised to use sunscreens following diagnosis, which may have confounded results. Following diagnosis of SCC, use of sunscreen was examined retrospectively in three age groups: 8–14, 15–19 and 20–24 years. Those in the 8–14 group who had used sunscreens seemed to have a slightly reduced risk of SCC (RR 0·61; 95% CI 0·82–4·4) not statistically significant. Those using sunscreen in the 15–19 age group had a relative risk of 1·9 (95% CI 0·82–4·4) and those in the 20–24 group had a risk of 0·99 (95% CI 0·44–2·2). No strong protective effect of sunscreens was found.

One cohort, Hunter et al. (1990)[48] and one case-control study by Kricker et al. (1995)[49] reported increased risks for BCC in sunscreen users. No significant association between sunscreen use and cancer risk was observed in one cohort and one case-control study of SCC[50], one of SCC and BCC of the skin or one case-control study of SCC of the vermilion border of the lip.[47] Confounding of sun sensitivity and exposure were present in these studies, as in previously described studies.

Kricker et al.[49] found that subjects who had used sunscreens for at least half the time spent in the sun 1–9 years prior to diagnosis had a higher relative risk for BCC than those who had never used sunscreens or had used them less than half the time (RR 1·8; 95% CI 1·1–2·9). This risk persisted after adjustment for age, sex, ability to tan and site of lesion. No change in RR was found for those who had used sunscreens more than half the time in the 1–9 years, prior to diagnosis (RR 1·1; 95% CI 0·69–1·7) in comparison to those who had not used sunscreens or who had used them for half the time. Few subjects had access to sunscreens 11–30 years before diagnosis.

Studies that have used intermediate end points such as incidence of solar keratoses as markers for basal and SCCs risk

Actinic (solar) keratoses are a risk factor for BCC and a precursor lesion for SCC. They are related to solar exposure and phenotype. The rate of development for SCC is low and many regress spontaneously, especially when exposure to UVR is reduced. These lesions have therefore been used as an intermediate endpoint in studies on the use of sunscreens in the prevention of SCC.[47,51] The Maryborough Trial in Australia[51] assessed whether the daily use of sunscreen had any effect in reducing the development of actinic keratoses in those already having these. This was a short-term study using a placebo and included body site examination and diaries to record the time of day patients applied sunscreen. Those using placebo had greater mean increase in the number of keratoses during the study (1·0 ± 0·3 SE) than those given sunscreen (0·6 ± 0·3; RR 1·5; 95% CI 0·81–2·2). Fewer new keratoses were found in the sunscreen group (1·6 versus 2·3 lesions per subject; RR 0·62; 95% CI 0·54–0·71). After controlling for sex and sun sensitivity, the likely remission of keratoses (those with keratoses at the start of study) was greater for the sunscreen group (25% versus 18% initial lesions regressing: RR 1·5, 95% CI 1·3–1·8.[51]

Comment on sunscreen use and BCC and SCC

There is no conclusive evidence that sunscreen protects against either SCC or BCC and there is some limited evidence to suggest that risk may increase with sunscreen use. However, these non-randomised studies had confounding variables that make it difficult to be conclusive about such evidence.

Although the Maryborough acitinic keratoses trial[51] was a short-term trial, the confounding factors were well accounted for. The study suggests that sunscreen can prevent the development of new actinic keratoses. Further research is required to provide conclusive evidence of these results.

Do multistrategy interventions increase intention to use sunscreens as a protective measure for reducing the risk of melanoma and non-melanocytic skin cancers?

A number of studies have assessed the effectiveness of targeted sun protection interventions combined with sunscreen use.[52-79] Sunscreen use is only one of many outcome measures in these multistrategic interventions targeted at specific groups or to communities in general but was reported separately. Seven studies[54,55,60,61,68,71,72] were conducted in schools; four at beaches[52,57,63,69]; two at pools[52,75] and three in other recreational settings.[62,65,67]; There were two studies in the workplace[69,72]; and two in clinical/medical settings.[58,61] There was one study in the tourist industry[53] and four multicomponent community studies.[56,66,70,73] Most studies were short term and aimed at improving sun-protection behaviour among specific high-risk groups, including children, young people, beachgoers, outdoor workers and patients with non-melanoma skin cancers.

In the main the studies used interactive educational presentations and communication strategies including peer-led programmes, role modelling, parental activities and materials aimed at increasing knowledge, including specific recommendations for sunscreen use. Interventions to enable policy change such as developing social and physical environments (shaded areas) for sun protection were the focus of three interventions.[52,60,73] Parental activities[62] and home activities[61] were the focus of two interventions. Medical interventions mainly used information giving to raise awareness of primary and secondary prevention of skin cancer.[56,58,60]

More complex community interventions used incentives for beach guards, booklets[52,56,61], primary and secondary prevention information and education,[66,73-76,79] and in schools.[54,55,67,71,73]

Twenty-two studies, quasirandomised and longitudinal studies reported on at least one outcome measure with regard to sunscreen use; proxy measures for behaviour were used in some studies (for example, the intention to use sunscreen). Eleven out of sixteen targeted interventions were successful in increasing knowledge and behaviour[52,54,56,59,61-64] and six were successful in increasing solar potection, either the use of shade, staying out of the sun or the use of clothing[52-59,62,64,68,73] and increased sunscreen use.[52,54,56-58,62,64,65,66-69] The duration and intensity of the intervention affected the success of the intervention. Successful interventions were longer, had multiple components or were supported by broader community initiatives.

Other reported successful educational intervention strategies were those intended to increase the perception of risk for developing skin cancer. Strategies that involved showing young people computer photoimages of their own faces with superimposed ageing and images of skin lesion were successful in improving both the frequency of sunscreen use and the application of sunscreen.[65]

An intervention for outdoor workers increased the use of sun protection but the use of sunscreen was not reported separately.[69] The impact of an intervention at swimming pools in which clients were given incentives and exposed to role modelling of lifeguards is unclear, although the authors reported that the sun-protection score was improved when two or more sun-protection measures were taken together, with no change in the mean quantity of free sunscreen used at pools.[52]

There have been six reported community interventions aimed at improving knowledge of skin cancer, encouraging the use of protective clothing and sunscreen use[74–79] Experience suggests that they require long-term funding, commitment and evaluation. Cross-sectional population surveys included the "Slip, Slap, Slop" and "SunSmart" campaigns in Australia[74,75]; "Sun Awareness" in Canada[76]; UVR index forecasting in the US[71]; the Melanoma and Skin Cancer Detection and Prevention programme in the US[72]; and the Falmouth Safe Skin Programme in the US.[77] These were aimed at improving community knowledge about skin cancer and sun protection, and included mass media components, distribution of educational leaflets, the development of school curriculum for sun protection and sometimes partnership working in locality settings. Five of these large-scale community interventions had a positive impact on sunscreen use at population level.[74–79] The UVR index study reported no effect on sunscreen use but sunscreen use was associated with increased awareness of weather forecasts.[71,72]

Comment on multifacet strategies to increase sunscreen use and sun protective behaviour

These multistrategic interventions are the most difficult to interpret collectively because of the plethora of outcome objectives. They remain difficult to design and require substantive formative research to appropriately determine specific behavioural outcome measures for each target group and for the selection of educational strategies for delivering the intervention. Those reporting indicate that interactive educational strategies are the most effective for increasing solar protection scores. Campaigns over time have the best outcome for increasing knowledge about skin cancer and use of sunscreens.

Implications for clinical practice

- There is little good evidence that sunscreens reduce the risk of cutaneous melanoma.
- There is some evidence that sunscreen use may inadvertently increase risk because it may encourage longer periods in the sun.
- There is no clear evidence that sunscreen use decreases the incidence of BCC.
- There is some evidence that sunscreen use can decrease the incidence of actinic keratoses and SCC.

Educational messages are needed to ensure:

- that sunscreens are not used as the first or only choice for skin cancer prevention
- that sunscreens are not used as a means of extending total sun exposure (i.e. sunbathing and suntanning).
- that sunscreens are not used as a substitute for clothes on body sites that are not usually exposed, such as the trunk and buttocks.
- the daily use of sunscreen with a high SPF (> than 15) on areas of the body that are not usually exposed areas is recommended for those in areas of high isolation who work outdoors or undertake regular outdoor leisure pursuits
- daily use of a sunscreen can reduce actinic keratoses and SCC.

In addition:

- Protecting children against solar exposure during childhood is more important than at any time in life.
- Using photo-protective clothing, hats and shade is essential. Parents, carers, schools and leisure organisations need to encourage and promote knowledge about sun-protective behaviour.
- Primary prevention interventions should first and foremost promote hats with as wide a brim as possible to protect the head, neck and face (see Chapter 22).

- Shade should be promoted as protective whenever possible, including avoiding outdoor activities between 11 am and 3 pm.

Recommendations for future research

- Future research should seek to understand the role of sunscreens in the prevention of skin cancers and the role of UVR in the causation of these diseases, the dose–response relationship, the dose rate and pattern of delivery on risk and the action spectrum for each effect.
- RCTs should be conducted in adults to evaluate whether a reduction in late-stage exposure to UVR can reduce the incidence of cutaneous melanoma and precursor lesions such as clinically atypical naevi.
- In children, studies are needed to evaluate whether a reduction in early-stage exposure to UVR can reduce the prevalence of acquired naevi, the precursor of cutaneous melanoma and SCC.
- Trials should ideally include a quantitative assessment of solar exposure and an evaluation of the various methods for reducing solar exposure – sunscreens, clothing and sun avoidance.
- As sunscreens are increasingly used on children, an evaluation of their safety for long-term use is needed.
- There is a need to evaluate whether the qualitative rating of the potential function of sunscreens against UVR, such as low, medium, high and ultra-high, rather than SPF, would promote appropriate use of sunscreens.
- There is a need to better understand the role of the mechanisms of skin cancer aetiology and how sunscreens might affect this. Intermediate endpoints (for example, naevi and biochemical markers of carcinogenesis such as DNA damage and *p53* mutations) could be studied to assess their relationship to sunscreen use.

- Researchers in health promotion need to develop qualitative and quantitative methods for measuring sunscreen use in order to identify major confounding variables such as sun sensitivity and sun exposure.
- There is a need to be able to measure, in the field, how much protection is provided by sunscreens at various sites on the skin.
- There is a need to understand how efficiently individuals use sunscreen. This would enable manufacturers to develop sunscreens that achieve adequate protection against UVR when in common use.

Conclusions

In the past 20 years, promoting the use of sunscreens has been the main focus of primary prevention for skin cancer together with photo-protective clothing and shaded areas. This summary demonstrates that health promoters across all settings, including primary care and hospital settings, need to re-think their sun protection promotion.

There is inadequate evidence in humans as to whether topical use of sunscreen has a preventative effect against cutaneous malignant melanoma and BCC of the skin and there is limited evidence for a protective effect against SCC of the skin. There is, however, good evidence that sunscreen prevents SCC of the skin induced in mice by solar-simulated radiation.

The review supports the hypothesis that the topical use of sunscreens reduces the risk of sunburn in humans and probably prevents SCC of the skin when used during intentional sunbathing. There is inconclusive evidence about the cancer preventive effects of topical use of sunscreens against BCC and cutaneous melanoma. It seems that sunscreen can extend intentional sun exposure (sunbathing and sun tanning) and that this increased exposure may subsequently increase the risk for cutaneous melanoma.

It is essential that the main educational message promoting long-term changes to attitude and behaviour in the sun should focus on the use of photo-protective clothing and shade; sunscreens should be promoted as an extra protective measure, after the use of clothing and shade. There should be very positive messages about the use of sunscreen including application and re-application at regular intervals. This will prevent individuals from having a false sense of security engendered by the use of sunscreens, particularly for intentional suntanning behaviour.

Promoting the use of photo-protective clothing and shade remains the most effective way to prevent against unintentional exposure. It is imperative that policy includes the development of shaded areas in communities and on beaches, even in temperate climes. Sunscreens may give a false sense of security about protection, putting individuals at increased risk for sun exposure and thus for cutaneous skin cancers.

Communication and appropriate efficacious delivery of messages intended to change behaviour remain the main goal point of long-term randomised studies across communities. This is very important as we face the threat of continued global warming. This will be a challenge for all in public health and health promotion.

References

1. Shaath NA. Evolution of modern sunscreen chemicals. In: Lowe NJ, Shaath NA, Pathak MA, eds. *Sunscreens, Development, Evaluation and Regulatory Aspects. 2nd edition. Cosmetic Science and Technology Series* 1997;**15**:3–33.

2. Bestak R, Barneston RS, Neath MR, Halliday GM. Sunscreen protection of contact hypersensitivity responses from chronic solar-simulated ultra irradiation correlates with the absorption spectrum of the sunscreen. *J Invest Dermatol* 1995:**105**;345–51.

3. Schulze R. Some tests and remarks regarding the problem of sunscreens that are found on the market (in German). *Parfum Kosmet* 1956;**37**:310–16.

4. Quinn AG, Diffey BL *et al.* Definition of the minimal erythema dose used for diagnostic phototesting. *Br J Dermatol* 1994;**131**:56–9.

5. Lock-Anderson J, Wulf HC Threshold level for measurement of UV sensitivity: Reproducibility of phototest. *Photodermatol Photoimmunol Photomed* 1996;**12**:154–61.

6. Janousek A. *Regulatory aspects of sunscreens in Europe.* In: Lowe NJ, Shaath NA, Pathak MA, eds. *Sunscreens, development, evaluation and regulatory aspects. 2nd edn: Cosmetic Science and Technology Series* 1997;215–25.

7. Fukuda M, Takata S. The evolution of recent sunscreens. In: Altmeyer P, Hoffmann K, Stuker M, eds. *Skin Cancer and UV Radiation.* Berlin: Springer-Verlag 1997:265–76.

8. Australian/New Zealand Standards. *Sunscreen products – Evalaution and Classification.* Homebush Standards, Australia; Wellington Standards; New Zealand, 1998.

9. Health Canada. *Regulatory Strategy for Pharmaceutical Products with Photo- Co-carcinogneic Potential.* Ottawa: Therapeutic Products Programme, 1999.

10. European Commission. Directive 76/78 Guidelines for testing of cosmetic ingredients (SCCMF), 1976.

11. Hill D, White V, Marks R *et al.* Melanoma prevention: Behavioural and non-behavioural factors in sunburn among and Australian urban population. *Prev Med* 1992;**21**:654–69.

12. McGee R, Williams S, Cox B, Elwood M, Bulliard JL. A community survey of sun exposure, sunburn and sun protection. *NZ Med J* 1995;**108**:508–10.

13. Melia J, Bulman A. Sunburn and tanning in a British population. *J Public Health Med* 1995;**17**:223–9.

14. Autier P, Dore AU JF, Cattaruzza MS *et al.* Sunscreen use, wearing clothes, and number of nevi in 6–7 year old European children. *J Natl Cancer Inst* 1998;**90**:1873–80.

15. Wulf HC, Stender IM, Lock-Andersen J. Sunscreens used at the beach do not protect against erythema: A new definition of SPF is proposed. *Photoderm Photoimmunol Photo Med* 1997;**13**:129–32.

16. Autier P, Dore JF, Negrier S *et al.* Sunscreen use and duration of sun exposure: A double blind randomised trial. *J Natl Cancer Inst* 1999;**91**:1304–9.

17. McCarthy EM, Ethridge KP, Wagner JF Jr. Beach holiday sunburn: The sunscreen paradox and gender differences. *Cutis* 1999;**64**:37–42.

18. Hill D, White V, Marks R, Borland R. Changes in sun-related attitudes and behaviours, and reduced sunburn prevalence in a population at high risk of melanoma. *Eur J Can Prev* 1993;**2**:447–56.

19. Baade PD, Balanda KP, Lowe JB. Changes in sun protection behaviours, attitudes and sunburn in a population with the highest incidence of skin cancer in the world. *Cancer Detect Prev* 1996;**20**:566–75.

20. Rivers JK, Gallagher RP. Public education projects in skin cancer: Experience of the Canadian Dermatology Association. *Cancer* 1995;**75**(Suppl.):661–6.

21. Miller RW, Rabkin CS. Merkel cell carcinoma and melanoma: Etiological similarities and differences. *Cancer Epidemiol Biomarkers Prev* 1999;**8**:153–8.

22. Lombard D, Neubauer TE, Canfield D, Winett RA. Behavioural community intervention to reduce risk of skin cancer. *J Applied Behav* 1991;**24**:677–86.

23. Gooderham MJ, Guenther L. Sun and the skin: Evaluation of a sun awareness program for elementary school students. *J Cutan Med Surg* 1999;**3**:230–5.

24. Cockburn J, Thompson S, Marks R, Jolley D, Schofield D, Hill D. Behavioural dynamics of a clinical trial of sunscreens for reducing solar keratoses in Victoria, Australia. *J Epidemiol Community Health* 1997;**51**:716–21.

25. IARC 2001 *Handbooks of Cancer Prevention. Vol. 5 Sunscreens*. Lyon, France: IARC Press.

26. Klepp O, Magnus K. Some environmental and bodily characteristics of melanoma patients. A case-control study. *Int J Cancer* 1979;**23**:482–6.

27. Graham S, Marshall J, Haughey B *et al.* An inquiry into the epidemiology of melanoma. *Am J Epidemiol* 1985:**122**: 606–19.

28. Herzfeld PM, Fitzgerald EF, Hwang SA, Stark A. A case-control study of malignant melanoma of the trunk among white males in upstate New York. *Cancer Detection Prev* 1993;**17**:601–8.

29. Beitner H, Norell SE, Ringborg U, Wennersten G, Mattson B. Malignant melanoma: Aetiological importance of individual pigmentation and sun exposure. *Br J Dermatol* 1990;**122**:43–51.

30. Elwood M, Gallagher RP. More about: Sunscreen use, wearing clothes and number of nevi in 6–7 year old European children. *J Natl Cancer Inst* 1999;**91**:1164–6.

31. Holman CDJ, Armstrong BK, Heenan PJ. Relationship of cutaneous melanoma to individual sunlight exposure habits. *J Natl Cancer Inst* 1986;**76**:403–14.

32. Holly EA, Kelly JW, Shpall SN, Chiu SH. Number of melanocytic nevi as a major risk factor for malignant melanoma. *J Am Acad Dermatol* 1987;**17**:459–68.

33. Osterlind A, Tucker MA, Stone BJ, Jenson OM. The Danish case-control study of cutaneous maligant melanoma. II. Importance of UV-light exposure *Int J Cancer* 1988;**42**:319–24.

34. Whiteman DC, Valery P, McWhirter W, Green AC. Risk factors for childhood melanoma in Queensland, Australia. *Int J Cancer* 1997;**70**:26–31.

35. Westerdahl J, Olsson H, Masback A, Ingvar C, Jonsson N. Is the use of sunscreens a risk factor for malignant melanoma? *Melanoma Res* 1995;**5**:59–65.

36. Rodenas JM, Delgado-Rodriguez M, Herranz M, Tercedor J, Serrano S. Sun exposure, pigmentary traits, and risk of cutaneous malignant melanoma: A case control study in a Mediterranean population. *Cancer Causes Control* 1996;**7**:275–83.

37. Espinoza-Arranz J, Sanchez-Hernandez JJ, Bravo Fernandez P, Gonzalez-Baron M, Zamora Aunon P. Cutaneous maligant melanoma and sun exposure in Spain. *Melanoma Res* 1999;**9**:199–205.

38. Autier P, Dore JF, Sciffers E *et al.* Melanoma and use of sunscreens: An EORTC case-control study in Germany, Belgium and France. *Int J Cancer* 1995;**61**:749–55.

39. Wolf P, Quehenberger F, Mulleger R, Stranz B, Kerl H. Phenotypic markers, sunlight-related factors and sunscreen use in patients with cutaneous melanoma: An Austrain case-control study. *Melanoma Res* 1998;**8**:370–8.

40. Westerdahl J, Ingvar C, Masback A, Olsson H. Sunscreen use and malignant melanoma. *Int J Cancer* 2000;**87**: 145–50.

41. Elwood M *et al.* More about: Sunscreen use, wearing clothes, and number of nevi in 6–7 year old European children. *J Natl Cancer Inst* 1999;**91**:1164–6.

42. Luther H, Altmeyer P, Garbe C, Ellwanger U, Jahn S, Hoffmann K, Sergerling M. Increase of melanocytic nevus counts in children during 5 years of follow up and analysis of associated factors. *Arch Dermatol* 1996;**132**:1473–8.

43. Pope DJ, Sorahan T, Marsden JR, Ball PM, Grimely RP, Peck LM, Benign pigmented nevi in children. *Arch Dermatol* 1992;**128**:1201–6.

44. Green A, Williams G, Nelae R *et al.* Daily sunscreen application and beta-carotene supplementation in prevention of basal cell and squamous cell carcinomas of the skin: A randomised controlled trial. *Lancet* 1999;**354**:723–9.

45. Green A, Williams G, Neale R, Battistutta D. Beta-carotene and sunscreen use. (Author's reply). *Lancet* 1999;**354**:2163–4.

46. Grodestein F. Speizer FE, and Hunter DJ. A prospective study of incident squamous cell carcinoma of the skin in the nurses' health study. *J Natl Cancer Inst* 1995;**87**:1061–6.

47. Pogoda JM, Preston-Martin S. Solar radiation lip protection and lip cancer risk in Los Angeles Country women. *Cancer Causes Control* 1996;**7**:458–63.

48. Hunter DJ, Colditz GA, Strampfer MJ, Rosner B, Willett WC, Speizer FE. Risk factors for basal-cell carcinoma in a prospective cohort of women. *Ann Epidemiol* 1990;**1**:13–23.

49. Kricker A, Armstrong BK, English DR, Heenana PJ. Does intermittent sun exposure cause basal-cell carcinoma? A case control study in Western Australia. *Int J Cancer* 1995;**60**:489–94.

50. English DR, Armstrong BK, Kricker A, Winter MG, Heenana PJ, Randell PL. Demographic characteristics, pigmentary and cutaneous risk factors for squamous cell carcinoma of the skin: A case control study. *Int J Cancer* 1998;**76**:628–34.

51. Thompson SC, Jolley D, Marks R. Reduction in solar keratoses by regular sunscreen use. *New Engl J Med* 1999;**329**:1147–51.

52. Dobinson S, Borland R, Anderson M. Sponsorship and sun protection practices in lifesavers. *Health Prom Int* 1999;**14**:167–75.

53. Segan CJ, Borland R, Hill DJ. Development and evaluation of a brochure on sun protection and sun exposure for tourists. *Health Educ J* 1999;**58**:177–91.

54. Gooderham MJ, Guenther L. Sun and the skin: Evaluation of a sun awareness program for elementary school students. *J Cutan Med Surg* 1999;**3**:230–5.

55. Hughes BR, Altman DG, Newton JA. Melanoma and skin cancer: Evaluation of a health education programme for secondary schools. *Br J Dermatol* 1993;**128**:412–17.

56. Putman GL, Yanagisako KL. Skin cancer comic book: Evaluation of a public education vehicle. *Cancer Detect Prev* 1982;**5**:349–56.

57. Robinson JK, Rademarker AW. Sun protection by families at the beach. *Arch Pediatr Adolescent Med* 1995;**152**:466–70.

58. Robinson JK, Rademaker AW. Skin cancer risk and sun protection learning by helpers of patients with non-melanoma skin cancer. *Prev Med* 1995;**24**:333–41.

59. Lombard D, Neubauer TE, Canfiled D, Winett RA. Behavioural community intervention to reduce the risk of skin cancer. *J Appl Behav* 1991;**24**:677–86.

60. Memelstein RJ, Riesenberg LA. Changing knowledge and attitudes about skin cancer risk factors in adolescents. *Health Psychol* 1992;**11**:371–6.

61. Buller DB, Callister M, Reichert T. Skin cancer prevention by parents of young children: Health information sources, skin cancer knowledge, and sun protection practices Oncol. *Nurs Forum* 1995;**22**:1559–6.

62. Glanz K, Chang L, Song V, Silverio R, Munecka L. Skin cancer prevention for children, parents, and caregivers: A field test of Hawaii's SunSmart program. *J Am Acad Dermatol* 1998;**384**:13–17.

63. Detweiler JB, Bedell BT, Salovey P, Pronin E, Rothman AJ. Message framing and sunscreen use: Gain-framed messages motivate beachgoers. *Health Psychol* 1999;**18**: 189–96.

64. Weinstock MA, Rossi JS, Redding CA, Maddock JE. Randomised trial of intervention for sun protection among beachgoers. *J Invest Dermatol* 1992;**110**:589.

65. Novick M. To burn or not to burn: Use of computer-enhanced stimuli to encourage application of sunscreens. *Cutis* 1997;**60**:105–8.

66. Dietrich AJ, Olson AL, Sox CH, Stevens M, Tosteson TD, Ahles TA. community based randomised trial encouraging sun protection for children. *Paediatrics* 1998;**102**:E64-E71.

67. Parrot R, Duggan A, Cremo J, Eckles A, Jones K, Steiner C. Commuicating about youth's sun exposure risk to soccer coaches and parents: A pilot study in Georgia. *Health Educ Behav* 1999;**26**:385–95.

68. Girgis A, Sanson-Fisher RW, Tripodi DA, Golding T. Evaluation of interventions to improve solar protection in primary schools. *Health Ed Q* 1993;**20**:275–87.

69. Girgis A, Sanson-Fisher RW, Watson A. A workplace intervention for increasing outdoor workers' use of solar protection. *Am J Public Health* 1994;**84**:77–81.

70. Lawler PE. Be sensible; Steps towards safety in the sun- An information handout. *Oncol Nursing Forum* 1989;**16**:424–7.

71. Reding DJ, Fischer V, Gunderson P, Lapper K. Skin cancer prevention: A peer education model. *Wisconsin Med J* 1995;**94**:77–81.

72. Friedman LC, Webb JA, Bruse S, Weinberg AD, Cooper HP. Skin cancer prevention and early detection intentions and behaviour. *Am J Prev Med* 1995;**11**:59–65.

73. Grant-Peterson J, Dietrich AJ, Sox CH, Winchell CW, Stevens MM. promoting sun protection in elementary schools and child care settings. The Sunsafe project. *School Health* 1999;**69**:100–7.

74. Hill D. White V, Marks R, Borland R. Changes in sun-related attitudes and behaviours, and reduced sunburn prevalence in a population at high risk of melanoma. *Eur J Cancer Prev* 1993;**2**:447–56.

75. Borland R, Hill D, Noy S. Being Sun Smart: Changes in community awareness and reported behaviour following a primary prevention programe for skin cancer control. *Behav Changes* 1990;**7**:126–35.

76. Rivers JK, Gallagher RP. Public education projects in skin cancer: Experience of the Canadian Dermatology Association. *Cancer* 1995;**75**(Suppl.):661–6.

77. Miller RW, Rabkin CS. Merkel cell carcinoma and melanoma: Etiological similarities and differences. *Cancer Epidemiol Biomarkers Prev* 1999;**8**:153–8.

78. Geller AC, Hufford D *et al.* Evalutation of the ultraviolet index: Media reactions and public response. *J Am Acad Dermatol* 1997;**37**:935–41.

79. Robinson JK, Rigel DS, Ammonete RA. Trends in sun exposure knowledge, attitudes and behaviours: 1986–1996. *J Am Acad Dermatol* 1997;**37**:179–86.

24

Cutaneous melanoma

Dafydd Roberts and Thomas Crosby

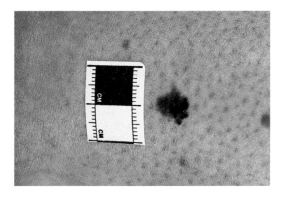

Figure 24.1   Cutaneous melanoma

Localised disease

Dafydd Roberts

Background

Malignant melanomas (MM) of the skin arise from melanocytes within the epidermis. After a variable period of time the tumour becomes invasive and penetrates the underlying dermis and subcutaneous fat. Once this occurs the tumour has potential for distant metastatic spread. MM may also rarely arise from other areas of the body including the meninges, retina, gastrointestinal tract, nasopharyngeal epithelium and vagina.

Incidence

The incidence of cutaneous MM, particularly thin curable lesions, has increased steadily over the past 30 years in all western countries and this

has been accompanied by a similar but less marked increase in mortality.[1] Whilst mortality has continued to rise in most countries, recent reports from Scotland, Canada, Australia and Wales suggest that mortality rates may have levelled off or declined in some groups, notably in women.[2-5] This may be the result of intensive public education campaigns leading to earlier detection of thinner lesions, with a better prognosis . The prevention of MM is an important topic and is dealt alongwith other skin cancers in Chapter 22. Early recognition of MM and surgical excision present the best opportunity for cure.

Prognosis

The prognosis of MM is related to a number of factors including sex, tumour site and ulceration, but the single most important guide to prognosis is the Breslow thickness.[6] This is a measure of the depth of invasion of the tumour from the granular layer of the epidermis. Lesions that are confined to the epidermis have no metastatic potential. Those that are less than 1 mm in depth have a very good prognosis, with 5-year survival rates of approximately 95%. Tumours deeper than 4 mm are associated with survival rates of about 50%. The involvement of regional lymph nodes with metastases at presentation further reduces survival rates to 25–50%.[7]

Diagnosis

The clinical diagnosis of classical MM is straightforward, but early changes may be subtle. Various clinical guides have been developed such as the ABCDE rule (A = asymmetry, B = irregular border, C = irregular colour, D = diameter >5 mm and E = elevation) and the seven-point checklist which may be useful as reminders of the main features of MM on clinical examination and history. The main clinical features are of a pigmented lesion with an irregular edge and irregular pigmentation, over 95% of patients giving a history of change in size, shape or colour, and fewer than 50% describing a change in sensation or bleeding of the lesion.[8,9] Dermatoscopy has gained ground as an aid to diagnosis, but training and experience are required to maximise its usefulness.[10]

Treatment objectives

The main aims of treatment are to detect the lesion as early as possible and to excise it with adequate margins but without mutilating the patient unnecessarily. Outcomes measured usually include both disease-free survival (i.e. until the first appearance of recurrence of the primary lesion or distant metastatic spread) and overall survival.

Searches

Medline was searched for the period 1966 to end of 2001. Citations found in review articles and other main articles found were also scrutinised for additional evidence.

QUESTIONS

What is the place of a diagnostic incisional biopsy?

Occasionally pigmented lesions that are clinically suspicious of being an MM may be considered to be too large or in a difficult anatomical site for complete immediate excision without extensive surgery. There is therefore a dilemma for the clinician as to whether an incisional biopsy of the lesion may be needed to confirm the diagnosis before more extensive surgery. Also, providing the biopsy is taken from a representative area of the melanoma, an incisional biopsy provides an indication of the depth of invasion of the lesion, thereby assisting the planning of the next course of appropriate treatment. There is some concern based on empirical reasoning that taking a biopsy of part of a malignant lesion might release some malignant cells into the bloodstream and local tissues, thereby worsening the eventual prognosis for that person.

Efficacy

There have been no randomised controlled trials (RCTs) of incisional versus excisional surgery. Retrospective studies of large numbers of patients have reported different results. A large study in 1985 of 472 patients with stage I cutaneous MM reported on the survival rate with different modalities of surgery. A total of 119 patients initially underwent an incisional or punch biopsy and 353 patients had their lesions excised. Survival in the two groups did not differ, regardless of the depth of invasion. Of 76 patients who had an incisional biopsy of a lesion <1·7 mm in depth none died. In the intermediate-thickness group (1·7–3·64 mm) there was a 35% mortality rate compared with 18% in the excision group, and in the thick-lesion group (>3·65mm) the mortality rates were 64% and 50% respectively. Cox regression analysis showed that the best predictors for outcome were tumour thickness and anatomical location, but not biopsy type.[11] In a further study of 1086 patients followed up for 5 years, 96 of these underwent an incisional biopsy initially. The mortality was 48·9% in the incisional-biopsy group (mean thickness 3·47 mm) and 39·2% in the wide-excision group (mean thickness 2·77 mm), compared with 33·9% in the narrow-margin group (mean thickness 2·34 mm). After correcting for tumour thickness there was no statistical difference in survival rates or local recurrence between those having an incisional biopsy and those who had their lesions fully excised initially.[12] A more recent and larger case-control study from Scotland of 5727 patients identified 265 patients who had undergone an incisional biopsy. These were matched to 496 controls. The survival analysis of time to recurrence and time to death revealed no differences between the groups.[13]

Drawbacks

Incisional biopsy runs the inherent risk of providing material that is not representative of the whole tumour; therefore errors may occur in assessing the depth of the tumour. One study reported that 38 of the 96 incisional biopsies on patients with cutaneous melanoma (40%) gave insufficient material to provide a full histological assessment of the lesion.[12] On the other hand, excising all pigmented lesions suspected of being a MM, regardless of their site and size, could lead to inappropriate surgery in some cases. One study reported the results of a retrospective series of patients with cutaneous melanoma limited to the head and neck. A total of 159 patients were followed up for a median period of 38 months, of whom 79 patients had their lesions fully excised, 48 had an incisional biopsy, and other procedures such shave excision or cryotherapy were carried out in a further 32. Thirty-one per cent of the patients who underwent an incisional biopsy died and 25% of the other biopsy group died, compared with 9% of those who had their lesions excised initially. As this was a retrospective study, the initial surface area of the lesions was not known. There were no significant differences between the three groups in the depth of invasion of the tumours or the sex of the patients, but a significantly higher proportion of the patients in the incisional biopsy and other-procedure groups had ulcerated tumours compared with the excision group.[14]

Comment

The evidence on incisional biopsy in MM remains controversial but the balance of observational evidence suggests that it is unlikely to influence prognosis adversely. Large studies have shown that, in general, incisional biopsies do not affect prognosis, except for the single study of melanoma of the head and neck, where there was a significant worsening in the survival of patients who underwent an incisional biopsy compared with those who had their lesions excised initially.[14] This study was, however, retrospective and no adjustment was made for ulceration of the tumours, which is known to worsen prognosis. Any future study should be prospective and the design of the study should ensure that study groups are randomised to balance for the various factors that may influence prognosis.

What are the surgical recommendations for excision margins for different Breslow thickness tumours?

The Breslow thickness represents the depth of invasion of cutaneous melanoma and is measured histologically from the granular layer to the deepest melanoma cells. It is the single best indicator of prognosis in primary cutaneous MM.[6] All of the trials so far performed in patients with MM have used the Breslow thickness of the tumour to categorise different patient groups. As a result of these trials, surgical margins of excision of MM have decreased significantly over the past 20 years.

Efficacy

The recommendations for surgical margins are based on three RCTs and have included patients with lesions of Breslow thickness up to 5 mm. The World Health Organization Melanoma Group randomised 612 patients with melanomas less than 2 mm in depth to surgical excision with either 1 cm or 3 cm margins.[15] The mean follow up period was 90 months and there was no difference in overall or disease-free survival between the two groups. A US Intergroup Study randomised 486 patients with intermediate thickness lesions (1–4 mm in depth, to either 2 cm or 4 cm margins.[16] The median follow up period was 6 years. The local recurrence rate was 0·8% for the 2 cm margin group and 1·7% for the 4 cm group. The overall survival rates over 5 years were 79·5% and 83·7%, respectively. The Swedish Melanoma Study Group randomised 769 patients with lesions of 0·8–2 mm in depth to either 2 cm or 5 cm margins, and have recently reported their long-term results with a median follow up period of 11 years.[17] The estimated relative hazard ratios for overall survival and relapse-free survival were 0·96 (95% confidence intervals (CI) 0·75–1·25) and 1·02 (CI 0·8–1·30), respectively. There was no significant difference in local recurrence rates or overall survival between the narrower and wider margins of excision in any of the trials.

A retrospective observational study of 278 patients with thick lesions (median thickness 6 mm) suggested that 2 cm margins were adequate and that wider margins did not improve local recurrence rates, disease-free survival or overall survival rates.[18]

Drawbacks

Excision with narrow surgical margins can often be performed in an out patient setting, whereas larger margins may require skin grafting and in patient treatment. The Word Health Organization Study demonstrated that skin grafting could be reduced by 75% with the 1 cm versus the 3 cm margins.[15] Some concern was expressed in the Intergroup Trial as three patients developed local recurrence as a first sign of relapse, all of whom had undergone a 1 cm excision margin for primary lesions between 1 mm and 2 mm in thickness.[16]

Comment

The evidence that narrow surgical margins are as beneficial as more extensive surgical treatment in terms of local recurrence and survival is reasonably strong. The studies have suggested that lesions <1 mm in depth can be safely treated with surgical margins of 1 cm and lesions equal to or >1 mm in depth can be safely treated with margins of 2 cm. There is also evidence from one observational study that 2 cm margins are also sufficient for thicker tumours.

MM <0·75 mm in depth have not been studied in any controlled trials, nor have lesions >4 mm in depth. Melanoma in situ, where the melanoma cells are confined to the epidermis, appear to have no potential for metastatic spread[19] and the current consensus based on empirical reasoning is that it is safe to excise such lesions with a margin of 5 mm of clinically normal skin to obtain a clear histological margin.[20]

How should patients with lentigo maligna or lentigo maligna melanoma be managed?

Lentigo maligna (LM) is the premalignant phase of lentigo maligna melanoma (LMM), where the malignant melanocytes are entirely confined to the epidermis. These usually occur on sun-exposed sites such as the face and neck. There is usually a prolonged premalignant phase before dermal invasion and the development of LMM. The lesions are difficulty to manage for several reasons. Patients with these lesions tend to be elderly, with other comorbidities that may limit extensive surgery. The lesions themselves may be large and occur close to important anatomical structures and therefore full surgical excision with suitable margins may be difficult or even impossible. In addition, histological changes within the epidermis may occur at some distance from the clinically obvious margins.[21]

Efficacy

LM and LMM will be considered separately.

Lentigo maligna

Surgery: There have been no RCTs of patients in this category. A comparative study of 42 cases of LM showed a recurrence rate of 9% (2/22) following surgical excision, compared with 35% (7/20) with other techniques such as radiotherapy, curettage and cryotherapy surgery, with a mean follow up period of 3·5 years (range 1 month to 11 years).[22] A further retrospective report of 38 cases of LM suggested cure rates of 91% (two recurrences) over a time period of 1–12 years (mean 3 years).[23] Mohs' micrographic surgery has also been evaluated in small numbers of patients, usually with excellent results. Twenty-six patients with LM were treated in one study, with no recurrences after a median follow up of 58 months.[24]

Cryotherapy: There have been no RCTs of cryotherapy for the treatment of LM. One study of 30 patients reported recurrence rates of 6·6% (two patients) in a follow up period of 3 years. Eleven patients who were observed for more than 5 years had no recurrences.[25] A further study of 12 patients showed a recurrence rate of 8·3% over a follow up period of 51 months.[26]

Radiotherapy: There have been no RCTs of radiotherapy for LM. One case series reported two recurrences in 68 patients with a 5-year follow up.[27] A further study showed an 86% cure rate in 36 patients at 5 years.[28]

Other treatments: There have been a few case reports on the use of various lasers in LM but the numbers are too small to be conclusive. A study of 5-fluorouracil cream showed 100% recurrence rate[29] and a similar study on topical retinoic acid showed no benefit.[30] Azelaic acid was reported to give recurrence rate of 22% in 50 patients, all of whom subsequently cleared with retreatment.[31]

Lentigo maligna melanoma

Surgery: Patients with LMM have not been included in any of the large randomised trials on surgical margins. However, it has been shown that the prognosis for patients with invasive LMM is the same as that for any other type of melanoma when matched for thickness.[32] Patients with LMM were included in a case series of Mohs' micrographic surgery, which found a 100% cure rate after 29 months and a 97% cure rate after 58 months.[24]

Radiotherapy: An uncontrolled follow up study of fractionated radiotherapy in both LM and LMM showed that of 64 patients with LM, none showed any signs of recurrence. Among 22 patients with LMM who also had the nodular part of the lesion excised, there were two recurrences. The mean follow up period was 23 months.[33]

Drawbacks

All of the treatment modalities including surgery, cryotherapy, radiotherapy and any other destructive treatment can result in scarring, and no studies have compared the long-term scars with any other methods described. Cryotherapy may lead to inadequate destruction of melanocytes extending down hair follicles and there have been subsequent reports of recurrences, sometimes amelanotic in type, after cryotherapy of these lesions. No reports have compared the short-term discomfort, pain or costs of these treatments.

Comment

In the absence of any controlled trials, it is not surprising that a recent survey of dermatologists has shown a wide variation in treatment modalities in use in the UK. An algorithm was devised on the basis of the current treatments for LM suggesting that surgical resection was the initial treatment of choice if possible, and Mohs' surgery when the margins were unclear. For those lesions that are not amenable to surgical resection, radiotherapy or cryotherapy may be suitable choices. There is an absence of information on the rate of progression of LM, and in the very old and infirm observation only may be considered appropriate.[34] As the prognosis of LMM is the same as any other MM when matched for Breslow thickness, the same surgical margins should be advised whenever possible until better evidence becomes available.

Does elective lymph node dissection improve outcome?

There is some evidence to show that lymph node dissection is beneficial when performed when there is evidence of metastatic spread. However, there is still some controversy about the place of elective lymph node dissection where there are no clinically involved lymph nodes.

Efficacy

Four RCTs have compared elective lymph node dissection with primary excision of the cutaneous lesion only. In all, 1718 people with no clinical evidence of lymph node metastases have been entered into the studies. None of these studies showed an overall survival benefit in patients receiving elective lymph node dissection. However, an unplanned subset analysis found non-significant trends in favour of elective lymph node dissection in those over the age of 60 years with intermediate thickness tumours.[35–38]

Drawbacks

Lymph node dissection is not without risk, lymphoedema being the most frequent complication, occurring in 20% in one study, temporary seroma occurred in 17%, wound infection in 9% and wound necrosis in 3%.[39]

Comments

In view of the lack of any clear benefits for elective lymph node dissection in the RCTs mentioned above, elective lymph node dissection has been largely abandoned in favour of sentinel lymph node biopsy (SLNB), which is considered separately.

What is the role of sentinel lymph node biopsy (SLNB)?

The technique of SLNB involves the identification and biopsy of the first-station lymph node draining an affected area. Its use in MM was pioneered by Morton.[40]

The SLN is found by injecting blue dye and/or radiolabelled colloid into the skin surrounding the primary lesion. The technique enables the identification of patients with micro-metastases affecting the regional lymph nodes and can successfully identify the sentinel node in up to 97% of cases. Patients so identified as having micro-metastases are submitted to a therapeutic lymph node dissection.

The technique is well established and is reproducible.[41] It is now regarded as an excellent indicator of prognosis and has therefore been incorporated into the new American staging system for MM (AJCC staging).[42] Gershenwald demonstrated that of 580 patients who underwent SLNB, 85 patients (15%) were positive and 495 were negative. This study showed that SLN status was the most significant prognostic factor with respect to disease-free and disease-specific survival. Although tumour thickness and ulceration influenced survival in SLN-negative patients, they provided no additional prognostic information in SLN-positive patients.[43] The psychological benefits of accurate staging for a patient have not been studied extensively but one small questionnaire study of 110 patients did show a slight psychological benefit in those who underwent SNLB, regardless of the result of the biopsy.[44]

Efficacy

No RCTs of SLNB accompanied by further treatment such as lymph node dissection or interferon therapy as an intervention (as opposed to SLNB as a pure staging procedure) could be found.

Drawbacks

Patients who do not undergo SLNB are treated by wide excision of the primary cutaneous melanoma. The additional surgery therefore entails some risk because a general anaesthetic is usually necessary and there are also additional costs, although these are difficult to quantify. About 3% of patients developed a seroma, and a further 3% developed a wound infection in one report of SLNB.[45]

Comment

SLNB is generally agreed to be useful as a staging procedure in patients with primary cutaneous melanoma, but no randomised trials have yet shown any therapeutic benefit in patients who have undergone SLNB. A randomised multicentre trial is now comparing survival after wide excision alone versus wide excision plus SLNB in patients with cutaneous melanoma (1 mm in depth or Clark level IV). The trial has been underway for 5 years and 11 000 patients had already been recruited by 1999.[41]

There are additional potential benefits of accurate staging in patients with positive results if adjuvant treatments such as interferon prove to be of value.

Are there any effective adjuvant treatments?

Once patients with MM develop distant metastatic disease the prognosis is poor. There is therefore a need to investigate additional or adjuvant treatments which may be given either after primary tumour resection in those with thicker lesions in patients who appear to have non-metastatic disease or after regional lymph node resection in those with established metastatic disease.

The role of adjuvant treatments, mainly in the form of interferon alfa-2b, is still controversial. Several studies have shown that interferon alfa has a biologically modifying effect on MM but the effect on overall survival has been variable. Side-effects are a major problem with patients receiving high-dose interferon alfa.

Efficacy

Trials have studied the role of interferon alfa in high- and low-dose regimens.

High-dose interferon

An early RCT of high-dose treatment (intravenous interferon alfa-2b 20 MU/day for 1 month, followed by 10 MU three times weekly for 11 months) in 287 people with lesions greater than 4 mm in depth at presentation showed a significant improvement in disease-free and overall survival compared with those treated with surgery alone. The overall survival in the interferon group was 3·1 years, compared with 2·8 years treated with surgery alone.[46] However, in a larger study of 642 patients there was no difference in the overall survival of patients with either high- or low-dose interferon alfa compared with no further therapy.[47] A recent study from the same authors compared high-dose interferon alfa-2b with vaccine treatment (GM2-KLH/QS-21) in patients with resected stage IIB–III melanoma of the skin.[48] A total of 880 patients were randomised equally between the two interferon alfa and vaccine groups. The trial demonstrated a significant treatment benefit for those receiving interferon alfa-2B in both relapse-free survival (hazard ratio 1·47, CI 1·14–1·90, $P = 0.0015$) and overall survival (hazard ratio 1·52, CI 1·07–2·15, $P = 0.009$). There was no control (observation only) arm so a direct comparison with no adjuvant treatment could not be made. However, based on comparisons with the observation arm of previous adjuvant trials, the outcome for patients receiving the vaccine seemed to be no worse than for similar patients receiving observation only. This study therefore seems to have confirmed the relapse-free survival and overall survival benefits of high-dose interferon reported earlier.[46]

Low-dose interferon

To date, two clinical trials have used low-dose subcutaneous interferon (3 MU three times weekly) in patients presenting with lesions greater than 1·5 mm in depth but with negative lymph nodes. In the first trial of 499 patients this regimen was continued for 18 months and compared with surgery alone. There was a significant extension of the relapse-free interval and a trend towards extension of overall survival.[49] The second trial randomised 311 patients to receive treatment for 12 months versus observation only, after surgical removal of the melanoma. At 41 months relapse-free survival was prolonged but overall survival was not.[50]

Drawbacks

Toxicity and withdrawal rates have been high in the high-dose interferon studies. In one study[46] there were two treatment-related deaths. In the latest study[48] 10% of patients discontinued treatment because of adverse advents, but there were no treatment-related deaths. The most frequent side-effects in patients receiving high-dose interferon alfa-2b were fatigue in 20%, granulocytopenia/leucopenia in over 50%, and liver abnormalities and neurological toxicity in about 30%.

In the low-dose interferon trials about 10% of people suffered significant toxicity as well as the milder nausea and flu-like symptoms experienced by most patients on the day of treatment.

Comments

From the information provided by the most recent trial,[48] interferon alfa-2b is the most effective adjuvant treatment now available, with a significantly improved prolongation in relapse-free survival and overall survival

compared with vaccine therapy in patients with resected high-risk melanoma. The rate of severe or very severe side-effects is high. Further studies are now underway combining interferon alfa-2b with other peptide vaccines as well as with polychemotherapy plus interleukin-2. Low-dose interferon alfa-2b may also have a disease-modifying effect, but as yet no benefit on overall survival has been shown.

Treatment with interferon is expensive, and attempts have been made to perform economic analyses of the different regimens used. In an

Key points – localised disease

- The incidence of cutaneous malignant melanoma continues to rise worldwide but there is evidence of a levelling of mortality in some groups as patients are presenting earlier.
- Incisional biopsy of a melanoma does not in general alter the prognosis adversely but may lead to problems in interpreting the histology.
- The main treatment for primary melanoma of the skin is surgical excision.
- There is good evidence from RCTs that the narrower margins used over the past 20 years are safe.
- All the treatments used for LM and LMM have poor evidence to support them and well-organised RCTs are needed in this area. Surgical excision probably represents the best treatment on current evidence.
- Elective lymph node dissection of uninvolved nodes does not improve prognosis in most patient groups.
- SLNB is a useful staging tool but there is no evidence as yet that it improves overall survival.
- Interferons used as adjuvant treatments can benefit some patient groups with MM, but further information is needed to clarify the optimum usage of this treatment.

analysis of the high-dose regimen, the estimated cost per life-year gained was US$13 700 over 35 years and US$32 600 over 10 years; the estimated cost of low-dose treatment per life-year gained was estimated to be US$1700 over a lifetime and US$6600 over 10 years. These costs were thought to be comparable to many other oncological treatments.[51,52]

References for localised disease

1. Armstrong BK, Kicker A. Cutaneous melanoma. *Cancer Surv* 1994;**19–20**:219–40.

2. Mackie RM, Hole D, Hunter JA *et al.* Cutaneous malignant melanoma in Scotland: incidence survival and mortality 1979–1994. *BMJ* 1997;**315**:1117–21.

3. Giles GG, Armstrong BK, Burton RC *et al.* Has mortality from melanoma stopped rising in Australia. Analysis of trends between 1931 and 1994. *BMJ* 1996;**312**:1121–5.

4. National Cancer Institute of Canada. Canadian Cancer Statistics 1997. National Cancer Institute of Canada: Toronto, 1997.

5. Holme SA. Malinovsky K, Roberts DL. Malignant melanoma in South Wales: changing trends in presentation (1986–98). *Clin Exp Dermatol* 2001;**26**:484–9.

6. Breslow A. Thickness, cross sectional areas and depth of invasion in the prognosis of cutaneous melanoma. *Ann Surg* 1970;**172**:902–8.

7. Balch CM, Soong SJ, Shaw HM *et al.* An analysis of prognostic factors in 8500 patients with cutaneous melanoma. In: Balch CM, Houghton Anilton GW, Sober AL Soong S, eds. *Cutaneous Melanoma, 2nd ed.* New York: Ellis Horwood, 1992.

8. Friedmann RJ, Rigel DS, Silverman M, Kopf AW. The continued importance of the early detection of malignant melanoma. *CA Cancer J Clin* 1991;**41**:201–26.

9. Healsmith MF, Bourke JF, Osborne JE, Graham Brown RAC. An evaluation of the revised seven-point checklist for the diagnosis of cutaneous malignant melanoma. *Br J Dermatol* 1994;**130**:48–50.

10. Nachbar F, Stolz W, Merkle T *et al.* The ABCD rule of dermatoscopy. High prospective value in the diagnosis of doubtful melanocytic skin lesions. *J Am Acad Dermatol* 1994;**30**:4:551–9.

11. Lederman JS, Sober AJ. Does biopsy type influence survival in clinical stage I cutaneous melanoma. *J Am Acad Dermatol* 1985;**13**:983–7.

12. Lees VC, Briggs JC. Effect of an initial biopsy on prognosis in stage I invasive cutaneous malignant melanoma; review of 1086 patients. *Br J Surg* 1991;**71**:1108–10.

13. Bong JL, Herd RM, Hunter JAA. Incisional biopsy and melanoma prognosis. *J Am Acad Dermatol* 2002;**46**:690–4.

14. Austin JR, Byers RM, Brown WD, Wolf P. Influence on biopsy on the prognosis of cutaneous melanoma of the head and neck. *Head Neck* 1996;**18**:107–17.

15. Veronesi U, Cascinelli N. Narrow excision (1cm margin); a safe procedure for thin cutaneous melanoma. *Arch Surg* 1991;**126**:438–41.

16. Balch CM, Urist MM, Karakousis CP *et al.* Efficacy of 2 cm surgical margins for intermediate-thickness melanomas (1–4 mm): result of a multi-institutional randomised surgical trial. *Ann Surg* 1993;**218**:262–7.

17. Cohn-Cedermark G, Rutqvist LE, Andersson R *et al.* Long term results of a randomised study by the Swedish Melanoma Study Group on 2 cm versus 5 cm resection margins for patients with cutaneous melanoma with a tumour thickness of 0·8 mm–2·0 mm. *Cancer* 2000;**89**: 1495–1501.

18. Heaton KM, Sussman JJ, Gershanwald JE *et al.* Surgical margins and prognostic factors in patients with thick (> 4mm) primary melanoma. *Ann Surg Oncol* 1998;**5**:322–8.

19. Guerry D IV, Synnestvedt M, Elder DE, Schultz D. Lessons from tumour progression; the invasive radial growth phase of melanoma is common, incapable of metastasis, and indolent. *J Invest Dermatol* 1993;**100**:3428–55.

20. Sober AJ, Tsu-yi Chang, Duvic M *et al.* Guidelines of care for primary cutaneous melanoma. *J Am Acad Dermatol* 2001;**45**:579–86.

21. Mackie RM. Melanocytic naevi and malignant melanoma. In: Champion RH, Burton JL, Burns DA, Breathnach SM, eds. *Textbook of Dermatology, 6th ed.* Oxford: Blackwell Science 1998;**Vol. 2**:1741–50.

22. Pitman GH, Kopf AW, Bart RS *et al.* Treatment of lentigo maligna and lentigo maligna melanoma. *J Dermatol Surg Oncol* 1979;**5**:727–37.

23. Coleman WP III, Davis RS, Reed RJ *et al.* Treatment of lentigo maligna and lentigo maligna melanoma. *J Dermatol Surg Oncol* 1980;**6**:476–9.

24. Cohen LM, McCall MW, Zax RH. Mohs' micrographic surgery for lentigo maligna and lentigo maligna melanoma: a follow up study. *Dermatol Surg* 1998;**24**: 673–7.

25. Kufflik EG, Gage AA. Cryosurgery for lentigo maligna. *J Am Acad Dermatol* 1994;**31**:75–8.

26. Bohler-Sommerregger K, Schuller-Petrovic S, Knobner R et al. Reactive lentiginous hyperpigmentation after cryosurgery for lentigo maligna. *J Am Acad Dermatol* 1992;**27**:523–6.

27. Arma-Szlachcic M, Ott F, Storck H. Zur Strahlentherapie der melanotischen Pracancerosen. *Hautartz* 1970;**21**: 505–8.

28. Tsang RW, Liu F, Wells W, Payne DG. Lentigo maligna of the head and neck; results of treatment by radiotherapy. *Arch Dermatol* 1994;**130**:1008–12.

29. Litwin MS, Kremetz ET, Mansell PW, Reed RJ. Topical treatment of lentigo maligna with 5-fluorouracil. *Cancer* 1995;**3**:721–33.

30. Rivers JK, McCarthy WH. No effect of topical tretinoin in lentigo maligna (letter). *Arch Dermatol* 1991;**127**:129.

31. Nazzoro-Porro M, Passi S, Zina G et al. Ten years' experience of treating lentigo maligna with topical azelaic acid. *Acta Derm Venereol* 1989;**143**(Suppl.):49–57.

32. Cox NH, Aitchison TC, Sirel JM, MacKie RM. Comparison between lentigo maligna melanoma and other histogenic types of malignant melanoma of the head and neck. Scottish Melanoma Group. *Br J Cancer* 1996;**73**:940–4.

33. Schmid-Wendtner MH, Brunner B, Konz B et al. Fractionated radiotherapy of lentigo maligna and lentigo maligna melanoma in 64 patients. *J Am Acad Dermatol* 2000;**43**:477–82.

34. Mahendran R, Newton-Bishop JA. Survey of UK current practice in the treatment of lentigo maligna. *Br J Dermatol* 2001;**144**:71–6.

35. Balch CN, Soong SJ, Bartolucci AA et al. Efficacy of an elective regional lymph node dissection of 1–4 mm thick melanomas for patients 60 years of age and younger. *Ann Surg* 1996;**224**:225–63.

36. Cascinelli N, Moradite A, Santinorrii M et al. Immediate or delayed dissection of regional nodes in patients with melanoma of the trunk: a randomised trial. WHO Melanoma Programme. *Lancet* 1998;**351**:793–6.

37. Sim PH, Taylor WF, Ivins JC et al. A prospective randomised study of the efficacy of routine elective lymphadenectomy in management of malignant melanoma: preliminary results. *Cancer* 1978;**41**:948–56.

38. Veronesi U, Adamus J, Bandiera DC et al. Inefficacy of immediate node dissection in stage I melanoma of the limbs. *N Engl J Med* 1977;**297**:627–30.

39. Baas PC, Schrafferdt KH, Koops H et al. Groin dissection in the treatment of lower extremity melanoma: short term and long term morbidity. *Arch Surg* 1992;**127**:281–6.

40. Morton DL, Wen D-R, Wong JH et al. Technical details of intra-operative lymphatic mapping for early stage melanoma. *Arch Surg* 1992;**127**:392–9.

41. Morton DL, Thompson JF, Essner R et al. Validation of the accuracy of intra-operative lymphatic mapping and sentinel lymphadenectomy for early-stage melanoma. *Ann Surg* 1999;**230**:453–65.

42. Balch CM, Buzard AC, Soong SJ et al. Final version of the American Joint Committee on Cancer staging system for cutaneous melanoma. *J Clin Oncol* 2001;**19**:3635–48.

43. Gershenwald JE, Thompson W, Mansfield PF et al. Multi-institutional melanoma lymphatic mapping experience: the prognostic value of sentinel lymph node status in 612 stage 1 or 11 melanoma patients. *J Clin Oncol* 1999;**17**:976–83.

44. Rayatt SS, Hettiaratchy SP. Having this biopsy gives psychological benefits (letter). *BMJ* 2000;**321**:1285.

45. Jansen L, Nieweg OE, Peterse JL, Hoefnagel CA, Ohnos RA, Kroon BBR. Reliability of sentinel lymph node biopsy for staging melanoma. *Br J Surg* 2000;**87**:484–9.

46. Kirkwood JM, Strawderman MH, Ernstoff MS et al. Interferon alfa-2b adjuvant therapy of high risk resected cutaneous melanoma: The Eastern Co-operative Oncology Group Trial. Est. 1684. *J Clin Oncol* 1996;**14**:7–17.

47. Kirkwood JM, Ibrahim JG, Sondak VK et al. High- and low-dose interferon alfa-2b in high-risk melanoma: first analysis of Intergroup trial 1690/S9111/C9190. *J Clin Oncol* 2000;**18**:2444–58.

48. Kirkwood JM, Ibrahim JG, Sosman JA et al. High-dose interferon alfa 2b significantly prolongs relapse-free and overall survival compared with the GM2-KLH/QS-21 vaccine in patients with resected stage IIb-III melanoma: results of Intergroup trial E1694/S9512/C509801. *J Clin Oncol* 2001;**19**:2370–80.

49. Grob JJ, Dreno B, de la Salmoniere P et al. Randomised trial of interferon alfa -2b as adjuvant therapy in resected primary melanoma thicker than 1·5 mm without clinically

detectable node metastases. French Co-operative Group on Melanoma. *Lancet* 1998;**351**:1905–10.

50. Perhamberger H, Peter Soyer H, Steiner A *et al.* Adjuvant interferon alfa-2b in resected primary stage II cutaneous melanoma. *J Clin Oncol* 1998;**16**:1425–9.

51. Hillner BE, Kirkwood JM, Atkins MB, Johnson ER, Smith TJ. Economic analysis of adjuvant interferon Alfa-2B in high risk melanoma based on projections from Eastern Cooperative Oncology Group 1684. *J Clin Oncol* 1997;**15**:2351–8.

52. Lafuma A, Dreno B, Delauney M *et al.* Economic analysis of adjuvant therapy with interferon alfa-2a in stage II malignant melanoma. *Eur J Oncol* 2001;**37**:369–75.

Metastatic malignant melanoma

Thomas Crosby

Metastatic, or stage IV, MM is a devastating disease. It is defined by dissemination of the cutaneous tumour to other organs or non-regional lymph nodes. The skin, subcutaneous tissues and lymph nodes are the first site of metastatic disease in 59% of patients. When haematogenous spread to liver, bone and brain occurs the natural history is that of one of the most aggressive of all malignant diseases.

For all patients with metastatic disease, the median survival is approximately 7 months; 25% will be alive after 1 year and only 5% of patients will be alive 5 years after diagnosis. Patients with a higher performance status (a numerical measure of physical fitness) and women have a better prognosis ($P = 0.001$ and $P = 0.056$, respectively).[1,2] Survival is also better in patients with a longer duration of remission after primary disease, fewer metastatic sites involved and in those with non-visceral disease (see Table 24.1).

The intention of treatment remains palliative in all but a few patients. A patient who is fit enough to tolerate systemic therapy will often choose active therapy despite the modest responses seen with such treatment. The aim of therapy should clearly be to optimise a patient's quality of survival, and must therefore take into account the morbidity and convenience of therapy.

QUESTIONS

Is there a preferred systemic therapy in metastatic melanoma?

Efficacy

A systematic review found no RCTs testing systemic therapy against best supportive care.[3] It is doubtful that such a trial will ever be done, given that there is great deal of evidence for albeit modest activity in patients with advanced disease.

Dacarbazine (DTIC, di-methyl triazeno imidazole carboxamide) has been the most tested single chemotherapeutic agent. With current anti-emetics, it is well tolerated and is considered by many to be the "gold standard" against which other therapies should be tested.[4–7] When used alone it gives partial response rates of about 20% (>50% regression for at least 4 weeks), complete responses (complete regression of measurable disease for at least 4 weeks) in 5–10% and long-term remissions in fewer than 2% of patients. It is usually given intravenously at 850–1000 mg/m^2 on day 1 every 3 weeks or 200 mg/m^2 on days 1–5 every 4 weeks. It is given with intravenous or oral 5-HT3 antagonist or dexamethasone as anti-emetics.

Temozolamide is a novel oral alkylating agent with a broad spectrum of antitumour activity. It has 100% oral bioavailability and good penetration of the blood–brain barrier and cerebrospinal fluid. Its efficacy is at least equal to that of dacarbazine in metastatic MM, median survival being 7·7 months with temozolamide

Table 24.1 Survival of patients with metastatic malignant melanoma

Prognostic factor	Median survival (months)
Number of metastatic sites	
1	7
2	4
3	2
Site of metastatic disease	
Cutaneous nodes	12·5
Lung	11
Brain, liver, bone	2–6

and 6·4 months with dacarbazine (hazard ratio 1·18, CI 0·92–1·52), and with improvement in some parameters of quality of life.[8] Given its similar mechanism of action to dacarbazine, it is not surprising that response rates are fairly similar but in a disease with such a poor prognosis, ease of administration and quality of life are clearly very important.

Drawbacks

The dose-limiting toxicities with such regimens are bone marrow suppression and nausea/vomiting, requiring hospital admission or threatening life in 20% and 5% of patients, respectively.[9,10]

Does combination chemotherapy help?

Efficacy

Many other drugs such as platinum agents, vinca alkaloids, nitrosoureas, and more recently, taxanes have been tried alone and in various combination regimens. Higher response rates have been claimed for some of these, but it remains unclear whether they offer significant improvement in quantitative or qualitative outcome over single-agent therapy. An example

of the false promise of such combinations was seen when a response rate of 55% was reported for the combination of dacarbazine, cisplatin, carmustine and tamoxifen,[11] which has become known as the Dartmouth regimen. However, a multicentre randomised trial comparing this regimen with single-agent dacarbazine found no survival advantage and only a small, non-significant increase in tumour response in an intention-to-treat analysis (see Table 24.2).[9]

Drawbacks

Bone marrow suppression, nausea/vomiting and fatigue were significantly more common with the combined therapies.[9]

Comment

Combination therapies should not be used routinely outside the context of clinical trials.

Do hormonal therapies help?

Efficacy

Tamoxifen, an oestrogen receptor-blocking agent widely used to treat breast cancer, has also been used, usually together with cytotoxic agents, and may modify the disease response to such drugs. An early study in 117 patients suggested a benefit for the addition of tamoxifen to single-agent dacarbazine (response rates 28% versus 12%, $P = 0·03$, median survival 48 weeks versus 29 weeks, $P = 0·02$).[12] Again, this was not confirmed in a four-arm study in 258 patients with metastatic MM. Response rates were 19% (CI 12–26) for patients receiving tamoxifen and 18% in the non-tamoxifen group (CI 12–25).[13]

Drawbacks

Anti-oestrogens can cause hot flushes, thromboembolic events, pulmonary embolism and endometrial cancer.

Table 24.2 Comparison of single-agent dacarbazine with the Dartmouth regimen of combination chemotherapy

	Dacarbazine	Dartmouth regimen
Response rate (%)	9·9	16·8
Median survival in months (95% CI)	7·7 (5·4–8·7)	6·3 (5·4–8·7)
1-year survival (%)	27	22

Comment

There is no consistent evidence to suggest a benefit for hormonal therapy.

Does immunotherapy help, used either alone or with cytotoxic therapy?

The immune system is important in metastatic MM, as evidenced by lymphoid infiltration into tumour and surrounding tissues, and well-reported spontaneous remissions.[4,5,7,14] This has led to attempts to modulate the immunological environment of tumours, usually by the use of cytokines, particularly interferon alpha[15] and interleukin-2,[16] given directly or by gene therapy. This has improved outcomes in other tumours.[17] Such therapy has single-agent response rates of 15–20% and it has been suggested that such therapy produces a higher rate of durable remissions.[15]

Efficacy

One meta-analysis has compared single-agent dacarbazine and combination chemotherapy with or without immunotherapy in metastatic MM.[18] Twenty RCTs were found, comprising 3273 patients. Although the addition of interferon alpha increased the response rate by 53% over dacarbazine alone, and dacarbazine combination therapy by 33% over single-agent therapy, there was no overall survival advantage for combination treatment.

Drawbacks

Interferons commonly cause malaise, fevers and flu-like symptoms. High-dose interferon alpha caused significant (greater than grade 3) myelosuppression in 24% of people, hepatotoxicity in 15% (including two deaths) and neurotoxicity in 28%.[19] With low-dose interferon, 10% of people suffered significant toxicity.[20]

Comment

Outside clinical trials, it is difficult to justify the additional toxicity with these complex regimens.

Implications for clinical practice

Treatment for malignant MM remains unsatisfactory. Response rates often appear encouraging in single-centre single-arm studies but when the treatments have been tested in larger, multicentre randomised trials, results have to date been very disappointing. Responses are usually partial (10–25% of patients), rarely complete (less than 10%) and are of short duration (median overall survival approximately 6 months).

Outside of clinical trials, standard therapy should remain as single-agent dacarbazine, with temozolamide for selected patients such as those in whom intravenous therapy may particularly interfere with quality of life and possibly those with predominantly cranial metastases.

Key points – metastatic malignant melanoma

- Metastatic malignant melanoma is a devastating disease; only 5% of patients survive for more than 5 years.
- No randomised trials have been performed comparing systemic therapy with no active treatment or placebo.
- Outside of clinical trials, single-agent chemotherapy with dacarbazine should be considered for the majority of these patients.

References for metastatic malignant melanoma

1. Balch CM, Reintgen DS, Kirkwood JM *et al.* Cutaneous melanoma. In: DeVita VT Jr, Hellman S, Rosenberg SA, eds. *Cancer: Principles and Practice of Oncology, 5th ed.* Philadelphia: Lippincot-Raven 1997:1947–94.

2. Unger JM, Flaherty LE, Liu PY *et al.* Gender and other survival predictors in patients with metastatic melanoma on Southwest Oncology Group Trials. *Cancer* 2001;**91**: 1148–55.

3. Crosby T, Fish R, Coles B, Mason MD. Systemic treatments for metastatic cutaneous melanoma. In: Cochrane Collaboration. *Cochrane Library.* Issue 2. Oxford: Update Software, 2002.

4. Balch CM, Houghton AN, Peters LJ. Cutaneous melanoma. In: Devita VT Jr, Hellman S, Rosenberg SA, eds. *Cancer: Principles and Practice of Oncology, 4th ed.* Philadelphia: JB Lippincott 1993:1612–61.

5. Cascinelli N, Clemente C, Belli F. Cutaneous melanoma. In: Peckham M, Pinedo HM, Veronesi U, eds. *Oxford Textbook of Oncology.* Oxford: Oxford University Press, 1995:902–28.

6. Pritchard KI, Quirt IC, Cowman DH *et al.* DTIC therapy in metastatic malignant melanoma: A simplified dose schedule. *Cancer Treat Rep* 1980;**64**:1123–6.

7. Taylor A, Gore M. Malignant melanoma. In: Price P, Sikora K, eds. *Treatment of Cancer, 3rd ed.* London: Chapman and Hall Medical, 1995;**37**:763–7.

8. Middleton MR, Grob JJ, Aaronson N *et al.* Randomised phase III study of temozolamide versus dacarbazine in the treatment of patients with advanced metastatic malignant melanoma. *J Clin Oncol* 2000;**18**:158–66.

9. Chapman PB, Einhorn LH, Meyers ML *et al.* Phase III multicenter randomised trial of the Dartmouth regimen versus dacarbazine in patients with metastatic melanoma. *J Clin Oncol* 1999;**17**:2745–51.

10. Falkson CI, Falkson G, Falkson HC. Improved results with the addition of interferon alfa-2b to dacarbazine in the treatment of patients with metastatic malignant melanoma. *J Clin Oncol* 1991;**9**:1403–8.

11. Del prete SA, Maurer LF, O'Donnell J *et al.* Combination chemotherapy with cisplatin, carmustine, dacarbazine, and tamoxifen in metastatic melanoma. *Cancer Treat Rep* 1984;**68**:1403–5.

12. Cocconi G, Bella M, Calabresi F *et al.* Treatment of metastatic malignant melanoma with dacarbazine plus tamoxifen. *N Engl Med J* 1992;**327**:516–23.

13. Falkson CI, Ibrahim J, Kirkwood JM, Coates AS, Atkins MB, Blum RH. Phase III trial of dacarbazine versus dacarbazine with interferon-alpha2b versus dacarbazine with tamoxifen versus dacarbazine with interferon-alpha 2b and tamoxifen in patients with metastatic malignant melanoma: An Eastern Cooperative Oncology Group Study. *J Clin Oncol* 1998;**16**:1743–51.

14. Rosenberg SA, Yang JC, Topalian SL *et al.* Treatment of 283 consecutive patients with metastatic melanoma or renal cell cancer using high-dose bolus interleukin-2. *JAMA* 1994;**271**:907–13.

15. Legha SS. The role of interferon alfa in the treatment of metastatic melanoma. *Semin Oncol* 1997;**24**:S24–31.

16. Legha SS, Gianin MA, Plager C *et al.* Evaluation of interleukin-2 administered by continuous infusion in patients with metastatic melnoma. *Cancer* 1996; **77**:89–96.

17. Atzpodien J, Kirchner H, Franzke A *et al.* Results of a randomised clinical trial comparing SC interleukin-2, SC alpha-2a-interferon, and IV bolus 5-fluorouracil against oral tamoxifen in progressive metastatic renal cell carcinoma patients. *Proc Am Assoc Clin Oncol* 1997;**16**:326.

18. Huncharek M, Caubet JF, McGarry R. Single agent DTIC versus combination chemotherapy with or without imunotherapy in metastatic melanoma: a meta-analysis of 3273 patients from 20 randomised trials. *Melanoma Res* 2001;**11**:75–81.

19. Kirkwood JM, Strawderman MH, Erstoff MS *et al.* Interferon alfa-2b adjuvant therapy of high-risk resected cutaneous melanoma: The Eastern Cooperative Oncology Group trial EST 1684. *J Clin Oncol* 1996;**14**:7–17.

20. Kleeberg UR, Brocker EB, Lejeune F. Adjuvant trial in melanoma patients comparing rIFN-alfa to rIFN-gamma to Iscador to a control group after curative resection high risk primary or regional lymph node metastasis (EORTC 18871). *Eur J Cancer* 1999;**35**(Suppl. 4):S82.

25
Squamous cell carcinoma

Nanette J Liégeois and Suzanne Olbricht

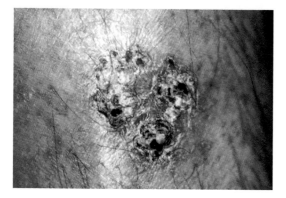

Figure 25.1   Squamous cell carcinoma arising on the leg of a 72-year-old man. With kind permission of Dr Suzanne Olbricht, Burlington

Background
Definition

Squamous cell carcinoma (SCC) is a form of skin cancer that originates from epithelial keratinocytes.[1] It is thought to arise as a focal intra-epidermal proliferation from precancerous lesions, including actinic keratoses, SCC *in situ*, Bowen's disease, bowenoid papulosis, erythroplasia of Queyrat and arsenical keratoses.[2] Without treatment, SCC may continue to grow, invade the dermis or subcutaneous tissues or metastasise.[3] This chapter focuses on interventions for localised, non-metastatic invasive SCC. The prevention of SCC is dealt with in Chapter 22.

Epidemiology

Since the 1960s, the overall incidence of SCC has been increasing annually.[4,5] In 1997, the Rochester Epidemiology Project in the US estimated the overall incidence of invasive SCC to be 106 per 100 000 people.[5] However, several population-based studies have shown that the risk of SCC appears to correlate with geographic latitude. The reported incidence of SCC is higher in tropical regions than in temperate climates, with an annual incidence approaching 1:100 in Australia.[6–9] Regional differences related to latitude have also been noted in the US.[4,10–13]

Sunlight exposure is an established independent risk factor for the development of SCC. SCC arises more commonly in the sun-exposed areas, including the head, neck and arms, but also occurs on the buttocks, genitals and perineum.[14] Other risk factors for SCC include older age, male sex, Celtic ancestry, increased sensitivity to sun exposure, increased number of precancerous lesions and immunosuppression.[4,15,16] Exposure to oral psoralens, arsenic, cigarette smoking, coal-tar products, UVA photochemotherapy and human papilloma virus have been associated with SCC. Genetic disorders that predispose to SCC include epidermodysplasia verruciformis, albinism and xeroderma pigmentosum.

Stasis ulcers, osteomyelitic sinuses, scarring processes such as lupus vulgaris, and vitiligo have been reported to increase the risk of SCC, but it is unclear how far the morphology of the underlying process delays the diagnosis.[15,16]

Pathogenesis

Several studies have shown that sun exposure, photo irradiation and ionising irradiation play a major role in the pathogenesis of SCC. DNA damage is a fundamental process that occurs in the development of cancer. Both UV light and ionising radiation are potent mutagens. Specifically, UVB light has been shown to produce pyrimidine dimers in DNA; these result in DNA point mutations during keratinocyte replication, which lead to abnormal cell function and replication.

In addition to direct DNA damage, genes involved in DNA repair have been implicated in the pathogenesis of SCC. The *p53* gene is mutated in most SCC cases, disabling normal p53 function, which is thought to be critical in suppressing the development of SCC by repairing of UV-damaged DNA.[17–20] Keratinocytes with *p53* mutations cannot repair the mutations induced by irradiation and subsequently proliferate to develop cancer.[17] Furthermore, mice with *p53* mutations develop skin tumours more readily. Mutations in *p53* can either be acquired (through multiple pathways including human papillomavirus, UV light, carcinogens) or inherited. People with xeroderma pigmentosum have a defective p53 pathway and develop numerous skin cancers; they cannot repair mutations induced by irradiation.[21]

Immunological status has also been implicated in the development of SCC. The rate of SCC in transplant recipients is high, particularly in those with a kidney or heart transplant.[22–25] How immunosuppression increases the risk is not known, but decreasing the immunosuppressive therapy helps to reduce the number of SCCs. Further studies are needed to determine how altered immune responses influence the development of SCC.

Prognosis
The prognosis of local recurrence, metastases and survival in SCC depends on the location of

disease and modality of treatment. The term "recurrence rate" at a post-treatment time point is preferable to "cure". The latter term wrongly suggests that no further recurrences occur after that point whereas in fact recurrence rate increases as the length of follow up increases. The overall local recurrence rate after excision of an SCC involving the sun-exposed areas is 8%, while the recurrence rates on the ear and lip are 19% and 11%, respectively.[26] The metastatic rate for primary SCC of the sun-exposed areas is 5%, while the rates for SCC on the external ear, lip and non-sun-exposed areas are 9%, 14% and 38%, respectively.[27] The 5-year overall survival rate associated with metastatic SCC of the skin has been estimated at 34%.[27]

Clinical factors that have been associated with an increased risk of local recurrence or metastases include treatment modality, size greater than 2 cm, depth greater than 4 mm, poor histological differentiation, location on the ear or non-sun-exposed areas, perineural involvement, location within scars or chronic inflammation, previously failed treatment and immunosuppression.[27]

Diagnostic tests
The diagnosis of SCC relies on the histopathological finding of atypical hyperproliferative keratinocytes compared with adjacent normal epidermis. Common findings include cytological and architectural disorganisation, decreased differentiation and atypical mitoses. SCC *in situ* is diagnosed when atypia is identified only in the epidermal compartment. Invasive SCC is distinguished from SCC *in situ* by the invasion of the dermis by epithelioid cells. SCC may also be classified according to the degree of differentiation, a clinically important specification since less differentiated tumours are associated with poor prognosis.

Aims of treatment and relevant outcomes

Treatment aims to remove or destroy the tumour completely and to minimise cosmetic and functional impairment. Success should therefore be measured by rates of recurrence or metastasis at fixed time points or survival analyses that document time to first recurrences in groups of patients. The morbidity of the procedure, as measured by short- and longer-term pain, infection, scarring, skin function and overall cosmesis should all be considered when choosing the appropriate treatment modality.[28,29] In addition, the cost and tolerance to the specific treatment modalities should be considered.

Methods of search

The following databases were searched:

- Medline 1966–2002
- Embase 1980–2002
- the Cochrane Skin Group Trials Register
- the Cochrane Database of Systematic Reviews and the Cochrane Central Register of Controlled Trials.

Search items included: SCC, squamous cell carcinoma, squamous cell cancer, skin neoplasms, xeroderma pigmentosum, non-melanoma skin cancers, non-melanoma skin cancer, transplant skin cancers.

QUESTIONS

The following questions relate to the treatment of an uncomplicated SCC on the leg of a 72-year-old man, as shown in Figure 25.1.

What are the effective therapeutic interventions for localised invasive SCC of the skin? How do the effective therapeutic interventions for SCC compare with each other? How do the cosmetic outcomes for these interventions compare?

Excision

Surgical excision remains the primary treatment for invasive SCC. Surgical excision of SCC is performed in the outpatient setting under local anaesthesia. Standard excision techniques involve the visual estimation of the tumour border and marking a predetermined margin. A steel blade is used to excise the tumour and closure is performed using complex layered, flap or graft technique. The histology of the tumour is examined in formalin-fixed sections.

Effectiveness

No large randomised controlled trial (RCT) has compared the effectiveness of surgical excision with any other treatment modality . No RCT has compared predetermined margin widths for the surgical removal of SCC.

Several case series demonstrate an excellent clearance of SCC lesions with surgical excision. Freeman et al.[30] reported 91 surgically excised SCC, with a follow up ranging from 1 to 5 years. Metastases developed in three of the 91 patients. The authors did not note the size or location of the tumours. For SCC less than 2 cm in diameter, surgical excision resulted in a 5-year cure rate of 96% (22 of 23 patients). For lesions greater than 2 cm, 83% (10 of 12) of patients were free of disease 5 years later.

While many authors report high cure rates for excision, with variable follow up, the recommendations for the width of the excision margin has ranged from 4 mm to 1 cm. In one prospective study, 141 SCC lesions were excised with incremental 1 mm margins and subclinical extension of tumours was examined using frozen tissue sectioning via Mohs' micrographic surgery (MMS).[31] With 4 mm surgical margins tumours less than 2 cm had a greater than 95% clearance, while tumours greater than 2 cm required at least 6 mm excision margins to achieve a greater than 95% clearance.

Drawbacks

Large tumours, or tumours in cosmetically complex areas such as near the eyelids or ears, often require an involved flap or graft technique for repair. The subsequent scar from surgical excision usually results in a hypopigmented line, and hypertrophic and keloidal changes may occur. SCC excision also requires removal of underlying fat as well as the tumour, which may disrupt normal vasculature, lymphatics or innervation. Since the surgical site is closed at the time of surgery and histology is performed on fixed tissues, the discovery of residual tumour may necessitate further surgical interventions.

Comment

Surgical excision remains the main definitive treatment option for SCC less than 2 cm in diameter. Caution is necessary when using this technique for larger SCC or lesions in cosmetically complex areas.

Mohs' micrographic surgery

MMS is a form of surgery that is performed in stages over several hours. The surgeon functions as a pathologist and extirpates the tumour and immediately evaluates the extirpated tissue, which is processed under frozen section. Before closure, the positive margins are removed in subsequent stages and final closure is performed once the tumour is declared fully removed by the attendant histopathologist. MMS is thought to be a highly curative procedure for non-melanoma skin cancers since immediate histopathological evaluation permits further tumour extirpation in successive stages. Although more tumour is removed from the positive margins in these stages, the remaining tissue is spared since only the tumour is removed, limiting potential damage to adjacent tissues.

Effectiveness

Although MMS is frequently used in the treatment of SCC, there are no RCTs comparing MMS with other treatments.

Mohs reported a 5-year cure rate of 95% for primary SCC.[32] In a case-series analysis, Rowe et al. found that MMS resulted in a lower rate of local recurrence compared with other treatment modalities.[27] Holmkvist and Roenigk report a cure rate for primary SCC of the lip of 92% after MMS for 50 patients in an 2·5 year average follow up.[33] Lawrence and Cottel reported only three local recurrences of SCC in 44 patients with perineural invasion treated by MMS in a 1-year follow up, and further noted that predicted survival was higher than previously published survival rates for surgical excision.[34–36]

Drawbacks

MMS is expensive and is not accessible to all patients. Full extirpation of the tumour may require multiple stages over a period of many hours. Patients who cannot lie down because of a comorbid condition may not tolerate the potentially lengthy procedure. In addition, the processing of the frozen sections is labour intensive and costs much more than conventional histology

Comments

MMS appears to have higher cure rates than other treatment modalities. Because it utilises sequential extirpation of tissue, it is more sparing of adjacent tissue. This provides a cosmetic advantage for tumours located in functionally critical areas. The procedure is performed in an outpatient setting and most patients tolerate it.[29] The technique avoids the delay associated with formalin-processed tissues and the need for multiple surgical procedures. For low-risk small-diameter SCC (minimally invasive or in a low-risk site), other treatment modalities should be considered as there is probably little to be gained in efficacy and much to lost in terms of cost and time.

Electrodesiccation and curettage

Electrodesiccation and curettage (ED&C) is frequently used in the treatment of SCC, particularly for *in situ* or minimally invasive lesions on the trunk or limbs. The tumour is prepared for ED&C and margins are marked. Taking advantage of the finding that skin tumours are usually more friable than the surrounding normal tissue, the sharp tip of a curette is used to debulk the tumour. Electric current through a fine-tipped needle is used to desiccate the base and destroy any residual tumour. This sequence is repeated several times and the eschar that remains is left to heal by secondary intention.

Effectiveness

ED&C is frequently used for SCC, but no RCTs have compared ED&C with other treatments. Several case series have examined the cure rate of ED&C for SCC lesions. Freeman et al.[30] treated 407 SCC lesions by ED&C over a 20-year period with follow up ranging from 1 to over 5 years. In patients with a greater than 5-year follow up, they found that ED&C cured 96% (46/48) of SCC less than 2 cm in diameter and 100% (9/9) of SCC greater than 2 cm in diameter. Of the 407 treated SCC lesions, 355 were less than 2 cm, suggesting choice of this technique for smaller SCC. Knox et al.[37] noted that only four SCC lesions recurred in 315 tumours treated with a follow up of 4 months to 2 years. SCC lesions in this study were all less than 2 cm and without significant invasion. Honeycutt and Jansen[38] treated 281 invasive SCC lesions by ED&C and reported three recurrences in a follow-up of up to 4 years. Of the patients who developed recurrences, two had had tumours greater than 2 cm.[38] Whelan and Deckers[39] treated 26 SCC lesions and reported a 100% cure rate in a 2–9 year follow up.

Drawbacks

The high cure rates obtained with ED&C in published case series probably reflect a selection bias for smaller and less invasive lesions. Cosmetically, the scar from ED&C is usually a hypopigmented sclerotic circle, as compared with a thin line from excision. Although the circular scar often contracts, hypertrophic changes can also occur that may make it difficult to recognise recurrent SCC. For SCC lesions on the face, particularly adjacent to critical tissues, contraction of resultant scars may distort or destroy the normal or functional anatomy. In addition, a surgeon performing ED&C at sites adjacent to vital or anatomically complex structures (such as the nose or eye) might limit the margins of destruction or be less aggressive in order to preserve native tissue; this is likely to diminish the effectiveness of this technique. Whelan and Deckers[39] found that the majority (65%) of lesions took 4 weeks to heal after ED&C, while in a separate study they found that the average time for healing was 5.1 weeks.[40] Prolonged healing compared with surgical excision should be considered, particularly for lesions on the legs. Daily wound care is an essential part of ED&C, and diligence is required to prevent infection.

Comment

ED&C appears to be effective for minimally invasive SCC lesions less than 2 cm in diameter. One clear advantage of ED&C over other modalities is that it is rapidly and easily performed by the experienced surgical clinician. Although the healing time may be increased, ED&C is an affordable, effective and rapid treatment option for SCC and should be considered for small or less invasive tumours. Adequate follow up is essential to recognise the rare recurrences.

Cryotherapy

Cryotherapy has been used for decades and is highly effective for treating small or minimally invasive SCC. The standard treatment protocol for cryotherapy consists of two cycles of freezing with liquid nitrogen lasting 1·5 minutes per cycle. The technique takes longer than ED&C but less time than surgical excision.

Effectiveness

No RCTs have compared the effectiveness of cryotherapy with other treatments. Several case series have examined the cure rate of cryosurgery in SCC. Over an 18-year period, Zacarian[41] treated 4228 skin cancers with cryotherapy, which included 203 SCC lesions. He noted a 97% cure rate in a follow up ranging from less than 3 months to over 10 years. Most recurrences (87%) occurred in the first 3 years. Zacarian further noted a healing time that ranged from 4 to 10 weeks. Kuflik[42] found a 96% 5-year cure rate for 52 SCC lesions. Holt[10] reported 34 SCC lesions treated with cryotherapy and a 97% cure after follow up ranging from 6 months to 5·5 years.

Drawbacks

Cryotherapy is usually initially complicated by oedema, followed by blister formation. After rupture, the resultant crust takes 4–10 weeks to heal.[41] Hypopigmentation is universal, with occasional hypertrophic scarring.[41] Atrophic scars can be seen on the face, and neuropathy has been reported.[41] Since cryotherapy rarely destroys deep tissues, significant invasion should be considered a relative contraindication.[41]

Patients with abnormal cold tolerance, cryoglobulinaemia, autoimmune deficiency or platelet deficiency should not be treated with cryotherapy.[41]

Comment

Cryotherapy is effective for treating minimally invasive SCC on the trunk or limbs. Caution is needed when treating SCC on the face, particularly near vital structures.

Key points

- Risk factors for recurrence of cutaneous SCC are treatment modality, size greater than 2 cm, depth greater than 4 mm, poor histological differentiation, location on the ear or mucosal areas, perineural involvement, location within scars or chronic inflammation, previously failed treatment and immunosuppression.
- The evidence base for treatment of cutaneous SCC is poor.
- None of the commonly used procedures has been tested in rigorous RCTs.
- Case series which have followed up patients with SCC treated by surgical excision, MMS, ED&C and cryotherapy all suggest 3–5-year cure rates of over 90%.
- Comparison of the cure rates between the existing main treatments is almost impossible as choice of treatment is probably based on likelihood of success (for example, only people with small uncomplicated SCCs are treated by non-surgical techniques).
- Based on the available case series, there is no evidence to suggest that any of the commonly used treatments for SCC are ineffective.
- Small (less than 2 cm tumours) at non-critical sites can probably be treated equally well by surgical excision with a 4 mm margin, ED&C or cryotherapy.
- Larger tumours, especially at sites where tissue sparing becomes vital, are probably best treated by MMS.
- RCTs are needed to inform clinicians about the relative merits of the various treatments currently used for people with SCC.
- Such trials will need to be large to exclude small but important differences, and they will need to accurately describe the sorts of people entered in terms of risk factors for recurrences. Follow up in such studies needs to be 5 years or longer.

Other treatment options

Many other treatment modalities such as radiotherapy, photodynamic therapy, oral retinoids and topical imiquimod have been or are being tried for SCC. These will be dealt with in the next edition of this book.

Clinical implications

In relation to the clinical scenario of an uncomplicated small SCC in an immunocompetent man, there is little in the evidence base to suggest that any one of the modalities above is "better" than the others. Choice of treatment will largely depend on the operator's preference, convenience to the patient, and cost. Surgical excision has the advantage of offering clear visualisation of the tumour margins whereas ED&C and cryotherapy might be more convenient.

References

1. Kirkham N. Tumors and cysts of the epidermis. In: Elder D, Eleritas R, Jaworsky C, Johnson B Jr, eds. *Lever's Histopathology of the Skin*. Philadelphia, Lippincott-Raven, 1997:685–746.

2. Lohmann CM, Solomon AR. Clinicopathologic variants of cutaneous squamous cell carcinoma. *Adv Anat Pathol* 2001;**8**:27–36.

3. Barksdale SK, O'Connor N, Barnhill R. Prognostic factors for cutaneous squamous cell and basal cell carcinoma. Determinants of risk of recurrence, metastasis, and development of subsequent skin cancers. *Surg Oncol Clin North Am* 1997;**6**:625–38.

4. Preston DS, Stern RS. Nonmelanoma cancers of the skin. *N Engl J Med* 1992;**327**:1649–62.

5. Gray DT, Suman VJ, Siu WPD *et al*. Trends in the population-based incidence of squamous cell carcinoma of the skin first diagnosed between 1984 and 1992. *Arch Dermatol* 1997;**133**:735–40.

6. Stenbeck KD, Balanda KP, Williams MJ *et al*. Patterns of treated non-melanoma skin cancer in Queensland – the region with the highest incidence rates in the world. *Med J Aust* 1990;**153**:511–15.

7. Magnus K. The Nordic profile of skin cancer incidence. A comparative epidemiological study of the three main types of skin cancer. *Int J Cancer* 1991;**47**:12–19.

8. Marks R, Staples M, Giles GG. The incidence of non-melanocytic skin cancers in an Australian population: results of a five-year prospective study. *Med J Aust* 1989;**150**:475–8.

9. Giles GG, Marks P, Foley P. Incidence of non-melanocytic skin cancer treated in Australia. *BMJ* (Clin Res Ed) 1988;**296**:13–17.

10. Holt PJ. Cryotherapy for skin cancer: results over a 5-year period using liquid nitrogen spray cryosurgery. *Br J Dermatol* 1988;**119**:231–40.

11. Scotto J, Kopf AW, Urbach F. Non-melanoma skin cancer among Caucasians in four areas of the United States. *Cancer* 1974;**34**:1333–8.

12. Schreiber MM, Shapiro SI, Berry CZ, Dahlen RF, Friedman RP. The incidence of skin cancer in southern Arizona (Tucson). *Arch Dermatol* 1971;**104**:124–7.

13. Serrano H, Scotto J, Shornick G, Fears TR, Greenberg ER. Incidence of nonmelanoma skin cancer in New Hampshire and Vermont. *J Am Acad Dermatol* 1991;**24**:574–9.

14. Dinehart SM, Pollack SV. Metastases from squamous cell carcinoma of the skin and lip. An analysis of twenty-seven cases. *J Am Acad Dermatol* 1989;**21**:241–8.

15. Johnson TM, Rowe DE, Nelson BR, Swanson NA. Squamous cell carcinoma of the skin (excluding lip and oral mucosa). *J Am Acad Dermatol* 1992;**26**:467–84.

16. Kwa RE, Campana K, Moy RL. Biology of cutaneous squamous cell carcinoma. *J Am Acad Dermatol* 1992;**26**:1–26.

17. Ziegler A, Jonason AS, Leffell DJ *et al*. Sunburn and p53 in the onset of skin cancer. *Nature* 1994;**372**:773–6.

18. Taguchi M, Watarabe S, Yashimak, Murakami Y, Sekiya T, Ikeda S. Aberrations of the tumor suppressor p53 gene and p53 protein in solar keratosis in human skin. *J Invest Dermatol* 1994;**103**:500–3.

19. Campbell C, Quinn AG, Ro YS, Angus B, Rees JL. p53 mutations are common and early events that precede tumor invasion in squamous cell neoplasia of the skin. *J Invest Dermatol* 1993;**100**:746–8.

20. Brash DE, Rudolf JA, Simon JA. A role for sunlight in skin cancer: UV-induced p53 mutations in squamous cell carcinoma. *Proc Natl Acad Sci USA* 1991;**88**: 10124–8.

21. Robbins JH. Xeroderma pigmentosum. Defective DNA repair causes skin cancer and neurodegeneration. *JAMA* 1988;**260**:384–8.

22. Hartevelt MM, Bavinck JN, Kootte AM, Vermeer BJ, Vandenbrouke JP. Incidence of skin cancer after renal transplantation in The Netherlands. *Transplantation* 1990;**49**:506–9.

23. Liddington, M, Richardson AJ, Higgins RM *et al.* Skin cancer in renal transplant recipients. *Br J Surg* 1989;**76**:1002–5.

24. Boyle J, Mackie RM, Briggs JD, Junior BS, Aitchison TC. Cancer, warts, and sunshine in renal transplant patients. A case-control study. *Lancet* 1984;(**1**)**8379**:702–5.

25. Dinehart SM, Chu DZ, Mahers AW, Pollack SV. Immunosuppression in patients with metastatic squamous cell carcinoma from the skin. *J Dermatol Surg Oncol* 1990;**16**:271–4.

26. Rowe DE, Carroll RJ, Day CL Jr, Long-term recurrence rates in previously untreated (primary) basal cell carcinoma: implications for patient follow-up. *J Dermatol Surg Oncol* 1989;**15**:315–28.

27. Rowe DE, Carroll RJ, Day CL Jr, Prognostic factors for local recurrence, metastasis, and survival rates in squamous cell carcinoma of the skin, ear, and lip. Implications for treatment modality selection. *J Am Acad Dermatol* 1992;**26**:976–90.

28. Motley R, Kersey P, Lawrence C. Multiprofessional guidelines for the management of the patient with primary cutaneous squamous cell carcinoma. *Br J Dermatol* 2002;**146**:18–25.

29. Drake LA, Dinehart SM, Goltz RW *et al.* Guidelines of care for Mohs micrographic surgery. *J Am Acad Dermatol* 1995;**33**:271–8.

30. Freeman RG, Knox JM, Heaton CL. The treatment of skin cancer: A statistical study of 1341 skin tumors comparing results obtained with irradiation, surgery, and curettage followed by electrodessication. *Cancer* 1964;**17**:535–8.

31. Brodland DG, Zitelli JA. Surgical margins for excision of primary cutaneous squamous cell carcinoma. *J Am Acad Dermatol* 1992;**27**:241–8.

32. Mohs FE. *Chemosurgery: Microscopically controlled surgery for skin cancer.* Springfield: Thomas CC, 1978.

33. Holmkvist KA, Roenigk RK. Squamous cell carcinoma of the lip treated with Mohs micrographic surgery: outcome at 5 years. *J Am Acad Dermatol* 1998;**38**:960–6.

34. Lawrence N, Cottel WI. Squamous cell carcinoma of skin with perineural invasion. *J Am Acad Dermatol* 1994;**31**:30–3.

35. Goepfert H, Dichtel WJ, Medina JE, Lindberg RD, Lura MD. Perineural invasion in squamous cell skin carcinoma of the head and neck. *Am J Surg* 1984;**148**:542–7.

36. Ballantyne AJ, McCarten AB, Ibanez ML. The extension of cancer of the head and neck through peripheral nerves. *Am J Surg* 1963;**106**:651–67.

37. Knox JM, Lyles TW, Shapiro EM, Martin RD. Curettage and electrodessication in the treatment of skin cancer. *Arch Dermatol* 1960;**82**:197–204.

38. Honeycutt WM, Jansen GT. Treatment of squamous cell carcinoma of the skin. *Arch Dermatol* 1973;**108**:670–2.

39. Whelan CS, Deckers PJ. Electrocoagulation for skin cancer: an old oncologic tool revisited. *Cancer* 1981;**47**:2280–7.

40. Whelan CS, Deckers PJ. Electrocoagulation and curettage for carcinoma involving the skin of the face, nose, eyelids, and ears. *Cancer* 1973;**31**:159–64.

41. Zacarian SA. Cryosurgery of cutaneous carcinomas. An 18-year study of 3,022 patients with 4,228 carcinomas. *J Am Acad Dermatol* 1983;**9**:947–56.

42. Kuflik EG, Gage AA. The five-year cure rate achieved by cryosurgery for skin cancer. *J Am Acad Dermatol* 1991;**24**:1002–4.

26
Basal cell carcinoma
Fiona Bath and William Perkins

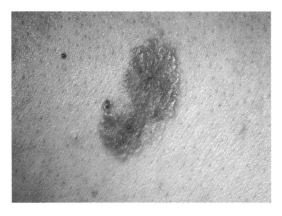

Figure 26.1 Superficial basal cell carcinoma (BCC)

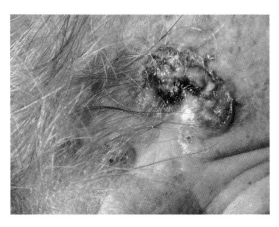

Figure 26.3 A morphoeic BCC

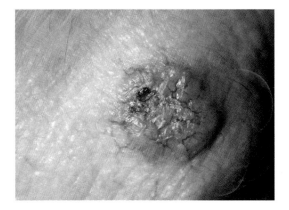

Figure 26.2 A nodular BCC

Background
Definition

Basal cell carcinoma (BCC) is defined as a slow-growing, locally invasive malignant epidermal skin tumour, which mainly affects Caucasians.[1]

Incidence/prevalence

BCC (or rodent ulcer) is the most common malignant cutaneous neoplasm found in humans.[1–3] For example, over 30 000 new cases are reported each year in the UK. This is likely to be an underestimate because of inconsistencies in registration of BCCs at regional cancer registries.[4] Many registries only register a person's first skin cancer, thus further underestimating the real burden of the problem.

The tumour may occur at any age but the incidence of BCC increases markedly after the age of 40 years. The incidence of BCC appears to be increasing in younger people, probably as a result of increased sun exposure.[5] The incidence rate (standardised using the European standard population) for new BCCs in the Trent Cancer Registry (UK) increased from 36·8 in 1985 to 71·3 for men, and from 25·6 to 52·0 in women (Trent Cancer Registry, written communication, September 2001). A total of 3826 new BCCs were registered in Trent in 2000 (80% of all non-melanoma skin cancers). A sustained rise in the incidence of BCC has been documented using a validated register in South Wales, UK.[6] Reliable national figures for BCC incidence are impossible to obtain because some cancer registries in the UK do not register BCCs. In the US, the incidence of BCC has doubled approximately every 14 years[7] and similar changes have occurred in Australia.[8]

Aetiology

Eighty-five per cent of all BCCs appear on the head and neck region.[9,10] Risk factors are fair skin, tendency to freckle,[11] degree of sun exposure,[12–14] excessive sunbed use, radiotherapy, phototherapy, male sex, and a genetic predisposition.[15] Naevoid BCC syndrome (Gorlin syndrome) is an autosomal dominantly inherited condition characterised by developmental abnormalities and the occurrence of multiple BCCs. Mutations in patients with naevoid BCC syndrome has been found on the patched gene located on chromosome 9, which appears to be crucial for proper embryonic development and for tumour suppression.[16]

Clinical patterns

As Figures 26.1–26.3 show, clinical appearances and morphology for BCC are diverse. They include nodular, cystic, ulcerated (rodent ulcer), superficial, morphoeic (scarring), keratotic and pigmented variants. Nodular BCC is the most common type (60%) in the UK. However, in other countries such as Australia, superficial BCC is the most common type.[17] Eighty-five per cent of all BCCs appear on the head and neck region,[9,10] visible areas where a good cosmetic and functional result is important.

Prognosis

Growth of BCC is a localised phenomenon in people with a competent immune system. BCCs tend to infiltrate surrounding tissues in a three-dimensional fashion through the irregular extension of finger-like outgrowths which may not be apparent clinically.[3,18] If left untreated, or if inadequately treated, the BCC can cause extensive local tissue destruction, particularly on the face. Neglected cases may even infiltrate bone and deeper structures such as the brain and cause death.[19] Death from BCC is extremely rare, but may occur in neglected cases and/or those with major underlying immunosuppression. The clinical course of BCC is unpredictable. A BCC can remain small for years with little tendency to grow, it may grow rapidly, or it may proceed by successive spurts of extension of tumour and partial regression.[20] Histological subtype (infiltrative, micronodular or morphoeic patterns), initial diameter and male sex have been shown to be the best independent predictors of BCC invasion.[21] It is unknown whether the phenotypic characteristics of people who present with clusters of BCCs or those who develop BCCs on truncal sites are also associated with increased growth once a BCC has established.

Diagnostic tests

The diagnosis is usually made clinically, with histological confirmation being made at the time of the intended definitive treatment, often surgical removal. Diagnostic biopsies are usually performed before treatments such as radiotherapy.

Aims of treatment

The three fundamental principles of treatment are to:

- eradicate the tumour
- preserve function
- produce an excellent or acceptable cosmetic result.

From a patient's perspective, the treatment should result in as little distress as possible in terms of pain, number of hospital visits and scarring. From a health provider's perspective, it is important to balance efficacy against cost.

Relevant outcomes

- Clearance of the lesion as measured by early treatment failure (within 6 months) and long-term recurrence of the lesion measured at 3–5 years since this is what would happen in practice.
- Adverse effects in terms of atrophy, scarring, changes in pigmentation and discomfort to the patient in terms of pain during treatment and afterwards.

Methods of search

The following databases were searched:

- Medline from 1966
- Embase from 1980
- BIDS ISI (Science Citation Index from 1981)
- The Cochrane Skin Group Trials Register
- The *Cochrane Library*, Cochrane Database of Systematic Reviews and Cochrane Central Register of Controlled Trials
- Mega Register of Controlled Trials on the Current Controlled Trials website and the National Research Register's MRC Clinical Trials Directory.

The search strategy used to locate RCTs included the search terms 1–29, as given in the *Cochrane Handbook*,[22] Appendix 5c.2.

Search terms included: BCC, Basal cell carcinoma, basal cell cancer, nodular BCC, naevoid BCC, Gorlin syndrome, rodent ulcer, Jacob's ulcer, basal cell epithelioma, basalioma, non-melanoma skin cancer which include squamous cell carcinoma and BCC, NMSC.

Pharmaceutical companies were contacted where appropriate for reviews or unpublished trials.

QUESTIONS

What are the effective therapeutic interventions for BCC of the skin? How do the therapeutic interventions for BCC compare with each other? How do the cosmetic outcomes for these interventions compare? Are these interventions cost-effective?

The first-line treatment of BCC is often surgical excision. Numerous alternatives are available and include: curettage, cryosurgery, laser, excision with predetermined margins, excision under frozen section control, Mohs' micrographic surgery (the use of horizontal frozen sections and mapping to determine tumour clearance), radiotherapy, topical therapy, intralesional therapy, PDT (the application of a cream to induce photodamage to the tumour using various light sources), immunomodulators (agents used to stimulate the immune system and work on eradicating the tumour) and chemotherapy. Surgical treatment requires access to a minor operating theatre and most other treatments are carried out in specialist centres. Although there is wide variety in the treatment modalities used in the management of BCC, and the vast majority of the tumours are probably treated successfully, little research is available which accurately compares these different treatment modalities.

Surgical excision

There are no large RCTs comparing surgical excision with a predetermined margin with any other intervention for BCC, despite the fact that this modality is probably the most frequent treatment. There are, however large case series, which demonstrate excellent "success" rates for this modality.[23]

Mohs' micrographic surgery is a technique whereby 100% of the surgical margin is examined by mapping horizontal frozen sections from successive excision layers until clearance is achieved. No RCTs have investigated the margin of excision that would be effective in the removal of BCC by surgical excision with predetermined margins. Proxy measures based on Mohs' micrographic surgical margins required to remove BCCs and histopathological studies of excised specimens have suggested that for small nodular or superficial BCC, a 4 mm margin of normal skin will clear 95% of tumours.[18,24] Larger margins are required for tumours greater than 20 mm and for morphoeic tumours.[18]

Surgical excision with frozen section margin control

One RCT of 347 patients compared surgical excision with frozen section margin control versus radiotherapy in primary BCC of the face less than 40 mm diameter.[25] As shown in Table 26.1, the main outcome measure was persistent or recurrent disease at 4 years. The secondary endpoint was the cosmetic result assessed by the patient, the dermatologist and three persons not involved in the trial.

Efficacy

The 4-year failure rate was 0·7% (95% confidence intervals (CI) 0·1–3·9%) in the surgery group and 7·5% (CI 4·2–13·1%) in the radiotherapy group. Cosmetic outcome as assessed by five observers over the 4 years of the study consistently favoured surgery (Petit 2000).[26] At 4 years the percentages of patients

assessed their cosmetic results as good in 87% after surgery and in 69% after radiotherapy.

Potential drawbacks

After radiotherapy, dyspigmentations and telangiectasia developed in more than 65% of the patients at 4 years. Radiodystrophy affected 41% of the patients at 4 years.

Comment

Concealment of allocation was clear and the paper showed evidence of an *a priori* sample size calculation; however, analysis was conducted per protocol. Several previous studies have reported cure rates and cosmetic results with surgery and radiotherapy; however, the above study was the first randomised trial giving an unbiased comparison of the two treatments.

Implications for practice

The trial shows that the failure rate was significantly lower in surgery than in radiotherapy for the treatment of BCC of the face for lesions less than 4 cm in diameter. Surgery may also be preferred for its cosmetic result.

Mohs' micrographic surgery

There are no RCTs comparing this with any other intervention, although large case series with 5-year follow up suggest that this modality has the highest cure rates for all types of BCC (0·5–1·3% depending on site).[27]

Cryotherapy

Three RCTs were found and are summarised in Table 26.2. One study of 93 patients compared radiotherapy with cryotherapy for primary BCC excluding lesions on the nose or pinna.[28] The aims of the study were to compare the control of the tumours with the two treatments, to assess the final cosmetic result and to compare the discomfort and inconvenience experienced by the

Table 26.1 Randomised controlled trials evaluating surgical excision in the treatment of basal cell carcinoma

Study	Method	Participants	Interventions	Outcomes	Notes
Avril *et al.* 1997[25] (France)	Single centre Randomisation by sequential sealed envelopes ITT	HP BCCs T1: 174, T2: 173 patients Histological type T1: 79 N, 52 ulcerated, 36 S and pagetoid, 7 sclerosing; T2: 74 N, 50 ulcerated, 41 S and pagetoid, 8 sclerosing Location T1: 53 nose, 36 eyelids, 36 forehead, 10 chin, 5 ear; T2: 49 nose, 42 cheek, 35 eyelids, 29 forehead, 12 chin, 6 ear	T1: surgery – resection of whole tumour with a free margin of at least 2 mm from visible borders; T2: radiotherapy – interstitial brachytherapy, superficial contract therapy or conventional therapy, chosen by radiotherapist according to tumour parameters and location and patient characteristics	FU: 3, 6, 12 months after end of treatment; then yearly until fourth year Rate of histologically confirmed persistent tumour or recurrence after 4 years Patients examined by dermatologists; photographs of scar taken at three standardised distances	Ex: BCC on scalp or neck, patients who had total removal of BCC at biopsy, with 5 or more BCCs, life expectancy <3 years

BCC, basal cell carcinoma; HP, histologically proven; BP, biopsy proven; MU, mega units; IFN, interferons; Ex, exclusion; T1/2/3, treatment groups 1/2/3; FU, follow up; 5-FU/epi, 5-fluorouracil/epinephrine; PC, phosphatidyl choline; PDT, photodynamic therapy; ALA, gamma-aminolevulinic acid; N, nodular; S, Superficial; M, morphea-like; PP, per protocol; ITT, intention to treat

patient. Cryotherapy consisted of two freeze–thaw cycles, freezing for 1 minute each time.

Radiotherapy versus cryotherapy
Efficacy
Recurrence rates at 1 year were 4% (2/49) in the radiotherapy group and 39% (17/44) in the cryotherapy group. At 2 years no further tumours had recurred in either group. The cosmetic results for the two modes of treatment were not significantly different.

Potential drawbacks
The degree of pain, discomfort, discharge and bleeding from the treated areas was the same in both groups. Only one patient from each group was seriously inconvenienced by their treatment. Hypopigmentation was more common than hyperpigmentation with both

modes of treatment (81% of those in the radiotherapy group and 88% of those in the cryotherapy group). Seven patient treated with radiotherapy developed some radiation telangiectasia. Hypopigmentation and telangiectasia tend to be lifelong. Five patients treated with cryotherapy developed milia – these all disappeared by 1 year.

Comments
The concealment of allocation was unclear and analysis was conducted per protocol. Their was no indication of the type of lesion.

Implication for clinical practice
Cryotherapy, although convenient and less expensive than radiotherapy, does not appear to have better cure rates than radiotherapy (especially for lesions >2 cm). Cosmetic effect

Table 26.2 Randomised controlled trials evaluating cryotherapy in the treatment of basal cell carcinoma

Study	Method	Participants	Interventions	Outcomes	Notes
Hall et al. 1986[28] (UK)	Single centre Method of randomisation not known PP	105 patients BP BCCs T1: 44, T2: 49 patients Sites: T1: 30 neck and face, 6 eyelids, 8 trunk. T2: 40 neck and face, 3 eyelids, 6 trunk	T1: cryotherapy using a Cry-Owen liquid nitrogen spray gun; all lesions treated with two freeze–thaw cycles, freezing for 1 minute each time, with a thaw time of at least 90 s T2: radiotherapy, (130 KV x rays)	FU: Recurrence of tumour and cosmetic appearance at 1, 6, 12, 24 months after treatment Tumour identified histologically	12 excluded: 5 died of other causes, 7 lost to FU Ex: recurrent tumours, lesions on nose or pinna, lesion near eye and vision in eye <6/18
Mallon and Dawber, 1996[29] (UK)	Single centre Method of randomisation not known PP	84 patients Mostly clinically proven BCCs Facial lesions ≤1·5 cm not extending >3 mm below skin were included. T1: 36, T2: 48 patients Mean age T1: 67, T2: 69 years	T1: single 30-second freeze–thaw cycle T2: double 30-second freeze–thaw cycle	FU: T1: 10 months to 7·1 years, T2: 1·2– 6·1 years Lesions assessed clinically	7 lost to FU, T1: 2, T2: 5
Thissen et al. 2000[30] (The Netherlands)	Single centre. Method of randomisation not known. PP	103 patients Some BP BCCs Lesions S or N, <2 cm diameter, localised anywhere on the head and neck	T1: surgery. T2: cryosurgery (no. 3 curette used to debulk the tumour; no. 1 used to remove remainder of BCC around the borders. Freezing: two freezing periods, each lasting 20 seconds)	FU: cosmetic and recurrence at 1 year Recurrence assessed clinically	Lost to FU: 3 in control group did not turn up for visits, 1 died (unrelated to treatment), 3 developed recurrent BCC (all T2)

See Table 26.1 for abbreviations.

for radiotherapy and cryotherapy are comparable. Variations in technique occur between different physicians and may account for differences in outcome. Lesions bigger than 2 cm diameter treated by cryotherapy recurred, but lesions bigger than 2 cm and treated with radiotherapy were controlled. It was concluded that cryotherapy does not offer a satisfactory alternative to radiotherapy in the treatment of BCC.

Varying number of freeze–thaw cycles

In a study of 84 patients, one freeze–thaw cycle of 30 seconds was compared with two freeze–thaw cycles of 30 seconds for low-risk facial BCCs.[29]

Efficacy

Recurrence rates were significant: 4·7% with two freeze–thaw cycles and 20·6% with one cycle at a median time of 18 months.

Potential drawbacks

No mention was made of adverse effects of the treatment.

Comments

Concealment of allocation was unclear and the analysis was conducted per protocol. Only common facial lesions of 1·5 cm or less were included and not all the lesions were biopsied. Variations in technique between different physicians may account for differences in outcome.

Implications for clinical practice

Facial lesions require a double freeze–thaw cycle with liquid nitrogen if the high cure rates in many reports of formal excision or radiotherapy are to be achieved. Although case series suggest that higher clearance rates can be achieved, particularly with low-risk tumours, more prospective evidence is required.

Cryotherapy versus surgical excision

A study of 96 patients[30] compared cryosurgery with surgical excision for BCC of the head and neck. The primary outcome was cosmetic result but recurrence rates in both groups were also compared. Recurrences were treated by surgical excision. Cosmetic results were judged by five independent professional observers and by the patients.

Efficacy

The recurrence rate for cryosurgery was 3/48 at 1 year whereas in the surgery group no recurrences developed at 1 year. Cosmetic results after surgical excision generally got significantly better evaluation as compared with cryosurgery for superficial and nodular subtypes localised in the head/neck region.

Comments

Concealment of allocation was unclear. The analysis was conducted per protocol, although the paper showed evidence of an *a priori* sample size calculation.

Potential drawbacks

Two patients (4%) developed secondary wound infections in the first and second week after surgery, for which systemic antibiotics were given. Ninety per cent of patients in the cryotherapy group complained of moderate-to-severe swelling of the treated area, followed by long-lasting leakage of exudates from the defect. After cryotherapy three patients (6%) had secondary wound infection, for which systemic antibiotics were given.

Implications for clinical practice

Surgical excision for nodular and superficial lesions smaller than 2 cm is cosmetically more acceptable than cryosurgery. Cryotherapy does not appear to be a satisfactory alternative to surgery for superficial or nodular lesions in the head and neck area of less than 2 cm in diameter.

Photodynamic therapy (PDT)

PDT is a non-ionising radiation treatment modality under development. It uses the interaction between visible light and tumour-sensitising agents to generate cell death. Two RCTs were identified, summarised in Table 26.3. No published trials have compared PDT against the standard treatment of surgical excision.

PDT versus cryotherapy

In a trial of 88 patients, PDT was compared with two freeze–thaw cycle cryotherapy for BCC.[31]

Efficacy

There was no significant difference in recurrence rates at 12 months. Histological recurrence rates

Table 26.3   Randomised controlled trials evaluating photodynamic therapy in the treatment of basal cell carcinoma

Study	Method	Participants	Interventions	Outcomes	Notes
Wang et al. 2001[31] (Sweden)	Single centre Randomised according to a stratified randomisation pattern in blocks of 10 patients PP	HP BCC 44 women; 44 men; age range 42–88 years Type: T1: 22 S, 25 N; T2: 17 S, 24 N Distribution: 47 trunk, 25 head and neck, 10 legs, 6 arms	T1: PDT (20% weight-based ALA/water-in-oil cream applied to lesion; irradiation 6 hr later. T2: cryosurgery (2 freeze–thaw cycles)	FU: 1, 4, 8 weeks, 3 months after treatment Last FU 12 months after first treatment Punch biopsy at 3 and 12 months	Ex: BCC on nose; M growth; porphyria; abdominal pain of unknown aetiology; photosensitivity; treatment of BCC with topical steroids type III or IV within the last month
Soler et al. 2000[32] (Norway)	Single centre Randomisation numbers in locked envelopes. The patients were randomly allocated on the treatment day to one of the two arms in blocks of four patients ITT	HP BCC 83 patients 245 lesions	All lesions in both groups topical 20% ALA, removed after 3 hours and light source applied: T1: laser light (630 nm); T2: broadband light	FU: 3, 6 months after treatment Outcomes: complete, partial or no response; cosmetic outcome and pain intensity during treatment and FU	

See Table 26.1 for abbreviations.

at 1 year were 25%(11 of 44) in the PDT group, compared with 15% (6 of 39) in the cryotherapy group, despite multiple retreatments in the PDT group. Scarring and tissue defect scored significantly better following PDT.

Potential drawbacks
More patients indicated pain and discomfort during and after treatment with PDT but the differences were not statistically significant.

Comments
Concealment of allocation was clear. However, analysis was conducted per protocol and no sample size calculation was given.

Implications for clinical practice
Although patient tolerability was greater and cosmetic outcomes were considered better in the PDT group, the efficacy data do not support the introduction of PDT for the treatment of BCC; further studies demonstrating greater efficacy are needed.

Laser versus broadband halogen light
A second RCT[32] of 83 patients compared the clinical and cosmetic outcome of superficial BCCs using either laser or broadband halogen light in PDT with topical 5-aminolevulinic acid (ALA).

Efficacy

At the end of the study (6 months), 86% in the laser group and 82% in the broadband halogen group were evaluated as complete responses by both investigators. The study showed no significant difference in cure rate ($P = 0.49$, 95% CI -7 to 14%) or cosmetic outcome ($P = 0.075$) between light exposure from a simple broad lamp with continuous spectrum (570–740 nm) or from a red-light laser (monochromatic 630 nm).

Potential drawbacks

Eighty-three per cent of patients receiving laser light and 76% of those receiving broadband halogen light PDT reported some discomfort during and after illumination. Sixty-eight per cent of the patients who received laser light and 74% of patients who received broadband halogen light reported some degree of discomfort (stinging, itching, pain, headache, sensation of warmth or blushing) during the first week of treatment. No serious adverse events were reported during the 6-month follow up.

Comments

Although 83 patients were involved, 245 superficial BCCs were included in the study, indicating more than one lesion per patient. Concealment of allocation was clear and analysis was carried out by intention to treat; however, no sample size calculation was included.

A further ongoing randomised trial aims to compare the efficacy of 5-ALA PDT following minimal debulking curettage with surgery for low-risk nodular BCCs and to compare pain and morbidity experienced by patients undergoing each procedure.[33]

Implications for practice

The results show that topical ALA-based PDT with a broadband halogen light source gives cure rates and cosmetic outcome similar to those obtained with a laser light source. Reduced costs, increased safety as well as the possibility of general use by dermatologists are other elements in favour of the lamp as a suitable light source.

PDT as a technique for treatment of BCC needs further research and/or modifications, given the poor outcomes reported.

Intralesional interferon therapy

Interferons are naturally occurring glycoproteins that exhibit antiviral, antitumour and immuno-modulatory activities. Four RCTs were found, summarised in Table 26.4.

Interferon alfa-2a and/or 2b
Efficacy

In the first trial,[34] 45 patients were randomised to receive 15 or 30 million units of interferon alfa-2a, -2b or both -2a and -2b. The aim of the study was to evaluate the effectiveness of the interferons alone and whether this effect might be increased by their combination.

Complete response at 8 weeks was similar at 66–73% in each treatment group. No significant differences were found between the groups in this respect.

Potential drawbacks

One drawback is pain at the injection site. All patients had flu-like syndrome (fever, chills, headaches, fatigue, myalgia) especially within the first 2 weeks after the initiation of interferon therapy.

Comments

Concealment of allocation was unclear; however, analysis was performed with intention to treat.

Implication for clinical practice

Combining interferon alfa-2a and -2b does not increase their effectiveness.

Table 26.4   Randomised controlled trials evaluating intralesional interferon in the treatment of basal cell carcinomas

Study	Method	Participants	Interventions	Outcomes	Notes
Alpsoy et al. 1996[34] (Turkey)	Single centre Method of randomisation not known ITT	45 patients HP BCC: T1: 15, T2: 15, T3: 15 patients Mean age T1: 58·7, T2: 63·6, T3: 60·3 years Histological types T1:12 N, 1 S, 2 M; T2: 11 N, 2 S, 2 M; T3: 11 N, 2 S, 2 M	T1: INF alfa-2a; T2: INF alfa-2b; T3: INF alfa-2a and-2b	FU: cytologic specimens taken 8 weeks after completion of therapy; all cases evaluated clinically and histologically	Ex: Recurrent lesions, genetic or naevoid conditions, deep tissue involvement
Cornell et al. 1990[35] (USA)	Multicentre (4) Randomisation by computer generated PP	T1. 123, T2: 42 patients. BP BCC Mean age T1: 56, T2: 57 years Histological type T1: 57 S, 66 N ulcerative; T2: 19 S, 23 N	T1: intralesional injections 1·5 million IU IFN alfa-2b; T2: vehicle for IFN preparation 3 alternate days/week for 3 consecutive weeks	FU: weekly after each of the three treatments then at 5, 9, 13 weeks after completion of treatment, then every 3 months to 52 weeks	Ex: Previously received therapy to test site, immunosuppressive or cytotoxic therapy (within previous 4 weeks), or exogenous IFN/IFN alfa-2b (Intron A), debilitating illness, lesion in perioral or central area of the face or penetrating to deep tissue
Edwards and Tucker 1990[36] (USA)	Single centre. Method of randomisation not known PP	T1: 33; T2: 32 patients BP BCC Age range 35–65 years Histological type: T1: 16 S, 17 N, T2: 15 S, 15 N	10 million IU zinc chelate IFN alfa-2b: T1: single injection; T2: one dose per week for 3 weeks	BCC measured, photographed before each treatment and at beginning of the 2nd, 8th, 12th and 16th week after the first injection Biopsy at week 16	Ex: thromboembolic disease, radiation therapy to the test site area, history of arsenic ingestion, pregnancy, immunosuppression, receiving non-steroidal anti-inflammatory drugs, M BCC, recurrent cancers, deeply invasive lesions, periorificial tumours, central facial BCC
Rogozinski et al. 1997[37] (Poland)	Single centre. Method of randomisation not known ITT	T1: 17, T2: 18 patients	T1: recombinant INF beta; T2: placebo	FU: 16 weeks after treatment and 2 years	

See Table 26.1 for abbreviations.

Interferon alfa-2b versus vehicle

Another trial of 165 patients[35] compared interferon alfa-2b, 1·5 million units three times weekly, for 3 weeks with vehicle in a 3:1 ratio of interferon-treated to placebo-treated patients.

Efficacy

Eighty-one per cent of interferon-treated patients were clinically and histologically cured at 52 weeks, compared with 20% of placebo recipients. The cure rate was independent of lesion type or size.

Potential drawbacks

Flu-like symptoms occurred more commonly in the interferon-treated group.

Comments

Concealment of allocation was clear; however, analysis was conducted per protocol. Interestingly, 20% of people treated with vehicle appeared to have histological cure at 1 year. Longer-term studies are needed to determine whether this is genuine.

Implications for clinical practice

Interferon alfa-2b could be considered for patients who are not candidates for simple surgery or desire non-surgical therapy. Interferon alfa-2b does not compare with current standards of surgical or radiotherapy cures and so cannot be recommended.

Number of dosages of interferon alfa-2b

In a third trial of 65 patients, a single dose of 10 million IU protamine zinc chelate interferon alfa-2b (a sustained-release preparation) was compared with the same dose weekly for 3 weeks.[36]

Efficacy

Histological cure rates at 16 weeks were 52% and 80% for one and three doses weekly, respectively. Cosmetic effect was graded by patients as follows: excellent 51%, very good 22%, good 14%, satisfactory 10% and poor 3%.

Potential drawbacks

All patients experienced at least one adverse reaction. Side-effects were similar for both single and repeated dosage groups, and were those common to interferon. Adverse reactions occurring in at least 20% of subjects were fever, rigors, myalgia, headache and nausea. Other side-effects included arthraglia, malaise, fatigue, diarrhoea, paraesthesias, somnolence, thirst, dizziness, vomiting, rashes and anorexia. Adverse reactions began on the day of treatment and generally lasted 5–8 hours, except for headaches which lasted about 1 day. Mild erythema was often present at the treatment site in the 16th study week.

Comments

Concealment of allocation was unclear and analysis was conducted per protocol. There was also a lack of any other active or standard treatment as comparator.

Implications for clinical practice

Refinement of the formulation to improve the release of interferon in order to help minimise side-effects has not been realised. A trial is needed to compare sustained-release formulation of interferon alfa-2b with standard interferon alfa-2b.

Interferon beta

Recombinant interferon beta, I million units three times weekly for 3 weeks has been compared with placebo in a trial of 35 patients.[37]

Table 26.5   Randomised controlled trials evaluating BEC-5 in the treatment of basal cell carcinoma

Study	Method	Participants	Interventions	Outcomes	Notes
Punjabi et al. 2000[38] (UK)	Multicentre Method of randomisation not known	94 patients BP BCCs Age 32–95 years	T1: BEC-5; T2: vehicle; twice daily under occlusion for 8 weeks	Patients reviewed every 2 weeks Repeat punch biopsy at 8 weeks on 84 patients	10 patients in T1 did not complete the study

See Table 26.1 for abbreviations.

Efficacy
At 2 years follow up, 47% in the treatment group showed complete response compared with none in the placebo group.

Potential drawbacks
Inflammation at the injection site was found in 11/16 patients in the treatment group and 4/18 receiving placebo.

Comment
Analysis was conducted per protocol; concealment of allocation is not known.

Implications for clinical practice
The paper suggests recombinant interferon beta as an alternative treatment for BCC, but the response rate for this trial is lower than in others – 47% is not a sufficiently good response rate to recommend a treatment.

BEC-5 cream
BEC-5 is a mixture of 0·005% solasodine glycosides found in solanaceous plants (aubergine). BEC-5 cream binds to endogenous ectins and shows preferential cytotoxicity to human cancer cells.

In a double-blind randomised trial, BEC-5 cream was compared with matching vehicle[38] (Table 26.5). Biopsy-proven lesions, excluding morpheic BCC, were treated twice daily under occlusion with BEC-5 or vehicle for 8 weeks.

Efficacy
There was a significant histological cure at week 8: 66% (41/62) in the BEC-5 group and 25% (8/32) in the vehicle group. Cure rates at 1-year follow up were also significant: 52% (32/62) in the BEC-5 group and 16% (5/32) in the placebo group.

Potential drawbacks
There were no major treatment-related adverse effects.

Comment
Concealment of allocation was unclear and analysis was conducted using intention to treat. The proportions of nodular and superficial BCCs was not clear from the published abstract.

Implications for clinical practice
Although significant differences were found between the groups, the cure rate is probably not sufficiently high compared with other treatments to recommend this method. Further trials are required to ascertain the true usefulness of this preparation.

5-Fluorouracil (5-FU)
The primary mechanism of action of 5-FU is thought to be inhibition of DNA synthesis

Table 26.6 Randomised controlled trials evaluating 5-fluorouracil (5-FU) in the treatment of basal cell carcinoma

Study	Method	Participants	Interventions	Outcomes	Notes
Ramgosa et al. 2000[40] (USA)	Single centre Method of randomisation not known ITT	13 patients, 17 BP non-S BCCs ≥ 0.7 cm greatest diameter	T1: 5% 5-FU in PC vehicle T2: 5% 5-FU in petrolatum base Applied am and pm for 4 consecutive weeks	FU: every 4 weeks for 16 weeks Final visit was biopsy of site	Ex: systemic disease, women of childbearing age, facial BCCs.
Miller et al. 1997[41] (USA)	Multicentre, randomised, open-label Method of randomisation not known PP	97 males, 25 females Single BP BCC Mean age 61 years Histological type: 38 S, 85 N Location: 9 head, 9 neck, 38 upper extremities, 11 lower extremities, 55 trunk Lesion area median 80 mm^2	6 treatment regimens with 5-FU/epi gel: T1: 1.0 ml once weekly for 6 weeks; T2: 0.5 ml once weekly for 6 weeks; T3: 1.0 ml twice weekly for 3 weeks; T4: 0.5ml twice weekly for 3 weeks. T5: 0.5 ml twice weekly for 4 weeks, T6: 0.5 ml three times weekly for 2 weeks	FU examinations of patients at 1, 4, 8, 12 weeks after last injection At each visit patient and investigator gave subjective evaluation of cosmetic appearance of lesion	Ex: high risk sites. Lesions with deep tissue involvement, basal cell naevus syndrome, hypersensitivities or allergies to 5-FU, sulfites, epinephrine, bovine collagen, history of autoimmune disease, pregnancy. Six patients were lost to follow up

See Table 26.1 for abbreviations.

by competitive inhibition of thymidylate synthetase.[39]

5-FU in phosphatidyl choline versus 5-FU in petrolatum

A double-blind randomised pilot study[40] of 5-FU 5% cream in phosphatidyl choline (PC) vehicle was compared with 5-FU 5% in petrolatum. Further details of this study are given in Table 26.6. PC was used as a vehicle to facilitate the penetration of 5-FU.

Efficacy

Histological cure at week 16 was 90% with the PC vehicle and 57% with the petrolatum-based cream. The patients also evaluated the treatment

site on each visit for cosmetic appearance. There was absolutely no difference detected in the clinical appearance and adverse effects between the two therapeutic arms of the study.

Comments

The study was not powered to detect any statistically significant differences in outcome between the groups, and concealment of allocation was unclear; however, analysis was conducted using intention to treat.

Potential drawbacks

Local irritation, erythema, ulceration and tenderness were common reactions but were well tolerated by the patients. Minimal itching and discomfort were experienced by some of the patients in both treatment arms.

Implications for clinical practice

The study may indicate an increase in short-term eradication of BCC using a PC-based vehicle compared with conventional petrolatum-based formulations of 5-FU. There was excellent cosmetic outcome in all treatment sites before excision at week 16. Further large-scale double-blind trials are needed to establish the efficacy of this treatment modality.

5-FU/epinephrine injectable gel

An open-label randomised study of 122 patients[41] tested the safety, tolerance and efficacy of six treatment regimens of 5-FU/epinephrine gel. Two doses and four treatment schedules were used (Table 26.6).

Efficacy

Overall, the average response rate for the six regimens was 91%, as defined by absence of any tumour on the basis of histological analysis of excised specimen A 100% complete response rate was observed in patients who received 5 ml 5-FU/epinephrine gel twice weekly for 4 weeks – a 92% response rate for superficial lesions and a 91% response rate for nodular lesions.

All regimens appeared to work well and there were no statistically significant differences between them. The various treatment regimens with higher doses and/or treatment frequency resulted in higher complete response rates than obtained in an earlier pilot study.[42] Cosmetic appearance of lesion site prior to excision at 3 months ranged from good to excellent.

Potential drawbacks

All patients had transient, moderate-to-severe stinging, burning or pain at the time of injection.

Local tissue reactions were confined to the treatment site and included erythema, swelling, desquamation, erosions and eschar in most patients. Hyperpigmentation was observed in 83% of patients but typically cleared up by follow up. Forty-seven per cent of patients had ulcerations at the treatment site. The lowest incidence and severity of reactions occurred with 0·5 ml 5-FU/epinephrine gel three times weekly for 2 weeks.

Comments

Analysis was per protocol. Concealment of allocation was unclear. No sample size calculation was shown.

Implication for clinical practice

High local drug concentrations can be maintained for longer with the epinephrine gel delivery of 5-FU. A trial of 5-FU/epinephrine gel versus surgical excision, monitoring adverse effects, is required to confirm the claim that response rates are comparable to surgery.

Imiquimod

Imiquimod is an immune response modifier. It induces cytokines that promote a TH1 lymphocyte or cell-mediated immune response.[43–45] These cytokines include interferon alpha and gamma, and interleukin (IL)-12. In animal studies, imiquimod has demonstrated broad antiviral and antitumor effects that are largely mediated by interferon alfa.[44] In humans, imiquimod 5% cream is safe and effective in the treatment of external anogenital warts.[47–48] We found six RCTs, summarised in Table 26.7.

Efficacy

One study of 35 patients evaluated the safety and efficacy of imiquimod 5% cream in the treatment of superficial and nodular BCC.[49,50]

Table 26.7 Randomised controlled trials evaluating imiquimod 5% cream in the treatment of basal cell carcinoma

Study	Method	Participants	Interventions	Outcomes
Beutner et al. 1999[49] (USA)	Single centre Randomisation to give 2:1 ratio of imiquimod cream to vehicle cream Method of randomisation not known ITT	Age range 37–81 years BP BCCs: T1: 7; T2: 4; T3: 4; T5: 5; T6: 11 patients Size: 0·5–2 cm² Mainly upper body Histological type: T1: 1 N, 2 S; T2: 1 N, 3 S; T3: 4 S; T4: 2 N, 3 S; T5: 2 N, 2 S; T6: 1 N, 10 S	Imiquimod 5% cream: T1: twice/day; T2: once/day; T3: three times/week; T4: twice/week; T5: once/week; T6: vehicle	FU: 6 weeks after treatment tumour site excised and examined histologically
Marks et al. 2001[51] (Australia and New Zealand)	Multicentre Method of randomisation not known ITT	72 male, 27 female HP S BCC; surface area 0·5–2 cm² Location: 32% upper limbs, 28% trunk, 40% head and neck	% imiquimod: T1: twice/day, T2: once/day, T3: twice/day for 3 days/week, T4: once/day for 2 days/week	FU: 1, 2, 4, 6 weeks Excision at week 6 Lost to FU: T2: 2 (pruritus) T3: 1 (cerebrovascular accident); T4: 1 (excision of nearby tumour)
Geisse et al. 2001[52] (USA)	Multicentre, randomised, blinded, vehicle-controlled dose–response Method of randomisation not known ITT	Single, primary BP S BCC (0·5–2·0 cm²)	Imiquimod for 12 weeks: T1: twice daily ; T2: once daily; T3: Mon–Fri; T4: Mon, Wed, Fri	FU: surgical excision 6 weeks after treatment
Sterry et al. 2001[53] (USA)	Multicentre, randomised open label, dose–response Method of randomisation not known ITT	93 patients, single, primary BP S BCC (0·5–2 cm²)	T1/T2: imiquimod 3 times/week for 6 weeks with (T1) and without (T2) occlusion; T3/T4: twice/week for 6 weeks, with (T3) and without (T4) occlusion	FU: surgical excision 6 weeks after treatment

(Continued)

Table 26.7 (*Continued*)

Study	Method	Participants	Interventions	Outcomes
Shumack et al. 2001[55] (USA)	Multicentre, randomised, open label, dose–response Method of randomisation not known ITT	99 patients, single, primary, BP N BCC (0·5–2 cm²)	Imiquimod for 6 weeks: T1: twice daily; T2: once daily; T3: twice daily 3 days/week for 6 weeks; T4: 3/week for 6 weeks	FU: surgical excision 6 weeks after treatment
Robinson et al. 2001[54] (USA)	Multicentre, randomised, blinded, vehicle-controlled dose–response Method of randomisation not known ITT	92 patients, single, primary BP N BCC (0·5–2 cm²)	Imiquimod for 12 weeks: T1 twice daily; T2: once daily; T3: Mon–Fri; T4. Mon, Wed, Fri	FU: surgical excision 6 weeks after treatment

See Table 26.1 for abbreviations.

This small trial suggested success rates similar to those of excision surgery, with the added advantage of no scarring.

In a phase II dose–response trial of imiquimod 5% cream applied for 6 weeks in 99 Australian patients with primary superficial BCC,[51] histological clearance (defined as patients with no histological evidence of BCC when the site of the treated lesion was excised 6 weeks after imiquimod treatment) rates were 100% (3/3), 88% (29/33), 73% (22/30) and 70% (23/33) for twice-daily, once-daily, six-times-weekly and three-times-weekly regimens, respectively.

Another similar multicentre RCT of 128 patients with superficial BCC compared imiquimod twice daily, once daily, 5 days/week and 3 days/week versus vehicle using the same endpoints.[52] Intention-to-treat analysis showed clearance rates of 100% (10/10), 87% (27/31), 81% (21/26) and 52% for the twice-daily, once-daily, 5 days/week and 3 days/week groups, respectively. Interestingly, there was a small vehicle response rate – 19% (6/32).

Another study[53] of 93 patients with superficial BCC found that occlusion increased the success rate for three-times-weekly application of imiquimod from 76% (19/25) to 87% (20/23).

Two further industry-sponsored trials[54,55] conducted in Australia and the US have evaluated imiquimod 5% cream for the treatment of nodular BCC. One[55] reported histological clearance rates of 71% (25/35) for once-daily treatment for 6 weeks. Another vehicle-controlled RCT[54] of 92 patients with nodular BCC who underwent treatment for 12 weeks using twice daily, once daily, 5 days/week or 3 days/week reported intention-to-treat histological clearance rates of 75% (3/4), 76% (16/21), 70% (16/23) and 60% (12/20), respectively, with a vehicle response rate of 13% (3/24).

This study suggested that longer treatment times (i.e. 12 weeks as opposed to 6 weeks) are needed to treat nodular tumours. This is what one might anticipate from a treatment that relies on percutaneous penetration – tumour depth may be an important predictor of treatment response.

Potential drawbacks

There may be some local skin reaction to the cream, including: redness, oedema, skin hardening, vesicles, erosion, ulceration, flaking and scabbing. These brisk inflammatory reactions, at least clinically, would be consistent with an acute immunologic reconstitution of the sun-damaged skin, resulting in an immunologically mediated elimination of malignant and premalignant cells. In all studies, local reactions were common, mostly mild or moderate, were well tolerated by patients, and declined in incidence and severity with less frequent dosing.[49–55]

Comment

Concealment of allocation was unclear for all the imiquimod trials; however, analysis was by intention to treat. There was no long-term follow up for recurrence. In all of these trials patients were able to apply the cream themselves, a distinct advantage in today's busy dermatology departments.

Implications for clinical practice

A long-term RCT of imiquimod 5% cream versus the best treatment currently available (surgery) is needed. If successful, topical imiquimod could become a useful treatment for superficial and low-risk BCCs and would allow dermatologists to concentrate on the high-risk BCCs.

Key points

- Despite the enormous amount of work involved in the treatment of BCC, there has been very little good-quality research on the efficacy of the treatment modalities used.
- Surgery and radiotherapy appear to be the most effective treatments. Other treatments might have some use, but none has been compared with surgery.
- The majority studies have been performed on low-risk BCCs, the results of which are probably not applicable to tumours of the morphoeic type shown in Figure 26.3. Specific trials or subgroup analyses are required for morphoeic tumours.
- Cryotherapy, although convenient and less expensive than surgery or radiotherapy, does not have better cure rates than surgery or radiotherapy (especially for lesions >2 cm). Cosmetic effect is better for surgery and comparable for radiotherapy.
- If cryosurgery is to be used, two freeze–thaw cycles are recommended for nodular and superficial facial lesions (Figures 26.1 and 26.2) if cure rates approaching equivalence to that of formal excision or radiotherapy are to be achieved.
- An RCT of PDT versus surgery is needed.
- Further studies for all of the interferon treatments and PDT that demonstrate greater efficacy are needed before they can be recommended.
- Broadband halogen light source may give cure rates and cosmetic outcome similar to laser light PDT with possible benefits of reduced costs, increased safety and ease of use.
- The efficacy of interferon alfa has not been directly compared with standard surgical treatment; inteferons are associated with significant side-effects, which may overshadow their usefulness, especially in the elderly. Interferon therapy requires several clinic visits.
- Increased short-term eradication of BCC using 5-FU in a phosphatidyl choline based vehicle to increase penetration should be compared with surgery, with long-term follow up.
- Preliminary studies suggest a high success rate (87–88%) for imiquimod in the treatment of superficial BCC using a once-daily regimen for 6 weeks and a useful (76%) treatment response when treating nodular BCC for 12 weeks. These results need to be confirmed in a long-term study (3–5 years) with excision surgery as a comparator.
- Studies comparing excision with predetermined margins versus Mohs' micrographic surgery in high-risk tumours would be useful.

References

1. Telfer NR, Colver GB, Bowers PW. Guidelines for the management of basal cell carcinoma. *Br J Dermatol* 1999;**141**:415–23.
2. Preston DS, Stern RS. Nonmelanoma cancers of the skin. *N Engl J Med* 1992;**327**:1649–62.
3. Miller SJ. Biology of basal cell carcinoma (part 1). *J Am Acad Dermatol* 1991;**24**:1–13.
4. Goodwin RG, Roberts, DL. Skin cancer registration in the United Kingdom. *Br J Dermatol* 2001;**145**(Suppl. 59):17.
5. Walberg P, Skog E. The increasing incidence of basal cell carcinoma. *Br J Dermatol* 1994;**131**:914–15.
6. Holme SA, Malinovszky K, Roberts DL. Changing trends in non-melanoma skin cancer in South Wales, 1988–98. *Br J Dermatol* 2000;**143**:1224–9.
7. Chuang TY, Popescu A, Su WP, Chute CG. Basal cell carcinoma: a population-based incidence study in Rochester, Minnesota. *J Am Acad Dermatol* 1990;**22**:413–17.
8. Marks R, Staples M, Giles GG. Trends in non-melanocytic skin cancer treated in Australia: the second national survey. *Int J Cancer* 1993;**53**:585–90.
9. Roenigk RK, Ratz JL, Bailin PL, Wheeland RG. Trends in the presentation and treatment of basal cell carcinomas. *J Dermatol Surg Oncol* 1986;**12**:860–5.
10. McCormack CJ, Kelly JW, Dorevitch AP. Differences in age and body site distribution of the histological subtypes

of basal cell carcinoma:a possible indicator of differing causes. *Arch Dermatol* 1997;**133**:593–6.

11. Gilbody JS, Aitken J, Green A. What causes basal cell carcinoma to be the commonest cancer? *Aust J Public Health* 1994;**18**:218–21.

12. Zaynoun S, Ali LA, Shaib J. The relationship of sun exposure and solar elastosis to basal cell carcinoma. *J Am Acad Dermatol* 1985;**12**:522–5.

13. Pearl DK, Scott EL. The anatomical distribution of skin cancers. *Int J Epidemiol* 1986;**15**:502–6.

14. Mackie RM, Elwood JM, Hawk JLM. Links between exposure to ultraviolet radiation and skin cancer. A report of the Royal College of Physicians. *J R Coll Phys Lond* 1987;**21**:91–6.

15. Schreiber MM, Moon TE, Fox SH, Davidson J. The risk of developing subsequent nonmelanoma skin cancers. *J Am Acad Dermatol* 1990;**23**:1114–18.

16. Johnson RL, Rothman AL, Xie J *et al.* Human homolog of patched, a candidate gene for the Basal Cell Nevus Syndrome. *Science* 1996;**272**:1668–71.

17. Staples M, Marks R, Giles G. Trends in the incidence of non-melanocytic skin cancer (NMSC) treated in Australia 1985–1995: are primary prevention programs starting to have an effect? *Int J Cancer* 1998;**78**:144–8.

18. Breuninger H, Deitz K. Prediction of subclinical tumour infiltration in basal cell carcinoma. *J Dermatol Surg Oncol* 1991;**17**:574–8.

19. Gussack GS. Schlitt M. Lushington A. Woods KE. Invasive basal cell carcinoma of the temporal bone. *Ear Nose Throat J* 1998;**68**:605–6;609–11.

20. Franchimont C. Episodic progression and regression of basal cell carcinomas. *Br J Dermatol* 1982;**106**:305–10.

21. Takenouchi T, Nomoto S, Ito M. Factors influencing the linear depth of invasion of primary basal cell carcinoma. *Dermatol Surg* 2001;**27**:393–6.

22. Clark M, Oxman AD eds. Optimat search strategy for RCTs. In: Cochrane Reviewers' Handbook 4.1 (updated June 2000). Cochrane Collaboration. Oxford, 2000: appendix 5c.

23. Dubin N, Kopf AW. Multivariate risk score for recurrence of cutaneous basal cell carcinoma. *Arch Dermatol* 1983;**119**:373–7.

24. Wolf DJ, Zitelli JA. Surgical margins for basal cell carcinoma. *Arch Dermatol* 1987;**123**:340–4.

25. Avril MF, Auperin A, Margulis A *et al.* Basal cell carcinoma of the face: surgery or radiotherapy? Results of a randomised study. *Br J Cancer* 1997;**76**:100–6.

26. Petit JY, Avril MF *et al.* Evaluation of cosmetic resulls of a randomised trial comparing surgery and radiotherapy in the treatment of basal cell carcinoma of the face. *Plas Reconstr Surg* 2000;**105**:2544-51.

27. Rowe DE, Carroll RJ, Day CL Jr. Long term recurrence rates in previously untreated (primary) basal cell carcinoma: implications for patient follow up. *J Dermatol Surg Oncol* 1989;**15**:315–28.

28. Hall VL, Leppard BJ, McGill J *et al.* Treatment of basal cell carcinoma: Comparison of radiotherapy and cryotherapy. *Clin Radiol* 1986;**37**:33–4.

29. Mallon E, Dawber R. Cryosurgery in the treatment of basal cell carcinoma. *Dermatol Surg* 1996;**22**:854–8.

30. Thissen MRTM, Nieman FHM, Ideler AHLB, Berretty PJM, Neumann HAM. Cosmetic results of cryosurgery versus surgical excision for primary uncomplicated basal cell carcinomas of the head and neck. *Dermatol Surg* 2000;**26**:759–64.

31. Wang I, Bendsoe N, Klinteberg CA *et al.* Photodynamic therapy *v* cryosurgery of basal cell carcinomas: results of phase III clinical trial. *Br J Dermatol* 2001;**144**: 832–40.

32. Soler AM, Angell-Petersen E, Warloe T *et al.* Photodynamic therapy of superficial basal cell carcinoma with 5–aminolevulinic acid with dimethylsulfoxide and ethylendiaminetetraacitic acid: A comparison of two light sources. *Photochem Photobiol* 2000;**71**:724–9.

33. Clark C. Randomised trial of minimal curettage and topical 5-aminolaevulinic acid (5-ALA) photodynamic therapy (PDT) compared with excision for the treatment of basal cell carcinomas with low recurrence risk. Ongoing trial. Photobiology Unit, Ninewells Hospital and Medical School, Tayside University Hospitals NHS Trust, Dundee UK.

34. Alpsoy E, Yilmaz E, Basaran E, Yazar S. Comparison of the effects of intralesional interferon alfa-2a, 2b and the combination of 2a and 2b in the treatment of basal cell carcinoma. *J Dermatol* 1996;**23**:394–6.

35. Cornell RC, Greenway HT, Tucker SB *et al.* Intralesional interferon therapy for basal cell carcinoma. *J Am Acad Dermatol* 1990;**23**:694–700.

36. Edwards L, Tucker SB. The effects of an intralesional sustained release formulation of interferon alfa2b on basal cell carcinomas. *Arch Dermatol* 1990;**126**:1029–32.

37. Rogozinski TT, Jablonska S, Brzoska J, Michalska I, Wohr C, Gaus W. Intralesional treatment with recombinant interferon beta is an effective alternative for the treatment of basal cell carcinoma. Double-blind, placebo-controlled study. *Przeglad Dermatol* 1997;**84**:259–63.

38. Punjabi S, Cook IJ, Kersey P *et al.* A double-blind, multicentric parallel group study of BEC-5 cream in basal cell carcinoma (BCC). *Eur Acad Dermatol Venereol* 2000;**14**(Suppl 1):47–60.

39. Fluorouracil. In: McEvoy GK, ed. *American Hospital Formulacy Service Drug Information.* Bethesda, MD: American Society of Hospital Pharmacists, 1993:573–7.

40. Romagosa R, Saap L, Givens M *et al.* A pilot study to evaluate the treatment of basal cell carcinoma with 5-fluorouracil using phosphatidyl choline as a transepidermal carrier. *Dermatol Surg* 2000;**26**:338–40.

41. Miller BH, Shavin JS, Cognetta A *et al.* Nonsurgical treatment of basal cell carcinomas with intralesional 5-fluorouracil/epinephrine injectable gel. *J Am Acad Dermatol* 1997;**36**:72–7.

42. Orenberg EK, Miller BH, Greenway HT. The effect of intralesional 5-fluorouracil therapeutic implant (MPI 5003) for treatment for basal cell carcinoma. *Acad Dermatol* 1992;**27**:723–8.

43. Testerman TL, Gerster JF, Imbertson LM *et al.* Cytokine induction by the immunomodulators imiquimod and S-27609. *J Leukoc Biol* 1995;**58**:365–72.

44. Slade HB, Owens ML, Tomai MA, Miller RL. Imiquimod 5% cream. *Exp Opin Invest Drugs* 1998;**7**:437–49.

45. Imbertson LM, Beaurline JM, Couture AM *et al.* Cytokine induction in hairless mouse and rat skin after topical application of the immune response modifiers imiquimod and S-28463. *J Invest Dermatol* 1998;**110**:734–9.

46. Beutner KR, Spruance SL, Hougham AJ, Fox TL, Owens ML, Douglas JM Jr. Treatment of genital warts with an immune response modifier imiquimod. *J Am Acad Dermatol* 1998;**38**:230–9.

47. Beutner KR 2, Tyring SK, Trofatter KR *et al.* Imiquimod, a patient applied immune response modifier for treatment of external genital warts. *Antimicrob Agents Chemother* 1998;**42**:788–94.

48. Edwards L, Ferenczy A, Eron L *et al.* Self-administered topical 5% imiquimod cream for external anogenital warts. *Arch Dermatol* 1998;**134**:25–30.

49. Beutner KR, Geisse JK, Helman D, Fox TL, Ginkel A, Owens ML. Therapeutic response of basal cell carcinoma to the immune response modifier imiquimod 5% cream. *J Am Acad Dermatol* 1999;**41**:1002–7.

50. Bavinck JN. Biological treatment of basal cell carcinoma. *Arch Dermatol* 2000;**136**:774–5.

51. Marks R, Gebauer K, Shumak S *et al.* Imiquimod 5% cream in the treatment of superficial basal cell carcinoma: results of a multicenter 6-week dose-response trial. *J Am Acad Dermatol* 2001;**44**:807–13.

52. Geisse JK, Marks R, Owens ML, Andres K, Ginkel AM. Imiquimod 5% cream for 12 weeks treating superficial BCC. Abstract P58 at 8th World Congress on Cancers of the Skin, Zurich, Switzerland 18th–21st July 2001.

53. Sterry W, Bichel J, Andres K, Ginkel AM. Imiquimod 5% cream for 6 weeks with occlusion treating superficial BCC. Abstract P61 at 8th World Congress on Cancers of the Skin, Zurich, Switzerland 18th–21st July 2001.

54. Robinson JK, Marks R, Owens ML, Andres K, Ginkel AM. Imiquimod 5% cream for 12 weeks treating nodular BCC. Abstract P57 at 8th World Congress on Cancers of the Skin, Zurich, Switzerland 18th–21st July 2001.

55. Shumak S, Marks R, Amies M, Andres K, Ginkel AM. Imiquimod 5% cream for 6 weeks treating nodular BCC. Abstract P55 at 8th World Congress on Cancers of the Skin, Zurich, Switzerland 18th–21st July 2001.

27
Primary cutaneous T-cell lymphoma

Sean Whittaker

Background
Definition

Primary cutaneous T-cell lymphomas (CTCL) represent a heterogeneous group of extranodal non-Hodgkin's lymphoma, of which mycosis fungoides/Sezary syndrome are the most common clinicopathological subtypes.[1] Mycosis fungoides is characterised by distinct clinical stages of cutaneous disease consisting of patches/plaques, tumours and erythroderma in which the whole skin is involved. Peripheral adenopathy may or may not be present. Sezary syndrome is defined by the presence of erythroderma, peripheral lymphadenopathy and a minimum number of Sezary cells within the peripheral blood. These clinicopathological entities are closely related pathogenetically but are distinct from other less common types of primary CTCL.

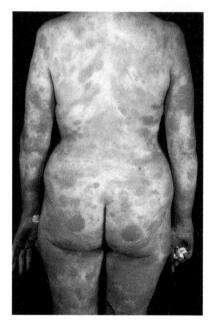

Figure 27.2   Plaque stage mycosis fungoides (IB/IIA)

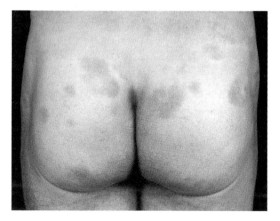

Figure 27.1   Patch stage mycosis fungoides (IA)

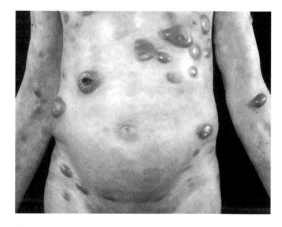

Figure 27.3   Tumour stage mycosis fungoides (IIB)

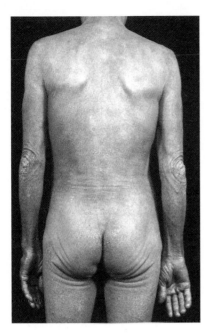

Figure 27.4   Erythrodermic mycosis fungoides (III)

Incidence/prevalence

The overall annual incidence of primary CTCL in the US in 1988 was 0·5–1·0 per 100 000 based on population data. However, the prevalence is much higher because most patients have low-grade disease and live long.[2] Males (2·1) and the black population are affected more commonly.[2,3] The incidence has increased during the past two decades but this almost certainly reflects improved diagnosis of earlier stages and possibly better registration, particularly in the US.[3]

Aetiology

The underlying aetiology is unknown. There is evidence for inactivation of key tumour suppressor genes and TH2 cytokine production by tumour cells in mycosis fungoides/Sezary syndrome, but no disease-specific molecular abnormality has yet been identified.[4] Primary CTCL must be distinguished from human T-lymphotropic virus type-1 (HTLV-I) associated adult T-cell leukaemia lymphoma (ATLL) in which skin involvement often closely mimics the clinicopathological features of mycosis fungoides/Sezary syndrome and may be the presenting feature.[1]

Prognosis

Most cases of primary CTCL are not curable. Independent prognostic features in mycosis fungoides include the cutaneous and lymph node stage of disease and age of onset (>60 years). The lymph node status and tumour burden within peripheral blood determine the prognosis in Sezary syndrome.[5,6] Serum lactate dehydrogenase and the thickness of the infiltrate in plaque-stage mycosis fungoides are also independent markers of prognosis.[7] Multivariate analysis indicates that an initial complete response (CR) to various therapies is an independent favourable prognostic feature, particularly in early stages of disease.[8–10] For mycosis fungoides, two staging systems are in regular use including a TNM (primary tumour, regional nodes, metastasis) system and a clinical staging specifically designed for CTCL (Box 27.1).[5] These staging systems can also be applied to Sezary syndrome, but neither system provides a quantitative method for assessing peripheral blood disease other than an additional B0 and B1 in the TNM system and this has prompted alternative approaches for Sezary syndrome.[6]

Table 27.1 summarises recent actuarial survival data for mycosis fungoides. The 5- and 10-year overall survival (OS) in mycosis fungoides are 80% and 57%, respectively, with disease-specific survival (DSS) rates of 89% and 75% at 5 and 10 years respectively.[8] Patients with very early stage disease (IA) are highly unlikely to die of their disease, with DSS rates of 100% and 97–98% at 5 and 10 years, respectively and risks of disease progression varying from 0% to 10% over 5–20 years.[8–11] In one study of 122 patients with stage IA disease median survival was not reached at 32·5 years.[9]

Box 27.1 TNM (primary tumour, regional nodes, metastasis) classification for mycosis fungoides (including "B" system for cutaneous T-cell lymphoma (CTCL) to incorporate Sezary syndrome)

Skin

T1 – limited patches/plaques (<10% of total skin surface)
T2 – extensive patches/plaques (>10% of total skin surface)
T3 – tumours
T4– erythroderma

Nodes

N0 — no clinical lymphadenopathy
N1 — clinically enlarged lymph nodes but histologically uninvolved
N2 — Lymph nodes not enlarged but histologically involved
N3 – Clincally enlarged lymph nodes and histologically involved

Visceral

M0 — no visceral involvement
M1 — visceral involvement

Blood

B0 — no peripheral blood Sezary cells (<5%)
B1 — peripheral blood Sezary cells (>5% of total lymphocyte count)

Clinical staging system for CTCL (mycosis fungoides)

Clinical Stages	T	N	M
IA	T1	N0	M0
IB	T2	N0	M0
IIA	T1–2	N1	M0
IIB	T3	N0—1	M0
III	T4	N0—1	M0
IVA	T1–4	N2–3	M0
IVB	T1–4	N0—3	M1

Stage IB patients have an OS rate of 73–86% at 5 years and 58–67% at 10 years, and DSS rates of 96% and 83% at 5 and 10 years respectively.[3,8,10] A median survival of 12·1–12·8 years should be expected for stage IB patients, with a risk of disease progression varying from 10% to 39%. The explanation for this marked variation in different studies of stage IB is unclear but it appears that patients with folliculotropic variants of mycosis fungoides have a worse prognosis than other patients with stage IB disease; this may reflect the depth of infiltrate, which perhaps makes skin-directed therapy less effective.[8]

Accurate data on stage IIA patients (patches/plaques and clinical adenopathy with no histological evidence of lymphoma) are scant, but this stage may be associated with a worse outcome – with OS rates of 49%, DSS rates of 68% and risks of disease progression of 65% at both 5 and 10 years. The lack of difference in outcome at 5 and 10 years in this study is unreliable since the data came from only 18 patients.[8] Of the 176 patients reported by Kim et al.[10] 56 (32%) had peripheral adenopathy (stage IIA) but in 23 of these 56 no histological assessment was made and therefore some of them could have had stage IVA disease. Nevertheless the OS rate is similar to stage IB disease at 5 years (73%), with a slight difference at 10 years (45% versus 58%), associated with a small difference in median survival of 10 years (stage IIA) compared with 12·8 years (stage IB) and overall risk of disease progression of 34% and 20%, respectively. Further studies of larger numbers of patients with stage IIA disease are needed to compare outcomes with those of stage IB patients.

Patients with tumour-stage disease (stage IIB) have OS rates of 40–65% at 5 years and 20–39% at 10 years,[3,8,9] and a median survival of 2·9 years in one study.[9] In one study DSS rates of 80% and

42% at 5 and 10 years, respectively, were reported for patients with stage IIB disease.[8] The survival data for patients with erythrodermic mycosis fungoides but no evidence of lymph node or peripheral blood involvement (stage III) are broadly similar to those for stage IIB disease, although median survival may be better (4·6 versus 3·6 years).[3,9,12] In contrast the OS and DSS rates at 5 and 10 years for stage IVA and IVB patients is poor (15–40% and 5–20% for stage IVA and 0–15% and 0–5% for stage IVB at 5 and 10 years, respectively) and a median survival of 13 months for both extracutaneous stages.[8,11,12]

The OS rates in CTCL based on stage of disease has led to suggestions that the staging system should be modified with four broad categories.[13] (i) Stage IA patients have a normal life expectancy but (ii) stage IB and IIA disease may have a similar prognosis, although the thickness of the infiltrate is an important prognostic factor in this group. Similarly (iii) the prognosis is similar for stage IIB and III disease, which is better than in patients with (iv) nodal or visceral disease (IVA/B). This proposal resembles that suggested by Sausville et al. in 1988.[14]

Patients with Sezary syndrome have an 11% 5-year survival, with a median survival of 32 months from diagnosis.[1] In contrast, other clinicopathological variants of CTCL are generally associated with an excellent long-term prognosis (100% 5-year survival in lymphomatoid papulosis and 90% in primary cutaneous CD30+ large cell anaplastic cutaneous lymphoma), with the exception of patients with subcutaneous panniculitis-like T-cell lymphomas and primary cutaneous natural-killer (NK)-like T-cell/NK cell lymphomas.[1]

Diagnostic tests
The diagnosis of different variants of primary CTCL is based on a critical assessment of the clinicopathological features. Repeated biopsies may be required to establish the diagnosis, and correlation between the histology and clinical features is essential. Immunophenotypic studies are required to identify different CTCL variants, and analysis of T-cell receptor genes in DNA extracted from skin biopsies can identify a T-cell clone, which helps to confirm the diagnosis. However T-cell clones are not always detected in early stages of mycosis fungoides because of a lack of sensitivity. Investigations including a CT scan of the chest, abdomen and pelvis to exclude systemic involvement and assessment of peripheral blood for Sezary cells and lymphocyte subsets are indicated in all patients, with the exception of those with early stages of mycosis fungoides (IA/IB) and lymphomatoid papulosis.[15] Bone marrow aspirate/trephine biopsies are indicated in CTCL variants but rarely in mycosis fungoides and Sezary syndrome.

Aims of treatment
The aim of treatment is to induce complete or partial remissions of disease and to prolong disease-free survival (DFS) and OS, while maintaining the patient's quality of life.

Relevant outcomes
- Severity of symptoms (pruritus, sleep disturbance, pain) and signs (erythema, scaling, fissuring, excoriation, oedema and thickness of plaques, presence of nodules, tumours, peripheral lymphadenopathy)
- Body surface area involvement
- Assessment of overall tumour burden, with histological assessment of skin and lymph nodes, staging CT scans and peripheral blood Sezary cell counts/lymphocyte subsets
- Establishment of molecular remission using T-cell receptor gene analysis of skin and peripheral blood
- Quality of life

Table 27.1 Published outcomes according to clinical stage in cutaneous T-cell lymphoma

	IA	IB	IIA	IIB	III	IVA	IVB	Overall	Reference	No. of patients	Median follow up (years)
Overall survival (%)											
5 years	99	86	49	65		40	0	80	Doorn et al. 2000[8a]	309	5·2
		84		52	57				Zackheim et al. 1999[3b]	489	4·7
	96	(78)		(40)	(40)				Kim et al. 1996[9c]	122	9·8
			73[d]						Kim et al. 1999[10d]	176	8
		73			45	17			Kim et al. 1995[12e]	106	10·5
						15	15		Coninck et al. 2001[11f]	112	8
10 years	84	61	49	27		20	0	57	Doorn et al. 2000[8]	309	5·2
	100	67		39	41				Zackheim et al. 1999[3]	489	4·7
	88	(60)		(20)	(20)				Kim et al. 1996[9]	122	9·8
		58	45[d]						Kim et al. 1999[10]	176	8
						5	5		Coninck et al. 2001[11]	112	8
Disease-free survival (%)											
5 years	100	96	68	80		40	0	89	Doorn et al. 2000[8]	309	5·2
10 years	97	83	68	42		20	0	75	Doorn et al. 2000[8]	309	5·2
	98								Kim et al. 1996[9]	122	9·8
Median survival (years)											
	NR[c]	12·1		2·9	3·6				Kim et al. 1996[9]	556	9·8
		12·8	10·0						Kim et al. 1999[10]	176	8
					4·6	13 mos			Kim et al. 1995[12]	106	10·5
						3 mos	13 mos		Coninck et al. 2001[11]	546	
Disease progression (%)											
5 years	4	21	65	32		70	100		Doorn et al. 2000[8]	309	5·2
10 years	10	39	65	60		70	100		Doorn et al. 2000[8]	309	5·2
20 years	0	10		36	41				Coninck et al. 2001[11]	546	

(Continued)

Table 27.1 (*Continued*)

	IA	IB	IIA	IIB	III	IVA	IVB	Overall	Reference	No. of patients	Median follow up (years)
Overall disease progression											
	9								Kim *et al.* 1996[9]	122	9·8
		20	34[d]						Kim *et al.* 1999[10]	176	8
FFR (%)											
5 years	50								Kim *et al.* 1996[9]	122	9·8
		36	9						Kim *et al.* 1999[10]	176	8
10 years	25 (50)[c]								Kim *et al.* 1996[9]	122	9·8
		31	3						Kim *et al.* 1999[10]	176	8

All overall (OS) survival curves were calculated using the Kaplan–Meier method.

[a]In the study by Doorn et al.[8] the presence of follicular mucinosis was an independent poor prognostic feature possibly related to depth of infiltrate in patients with stage IB disease (disease-free survival of 81% and 36% and OS of 75% and 21% at 5 and 10 years, respectively). A lack of a complete response to initial therapy was also associated with a poor outcome ($P<0.001$) in a multivariate analysis as well as increasing clinical stage and the presence of extracutaneous disease. A different staging system was used in this study (Hamminga et al. *Br J Dermatol* 1982;**107**:145–55) but for the purposes of this table the staging has been altered to be consistent. This study is the only one to provide comprehensive disease-specific survival (DSS) data for different stages of mycosis fungoides. Only three patients had stage IVB disease and only 18 patients each had stage IIA and IVA disease. Therefore the results for these stages must be interpreted cautiously.

[b]In the study by Zackheim et al.[3] black patients had a relatively more advanced stage of disease than white patients. The TNM classification was used in this study. Lymph node stage had an unfavourable impact on survival but this trend did not reach significance for *each individual* T stage because of a lack of sufficient power (an estimated 1700 subjects required) and IIA/IVA patients were not designated separately. Similar considerations apply to peripheral blood involvement. Similar outcomes for patients with stage IIB (T3) and III (T4) disease is consistent with other studies but this might reflect a lack of lymph node staging data included in this study.

[c]The 1996 study by Kim et al.[9] primarily included data on 122 patients with stage IA disease, but survival data on 556 patients with all stages were also included to give the values in parentheses. The freedom from relapse (FFR) data at 5 and 10 years are confusing because the text states that the FFR at 10 years was 25% but the figure indicates that it remains at approximately 50%, as for FFR at 5 years. The median survival for stage IA patients was not reached at 32·5 years. NR, not reached

[d]In the 1999 study by Kim et al.[10] OS at 20 years for stage IB and IIA patients was 27%. DSS was better for patients <58 years of age ($P<0.03$). In 23 of the 56 patients with palpable lymphadenopathy, no histological assessment was made and these patients were assumed to have reactive/dermatopathic nodes (IIA). This might account for the lack of difference in OS at 5 years between stage IB and IIA patients, although there appears to be a difference in OS at 10 years.

[e]In the 1995 study by Kim et al.[12] the OS and median survival data was calculated from the date of initial treatment, which was usually within 3 months of diagnosis. This study also stratified patients into three groups according to the presence of none, one, or two or three poor prognostic parameters, namely: age at presentation (>65 years), the presence of clinical adenopathy, and B1 stage, producing varied median survivals of 10·2 years (no factors), 3·7 years (one factor) and 1·5 years (two or three factors) $P<0.005$.

[f]The study by Connick et al.[11] included 112 patients with extracutaneous disease at presentation or with progression and 434 patients with only cutaneous disease, giving the 546 patients listed in the table for median survival and disease progression.

Several recent trials have used various scoring systems involving computed measures of the above but most studies included in this review define responses in terms of simple clinical observation with CR defined as complete resolution of clinically apparent disease (based in CTCL usually on cutaneous signs of disease) for at least 4–6 weeks. Partial response (PR) is usually defined as >50% reduction of clinical disease or tumour burden, although some studies in CTCL have defined this as >25% reduction in tumour burden. More importantly, most studies do not include a validated scoring system, which effectively makes any interpretation of PR impossible. Similar considerations apply to assessment of stable disease (SD), defined usually as <50% improvement, and progressive disease (PD), defined as >25% increase in tumour burden. For most studies in CTCL, PD is defined as a deterioration in clinical stage of disease.

Methods of search

Systematic reviews, controlled clinical trials and clinical trials were located by searching the *Cochrane Library* (1999–2001) and Medline (1985–2001). Because of a limited number of randomised clinical trials (RCTs) and the overall low incidence of CTCL, some small studies are included and the limitations of such studies are discussed.

QUESTIONS

What are the effects of topical therapy in mycosis fungoides?

Topical corticosteroids
Efficacy

No systematic reviews or RCTs were identified. One large open uncontrolled study of 79 patients with mycosis fungoides (stage T1/T2) who were treated with class I to III (potent/moderate potency) topical corticosteroids twice daily for 3–4 months and under occlusion showed complete clinical remission in 63% and PR in 31% of stage T1 patients and CR and PR in 25% and 57%, respectively, for patients with stage T2.[16] CR was confirmed histologically in seven patients but the median duration of CR was not documented.

Drawbacks

Reversible depression of serum cortisol levels occurred in 13% of patients and skin atrophy in one patient.

Comment

Lack of controlled studies and short median follow up of 9 months weakens the impact of results. No evidence of impact on DSS or OS was reported. However, it does appear that topical corticosteroids, especially class 1 (potent) compounds, are effective at temporarily clearing patches and plaques in some patients with early stage IA/IB mycosis fungoides.

Topical mechlorethamine (nitrogen mustard)
Efficacy

No RCTs were found. A retrospective review of 123 patients treated at one institution (1969–85) with whole-body once-daily application of topical mechlorethamine, (10–20 mg/ml; aqueous preparation from 1968 to 1980 and ointment base from 1980 to 1985) until maximum response reported CR rates of 51% in IA, 26% in IB, 0% in IIB and 22% in stage III disease.[17] There were no differences in outcome with the aqueous or ointment base. Fifty patients had received total skin electron beam (TSEB) therapy before topical mechlorethamine. Relapse occurred in 56% of patients who achieved CR, despite continued maintenance treatment for 1–2 years.[17]

A study of 117 patients reported CR in 76% with stage I disease, 45% with stage II and 49% with stage III patients within 2 years of therapy (median response duration of 45 months).[18] Patients in this study were allowed local radiotherapy for tumours and these were not excluded as responders. Overall 5-year survival for all patients in this study was 89%.

In a retrospective review of 331 patients (all stages; 1968–82) treated with topical mechlorethamine daily and with maintenance therapy daily or alternate days for at least 3 years for those with a CR, a complete remission lasting 4–14 years was observed in 20% but was confined to those with stage IA–IB.[19] However, patients in this series were allowed other therapies including radiotherapy, TSEB, phototherapy and methotrexate to achieve a response. Subsequent relapse occurred in only 17% of these patients within 8 years of withdrawing therapy, suggesting that some patients with very early stage disease may have achieved a cure. Response rates were highest in early stages of disease (IA: 80%; IB: 68%; IIA: 61%; IIB: 49%; III: 60%; IVA:13%; IVB: 11%). Stage-specific 5/10 year survival rates were 94/89% (IA), 85/83% (IB), 82/67% (IIA), 59/31% (IIB), 75/49% (III), 20/13% (IVA) and 11/0% (IVB).[19]

Drawbacks

Topical mechlorethamine may cause an irritant reaction and up to 40% of patients develop contact hypersensitivity. This is less common with the ointment (0·01–0·02%). The aqueous solution (10–20 mg in 40–60 ml water) is less stable than the ointment. Mechlorethamine (nitrogen mustard) is carcinogenic and secondary cutaneous malignancies (non-melanoma skin cancer) have been attributed to long-term use of topical mechlorethamine (8·6-fold and 1·8-fold increased risk for squamous cell carcinoma and basal cell carcinoma respectively). Home use is acceptable, with patients applying topical treatment overnight; however, partners should avoid contact,

especially if pregnant. Appropriate protection for staff members applying topical therapy in the hospital setting is required although no toxic effects have been reported.[20]

Comments

Mechlorethamine is an effective topical therapy for early-stage (patches/thin plaques) mycosis fungoides. However, interpretation of the studies is confounded by the use of other therapeutic modalities for most patients and the retrospective nature of the studies. Duration of response varies, and the efficacy of maintenance therapy (6–18 months) and whole-body application remains unclear, but some patients with stage IA disease may be cured. The survival data reported for topical mechlorethamine are similar to those previously published for patients with early-stage disease (Table 27.1). Any clinical efficacy of topical mechlorethamine therapy after TSEB therapy has to be confirmed. Almost all patients with stage IA mycosis fungoides have a normal life expectancy and so controlled trials are required.

Topical carmustine (BCNU)
Efficacy

A retrospective review of therapy in 143 patients revealed CRs in 86% of stage IA patients, 47% in stage IB patients, 55% in stage IIA patients, 17% in stage IIB patients, 21% in stage III patients and 0% in stage IV patients.[21] Median time to CR was 11·5 weeks. Alternate day or daily treatment with 10 mg BCNU in dilute (95%) alcohol (60 ml) or 20–40% BCNU ointment can be used.

Drawbacks

Contact hypersensitivity is uncommon (10%) but bone marrow suppression is common (30%). The risk of secondary cutaneous malignancies may be lower than with mechlorethamine. Total doses should not exceed 600 mg per course, and repeated courses may be required. Maintenance therapy should be avoided. The ointment is more stable than the alcohol solution (3 months).

Comments

Limited data suggest that topical carmustine is clinically effective but is more extensively absorbed than mechlorethamine and therefore has a significant risk of bone marrow suppression. It may help in patients with early-stage disease who show an irritant or allergic contact reaction to mechlorethamine. Comparative trials are needed.

Topical retinoids
Efficacy

No RCTs were found. A phase I/II open study of 0.1–1% bexarotene (Targretin) gel as incremental doses in 67 patients with stage IA/IB/IIA disease (initially alternate day treatment, increasing to a maximum of four-times daily treatment if tolerated) showed a response rate of 63%, with 21% of patients showing a complete clinical response.[22] Median time to and duration of response were 20 and 99 weeks, respectively.

Drawbacks

Bexarotene 1% gel twice daily was well tolerated. Mild/moderate pruritus, burning pain and rash (12% irritant contact dermatitis) were common.

Comment

The lack of a placebo control makes interpretation difficult but the US Food & Drug Administration (FDA) has approved 1% Targretin gel for the treatment of patients with stage IA/IB disease. Further studies are required.

Topical peldesine (BCX-34)

Peldesine is an inhibitor of purine nucleoside phosphorylase, an enzyme involved in purine degradation within lymphocytes.

Efficacy

One RCT has compared topical application of peldesine twice daily to the entire skin surface for 24 weeks with a placebo (vehicle control) in 90 patients with stage IA/IB mycosis fungoides.[23] Partial or complete clinical responses occurred in 28% of patients treated with peldesine and 24% of patients treated with placebo ($P = 0.677$).

Drawbacks

A minority of patients noted minor pruritus and rash.

Comment

This is the only published placebo-controlled trial in CTCL. Although no significant efficacy is apparent, the results indicate a high placebo therapeutic response (mostly PR), which should be considered when interpreting the efficacy of different topical therapies in early-stage mycosis fungoides. This study also emphasises the importance of developing a validated scoring system to assess PR.

What are the effects of phototherapy in mycosis fungoides/Sezary syndrome?

Phototherapy
Efficacy

No RCTs were found. Broadband UVB (290–320 nm) phototherapy with maintenance therapy produced CR in 83% of 35 patients with early-stage disease (IA/IB) with a median response time of 5 months and median response duration of 22 months.[24]

Narrowband UVB (TL-01; 311–313 nm) also produces CR in 75% of patients (6/8 cases with early patch-stage (IA) disease) with a mean duration of response of 20 months.[25]

High-dose UVA1 phototherapy (340–400 nm; 100 J/cm^2 on a 5 day per week basis) has been used in 13 patients (8 stage IB, four stage IIB and one stage III) until maximal response. Eleven of the 13 patients showed a CR, defined as a complete resolution of cutaneous lesions (mean number of sessions 22; cumulative dose 2149 J/cm^2) and seven patients remained in CR after a mean follow up of 7·2 months.[26]

Drawbacks

One drawback is UV-induced erythema. In addition, high cumulative doses of UVA contribute to an increased risk of non-melanoma skin cancer.

Comments

UVB phototherapy is an effective therapy for early patch and thin plaques but duration of disease-free remission varies and treatment probably does not affect long-term survival rates. UVA1 penetrates more deeply than UVB and PUVA but whether this is clinically relevant has not yet been established. No adequate comparative studies between different forms of phototherapy and PUVA have been published.

PUVA photochemotherapy
Efficacy

No RCTs were found. An open study of 82 patients treated with PUVA and followed for up to 15 years reported an overall CR rate of 65% (79% for stage IA, 59% for stage IB and 83% for stage IIA disease) and mean cumulative doses of 134 J/cm^2 (IA), 140 J/cm^2 (IB) and 240 J/cm^2 (IIA), with median time to CR of 3 months.[27] Few patients with more advanced disease were treated, making interpretation of results for patients with stage >IIA difficult. In this study, 67% of stage IA, 41% of stage IB and 67% of stage IIA patients were free of disease at 2 years but maintenance PUVA was given to most patients.[27] Survival rates at 5 and 10 years were 89% for stage IA, 78% for stage IB and, surprisingly, 100% for stage IIA.

A further open study of PUVA in 82 patients with CTCL showed CR in 62% of patients, with 88% CR in stage IA (mean cumulative PUVA dose 160 J/cm^2), 52% in stage IB (498 J/cm^2) and 46% in stage III disease (178 J/cm^2). No responses were seen in stage IIB patients. The maximum duration of response was 68 months; 38% of complete responders relapsed despite maintenance PUVA.[28]

Although maintenance therapy has been recommended for responders, a further open study has shown that 56% of stage IA and 39% of stage IB patients with CR had no recurrence of CTCL during a maximum period of 44 months follow up, despite no maintenance therapy.[29]

Drawbacks

Nausea, phototoxic reactions and skin carcinogenesis are well-recognised adverse effects. The risk of non-melanoma skin cancer is directly related to the cumulative dose and total number of sessions.

Comments

Despite the lack of controlled trials, PUVA remains one of the most useful skin-directed therapies for early stages of mycosis fungoides. RCTs comparing PUVA with TL-01 and topical mechlorethamine would be helpful in early-stage disease (IA/IB). Duration of response and DFS/OS data are also urgently required. The role of maintenance therapy is unclear but high cumulative doses entail a significant risk of squamous cell carcinoma. DFS and OS rates in patients treated with topical chemotherapy, phototherapy and TSEB are difficult to compare without RCTs, but there appears to be little difference in early-stage disease, which emphasises the urgent need for RCTs.

Combination regimens involving photochemotherapy
Efficacy

An RCT has compared PUVA, 2–5 times weekly, plus alfa interferon, 9 MU three times weekly, with alfa interferon plus acitretin, 25–50 mg/day, in 98 patients (maximum duration of treatment in both groups 48 weeks).[30] In 82 patients with stage I/II diseases, CR rates were 70% in the PUVA/interferon group compared with 38% in the interferon/acitretin group (P<0·05). Responses were assessed on the basis of clinical observation only. Time to response was 18·6 weeks in the PUVA/interferon, compared with 21·8 weeks in the interferon/acitretin group (P = 0·026) but no data on duration of response was reported. Total cumulative doses of alfa interferon were similar in both groups.

An open study of 69 patients compared PUVA and acitretin with PUVA alone in mycosis fungoides.[31] This showed that the cumulative dose of PUVA to achieve a CR was lower in the combined-treatment group, although the overall CR was similar in the two groups (73% and 72%, respectively). No data on duration of response was documented.[31]

Phase I and II studies of PUVA (three times weekly) combined with variable doses of alfa interferon (maximum tolerated dose of 12 MU/m^2 three times weekly) in 39 patients with mycosis fungoides (all stages) and Sezary syndrome have reported an overall response (OR) rate of 100%: 62% showing CR and 28% PR. (CR rates

were 79% in stage IB patients, 80% in IIA patients, 33% in stage IIB patients, 63% in stage III patients and 40% in stage IVA patients).[32] PUVA was continued as a maintenance therapy indefinitely while alfa interferon was continued for 2 years or until disease progression or withdrawal due to adverse effects. The median response duration was 28 months, with a median survival of 62 months.[32]

Drawbacks

These were as for PUVA, alfa interferon and acitretin alone. In the RCT[30] similar rates of mild/moderate adverse effects were noted in both groups but more patients discontinued treatment in the interferon/acitretin group because of adverse effects.

Comments

This RCT is one of very few in CTCL and it shows that combined PUVA and interferon alfa is more effective than interferon alfa or acitretin in early stage I/II disease. Weaknesses of this study are the lack of a validated scoring system to assess tumour burden and lack of evidence that outcome was assessed blind to allocation status. In addition, data regarding the duration of response and DFS/OS are urgently required. The trial comparing PUVA alone with PUVA plus acitretin[31] suggests a reduction in mean cumulative dose of PUVA to CR, which would be helpful; disappointingly, however, there is no evidence for increased overall efficacy in the retinoid-PUVA group. The combination of alfa interferon and PUVA appears to be highly effective in all stages of CTCL. An RCT comparing PUVA alone with PUVA plus alfa interferon has recently closed (2001) and the results are awaited.

What are the effects of immunotherapy in mycosis fungoides/Sezary syndrome?

Interferon alfa
Efficacy
No RCTs of alfa interferon in CTCL have been reported, except as combination therapy (see above).

In an open study, 20 heavily pretreated patients (stage IB-III) were given maximum tolerated doses of alfa interferon (50 MU/m² intramuscularly three times weekly) for 3 months.[33] An OR rate of 45% was reported, with a median response duration to maximum tolerated doses of alfa interferon of 5 months.

A subsequent non-randomised study revealed response rates of 64% in 22 patients (stage IA–IVA) with an overall CR rate of 27%.[34] Objective responses were greater in the group treated with an escalating-dose schedule of alfa interferon (36 MU/day) compared with those on a low-dose regimen (3 MU/day) for 10 weeks (78% versus 37%) but overall numbers were too small for statistical comparison.

An open study of 43 patients treated with escalating doses (3–18 MU daily) of alfa interferon showed an OR rate of 74%, with a CR rate of 26%.[35] Responses were more common in those who had not had prior treatment and in those with stage I/II (88%) than in those with stage III/IV (63%) disease. DFS was 21% at 55 months.

A phase II study of intermittent high-dose interferon alfa-2a given on days 1–5 every 3 weeks (mean dose 65·5 MU/m²/week) showed a response rate of 29%, with only one CR in 24 patients with advanced (IVA/B) refractory CTCL.[36] Dose reductions were necessary and no improved responses were seen in those patients receiving dose escalation.

In an open study, 45 patients with CTCL, including 13 patients with Sezary syndrome, received low-dose alfa interferon (6–9 MU daily) for 3 months and those responding were continued on alfa interferon alone while non-responders were given alfa interferon plus acitretin, 0·5 mg/kg/day.[37] After 12 months' therapy 62% achieved PR or CR, including 11 patients on combined therapy. However, this study design does not exclude the possibility that the response in the alfa interferon non-responder group was due to a delayed efficacy from continued alfa interferon therapy after 3 months.

Intralesional alfa interferon (1–2 MU three times weekly for 4 weeks) can induce complete regression of individual plaques (10 of 12 sites) compared with placebo-treated sites (1 of 12 sites).[38]

Drawbacks
Dose-limiting toxicity of alfa interferon includes reversible haematological abnormalities, hepatitis, weight loss, headache, depression, and flu-like symptoms consisting of fever, myalgia, lethargy and anorexia.

Comments
The clinical efficacy of alfa interferon in all stages of CTCL is supported by the CR rates seen in these uncontrolled studies and it appears that higher doses are more effective, but dose-limiting toxicity is a problem. Critical questions remain about the effect on DFS and OS and the role of combined therapy with PUVA. RCTs are required to address these issues.

Interferon gamma
Efficacy
No RCTs were found. A phase II trial of imtramuscular gamma interferon in 16 CTCL patients with escalating doses to a maximum of

0·5 mg/m^2 daily reported objective PR of 31%, with a median duration of 10 months.[39]

Drawbacks
As for alfa interferon.

Comments
The lack of CR is disappointing. Further studies are required but are a low priority.

Interleukins
Efficacy
No RCTs were found. Interleukin (IL)-2 (20 MU/m^2 every 2 weeks for 6 weeks and then monthly for 5 months) produced responses in five of seven CTCL patients, including CR in three.[40]

In a phase I dose-escalation study of subcutaneous IL-12 (50–300 ng/kg) twice weekly for up to 24 weeks, objective responses were noted in five CTCL patients (4/5 with stage IB disease; 1/3 with Sezary syndrome).[41] Two patients with stage IB disease had a CR within 7–8 weeks, which was confirmed histologically. Intralesional therapy was also effective for individual tumours in two patients with stage IIB disease, but both developed progressive disease.[41]

Drawbacks
Side-effects were minor and included flu-like symptoms, mild transient liver function abnormalities and depression.

Comments
RCTs are required to establish whether IL-2 and IL-12 have any therapeutic role in CTCL.

Extracorporeal photopheresis
Efficacy
No RCTs were reported. A systematic review (1987–98) of response rates and outcomes in open non-randomised and mostly retrospective studies of extracorporeal photopheresis (ECP) in erythrodermic CTCL (stage III/IVA) showed an OR rate of 35–71%, with CR rates of 14–26%.[42] Responses have been assessed mostly using a similar scoring system to that devised for the original study.[43]

A further retrospective study of 34 patients with mostly erythrodermic CTCL (22 stage IV, 10 stage III, and 2 stage I) reported an OR rate of 50%, with 18% achieving CR.[44] Response was restricted to those with erythrodermic disease. This study involved a modified "accelerated" treatment schedule consisting of nine (as opposed to six) collections during each cycle and an increase to twice-monthly treatment if there was a lack of response.

Other studies have reported minor responses (25–50% improvement) but this would not satisfy accepted criteria for PR. ECP is generally administered on two consecutive days (one cycle) each month and it is accepted that at least six cycles are required to assess response. Survival data have been reported in four studies of erythrodermic disease, with median survivals of 39–100 months from diagnosis.[45–48]

A randomised crossover study comparing ECP with PUVA in patients with non-erythrodermic (stage IB–IIA) mycosis fungoides has shown no clinical efficacy for ECP in early stages of the disease compared with PUVA.[49] In contrast, other uncontrolled studies have reported successful responses in patients with non-erythrodermic disease.

A 9-year retrospective study of ECP alone in 37 patients (68% stage IB, 5% stage IIB, 27% stage III) showed a CR rate of 14% and a PR rate of 41%, with an improved response rate in resistant patients with the addition of alfa interferon.[50]

A prospective open non-randomised study of 14 patients with non-erythrodermic mycosis fungoides (stage IIA/IIB) treated with combined alfa interferon (maximum tolerated dose of 18 MU three times weekly) and ECP for 6 months showed a CR in four and a PR in three (OR 50%) but this design does not exclude responses to alfa interferon alone.[51]

A non-randomised retrospective study in erythrodermic disease (stage III/IVA) (1991–1996) showed that six of nine patients treated with alfa interferon plus ECP showed a response (with four CRs) while only one of 10 patients treated with ECP alone achieved a CR. In the patients achieving a CR, lymph node disease also resolved.[52] In contrast, the combination of alfa interferon plus ECP failed to produce significant clinical responses in six patients with Sezary syndrome,[53] although isolated case reports have described patients with Sezary syndrome in whom a complete clinical and molecular remission has been achieved with this combination.[54,55]

A retrospective non-randomised study (1974–97) has compared DSS and OS in 44 patients with erythrodermic CTCL treated with either TSEB alone or TSEB and adjuvant or neoadjuvant ECP (see below).

Drawbacks
ECP is well tolerated. Mild lymphopenia and anaemia can occur with long-term therapy. High cost and lack of availability means that ECP will remain confined to specialist centres.

Comments
Controlled trials are urgently required to compare ECP with standard single-agent chemotherapy regimens in erythrodermic disease and specifically in Sezary syndrome. Some previous studies have not clearly defined their diagnostic criteria for erythrodermic CTCL and others have included patients with non-erythrodermic disease. Combination therapy with ECP and alfa interferon is frequently used but the existing studies do not exclude a beneficial response to alfa interferon alone. An RCT to address this important issue is currently being considered by the European Organisation for the Research and Treatment of Cancer (EORTC). Studies suggest that ECP requires a minimum tumour burden within peripheral blood[56] and the only RCT of ECP in non-erythrodermic, early-stage disease suggests that it is not effective.

Thymopentin
Efficacy
In a phase II trial, 20 patients with Sezary syndrome were treated with 50 mg intravenous thymopentin (TP-5), a synthetic pentapeptide, three times weekly for a mean of 16 months. The OR rate was 75%, with 8 CRs and seven PRs and a median duration of 22 months. Four-year survival was 54%.[57]

Drawbacks
Thymopentin was well tolerated. Mild hypersensitivity reactions during the infusion were noted.

Comments
The mechanism of action of thymopentin remains unclear. The OR rate is very high but the lack of subsequent reports is surprising and further studies are required to confirm this data.

Ciclosporin
Efficacy
A phase II trial of ciclosporin, 15 mg/kg/day, in 16 patients with refractory T-cell lymphomas, including 11 CTCL (all stage IVA/B), revealed only two responses in CTCL, with eight CTCL patients developing progressive disease; there

was one drug-related death.[58] The two patients showing a PR had a rapid relapse of disease when treatment was discontinued.

Drawbacks
High doses of ciclosporin are poorly tolerated and frequent dose reductions are required. Hypertension, renal toxicity and infection were common.

Comments
This study suggests that ciclosporin is not effective in CTCL and anecdotal reports suggest that ciclosporin can actually cause rapid disease progression in CTCL.

> What are the effects of systemic retinoids in mycosis fungoides/Sezary syndrome?

Etretinate/acitretin/isotretinoin
Efficacy
A systematic review (1988–94) of open studies of oral retinoids in CTCL (mycosis fungoides and Sezary syndrome) showed an overall mean response rate of 58% and a CR rate of 19%, with a median duration of response of 3–13 months.[59]

A non-randomised study of 68 patients with various stages of mycosis fungoides and Sezary syndrome compared 13-*cis*-retinoic acid with etretinate and showed similar efficacy and toxicity (isotretinoin: CR 21%; PR 38%; etretinate: CR 21%; PR 46%).[60] A phase II study of isotretinoin in 25 patients with mycoses fungoides (IB–III) showed an OR rate of 44%, three patients achieving a CR, and a median response duration of 8 months using high doses (2 mg/kg/day).[61]

An RCT comparing PUVA and alfa interferon with PUVA and acitretin showed a significantly better response rate for PUVA and alfa interferon[30] (see above).

Drawbacks
Adverse events included mucocutaneous erosions and xerosis, hyperlipidaemia, hepatotoxicity and teratogenicity.

Comments
Acitretin and etretinate have some efficacy in the early stages of disease, but are no better and probably less effective than, for example, PUVA and alfa interferon.

Bexarotene
Bexarotene is a new retinoid capable of binding to the RXR as opposed to the RAR retinoid receptor. This drug has antiproliferative and pro-apoptotic properties.

Efficacy
No RCTs were found. A phase II open trial compared two doses (6·5 mg/m^2/day and 650 mg/m^2/day) of oral bexarotene in 58 patients with refractory stage IA–IIA CTCL.[62] The optimal dose was 300 mg/m^2/day in terms of response and tolerability. Objective responses of 20%, 54% and 67% were noted at the 6·5, 300 and 650 mg/m^2/day doses, respectively. Rates of disease progression were 47%, 21% and 13%, respectively. Median duration of response at the highest dose level was 516 days. In late stages of disease (stage IIB–IVB) OR rates of 45% (at 300 mg/m^2/day) and 55% (at doses >300 mg/m^2/day) have been reported with a relapse rate of 36% and projected median duration of response of 299 days.[63]

Drawbacks
Reversible adverse effects included hyperlipidaemia, central hypothyroidism, leucopenia, headache and asthenia as well as other retinoid adverse effects.

Comments
These studies suggest a therapeutic efficacy for bexarotene in all stages of CTCL

but comparisons with other therapies and data on effects on DFS and OS in later stages of disease are required. An EORTC RCT comparing PUVA with PUVA and bexarotene in stage IB is due to start enrolment shortly.

What are the effects of antibody and toxin therapies in mycosis fungoides/Sezary syndrome?

Anti-CD4 monoclonal antibody
Efficacy
In a phase I/II trial seven patients with mycosis fungoides were treated with a chimeric (murine/human) anti-CD4 monoclonal antibody with successive increasing doses (10, 20, 40 and 80 mg) twice weekly for 3 weeks. All patients showed some clinical response, with one CR and two PR, but these were all short lived (median duration of 2 weeks).[64]

A subsequent study from the same group showed PR in 7/8 patients given higher doses (50–200 mg), with median freedom from progression of 28 weeks.[65]

Drawbacks
Treatment was well tolerated with no acute toxicity. There is a marked but temporary suppression of T-cell proliferative responses to phytohaemaglutinin. There is no documented depletion of CD4 counts. The immunogenicity of the antibody is unclear.

CAMPATH-1H
Efficacy
As part of a phase II trial in advanced low-grade non-Hodgkin's lymphoma, eight patients with mycoses fungoides received 30 mg intravenous CAMPATH-1H three times weekly for a maximum of 12 weeks.[66] Fifty per cent of CTCL patients achieved a response, with two (25%) showing CR. No details of duration of response were provided.

Drawbacks
Severe neutropenia and opportunistic infections were common.

Comments
CAMPATH-1H is a humanised anti-CD52 antibody which binds to all lymphocytes. This study suggests that patients with CTCL show the highest response rate but infectious complications leading to death do occur. Further studies are justified.

Denileukin diftitox (diphtheria IL-2 fusion toxin)
Efficacy
A phase III open uncontrolled study of denileukin diftitox in 71 patients with stage IB–IVA CTCL has shown an OR rate of 30%, with 10% showing a complete clinical response.[67] Only CTCL cases with biopsies showing >20% CD25+ (IL-2R) lymphocytes were enrolled. Median duration of response was 6·9 months. No difference in response rates or duration of response was noted between 9 and 18 micrograms/kg/day. The development of anti-denileukin diftitox antibodies apparently did not affect response rates.

Drawbacks
Adverse effects include flu-like symptoms, acute infusion-related hypersensitivity effects, a vascular leak syndrome and transient elevations of hepatic enzymes.

Comments
This uncontrolled study suggests that CD25+ CTCL can respond to this new fusion toxin but

the duration of response is short. However, patients recruited for this trial were heavily pretreated, suggesting that this is likely to be a useful additional therapy for CTCL patients with resistant disease, despite potential adverse effects. A randomised placebo-controlled trial in patients with stage IB/IIB/III mycosis fungoides who have undergone fewer than three previous treatments is ongoing.

Ricin-labelled anti-CD5 immunoconjugate (H65-RTA)
Efficacy
A phase I trial of H65-RTA in 14 patients with resistant CTCL revealed a maximum tolerated dose of 0·33 mg/kg/day and PR in only four patients of short duration (3–8 months).[68]

Drawbacks
Acute hypersensitivity effects and vascular leak syndrome were noted.

Radioimmunoconjugate (90Y-T101)
Efficacy
A phase I trial of this radioimmunoconjugate (which also targets CD5+ lymphocytes) in 10 patients (CD5+) with haematological malignancies, of whom eight patients had CTCL, showed PR in three CTCL patients with a median response duration of 23 weeks.[69] Biodistribution studies showed good uptake into skin and involved lymph nodes.

Drawbacks
Bone-marrow suppression was observed. T cells recovered within 3 weeks but B-cell suppression persisted after 5 weeks.

Comments
This is an interesting phase I study because CTCL is a radiosensitive tumour. Further studies are required.

What are the effects of radiotherapy in mycosis fungoides/Sezary syndrome?

Superficial radiotherapy
Efficacy
No systematic reviews or RCTs were identified. Dose–response studies have clearly established that localised superficial radiotherapy is an effective palliative therapy for individual lesions in mycosis fungoides.[70] A retrospective study of palliative superficial radiotherapy used to treat 191 lesions from 20 patients with mycosis fungoides showed CRs of 95% for plaques and small (<3 cm) tumours and a CR of 93% for large tumours (>3 cm), irrespective of dose. However in-field recurrences within 1–2 years were more common for those lesions treated with lower doses (42% for <1000 cGy, 32% for 1000–2000 cGy, 21% for 2000–3000 cGy and 0% for >3000 cGy).

Drawbacks
Superficial radiation is well tolerated. Mild erythema and occasional erosion have been reported. Use of low-dose/energy (400 cGy in 2–3 daily fractions at 80–150 Kv) is therapeutically effective and allows treatment of overlapping fields and lower limb sites.

Comments
CTCL is a highly radiosensitive malignancy, and localised superficial radiotherapy is an invaluable palliative therapy for patients with all stages of mycosis fungoides. Treatment should be palliative except for patients with solitary localised disease where "cure" is possible. Although in-field recurrence rates were very low for lesions treated with >3000 cGy, the number of lesions treated with this dose was very low compared with the other groups and this form of therapy is only palliative in mycosis fungoides because disease is multifocal. Therefore the use of high-dose fractionation regimens for individual

lesions should be avoided in mycosis fungoides because CR rates are similar to those for low-dose regimens (see above) and recurrent disease adjacent to previously treated fields can be treated with overlapping fields if necessary. However, treatment of disease on the lower legs can be difficult in view of a higher risk of radiation necrosis with repeated treatments.

Total skin electron beam therapy (TSEB)
Efficacy
A systematic review (meta-analysis) of open uncontrolled and mostly retrospective studies of TSEB as monotherapy for 952 patients with all stages of CTCL has established that the rate of CR is dependent on stage of disease, skin surface dose and energy, with CR rates of 96% in stage IA/IB/IIA disease, 36% in stage IIB disease and 60% in stage III disease.[71] Greater skin surface dose (32–36 Gy) and higher energy (4–6 MeV electrons) were significantly associated with a higher rate of CR; 5-year relapse-free survivals of 10–23% were noted.[71]

An RCT has compared TSEB with topical mechlorethamine in 42 patients, with similar rates of CR and duration of response in both groups in early stages of disease but better ORs in later stages of disease with TSEB.[72]

A retrospective study of TSEB (median dose 32 Gy; median treatment time 21 days) as monotherapy for 45 patients with erythrodermic CTCL (28 stage III, 13 stage IVA, 4 stage IVB) showed a 60% CR rate, with 26% disease free at 5 years.[73] Overall median survival was 3·4 years, which was associated significantly with an absence of peripheral blood involvement (stage III disease). Higher rates of CR (74%) and disease-free progression (36%) were noted in those patients receiving a more intense regimen (32–40 Gy and 4–6 MeV).

A retrospective study of 66 CTCL patients (1978–96) treated with 30 Gy in far fewer fractions (12 fractions over 40 days) showed a CR rate of 65% with progression-free survival of 30% at 5 years and 18% at 10 years.[74] Responses and specifically 5-year OS were highest in those with early-stage disease (79–93% for IA/IB/III compared with 44% for IIB/IVA/B).

Although it has been recommended that TSEB can only be given once in a lifetime, several reports have described multiple courses in CTCL.[75,76] A retrospective analysis of 15 patients (1968–90) with mycosis fungoides who received two courses of TSEB reported a mean dose of 32·6 Gy for the first course and 23·4 Gy for the second, with a mean interval of 41·3 months. No additional toxicities were noted but the CR rate for the second course was lower (40% compared with 73%).[75] A further retrospective study of 14 patients with CTCL revealed a mean dose of 36 Gy for the first (93% CR) and 18 Gy for the second course (86% CR).[76] In this series five patients received a third course (total dose 12–30 Gy). The median duration of response was 20 months for the first and 11·5 months for the second course. No additional toxicities were reported. In both of these studies the fractionation regimens employed may have been critical for tolerability (1 Gy per day at 6 MeV over 9–12 weeks).

Combination TSEB regimens
An RCT in 103 CTCL patients comparing TSEB and multi-agent chemotherapy (CAVE) with sequential topical therapy including superficial radiotherapy and phototherapy revealed a higher CR rate in the TSEB/chemotherapy group (38% compared with 18%; $P = 0·032$) but after a median follow up of 75 months DFS and OS did not differ significantly.[77]

A retrospective non-randomised study comparing TSEB (32–40 Gy) alone with TSEB followed by

ECP (given 2 days monthly for a median of 6 months) in 44 patients with erythrodermic CTCL (57% stage III, 30% stage IVA, 13% stage IVB/overall 59% had haematological involvement B1) has reported an overall CR rate of 73% after TSEB, with a 3-year DFS of 49% for 17 patients who received only TSEB (OS 63%) and 81% for 15 patients who received TSEB followed by ECP (OS 88%).[78] A multivariate analysis suggested that the combination of TSEB and ECP was significantly associated with a prolonged disease-free and cause-specific survival when corrected for peripheral blood involvement (B1) and stage of disease.

Drawbacks

Adverse effects of TSEB include radiation-induced secondary cutaneous malignancies, telangiectasia, pigmentation, anhidrosis, pruritus, alopecia and xerosis. Treatment is generally only given once in a lifetime, but several reports suggest that multiple therapies may be tolerated (see above).

Comments

Although these studies are uncontrolled and mostly retrospective, the response rates indicate that TSEB is highly effective for CTCL. The lack of a long-term response in early-stage disease suggests that TSEB should be reserved for later stages of disease, particularly as an RCT has indicated that responses are similar for TSEB and topical mechlorethamine. Meta-analysis of observational data indicates that higher dosage regimens are more effective (32–40 Gy with 4–6 MeV).

Although an RCT in CTCL indicates that combined TSEB and chemotherapy is no more effective than sequential skin-directed therapy, a further trial comparing TSEB alone with TSEB and chemotherapy in late stages of disease (stage IIB) would be helpful. The current data on

long-term DFS and OS in erythrodermic CTCL suggest that TSEB is effective, particularly if combined with ECP, but this requires confirmation in an RCT.

> What are the effects of single-agent chemotherapy in mycosis fungoides/Sezary syndrome?

Single-agent chemotherapy regimens
Efficacy

No RCTs have been reported. A systematic review of uncontrolled open studies of single-agent regimens in 526 CTCL patients (1988–1994) revealed OR rates of 62%, with a CR rate of 33% and median response durations of 3–22 months.[59] These therapies included alkylating agents (chlorambucil and cyclophosphamide), antimetabolites (methotrexate), vinca alkaloids and topoisomerase II inhibitors.

Drawbacks

As with all chemotherapy regimens, infection and myelosuppression are significant risks.

Comments

The lack of controlled studies makes interpretation difficult but single-agent regimens may have similar efficacy to combination regimens (see below) but with lower toxicity and therefore may be preferable as palliative therapy in late stages of mycosis fungoides and Sezary syndrome, especially as durable responses and cures are rarely, if ever, achieved. RCTs are urgently required.

Methotrexate
Efficacy

No RCTs were identified. A retrospective report of low-dose methotrexate in 29 patients with erythrodermic CTCL (III/IVA) has shown a 41%

complete remission rate, with an OR of 58%.[79] Median freedom from treatment failure was 31 months and OS was 8·4 years. Weekly doses ranged from 5 to 125 mg for a median duration of 23 months. A majority (62%) of patients satisfied criteria for a diagnosis of Sezary syndrome.

Drawbacks

Adverse effects included reversible abnormalities of liver function, mucositis, cutaneous erosions, reversible leucopenia and thrombocytopenia, nausea, diarrhoea and, in one case, pulmonary fibrosis.

Comments

Although these data are uncontrolled, the OS in this cohort is surprisingly good. A randomised study comparing methotrexate with other single-agent chemotherapies in erythrodermic CTCL would be worthwhile.

Purine analogues
Efficacy

No RCTs were found. A systematic review of purine analogues in CTCL (1988–94) revealed overall and CR rates, respectively, of 41% and 6% for deoxycoformycin (n = 63), 41% and 19% for 2-chlorodeoxyadenosine (n = 27), and 19% and 3% for fludarabine (n = 31).[59] Most of these studies included some patients with peripheral T-cell lymphomas. No comparative studies were available.

A prospective open study of deoxycoformycin in 28 heavily pretreated patients, of whom 21 had CTCL (14 Sezary syndrome, seven stage IIB) revealed an OR rate of 71%, with 25% CR and 46% PR (OR: 10/14 patients with Sezary syndrome; four CR, and 4/7 stage IIB patients; one CR). Response was short lived (median duration of 2 months for stage IIB disease and 3·5 months for Sezary syndrome) except in two

cases of Sezary syndrome with remissions for 17 and 19 months. The regimen consisted of starting doses of 3·75–5·0mg/m^2/day for 3 days every 3 weeks. A dose escalation to 6·25 mg/m^2/day was rarely possible because of toxicity.[80]

Two recent open studies of deoxycoformycin in CTCL (27 mycosis fungoides and 37 Sezary syndrome) patients have shown OR rates ranging from 35% to 56%, with CR rates from 10% to 33% and a reported median disease-free interval of 9 months in one of the studies.[81,82] Interestingly, responses were better in Sezary syndrome than mycosis fungoides. The usual schedule for deoxycoformycin consists of a once-weekly intravenous dose of 4 mg/m^2 for 4 weeks and then every 14 days for either 6 months or until maximal response.

Combination therapy consisting of deoxycoformycin and alfa interferon in CTCL has shown OR and CR rates of 41% and 5%, respectively.[83]

A recent phase II trial of 2-chlorodeoxyadenosine in 21 refractory CTCL patients (mycosis fungoides IIB/IV and Sezary syndrome) revealed an OR rate of 28%, with 14% CR (median duration of 4·5 months) and 14% PR (median duration of 2 months).[84]

Drawbacks

Side-effects include nausea, infections (especially herpetic), CD4 lymphopenia, renal toxicity, hepatotoxicity and myelosuppression (especially for 2-chlorodeoxyadenosine and fludarabine).

Comments

Purine analogues are attractive therapeutic candidates for CTCL because they are potent inhibitors of the enzyme adenosine deaminase, which preferentially accumulates in lymphoid cells, such that these drugs are selectively lymphocytotoxic independently of cell division. Although efficacy in CTCL is moderate, most of these patients were heavily pretreated and relatively chemoresistant. Patients with Sezary syndrome appear to respond better than those with late stages of mycosis fungoides. Purine analogues are appropriate as monotherapy, especially in Sezary syndrome, but response duration may be short. Comparative trials with other single-agent regimens in Sezary syndrome are required.

Gemcitabine
Efficacy

A phase II prospective trial (1200 mg/m^2 weekly for 3 weeks each month for a total of three cycles) in 44 previously treated patients with CTCL (30 mycosis fungoides patients with stage IIB or III disease) reported a PR rate of 59% and a CR rate of 12%, with median durations of 10 and 15 months, respectively.[85]

Drawbacks

Treatment was well tolerated and only mild haematological toxicity was noted.

Comments

Gemcitabine is a new pyrimidine antimetabolite which appears to be well tolerated in heavily pretreated patients with advanced stages of mycosis fungoides. Further trials are required.

Doxorubicin
Efficacy

An open study of pegylated liposomal doxorubicin, 20 mg/m^2 monthly to a maximum of 400 mg or eight cycles, in 10 patients with various stages of mycosis fungoides revealed a CR in six and PR in two patients, with a median response duration of 15 months.[86]

Drawbacks

Mild haematological toxicity was reported.

Comments

An EORTC phase II trial in advanced stages of mycosis fungoides (>IIB) is due to start enrolment shortly.

What are the effects of multiagent chemotherapy regimens in mycosis fungoides/Sezary syndrome?

Combination chemotherapy
Efficacy

An RCT in 103 CTCL patients comparing TSEB and multiagent chemotherapy (CAVE) with sequential topical therapy including superficial radiotherapy and phototherapy revealed a higher CR rate in the TSEB/chemotherapy group (38% compared with 18%; $P = 0.032$ with OR rates of 90% and 65%, respectively) but after a median follow up of 75 months there was no significant difference in DFS or OS.[77]

A systematic review of all systemic therapy in CTCL (mycoses fungoides and Sezary syndrome, 1988–94) showed an OR rate of 81% in 331 patients treated with various different combination chemotherapeutic regimens, with a CR rate of 38% and response duration ranging from 5 to 41 months, with no documented cures for patients with late stages of disease (IIB–IVB).[59]

Recent prospective non-randomised studies of different multiagent chemotherapy regimens have revealed similar OR rates. A third-generation anthracycline (idarubicin) was used in combination with etoposide, cyclophosphamide, vincristine, prednisolone and bleomycin (VICOP-B) to treat 25 CTCL patients (eight stage IIB, 13 IVA, four stage IVB) for 12 weeks. OR rates of 80%, with 36% CR, were documented, although

10 patients had not received any previous therapy. The two patients with Sezary syndrome did not respond and the median duration of response in patients with mycoses fungoides was 8·7 months. Stage IIB patients had a median duration of response of 22 months but four previously untreated patients received additional TSEB therapy after completion of chemotherapy.[87]

A combination of etoposide, vincristine, doxorubicin, cyclophosphamide and prednisolone (EPOCH) was used to treat 15 patients with advanced, refractory CTCL (six with Sezary syndrome; four with stage-IVB mycoses fungoides, one with adult T-cell lymphoma and four with large cell anaplastic lymphoma). After a median of five cycles, 27% had a CR and 53% achieved a PR (OR rate 80%) with an overall median survival of 13·5 months.[88]

Drawbacks
Multi-agent chemotherapy regimens are associated with very high rates of toxicity and considerable morbidity, including nausea, anorexia, infection, hepatotoxicity and myelosuppression. Patients with CTCL are at high risk of septicaemia, and therapy-related mortality with combination chemotherapy is a significant risk.

Comments
Patients with late stages of CTCL (IIB–IVB) will require treatment with a chemotherapy regimen, although response duration is short. In the RCT,[77] OS/DFS was similar to that in those treated with skin-directed therapy although in this study patients with early stage disease were also included. The individual patient's quality of life should always be considered before embarking on very toxic regimens with limited efficacy. Single-agent regimens (see above) appear to have similar efficacy, although studies involving a comparison between single agent and multi-agent

regimens, with or without TSEB, are required. To date there have been no studies assessing the use of biochemotherapy in CTCL although subsequent treatment with immunotherapy for patients achieving a response with chemotherapy should be considered.

Myeloablative chemotherapy with autologous/allogeneic peripheral blood/bone-marrow stem-cell transplantation
Efficacy
No systematic reviews or RCTs were identified. Most studies were based on small numbers of patients High-dose chemotherapy with TSEB and total-body irradiation (TBI) in four and three patients with mycoses fungoides (two patients had both TSEB and TBI) followed by autologous bone marrow transplantation in six patients (three stage IIB, one stage IVA, two stage IVB) produced five complete clinical responses but disease relapse occurred within 100 days in three patients.[89] The other two patients, who had both received a combination of carmustine-etoposide-cisplatin chemotherapy, were disease free at almost 2 years (666 and 631 days post-transplant).

High-dose chemotherapy combined with either TSEB or TBI and followed by autologous peripheral blood stem cell transplantation in patients with stage IIB/IVA mycosis fungoides revealed CRs in eight patients and durable clinical responses in four patients (median DFS 11 months).[90]

Isolated case reports of high-dose chemotherapy with TBI followed by allogeneic bone-marrow or stem-cell transplantation have shown excellent long-term complete remissions in stage IIB mycosis fungoides (CR for total of 17 months at time of report) and Sezary syndrome.[91,92]

Drawbacks

Myeloablative therapy is associated with a high incidence of toxicity and systemic infections. Significant mortality, especially with allogeneic transplantation, occurs.

Comments

Controlled trials comparing autologous transplantation with standard chemotherapy in late stages of mycosis fungoides are required, as conducted in systemic follicular B-cell lymphoma. The mortality rate associated with allogeneic transplantation makes this a less attractive approach but the use of mini-allogeneic procedures to induce a graft-versus-tumour effect would be worth investigating.

Key points

Implications for practice

- Although there are few well-designed RCTs in CTCL, there is convincing evidence that several skin-directed therapies have a significant therapeutic effect. However, there is a fundamental lack of data on the impact of different therapies on DFS and OS, which will only become clearer when the results of key RCTs in different stages of disease become available.
- In addition, patients with early-stage disease can have a normal life expectancy, and so aggressive therapies with a significant mortality and morbidity should be avoided in these patients, especially when the chance of a cure is very low.
- Patients with early-stage disease (IA/IB/IIA) should be offered skin-directed therapies such as topical mechlorethamine, phototherapy, PUVA and superficial radiotherapy. Alfa interferon should be considered for patients with persistent or recurrent stage IB/IIA disease. Some patients with stage IA disease may not require any specific therapy.

- Patients with late stages of disease (IIB/IV) should be offered TSEB, single-agent palliative chemotherapy and multi-agent chemotherapy, according to performance status.
- Patients with erythrodermic disease should be offered photopheresis, immunotherapy and single-agent chemotherapy as palliative therapy aiming to improve quality of life. TSEB therapy may be indicated for erythrodermic disease when there is a lack of significant peripheral blood tumour burden.

Recommendations for the future

- New topical therapies should be assessed in the context of well-designed clinical trials comparing them with topical mechlorethamine.
- The role of new immunotherapies and retinoids in early stage (IB/IIA) disease should involve comparative RCTs with standard therapies such as PUVA.
- TSEB therapy with or without adjuvant immunotherapy and chemotherapy should be reserved for patients with late stages of disease, preferably in the context of clinical trials.
- There is an urgent need for more effective therapy for late-stage disease and this should be based on appropriate RCTs involving new immunotherapies, adjuvants, single- and multi-agent chemotherapies and both (mini)allogeneic and autologous transplants in selected individuals.

References

1. Willemze R, Kerl H, Sterry W *et al.* EORTC classification for primary cutaneous lymphomas A proposal from the cutaneous lymphoma study group of the European organisation for research and treatment of cancer. *Blood* 1997;**90**:354–71.
2. Weinstock M, Horm J. Mycosis fungoides in the United States: increasing incidence and descriptive epidemiology. *JAMA* 1988;**260**:42–6.

3. Zackheim H, Amin S, Kashani-Sabet M, McMillan A. Prognosis in cutaneous T-cell lymphoma by skin stage: long term survival in 489 patients. *J Am Acad Dermatol* 1999;**40**:418–25.

4. Siegel R, Pandolfino T, Guitart J, Rosen S, Kuzel T. Primary cutaneous T-cell lymphoma: review and current concepts. *J Clin Oncol* 2000;**18**:2908–25.

5. Bunn P, Lamberg S. Report of the committee on staging and classification of cutaneous T-cell lymphomas. *Cancer Treat Rep* 1979;**63**:725–8.

6. Scarisbrick J, Whittaker S, Evans A *et al.* Prognostic significance of tumour burden in the blood of patients with erythrodermic primary cutaneous T-cell lymphoma. *Blood* 2001;**97**:624–30.

7. Marti L, Estrach T, Reverter J, Mascaro J. Prognostic clinicopathologic factors in cutaneous T-cell lymphoma. *Arch Dermatol* 1991;**127**:1511–16.

8. Doorn R, Van Haselan C, Voorst Vader P *et al.* Mycosis fungoides: Disease evolution and prognosis of 309 Dutch patients. *Arch Dermatol* 2000;**136**:504–10.

9. Kim Y, Jensen R, Watanabe G, Varghese A, Hoppe R. Clinical stage IA (limited patch and plaque) mycosis fungoides. *Arch Dermatol* 1996;**132**:1309–13.

10. Kim Y, Chow S, Varghese A, Hoppe R. Clinical characteristics and long-term outcome of patients with generalised patch and/or plaque (T2) mycosis fungoides. *Arch Dermatol* 1999;**135**:26–32.

11. Coninck E, Kim Y, Varghese A, Hoppe R. Clinical characteristics and outcome of patients with extracutaneous mycosis fungoides. *J Clin Oncol* 2001;**19**:779–84.

12. Kim Y, Bishop K, Varghese A, Hoppe R. Prognostic factors in erythrodermic mycosis fungoides and the Sezary syndrome. *Arch Dermatol* 1995;**131**:1003–8.

13. Kashani-Sabet M, McMillan A, Zackheim H. A modified staging classification for cutaneous T-cell lymphoma. *J Am Acad Dermatol* 2001;**45**:700–6.

14. Sausville E, Eddy J, Makuch R, Fischmann A *et al.* Histopathologic staging at initial diagnosis of mycosis fungoides and the Sezary syndrome. Definition of three distinctive prognostic groups. *Ann Intern Med* 1988;**109**:372–82.

15. Bunn P, Huberman M, Whang-Peng J *et al.* Prospective staging evaluation of patients with cutaneous T-cell lymphomas. *Ann Intern Med* 1980;**93**:223–30.

16. Zackheim H, Kashani-Sabet M, Amin S. Topical corticosteroids for mycosis fungoides. *Arch Dermatol* 1998;**134**:949–54.

17. Hoppe R, Abel E, Deneau D, Price N. Mycosis fungoides: management with topical nitrogen mustard. *J Clin Oncol* 1987;**5**:1796–1803.

18. Ramsey D, Ed M, Halperin P *et al.* Topical mechlorethamine therapy for early stage mycosis fungoides. *J Am Acad Dermatol* 1988;**19**:684–91.

19. Vonderheid E, Tan E, Kantor A *et al.* Long term efficacy, curative potential and carcinogenicity of topical mechlorethamine chemotherapy in cutaneous T-cell lymphoma. *J Am Acad Dermatol* 1989;**20**:416–28.

20. Zachariae H, Thestrup-Pedersen K, Sogaard H. Topical nitrogen mustard in early mycosis fungoides. *Acta Derm Venereol* 1985;**65**:53–8.

21. Zackheim H, Epstein E, Crain W. Topical carmustine (BCNU) for cutaneous T-cell lymphoma: a 15-year experience in 143 patients. *J Am Acad Dermatol* 1990;**22**:802–10.

22. Breneman D, Duvic M, Kuzel T, Yocum R, Truglia J, Stevens V. Phase I and I trial of Bexarotene gel for skin directed treatment of patients with cutaneous T-cell lymphoma. *Arch Dermatol* 2002;**138**:325–32.

23. Duvic M, Olsen E, Omura G *et al.* A phase III, randomised, double-blind, placebo-controlled study of peldesine (BCX-34) cream as topical therapy for cutaneous T-cell lymphoma. *J Am Acad Dermatol* 2001;**44**:940–7.

24. Ramsey D, Lish K, Yalowitz C, Soter N. Ultraviolet-B phototherapy for early stage cutaneous T-cell lymphoma. *Arch Dermatol* 1992;**128**:931–3.

25. Clark C, Dawe R, Evans A, Lowe G, Ferguson J. Narrowband TL-01 phototherapy for patch stage mycosis fungoides. *Arch Dermatol* 2000;**136**:748–52.

26. Zane C, Leali C, Airo P *et al.* "High dose" UVA1 therapy of widespread plaque-type, nodular and erythrodermic mycosis fungoides. *J Am Acad Dermatol* 2001;**44**:629–33.

27. Hermann J, Roenigk H, Hurria A *et al.* Treatment of mycosis fungoides with photochemotherapy (PUVA): long term follow-up. *J Am Acad Dermatol* 1995;**33**:234–42.

28. Roenigk H, Kuzel T, Skoutelis A *et al.* Photochemotherapy alone or combined with interferon alpha in the treatment of cutaneous T-cell lymphoma. *J Invest Dermatol* 1990;**95**:198–205S.

29. Honigsmann Brenner W, Rauschmeier W, Konrad K, Wolff K. Photochemotherapy for cutaneous T cell lymphoma. *J Am Acad Dermatol* 1984;**10**:238–45.

30. Stadler R, Otte H, Luger T *et al.* Prospective randomised multicentre clinical trial on the use of interferon alpha-2a plus acitretin versus interferon alpha-2a plus PUVA in patients with cutaneous T-cell lymphoma stages I and II. *Blood* 1998;**10**:3578–81.

31. Thomsen K, Hammar H, Molin L *et al.* Retinoids plus PUVA (RePUVA) and PUVA in mycosis fungoides plaque stage. *Acta Derm Venereol* 1989;**69**:536–8.

32. Kuzel T, Roenigk H, Samuelson E *et al.* Effectiveness of interferon alfa-2a combined with phototherapy for mycosis fungoides and the Sezary syndrome. *J Clin Oncol* 1995;**13**:257–63.

33. Bunn P, Ihde D, Foon K. The role of recombinant interferon alpha-2a in the therapy of cutaneous T-cell lymphomas. *Cancer* 1986;**57**:1689–95.

34. Olsen E, Rosen S, Vollmer R *et al.* Interferon alfa-2a in the treatment of cutaneous T-cell lymphoma. *J Am Acad Dermatol* 1989;**20**:395–407.

35. Papa G, Tura S, Mandelli F *et al.* Is interferon alpha in cutaneous T-cell lymphoma a treatment of choice? *Br J Haematol* 1991;**79**:48–51.

36. Kohn E, Steis R, Sausville E, Veach S *et al.* Phase II trial of intermittent high-dose recombinant interferon alfa-2a in mycosis fungoides and the Sezary syndrome. *J Clin Oncol* 1990;**8**:155–60.

37. Dreno B, Claudy A, Meynadier J *et al.* The treatment of 45 patients with cutaneous T-cell lymphoma with low doses of interferon-alpha 2a and etretinate. *Br J Dermatol* 1991;**125**:456–9.

38. Vonderheid E, Thompson R, Smiles K, Lattanand A. Recombinant interferon alpha-2b in plaque phase mycosis fungoides. Intralesional and low dose intramuscular therapy. *Arch Dermatol* 1987;**123**:757–63.

39. Kaplan E, Rosen S, Norris D *et al.* Phase II study of recombinant interferon gamma for treatment of cutaneous T-cell lymphoma. *J Natl Cancer Inst* 1990;**82**:208–12.

40. Marolleau J, Baccard M, Flageul B *et al.* High dose recombinant interleukin-2 in advanced cutaneous T-cell lymphoma. *Arch Dermatol* 1995;**131**:574–9.

41. Rook A, Wood G, Yoo E *et al.* Interleukin-12 therapy of cutaneous T-cell lymphoma induces lesion regression and cytotoxic T-cell responses. *Blood* 1999;**94**:902–8.

42. Russell Jones R. Extracorporeal photopheresis in cutaneous T-cell lymphoma. Inconsistent data underline the need for randomised studies. *Br J Dermatol* 2000;**142**:16–21.

43. Edelson R, Berger C, Gasparro F *et al.* Treatment of cutaneous T-cell lymphoma by extracorporeal photochemotherapy. *N Engl J Med* 1987;**316**:297–303.

44. Duvic M, Hester J, Lemak N. Photopheresis therapy for cutaneous T-cell lymphoma. *J Am Acad Dermatol* 1996;**35**:573–9.

45. Heald P, Rook A, Perez M *et al.* Treatment of erythrodermic cutaneous T-cell lymphoma with extracorporeal photopheresis. *J Am Acad Dermatol* 1992;**27**:427–33.

46. Zic J, Stricklin G, Greer J *et al.* Long term follow up of patients with cutaneous T-cell lymphoma treated with extracorporeal photochemotherapy. *J Am Acad Dermatol* 1996;**35**:935–45.

47. Gottleib S, Wolfe J, Fox F *et al.* Treatment of cutaneous T-cell lymphoma with extracorporeal photopheresis monotherapy and in combination with recombinant interferon-alpha: a 10 year experience at a single institution. *J Am Acad Dermatol* 1996;**35**:946–57.

48. Fraser-Andrews E, Seed P, Whittaker S, Russell Jones R. Extracorporeal photopheresis in Sezary syndrome: no significant effect in the survival of 44 patients with a peripheral blood T-cell clone. *Arch Dermatol* 1998;**134**:1001–5.

49. Child F, Mitchell T, Whittaker S, Watkins P, Seed P, Russell Jones R. A randomised cross-over study to compare PUVA and extracorporeal photopheresis (ECP) in the treatment of plaque stage (T2) mycosis fungoides. *Br J Dermatol* 2001;**145**(Suppl. 59):16.

50. Bisaccia E, Gonzalez J, Palangio M, Schwartz J, Klainer A. Extracorporeal photochemotherapy alone or with adjuvant therapy in the treatment of cutaneous T-cell lymphoma: A 9 year retrospective study at a single institution. *J Am Acad Dermatol* 2000;**43**:263–71.

51. Wollina U, Looks A, Meyer J *et al.* Treatment of stage II cutaneous T-cell lymphoma with interferon alfa-2a and extracorporeal photochemotherapy: a prospective controlled trial. *J Am Acad Dermatol* 2001;**44**:253–60.

52. Dippel E, Schrag H, Goerdt S, Orfanos C. Extracorporeal photopheresis and interferon-α in advanced cutaneous T-cell lymphoma. *Lancet* 1997;**350**:32–3.

53. Vonderheid E, Bigler R, Greenberg A, Neukum S, Micaily B. Extracorporeal photopheresis and recombinant interferon alfa-2b in Sezary syndrome. *Am J Clin Oncol* 1994;**17**:255–63.

54. Haley H, Davis D, Sams M. Durable loss of a malignant T-cell clone in a stage IV cutaneous T-cell lymphoma patient treated with high-dose interferon and photopheresis. *J Am Acad Dermatol* 1999;**41**:880–3.

55. Yoo E, Cassin M, Lessin S, Rook A. Complete molecular remission during biologic response modifier therapy for Sezary syndrome is associated with enhanced helper T type I cytokine production and natural killer cell activity. *J Am Acad Dermatol* 2001;**45**:208–16.

56. Evans A, Wood B, Scarisbrick J et al. Extracorporeal photopheresis in Sezary syndrome: hematologic parameters as predictors of response. *Blood* 2001;**98**:1298–301.

57. Bernengo M, Appino A, Bertero M et al. Thymopentin in Sezary syndrome. *J Natl Cancer Inst* 1992;**84**:1341–6.

58. Cooper D, Braverman I, Sarris A et al. Cyclosporine treatment of refractory T-cell lymphomas. *Cancer* 1993;**71**:2335–41.

59. Bunn P, Hoffman S, Norris D, Golitz L, Aeling J. Systemic therapy of cutaneous T-cell lymphomas (mycosis fungoides and the Sezary syndrome). *Ann Intern Med* 1994;**121**:592–602.

60. Molin L, Thomsen K, Volden G et al. Oral retinoids in mycosis fungoides and Sezary syndrome: a comparison of isotretinoin and etretinate. *Acta Dermatol Venereol* 1987;**67**:232–6.

61. Kessler J, Jones S, Levine N et al. Isotretinoin and cutaneous helper T-cell lymphoma (mycosis fungoides). *Arch Dermatol* 1987;**123**:201–4.

62. Duvic M, Martin A, Kim Y et al. Phase 2 and 3 clinical trial of oral Bexarotene (Targretin capsules) for the treatment of refractory or persistent early stage cutaneous T cell lymphoma. *Arch Dermatol* 2001;**137**:581–93.

63. Duvic M, Hymes K, Heald P et al. Bexarotene is effective and safe for treatment of refractory advanced-stage cutaneous T-cell lymphoma: multinational phase II–III trial results. *J Clin Oncol* 2001;**19**:2456–71.

64. Knox S, Levy R, Hodgkinson S et al. Observations on the effect of chimeric anti-CD4 monoclonal antibody in patients with mycosis fungoides. *Blood* 1991;**77**: 20–30.

65. Knox S, Hoppe R, Maloney D et al. Treatment of cutaneous T-cell lymphoma with chimeric anti-CD4 monoclonal antibody. *Blood* 1996;**87**:893–9.

66. Lundin J, Osterborg A, Brittinger G et al. CAMPATH-1H monoclonal antibody in therapy for previously treated low-grade non-Hodgkin's lymphomas:a phase II multicenter study. European study group of CAMPATH-1H treatment in low-grade non-Hodgkin's lymphoma. *J Clin Oncol* 1998;**16**:3257–63.

67. Olsen E, Duvic M, Frankel A et al. Pivotal phase III trial of two dose levels of Denileukin Diftitox for the treatment of cutaneous T-cell lymphoma. *J Clin Oncol* 2001;**19**:376–88.

68. LeMaistre C, Rosen S, Frankel A et al. Phase I trial of H65-RTA immunoconjugate in patients with cutaneous T-cell lymphoma. *Blood* 1991;**78**:1173–82.

69. Foss F, Raubitscheck A, Mulshine J et al. Phase I study of the pharmacokinetics of a radioimmunoconjugate, 90Y-T101, in patients with CD5-expressing leukaemia and lymphoma. *Clin Cancer Res* 1998;**4**:2691–700.

70. Cotter G, Baglan R, Wasserman T, Mill W. Palliative radiation treatment of cutaneous mycosis fungoides: a dose response. *Int J Radiat Oncol Biol Phys* 1983;**9**:1477–80.

71. Jones G, Hoppe R, Glatstein E. Electron beam treatment for cutaneous T-cell lymphoma. *Haematol Oncol Clin North Am* 1995;**9**:1057–76.

72. Hamminga B, Noordijk E, Van Vloten W. Treatment of mycosis fungoides: total skin electron beam irradiation v topical mechlorethamine therapy. *Arch Dermatol* 1982;**118**:150–3.

73. Jones G, Rosenthal D, Wilson L. Total skin electron beam radiation for patients with erythrodermic cutaneous T-cell lymphoma (mycosis fungoides and the Sezary syndrome). *Cancer* 1999;**85**:1985–95.

74. Kirova Y, Piedbois Y, Haddad E et al. Radiotherapy in the management of mycosis fungoides: indications, results, prognosis. Twenty years experience. *Radiother Oncol* 1999;**51**:147–51.

75. Becker M, Hoppe R, Knox S. Multiple courses of high dose total skin electron beam therapy in the management of mycosis fungoides. *Int J Radiat Oncol Biol Phys* 1995;**30**:1445–9.

76. Wilson L, Quiros P, Kolenik S et al. Additional courses of total skin electron beam therapy in the treatment of patients with recurrent cutaneous T-cell lymphoma. *J Am Acad Dermatol* 1996;**35**:69–73.

77. Kaye F, Bunn P, Steinberg S *et al.* A randomised trial comparing combination electron beam radiation and chemotherapy with topical therapy in the initial treatment of mycosis fungoides. *N Engl J Med* 1989;**321**:1748–90.

78. Wilson L, Jones G, Kim D *et al.* Experience with total skin electron beam therapy in combination with extracorporeal photopheresis in the management of patients with erythrodermic (T4) mycosis fungoides. *J Am Acad Dermatol* 2000;**43**:54–60.

79. Zackheim H, Kashani-sabet M, Hwang S. Low dose methotrexate to treat erythrodermic cutaneous T-cell lymphoma:results in twenty-nine patients. *J Am Acad Dermatol* 1996;**34**:626–31.

80. Kurzrock R, Pilat S, Duvic M. Pentostatin therapy of T-cell lymphomas with cutaneous manifestations. *J Clin Oncol* 1999;**17**:3117–21.

81. Deardon C, Matutes E, Catovsky D. Pentostatin treatment of cutaneous T-cell lymphoma. *Oncology* 2000;**14**:37–40.

82. Ho A, Suciu S, Stryckmans P *et al.* Pentostatin in T-cell malignancies. Leukaemia cooperative group and the European Organisation for Research and Treatment of Cancer. *Semin Oncol* 2000;**27**:52–7.

83. Foss F, Ihde D, Breneman D *et al.* Phase II study of pentostatin and intermittent high dose recombinant interferon alfa-2a in advanced mycosis fungoides/Sezary syndrome. *J Clin Oncol* 1992;**10**:1907–13.

84. Kuzel T, Hurria A, Samuelson E *et al.* Phase II trial of 2-chlorodeoxyadenosine for the treatment of cutaneous T-cell lymphoma. *Blood* 1996;**87**:906–11.

85. Zinzani P, Baliva G, Magagnoli M *et al.* Gemcitabine treatment in pretreated cutaneous T-cell lymphoma:

experience in 44 patients. *J Clin Oncol* 2000; **18**:2603–6.

86. Wollina U, Graefe T, Kaatz M. Pegylated doxorubicin for primary cutaneous T-cell lymphoma: a report on ten patients with follow-up. *J Cancer Res Clin Oncol* 201;**127**:128–34.

87. Fierro M, Doveil G, Quaglino P, Savoia P, Verrone A, Bernengo M. Combination of etoposide, idarubicin, cyclophosphamide, vincristine, prednisone and bleomycin (VICOP-B) in the treatment of advanced cutaneous T-cell lymphoma. *Dermatology* 1997;**194**:268–72.

88. Akpek G, Koh H, Bogen S, O'Hara C, Foss F. Chemotherapy with etoposide, vincristine, doxorubicin, bolus cyclophosphamide and oral prednisone in patients with refractory cutaneous T-cell lymphoma. *Cancer* 1999;**86**:1368–76.

89. Bigler R, Crilley P, Micaily B *et al.* Autologous bone marrow transplantation for advanced stage mycosis fungoides. *Bone Marrow Transplant* 1991;**7**:133–7.

90. Olavarria E, Child F, Woolford A *et al.* T-cell depletion and autologous stem cell transplantation in the management of tumour stage mycosis fungoides with peripheral blood involvement. *Br J Haematol* 2001; **114**:624–31.

91. Burt R, Guitart J, Traynor A *et al.* Allogeneic hematopoietic stem cell transplantation for advanced mycosis fungoides: evidence of a graft-versus-tumour effect. *Bone Marrow Transplant* 2000;**25**:111–13.

92. Molina A, Nademanee A, Arber D, Forman S. Remission of refractory Sezary syndrome after bone marrow transplantation from a matched unrelated donor. *Biol Blood Marrow Transplant* 1999;**5**:400–4.

28

Actinic keratoses and Bowen's disease

Seaver L Soon, Elizabeth A Cooper, Peterson Pierre, Aditya K Gupta and Suephy C Chen

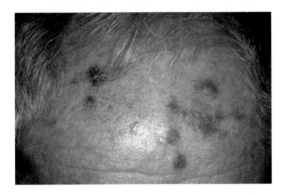

Figure 28.1 Actinic keratoses

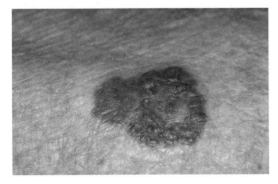

Figure 28.2 Bowen's disease

Background
Definition
Actinic keratoses (AK), also known as solar keratoses, and Bowen's disease (BD) are precursors of invasive squamous cell carcinoma (SCC). Whereas AK is precancerous, BD represents intraepidermal *(in situ)* SCC.[1] AK generally presents as multiple, erythematous scaly papules, and is termed actinic cheilitis if the lips are involved. BD usually presents as a solitary, well demarcated, erythematous plaque of varying size with irregular borders and a crusted, scaling or fissured surface.[2]

AK arises on areas of intense ultraviolet light exposure, with over 80% developing on the head and neck, forearms and hands.[3,4] A male predominance is observed.[5,6] The distribution of BD varies, demonstrating predominance on the lower legs in women and the head and neck in men in the UK and Australia.[7,8] Australia and Denmark feature a marginal propensity for women (56%) and occurrence on the head and neck (44–54%).[8,9] Approximately one-third of patients with BD have other non-melanoma skin cancer at diagnosis.[9]

Incidence/prevalence
The exact incidence and prevalence of AK and BD is unknown. Both increase in prevalence with advancing age.[8,10–12] AK may occur in children with albinism and xeroderma pigmentosum.[13]

Aetiology
Chronic solar damage is the principal aetiological factor in AK and BD.[8,14–16] People

with light complexions, blue eyes and childhood freckling are at highest risk given their innate lack of protective pigment.[3] Individuals with compromised immunity, such as organ-transplant recipients, with diminished or absent melanin, such as albinos, with decreased capacity to repair ultraviolet-induced damage, such as persons with xeroderma pigmentosum, all demonstrate increased risk for AK. Risk factors for BD include arsenic exposure,[17–20] immunosuppression,[21] and human papillomavirus (HPV), particularly HPV-16 in anogenital lesions.[22,23]

Prognosis

Although precancerous,[24,25] the probability of a given AK undergoing malignant transformation is unknown.[13] Reported risk of progression to SCC for individual lesions ranges from 0·025 to 16% per year.[26] The 10-year risk of malignant transformation of at least one AK on a given patient is 10·2%.[27] The relative risk of malignant transformation depends ultimately on factors related to the AK itself (for example, thickness), as well as patient characteristics (for example, drug therapy, degree of pigmentation, immune status).[5] However, another aspect that may confound estimation of the prognosis of AK is in the spontaneous regression rate. A recent study from Queensland[28] reported a spontaneous regression rate of 85% (95% CI: 75–96%) in subjects with prevalent AK (AK diagnosed on a person during their first examination) and 84% (95% CI: 72–96%) in persons with incident AK (AK appearing for the first time during the study). However, the distribution of lesions per person was highly skewed, with 12% of subjects having 65% of the total number of AK.

BD is associated with an excellent prognosis, related to the disease's indolent nature and its favourable response to a range of therapy. Retrospective studies demonstrate an approximate 3% progression rate to SCC,[29,30]

which is further associated with an approximate 33% metastasis rate.[31] Contrary to findings of earlier reports,[32–35] a meta-analysis of 12 studies in 1989 determined no significant association between BD and internal malignancy.[36]

Aims of treatment

Aims of treatment are to achieve clinical and histological clearance, prevent recurrence, prevent progression to invasive SCC and to minimise adverse effects of treatment.

Relevant outcomes

- Short-term clinical and histological clearance
- Recurrence rates
- Adverse effects of treatment

Methods of search

To identify studies of 5-fluorouracil (5-FU) and cryotherapy in patients with AK, we reviewed Medline, Embase and CancerLit from 1966 to October 1999 and proceedings from the American Association of Dermatology meetings (1997–2000). We searched non-5-FU and non-nitrogen therapies by name and type, as well as the term "actinic keratosis treatment". We scrutinised review articles for treatments not detected through database searches.

To locate articles on interventions for BD, we searched Medline (1966–2001) and Embase (1988–2001). We limited our topic to non-anogenital BD and to English publications since translators were not readily available for this unfunded endeavour. We reported numbers of patients as well as number of lesions treated wherever information was available.

Since few randomised controlled trials (RCTs) were found, uncontrolled trials were included in this report. Evidence was graded using the quality of evidence scale employed by the British Association of Dermatology guidelines, and derived from the US Task Force on Preventative Care Guidelines.[37,38]

Box 28.1 Quality of evidence scale employed by the British Association of Dermatology guidelines, derived from the US Task Force on Preventative Care Guidelines.[37,38]

I Evidence obtained from at least one properly designed RCT

II-i Evidence obtained from well-designed control trials without randomisation

II-ii Evidence obtained from well-designed cohort or case-control analytical studies, preferably from more than one centre or research group

II-iii Evidence obtained from multiple time series with or without the intervention. Dramatic results in uncontrolled experiments could also be included

III Opinions of respected authorities based on clinical experience, descriptive studies or reports of expert committees

IV Evidence inadequate owing to problems of methodology (for example sample size, length or comprehensiveness of follow up or conflicts in evidence)

derived from the US Task Force on Preventative Care Guidelines.[37,38] We have only presented data from the best quality studies; for example, data from comparative studies is presented preferentially over data from case series when both exist for a given intervention. The grading system is given in Box 28.1.

QUESTIONS

What are the effects of non-drug therapy?

Cryotherapy

Studies of varying quality investigated the efficacy of cryotherapy for AK and BD.

Actinic keratoses

Quality of evidence: III

We found one systematic review[39] but no RCTs. The systematic review found only one study with quantifiable results.[40]

Benefits

A total of 1018 lesions in 70 patients were treated; the majority had biopsy confirmation of their diagnosis. Clinical follow up after treatment ranged from 1 to 8·5 years. Twelve recurrences were reported for a success rate of 98·8% during a follow up period of 1–8·5 years. However, not all lesions were followed uniformly after 1 year.

Harms

Discomfort during application of the cryogen is the norm but the procedure is usually well tolerated by patients, and complications are rare. Blisters, scarring, textural skin changes, infection and hyper- or hypopigmentation may occur.[41]

Comment

Given the popularity of cryotherapy for treating AK, it is surprising that there is only one study with quantifiable results. All other papers are qualitative. Future studies for new therapeutic modalities should include cryotherapy as a comparison arm since cryotherapy is considered by many dermatologists to be standard care, but also to further quantify its efficacy.

Bowen's disease

Quality of Evidence: II-i

We found no systematic reviews and no RCTs. One unblinded controlled trial compared cryotherapy (n = 36) with curettage (n = 44),[42] and one retrospective comparative study compared cryotherapy (n = 82) with external beam radiotherapy (n = 59).[43]

Benefits

Complete clinical clearance was comparable between cryotherapy (94% with one treatment and 100% with two) and curettage (100% after one treatment). Clinical clearance in the trial was not defined objectively, and probably refers to dermatologists' subjective assessment. The time point for assessment of clinical clearance was 1 week following treatment. Healing was defined as complete when the post-procedural eschar had dropped off and, apart from erythema, the underlying skin appeared normal. Overall, average time to healing was 60 days. Healing was significantly prolonged for lower-leg lesions treated by cryotherapy compared with curettage (90 versus 30 days, $P<0.001$). No difference in healing time was observed for other sites. Recurrence rates were less (12% versus 50%, $P = 0.04$) and time to recurrence longer ($P = 0.0087$) for curettage.[42] Compared with radiotherapy, higher recurrence occurred in the cryotherapy group (6%, one as invasive SCC, versus 0%).[43]

Harms

Complications of cryotherapy include pain, poor healing and infection, requiring antibiotics.[42] Patients were 10·4 times more likely to report pain with cryotherapy ($P<0.001$), and were 5·5 times more likely to report pain on the lower leg compared with other body sites, irrespective of treatment method ($P<0.016$).[42] Poor healing occurred in 2% of patients who received cryotherapy in this retrospective comparison study.[43] Poor healing was defined as a residual ulcer requiring salvage surgery, that ceased to show signs of continuing reduction in diameter, or considered by the dermatologist to be progressing poorly over at least 3 months. Biopsy of these poor-healing lesions revealed residual tumour. The authors speculate that failure to heal may suggest residual BD, and may be an indication for surgical excision.

Comment

These studies report high clearance rates with liquid-nitrogen cryotherapy, although poor healing and discomfort related to the procedure may limit its utility in BD of such sites as the lower legs. In relation to the study comparing cryotherapy and curettage, methodological limitations include deviation from an ITT analysis and use of non-random allocation. The former omission would tend to overestimate the efficacy of the intervention, whereas the latter would tend to weaken the validity of the results, as there is no assurance that known and unknown confounders are homogeneously distributed between the comparison groups.

Laser treatment

Studies investigating laser therapy for AK and BD highlight its capacity to selectively vaporise the epidermis and upper papillary, yielding minimal scar formation. We found no systematic reviews and no RCTs for either AK or BD.

Actinic keratoses

Quality of evidence: II-iii

Two uncontrolled trials investigated the use of the Er:YAG laser to treat AK.[44,45] Both reports had small sample sizes and used different energy rates. The first report treated only eight lesions, with a follow up period of 12–15 months.[44] The second report provided full-face laser resurfacing for four of five patients (n = 121 lesions), with a follow up of 3 months.[45]

Benefits

The two studies report 93%[45] to 100%[44] clearance of the AK lesions at 12–15-month follow up.

Harms

Laser treatment is associated with exudation, crusting and erythema following treatment. Re-epithelialisation occurs 7–10 days after treatment, but erythema may persist for 3 weeks or more. General use of the Er:YAG laser noted in the second report found no hypo- or hyperpigmentation following treatment.

Comments

Treatment appeared to be well tolerated, both in individual lesion treatment[44] and in full- or partial-facial resurfacing.[45] The first study indicated that skin may remain clear of lesions for up to a year after laser treatment, but larger studies with longer follow up would be required for confirmation of this effect. Laser resurfacing was performed only for Fitzpatrick skin types I and II. Use of laser treatment on patients with darker skin tones may be associated with a higher risk of hypo- or hyperpigmentation. Further studies should be performed before Er:YAG laser treatment can become a routine treatment for AK.

Bowen's disease

Quality of evidence: II-iii

Two small uncontrolled trials reported the use of CO_2 laser therapy for BD of the digits.[46,47] The first report[46] described treatment of five lesions with a 36-month follow up; the second report[47] described treatment of six lesions with an 84-month follow up.

Benefits

Both studies reported 100% clearance within 10–24 days following the procedure. Determination of clearance in both studies was based on clinical criteria and, in cases deemed necessary by the supervising dermatologist, by histological criteria. Biopsies showed only slightly thinned epidermis and mild superficial fibroplagia of the papillary dermis.[46,47] Recurrence rates varied between 0% at 84 months[47] to 20% (one of five patients) at 5 months. (After retreatment by electrodesiccation and curettage, no recurrence was observed at 20 months.)[46] The disparate recurrence rates may be related to differences in energy settings and in the width of clinically normal margins included in the treatment area. No impairment in digital function was noted in either study.

Harms

Exudation, crusting and erythema may follow laser treatment. Re-epithelialisation occurs 7–10 days after treatment, but erythema may persist for 3 or more weeks. One Er:YAG laser study[45] found no post-therapeutic dyspigmentation. The CO_2 laser studies report hypopigmentation, mild cutaneous atrophy and nail dystrophy.[46,47]

Comment

CO_2 lasers may be particularly useful in the treatment of digital BD lesions. Clearance rates in the small uncontrolled trials were high, with acceptable recurrence rates during follow up periods of sufficient duration. The suitability of CO_2 laser therapy for digital BD relates principally to two properties. First, CO_2 laser has the ability to vaporise the epidermis and the upper papillary dermis, leading to healing with minimal scar formation. This feature is desirable in mobile areas such as the fingers where cicatricial contracture following excision may lead to functional impairment. Second, the concern that CO_2 lasers may not penetrate to a sufficient depth to eradicate perifollicular BD is obviated by the paucity of hair on the fingers. The risk of recurrence secondary to perifollicular involvement is therefore less of a concern in digital lesions than in lesions at other body sites. CO_2 lasers may thus be helpful for digital lesions where more conventional and less costly therapies have failed.

Radiotherapy

We found no systematic reviews or RCTs for either AK or BD.

Actinic keratoses

Quality of evidence: IV

We found only one case report using radiotherapy for AK.[48]

Benefit

One person with a large AK recalcitrant to 5-FU responded to fractionated radiotherapy.[48]

Comment

Given the availability of other therapeutic modalities, radiotherapy should be reserved for AK recalcitrant to conventional therapies.

Bowen's disease

Quality of evidence: II-iii

We found one comparative study comparing the effect of radiotherapy with cryotherapy on lower-leg lesions,[43] as reported above.

Benefits

Radiotherapy was more effective than cryotherapy in terms of recurrence (0% versus 6%).[43] Skin cosmesis following radiotherapy is reported as "good" to "excellent" in the majority of patients in uncontrolled trials, with only 5–15% of irradiated skin considered "fair" to "unsatisfactory".[49,50]

Harms

The 100% clinical clearance and 0% recurrence rate was offset by poor healing in 20% of lesions.[43] Poor healing in this study was defined as a residual ulcer requiring salvage surgery, that ceased to show signs of continuing reduction in diameter, or considered by the dermatologist to be progressing poorly over at least 3 months Other reported adverse effects from uncontrolled studies included minor pain and burning during the procedure,[51,52] short-term hypopigmentation,[52] radiation dermatitis and radionecrosis.[51] Poor healing, including radionecrosis, appear to be associated with older age, an irradiation field diameter >4 cm, and a total dose >3000 cGy.[43,51]

Comment

As noted by the authors of this retrospective comparative study of radiotherapy and cryotherapy, the conclusions must be considered in light of the non-comparability of the groups. This study was retrospective, and shows a selection bias inasmuch as the severity and extent of a lesion often determines its initial therapy. A higher proportion of broad and thick lesions were thus treated in the radiotherapy group. Considering the radiotherapy group alone, however, may be informative in that poor healing was significantly related to age >90 years, a field irradiation diameter >4 cm, and a radiotherapy dose >3000 cGy. In view of their risk for poor healing, the authors suggested that patients meeting these criteria require cautious consideration in determining their candidacy for radiotherapy.

Chemical peels

Chemical peels have only been investigated for AK.

Quality of evidence: II-I

We found no systematic reviews or RCTs. We found two comparative studies[53,54] (with one follow up study[55]) using trichloroacetic acid (TCA). Pretreatments included topical tretinoin (0·05%, increasing to 0·1%) for the first study,[53] and Jessner's solution for the second study.[54,55] The concentrations of TCA varied from 35% to 40%.

The first study[53] was reportedly randomised. However, all patients pretreated with tretinoin previously received topical therapies in addition to cryotherapy, whereas all patients without tretinoin pretreatment previously received only cryotherapy. This study reported a 6-month follow up. In the second study, a split-face design was used. One side of the face received a TCA chemical peel after pretreatment with Jessner's solution, and the other side received 5% topical 5-FU twice daily for 3 weeks. Despite a small sample size, follow up was reported at 12 months[54] and 32 months.[55]

Benefits

No significant difference was observed for pretreatment with topical tretinoin before 40% TCA: AK was reduced by 20–75% in both groups. They used a reduction in the appearance of lesions, which was not necessarily a reduction in number of lesions. Scores for photodamage decreased, and telangiectasias improved with tretinoin pretreatment. Jessner's solution followed by TCA did not differ significantly from topical 5-FU: both yielded a 75% reduction in number of lesions that persisted for 12 months. Analysis of eight patients at 32-month follow up showed three (37%) had more lesions than at baseline, but that three patients maintained a 50% reduction from baseline.

Patients were extremely pleased with the cosmetic results of TCA facial peels, and scored improvement significantly higher than did the clinicians. Patients preferred the facial peel to 5-FU because of the convenient single application and the shorter duration of adverse effects.

Harms

The medium-depth facial peel procedures were associated with erythema lasting generally 10 days to 2 weeks. Mild desquamation was noted.

Comments

Facial peel with TCA appears to be a viable option if the patient is not a good candidate for cryotherapy (i.e. widespread facial AK), or is intolerant to other topicals applied over the long term, such as 5-FU.

Dermabrasion

Dermabrasion was investigated only for AK.

Quality of evidence: II-i

We found one unblinded comparative study[56] comparing recurrence rates for dermabrasion, 50% phenol chemical peels and 1% topical 5-FU. Methodological problems included small sample size, varying follow up periods, lack of data on initial elimination rate, and lack of explicit evaluation criteria for remission or recurrence.

Benefits

Dermabrasion yielded longer time to recurrence than facial peel, but shorter times than 5-FU. However, no statistical data was presented.[56]

Harms

No information on adverse events was reported in the unblinded study. One case series of dermabrasion of the scalp[57] reported a conspicuous line marking the periphery of abrasion at postoperative week 6–8.

Comments

This small study concluded that topical 5-FU was more effective and easier to use than dermabrasion. Although dermabrasion may produce longer-term clearance than chemical peels, the case series[57] indicated a risk of scarring. Although larger studies are necessary to make definitive conclusions, it would appear that the indication for dermabrasion as a primary therapeutic modality for AK is minimal.

Surgery and electrodesiccation and curettage

Surgery is commonly used for BD but not for AK, presumably because less invasive interventions are available for the latter.

Quality of evidence: II-iii

We found no systematic reviews or RCTs. We found one small retrospective uncontrolled trial investigating surgical excision (n = 4)[58] and two large retrospective uncontrolled trials for electrodesiccation and curettage (ED&C) (n = 20,[58] n = 83[49]).

Benefits

Although surgical excision appeared to clinically clear all four cases, two cases recurred.[58] The author did not report time to recurrence. ED&C[49,58] resulted in complete clinical clearance ranging from 80% to 90%, with recurrences ranging from 10% to 20% during a follow up period up to 18 years. Again, time to recurrence was not reported in either study.

Harms

No harms were reported with ED&C or with surgical excision, other than the understood risks of bleeding, infection, and local anaesthesia associated with minor surgery.

Comment

Surgical excision is commonly reported as the treatment of choice for BD, although no RCTs and only this small series were found to support its use. The unmatched efficacy ascribed to surgical excision probably relates to the notion that excision of an *in situ* neoplasm is, by definition, curative. The predominance of BD in elderly populations and its slow progression to SCC suggest that additional outcomes such as healing, scarring and patient preferences should be considered in determining the choice of treatment. The large series investigating ED&C demonstrated high efficacy, with tolerable recurrence rates during a sufficiently long follow up. ED&C may thus be a highly useful procedure for patients with small solitary lesions.

Miscellaneous

One uncontrolled trial[59] examined the use of hyperthermic pocket warmers applied with direct pressure to BD lesions in eight patients every day for 4–5 months. Complete histological clearance was seen in three cases, isolated tumour cells remained in three cases, and two cases showed no change.

Comment

Although non-invasive and innovative, the low efficacy, troublesome nature of the therapy for the patient, and poor level of evidence provided by uncontrolled studies suggest that hyperthermic pocket warmer therapy be considered only in patients who refuse more conventional therapy.

What are the effects of topical therapy?

Topical retinoids

Topical retinoids were reported only for AK.

Quality of evidence: I

We found two double-blind RCTs investigating topical retinoids for AK.[60,61] The first study compared tretinoin cream (n = 25) with Ro 14-9706 (arotinoid methyl sulphone cream) (n = 25) using a split-face design.[60] The second study was a parallel-group multicentre trial comparing 0·1% isotretinoin (n = 41) with placebo (n = 47).[61]

Benefit

Reductions in the number of AK lesions by 30% and 38% were reported for tretinoin and Ro 14-9706, respectively. Complete clearance of all lesions occurred in 8% of patients using tretinoin.[60] Compared with placebo, 0·1% topical isotretinoin significantly reduced the number of facial lesions (65% versus 45%, $P < 0·005$).[61]

Harms

Severe local skin irritation was associated with topical tretinoin whereas the irritation was mild to moderate with isotretinoin. No significant changes in laboratory parameters were observed.

Comments

Although some reduction in AK counts and size has been noted, few patients (8%) had complete clearance of lesions, which should be the goal of effective AK treatment. The relatively high rate of reduction noted with placebo use indicates either that the study was flawed or that topical retinoids may not sufficiently enhance the clearance of AK lesions to be used as standard treatment for AK.

5-Fluorouracil

Topical chemotherapy with 5-FU interferes with DNA and RNA synthesis. It is indicated for diffuse, ill-defined AK where treatment of individual lesions is impractical or impossible. It is also used in BD.

Actinic keratoses

Quality of evidence: I

We found one systematic review[39] and one double-blind RCT comparing 5% 5-FU (n = 30) with masoprocol (n = 27).[62] Details of masoprocol are described below.

Benefits

The systematic review[39] found marked heterogeneity in the concentration of 5-FU and drug vehicle, ranging from 1% in propylene glycol[63,64] or 1% cream,[65] to 3% ointment,[66] to 5% solution,[67,68] ointment,[69–73] or cream.[54,55,74,75] Combination therapies have also been reported.[68,76] To complicate issues further,

variation in treatment site and outcomes was noted. An attempt to combine studies using meta-analysis techniques[39] revealed that only three studies could be combined.[70–72] This combination showed that overall efficacy (treatment period of 2–8 weeks and follow up period of 3–18 months) of 5% 5-FU ointment ranged from 79% (95% CI: 72–87%) using patient-level data (by pooling individual subjects' data) to 84% (77% to 91%) using study-level data (by using the reported effect size from each study, weighted by the reported variance).[39] In the RCT, the authors demonstrated a significantly higher percentage reduction in the number of lesions ($P<0.0001$) and improvement in the investigators' global assessment ($P< 0.001$).

Harms

5-FU is associated with pain, inflammation, and erosions.[63,77]

In the RCT, 5-FU produced significantly more necrosis ($P<0.007$), erosions ($P<0.001$), pain ($P<0.001$), erythema ($P = 0.016$) and contact dermatitis ($P = 0.016$) than masoprocol.[62]

Comments

Although 5-FU has a high efficacy rate, one should note that it is associated with a high degree of morbidity, including pain, inflammation, and erosions. Thus, if patients are unable to tolerate these side-effects, we would expect the cure rate to drop off dramatically.

Of methodological note, the authors in the RCT did not perform an ITT analysis. If the subjects who dropped out of the study were included in the denominator, as prescribed in an ITT analysis, the efficacy rate (by investigator global assessment of cure) of 5-FU falls from 77% to 67% while that of masoprocol falls from 23% to 20%. Despite the lack of ITT analysis, however, the difference between 67% and 20% undoubtedly reaches statistical significance.

Bowen's disease
Quality of evidence: II-i

We found no systematic reviews and no RCTs. We found one small unblinded quasi-randomised controlled trial comparing topical 5% 5-FU cream with intralesional interferon alfa-2b (1 000 000 units/injection) for both BD and AK.[78] The treatment-allocation method was not specified. Ten lesions of BD and AK were allocated to each group, and clinical clearance and histological change were assessed at 1 and 2 months' follow up. We found five uncontrolled trials addressing the therapeutic efficacy of 5-FU.[49,58,79–81]

Benefits
Clinical clearance in the 5-FU group was superior to the interferon alfa-2b group (100% versus 90%) at 8-week assessment. A statistically significant difference in histological response to treatment was further noted at 4 and 8 weeks in favour of interferon ($P<0.05$).[78] This trial failed to specify the number of BD lesions in each treatment group; consequently, the reported data prevents conclusions for BD independent of AK.

In the uncontrolled trials, clinical clearance rates were generally high, ranging from 87%[80] to 100%.[49] It is noteworthy that, of studies with sufficient follow up to document recurrence (12–24 months), one study reported a significantly higher recurrence rate (20%)[81] than other studies (0% and 8%).[49,58,80] The largest uncontrolled trial (n = 41) used 5-FU (in 1–3% in propylene glycol) applied twice daily for 2–3 months.[58] Clinical clearance rate in this study was 93%, with an 8% recurrence rate during a median follow up of 8 years (range: 6–121 months). The authors

suggest that at least 2.5% 5-FU in propylene glycol is required for extrafacial sites.

The base in which 5-FU is delivered significantly affects its activity: 20% 5-FU in an ointment base, 5% 5-FU in a cream base, and 1% 5-FU in propylene glycol provide approximately equivalent cytotoxic activity.[72,77,82,83] Several studies investigated ways to enhance 5-FU activity. Iontophoresis does not appear to improve 5-FU activity when compared with 5-FU alone.[49,58,80,81] Application under occlusion, pretreatment with keratolytic agents, or deliberate exposure to sunlight (photosensitivity effect of 5-FU) are anecdotally reported as enhancement techniques.[58]

Harms
Expected side-effects include pain, pruritus, burning at the site of application, erythema, inflammation and erosions.[41] Some authors suggest application of the medication 4 times daily to reduce the duration of treatment,[84] while others advocate pulse therapy once or twice weekly to decrease the intensity of discomfort.[85] Although compliance with the latter regimen is higher, cure rates may be lower.[86] Lower-leg ulceration has been reported with 5% 5-FU cream,[81] and allergic reaction to 5-FU has been reported in conjunction with iontophoretic therapy.[79]

Comment
Although the studies have significant methodological limitations, 5-FU appears to be of likely benefit in treating BD. As with AK, if patients are unable to tolerate the side-effects of 5-FU, then we would expect the cure rate to drop off dramatically.

The quasi-randomised controlled trial comparing 5-FU with interferon suffers from two methodological limitations in addition to the non-randomised allocation. No data are presented regarding the proportion of BD and AK in each treatment group, thus conclusions regarding therapeutic efficacy can only be generalised to BD and AK in aggregate. Furthermore, the significant difference in histological response in favour of interferon does not correlate with the higher efficacy of 5-FU in terms of clinical clearance. Thus, histological response may have been used as a surrogate outcome for clinical response and should be viewed accordingly in clinical decision making.

It is impossible to draw definitive conclusions from uncontrolled trials. However, it is worth noting that the disparity in recurrence rates may relate to different therapeutic regimens: the study reporting a higher recurrence employed weekly topical pulse therapy for a minimum of 12 weeks, whereas most other studies used once- or twice-daily applications for 2–16 weeks.[58,78,79]

Imiquimod

The immunomodulator imiquimod is one of the newest treatments studied for use in AK and BD. We found no systematic reviews or RCTs for either AK or BD.

Actinic keratoses

Quality of evidence: IV

We found a case series of six patients with AK with up to 10 scalp lesions treated with topical imiquimod for 6–8 weeks.[87]

Benefit

All AK lesions resolved histologically as well as clinically; follow up is ongoing, ranging from 2 to 12 months at the time of publication.

Comment

Although the case series appears promising, there is not enough evidence to make recommendations for the use of imiquimod for treatment of AK.

Bowen's disease

Quality of evidence: III

We found two uncontrolled trials, the first following 16 lesions of the lower limbs with once-daily application of imiquimod cream for 16 weeks[88] and the second using imiquimod cream and oral sulindac, 200 mg twice daily, for 16 weeks in five immunocompromised patients.[89]

Benefits

The first study reported a 93% (15 of 16 patients) treatment response, evidenced by no residual tumour on histology, although six subjects withdrew prematurely because of local skin reactions and were not included in the final analysis.[88] An ITT analysis showed that 87·5% (14 of 16 patients) had no residual tumour. All immunocompromised patients showed complete clinical response within 4 weeks of therapy and histological response at 20 weeks after initiation of therapy.[89]

Harms

The case series for AK reported mild erythema in all patients In uncontrolled trials in BD, adverse events included marked local skin irritation requiring discontinuation of therapy, superinfection requiring antibiotics, satellite lesions in adjacent sun-damaged areas.[88]

Comments

Imiquimod 5% cream appears to be an efficacious treatment for BD of the lower limbs, particularly for large lesions on the lower extremity, such as the shin, where poor healing is of particular concern. The dosing schedule and length of treatment require further evaluation in RCTs.

Photodynamic therapy (PDT)

PDT involves activation of a photosensitiser, usually a porphyrin derivative, by visible light. A common photosensitiser is topical aminolaevulinic acid (ALA).

Actinic keratoses

Quality of evidence: I

We found no systematic reviews and three RCTs.

One compared 0%, 10%, 20% or 30% 5-ALA with placebo in a dose-ranging study using a 630 nm light source and a 3-hour incubation time.[90] Another RCT tested a recent formulation of ALA, the Levulan Kerastick topical solution, (n = 180) with placebo (n = 61) using a 14–18 hour incubation time and illumination with BLU-U blue light (417 nm).[91] The third study compared treatment of hand lesions with a 4-hour incubation with 20% 5-ALA and 580–740 nm light against topical 5% 5-FU.[92]

Benefits

All concentrations of 5-ALA were significantly better than placebo using the 630 nm light source ($P<0.001$).[90] Thirty per cent 5-ALA showed the highest rates of complete and partial response at assessment 8 weeks after light treatment (61% and 26%, respectively) compared with 20% 5-ALA (complete response about 50%). Partial response was defined as 50–100% reduction in lesion area, and complete response was considered as no palpable or visible lesions. Facial and scalp lesions had better rates of complete clearance than trunk and extremity lesions (30% ALA: 91% versus 45%; 20% 5-ALA: 78% versus 38%). Levulan Kerastick topical solution showed higher complete response (66% versus 13%) and 75% clearance rates (77% versus 23%) at 8 weeks than placebo[91] Use of 580–740 nm light with 5-ALA for lesions on hands was not significantly

different from 5-FU (73% versus 70% reduction).[92] Complete clearance was not observed in either group.

Harms

Most patients experienced a stinging or burning sensation during photoirradiation, which generally ceased on completion of phototherapy. Treated lesions typically became erythematous and oedematous following treatment. Healing occurred over 2–4 weeks.

Comments

PDT has produced a reduction of AK lesions using a wide variety of light sources, and occluded incubation periods with 5-ALA. A 20% concentration has been used most frequently, but other concentrations (10%, 30%) have also been used effectively. However, in the US only a 20% ALA HCl topical solution used in conjunction with the blue light PDT illuminator is approved for the treatment of AK. Although the healing process is somewhat lengthy, it is comparable to the events experienced by patients following 5-FU and other topical regimens. As treatment takes place over 2 days, rather than many weeks with topical formulations, PDT may be more convenient for the patient willing to undergo the process; however, long-term efficacy has not been established. Moreover, PDT has not been effective in treating hyperkeratotic lesions.

Bowen's disease

Quality of evidence: I

We found no systematic reviews, one RCT and one unblinded controlled trial. The RCT investigated 61 lower leg lesions to compare the efficacy of green light and red light wavelengths after incubation with 20% 5-ALA for 4 hours.[93] The follow up period was 12 months. The unblinded, controlled trial investigated 40 lesions to determine the relative efficacy of 20% 5-ALA cream and a modified portable desktop lamp against cryotherapy.[94] The method of randomisation in this study was not specified. The follow up period was 12 months.

Benefits

Lesions receiving red light showed significantly greater clinical clearance rate determined by dermatologist examination (94% versus 76%, $P = 0.002$) and lower recurrence (6% versus 38%) compared with green light (odds ratio 0.13; 95% CI 0.04–0.48). Punch biopsies were performed in cases where there was uncertainty about clinical clearance or recurrence. The authors attribute this difference to the reduced depth of tissue penetration by green light, postulating that peri-appendageal BD (which may extend up to 3 mm in depth) may survive ALA-PDT using less penetrating wavelengths. No ulceration, infection, scarring or photosensitivity reactions were reported in either group. There was no significant difference in pain between groups, and the majority of patients reported "none" to "moderate" pain.

In the unblinded controlled trial, a significant difference that a lesion of any size would clear after the first treatment with PDT compared with the first treatment with cryotherapy was observed ($P < 0.01$). However, there was no significant difference in the overall clearance rates between treatments following three treatments of cryotherapy ($P = 0.08$).[94] Clinical clearance at 12-month follow up was 90% in the cryotherapy group and 100% in the PDT group.

Harms

Adverse effects of PDT include treatment-induced pain requiring anaesthesia in up to 25% of lesions,[95–97] skin fragility and dyspigmentation,[97–99] permanent hair loss,[98] toxic reactions to ALA cream,[96] and photosensitivity reaction.[95]

Comments

PDT appears promising for BD but there were two major flaws in the study design. First, investigators were not blinded to the type of light used, thus potentially introducing bias. Although more objective outcomes such as clinical clearance and recurrence are unsusceptible to bias related to lack of blinding, the validity of the results concerning treatment-related pain may be improved with blinding. The analysis did not follow an ITT analysis, as 13% of initially randomised lesions (nine of 61) were excluded from the final analysis, thus risking overestimation of efficacy and underestimation of recurrence.

Masoprocol

Masoprocol (meso-nordihydroguariaretic acid) is a potent 5-lipoxygenase inhibitor with antitumour properties, investigated for use in AK.[100]

Quality of evidence: I

We found two double-blind RCTs.[62,100] The first study[101] compared masoprocol (n = 113) with topical placebo (n = 41), and the second study[62] compared masoprocol (n = 27) with topical 5% 5-FU (n = 30). Both studies reported 1-month follow up following end of treatment.

Benefits

Masoprocol produced a larger median percentage reduction in the number of AK lesions than placebo (71.4% versus 4.3%, respectively; $P < 0.0003$), and an 11% (12/113) cure rate on a per-patient basis.[100] Masoprocol produced a 78% reduction in AK lesions compared with a 98% reduction with 5-FU ($P < 0.0001$). Cure rates of masoprocol and 5-FU on a per-patient basis were 22% (5/23) and 77% (20/26), respectively.

Harms

Erythema occurred at rates of 53% and 22% with masoprocol and placebo, respectively, and flaking occurred at rates of 53% versus 4%, with masoprocol and placebo, respectively. Itching, burning, oedema, tightness, and dryness and bleeding of the skin were also reported with masoprocol.[100] Compared with 5-FU, masoprocol caused significantly fewer and less severe adverse effects, including, necrosis, erosion and erythema.[62] One report[101] described the potential for masoprocol to induce potent sensitisation (allergic contact dermatitis). The two clinical studies reported here did not exclude the possibility of allergic contact dermatitis with masoprocol.

Comments

Masoprocol produces significant reduction in AK lesions, and some patients had complete clearance of AK, although 5-FU appears to provide higher rates of cure on a per-patient basis. Masoprocol may provide an alternative for those who cannot tolerate 5-FU. Long-term efficacy for masoprocol has yet to be established.

Miscellaneous topical therapies

A variety of other topical therapies have been assessed as treatment for actinic lesions, with varied success. These include Solaraze™ (3% diclofenac sodium in 2·5% hyaluronan gel) Curaderm (0·005% solasodine glycosides (BEC), 10% salicylic acid, 5% urea, 0·1% melaleuca oil, 0·05% linolenic acid in cetomacrogol-based cream) and the nucleoside tubercidin (7-deaza-adenosine).

Quality of evidence: IV

We found no systematic reviews for any of these three topical therapies. We found one RCT for Solaraze™, but only the abstract was accessible. Although complete and partial responses were reported, neither was defined; time of final assessment was also not defined.[102] In an open-label study,[103] the responses in 29 patients were graded on a seven-point scale, ranging from "complete response" to "much worse", 30 days after treatment. The parameters used to determine this response grading, the degree of change required to increase or decrease a grading, as well as location of lesions, were not specified. Clearance rates for 90-day treatment are also available from two placebo-controlled trials reported in the package insert for Solaraze, but details of the trials were unavailable to us.

A case series used tubercidin to treat five patients with facial and scalp AK lesions.[104]

A single open-label trial treated 56 AK lesions using Curaderm,[105] with follow up at 3 months post-treatment.

Benefits

Diclofenac sodium is a non-steroidal anti-inflammatory drug which has been examined for use in treatment of AK, with some success.[102,103]

Curaderm has been reported to completely cure (clinically and histologically) AK lesions in a mean time of 2·9 weeks (range 1–4 weeks) in an open-label Australian trial.[105] However, no recent literature on this treatment was found in any searches, and no North American use has been reported.

The nucleoside tubercidin interferes with glycolysis and inhibits synthesis of DNA, RNA and proteins. Tubercidin was not effective in a case series of five patients with facial and scalp AK.[104] Four of the patients showed no response of lesions to tubercidin after 4 weeks of treatment.

Harms

Mild-to-moderate skin reactions occurred with diclofenac: 29% versus 5% with placebo ($P = 0.0002$) in the RCT,[102] 72% in the open-label trial,[103] and 86% in the trials reported in the package insert.

The one patient who had complete resolution with tubercidin had marked facial erythema. Curaderm produced itching and burning sensations in lesions during treatment but no abnormal haematological, biochemical or urinalytic parameters were noted.

Comments

Topical treatments, which the patient can apply in the comfort of their home, are more convenient than treatments that must be administered by a physician, and in general are more convenient than cryotherapy in treating multiple lesions. However, many treatments require further study to confirm the efficacy compared with the standard treatments with liquid-nitrogen cryotherapy and 5-FU.

What are the effects of intralesional or oral medication?

Oral retinoids
Actinic keratoses
Quality of evidence: I

We found two double-blind placebo-controlled RCTs investigating the reduction in AK lesion size and overall grade (based on number, diameter, thickness and hyperkeratosis).[106,107] Both studies used a crossover design and followed lesions from 2 to 18 months.

Benefits

Oral etretinate (Tegison) reduced the lesion size in 82–86% of patients in the first study,[106] both when etretinate was the primary drug (19/22, followed by placebo) or when etretinate was used after crossover from placebo (18/22). Placebo reduced lesion size in only 4·3% (1/23) of patients who used placebo before etretinate. Use of placebo following etretinate resulted in no change in lesions for 95% of subjects (18/19).

In the second study,[107] etretinate improved the overall grading of lesions in 89–100% of patients (8/9 subjects using etretinate before placebo and 6/6 subjects using etretinate after placebo use). Placebo improved lesion gradings in 17% of subjects who used placebo before crossing over to etretinate (1/6). For those subjects who crossed over to placebo from etretinate, only 11% had any further improvement (1/9).

Harms

Dry lips and mouth may occur in a high proportion of patients using etretinate, although symptom alleviation occurs with dose reduction. Transient elevations of serum cholesterol and triglycerides, and one case of drug-related hepatitis were reported.[107]

Comments

Rates of reduction in lesion size and grading appear to be significantly better for etretinate than placebo. However, one should be careful of crossover study designs, where a big carry-over effect is likely. If insufficient time is allowed for the etretinate to "wash-out" in those arms where etretinate was given before placebo, then the effects of etretinate were probably confounding the results of the placebo. Long-term efficacy has not been established, but it is unlikely that the long-term efficacy will reflect the efficacy rates reported in the studies, since they reported reduction in AK size. If the AK lesions are not eradicated, they will surely regrow; moreover, even if a particular AK lesion is eradicated, it does not prevent new ones from forming.

Bowen's disease
Quality of evidence: IV

One uncontrolled trial[108] examined the use of aromatic retinoid tablets, 1 mg/kg daily, over a period of 2–7 months in five patients with multiple BD secondary to chronic arsenism.

Benefit
Residual tumour cells were found all patients.

Interferon
Actinic keratoses
Quality of evidence: I

We found one double-blind placebo-controlled parallel-group RCT each for intralesional interferon alfa[109] and topical interferon gel (Intron A; unterferon alfa-2b).[110] The studies involved 16–23 patients, with a post-treatment follow up period of 1–2 months. No indication of complete cure on a per-patient basis was indicated.

Benefit
High-dose interferon given intralesionally three times weekly for 2–3 weeks produced complete cure in 47–93% of lesions treated.[109] No complete cures were produced with topical interferon gel, and only 9% (n = 35 lesions) of lesions showed marked (>75%) improvement.[110]

Comment
While high doses of intralesional interferon appears promising, it is unlikely that the topical formulation will be of much benefit. However, intralesional interferon should be reserved for those patients who cannot use more conventional and economical therapies.

Bowen's disease
Quality of evidence: II-i

We found one small unblinded quasi-randomised controlled trial comparing topical 5-FU (5% cream) with intralesional interferon alfa-2b (1 000 000 units/injection) in the treatment of BD and AK, as reported above.[78]

Benefit
The 5-FU group showed 100% clinical clearance whereas the interferon group showed 90% clinical clearance at the 8-week assessment. The study did not differentiate between BD and AK.

Comment
Intralesional interferon may be a good option for BD in those not responsive to more conventional and economical therapies.

Bleomycin
There is one successful anecdotal report using intralesional bleomycin for BD.[111]

Clinical scenarios
Scenario 1
An elderly man with recurrent AK has 30 lesions on his sun-damaged head. How would you approach his problem?

The most likely therapy that a dermatologist would offer is cryotherapy since it is easy for the clinician, relatively well tolerated by the patient, and if the patient has medical insurance, inexpensive for the patient. However, only one study has quantified the efficacy of cryotherapy.

Therapies for which there is more substantial evidence are oral retinoids and topical 5-FU. However, the elderly patient may not tolerate the side-effects of these therapies. The clinician may then offer either topical retinoids or chemical peels. PDT and masoprocol, while likely to be beneficial according to the evidence, are not yet widely available. Similarly while intralesional interferon is likely to be beneficial, injection into the lesions is unlikely to be tolerated by the patient.

Scenario 2

A woman in her 50s presents with a large biopsy-proven BD lesion on her ankle. What would you do?

While there are no studies demonstrating strong evidence for beneficial therapies, several therapies are likely to beneficial on the basis of the evidence presented. Cryotherapy and ED&C are both likely to be beneficial and the patient may feel reassured about these therapies because they are destructive and are performed by the clinician. While PDT is also likely to be beneficial, it is not widely available. Topical 5-FU is also likely to be beneficial and can be used in patients who are either very compliant and/or would not otherwise tolerate a more invasive procedure. Intralesional interferon is also likely to be beneficial but will probably be a second-line agent because of its cost.

Implications for clinical practice
Spontaneous regression rates

As discussed in the background section, the prognosis of AKs without treatment is confounded by the spontaneous regression rate. A study from Queensland[28] reported a spontaneous regression rate of 85% (95% CI: 75–96%) in subjects with prevalent AK (AK diagnosed on a person during their first exam) and 84% (95% CI: 72–96%) in persons with incident AK (AK appearing for the first time during the study).

We (PP and SC) compared the efficacy of 5% 5-FU with a range of plausible spontaneous regression rates of AK.[39] While we could not pinpoint the exact threshold of spontaneous regression rate above which 5-FU would be less effective than no therapy, we find it intriguing that the natural regression rate of AK can be such that the efficacy of a therapeutic modality may appear to be less than no therapy. Assuming the efficacy of 5-FU ointment to be 79%, we

calculated that if the spontaneous AK regression rates were above 75%, no therapy may be better than using 5-fluorouracil.

Of note, standard care is to always treat AK because we cannot predict which cases will resolve spontaneously and which will progress to cancers. To explore this idea more fully, we propose future studies to directly compare three strategies: 5-FU, cryotherapy and no therapy.

Implications for future studies

General points that future investigators should bear in mind include using a double-blind randomised study design wherever possible, in order to minimise bias and confounding factors. If investigators wish to use a crossover study design, extreme care must be taken because of the potentially long wash-out periods for most AK therapies. Lastly, investigators should report results of ITT analysis. Without taking into account those subjects who drop out of the study, results can be misleading.

While any given individual AK lesions has a high probability of resolving spontaneously, a patient with extensive involvement most probably has a much lower probability of all his/her AK lesions resolving spontaneously – an issue unique to AK. Thus, studies should either take into account the high correlation of multiple AK lesions if they choose to use number of lesions as their unit of analysis, or results should be stratified by severity of AK if persons cleared is used as the unit of analysis. The later outcome is likely to be of more interest because it is clinically more relevant.

Another precaution unique to AK studies is to ensure that the outcome measure is reliable. Weinstock et al.[112] reported their experience in counting numbers of AK lesions, a commonly used technique. They found the outcome measure to be unreliable, most likely because of

Table 28.1 Summary of therapies for actinic keratoses (AK) and Bowen's disease (BD). Unless indicated, all interventions listed pertain to both AK and BD

- We designated therapies to be "beneficial" if they met the Quality of Evidence level I (see Box 28.1) and had an efficacy of at least 75%.
- Therapies were "likely to be beneficial" if they met the Quality of Evidence levels II-i or II-ii and had an efficacy of at least 60%.
- Therapies were of "unknown effectiveness" if the Quality of Evidence level was II-iii, III or IV. Therapies were "unlikely to be beneficial" if they met a quality of evidence level of I and had an efficacy rate of less than 30%.

Beneficial	Likely to be beneficial	Unknown effectiveness	Unlikely to be beneficial
Actinic keratoses			
• Oral retinoids	• Topical retinoids	• Cryotherapy	• Topical interferon
• Topical 5-FU	• Chemical peels	• Laser	
	• PDT	• Radiotherapy	
	• Masoprocol	• Dermabrasion	
	• Intralesional interferon	• Topical imiquimod	
		• Diclofenac	
		• Tubercidin	
		• Curaderm	
Bowen's disease			
• None	• Cryotherapy	• Laser	• None
	• ED&C	• Radiotherapy	
	• PDT	• Topical imiquimod	
	• Intralesional interferon	• Oral retinoids	
	• Topical 5-FU	• Intralesional bleomycin	

ED&C, electrodessication and curettage; 5-FU, 5-fluorouracil; PDT, photodynamic therapy

the spectrum of clinical features. Discussion of discrepancies among investigators enhanced the reliability of the counts, but substantial variation remain. Thus, investigators should test the reliability of their outcome measure before proceeding with the therapeutic part of a study.

Key points

- The likely benefits of the various therapies proposed for AK and BD are summarised in Table 28.1.
- We found good evidence to suggest that oral retinoids and topical 5-FU may be beneficial in the treatment of AK.

- The evidence supporting the efficacy of most therapies is insufficient or limited.
- Studies were not consistent in choosing their unit of analyses. Some used number of lesions, other used persons cleared, and others used both as their unit of analyses. Readers should determine which unit is most relevant to their practice.
- The evidence for treatment of BD is generally of poor quality.
- Choice of therapy in BD should consider location of lesions, particularly the lower legs and the digits, where healing may be complicated.
- ED&C, 5-FU, and cryotherapy are acceptable first-line agents for BD, given the available evidence.

- ED&C may be superior to cryotherapy for lower-leg lesions.
- There appears to be good evidence for the superior efficacy of red light over green light in ALA-PDT.

References

1. Bowen J. Precancerous dermatoses: a study of two cases of chronic atypical epithelial proliferation. *J Cutan Dis* 1912;**30**:241–55.

2. Lee M, Wick M. Bowen's disease. *Cancer J Clin* 1990;**40**:237–42.

3. Frost C, Green A. Epidemiology of solar keratoses. *Br J Dermatol* 1994;**131**:455–64.

4. Vitasa B, Taylor H, Strickland P *et al.* Association of non-melanoma skin cancer and actinic keratosis with cumulative solar ultraviolet exposure in Maryland watermen. *Cancer* 1990;**65**:2811–17.

5. Schwartz R. The actinic keratosis. A perspective and update. *Dermatol Surg* 1997;**23**:1009–19.

6. Marks R, Jolley D, Dorevitch A *et al.* The incidence of non-melanocytic skin cancers in an Australian population: results of a five-year prospective study. *Med J Aus* 1989;**150**:475–8.

7. Eedy D, Gavin G. Thirteen-year retrospective study of Bowen's disease in Northern Ireland. *Br J Dermatol* 1987;**117**:715–20.

8. Kossard S, Rosen R. Cutaneous Bowen's disease. *J Am Acad Dermatol* 1992;**27**:406–10.

9. Thestrup-Pederson K, Ravnborg L, Reymann F. Morbus Bowen. *Acta Derm Venereol* 1988;**68**:236–9.

10. Holman C, Armstrong B, Evans P *et al.* Relationship of solar keratoses and history of skin cancer to objective measures of actinic skin damage. *Br J Dermatol* 1984;**110**:129–38.

11. Green A, Beardmore G, Hart V *et al.* Skin cancer in a Queensland population. *J Am Acad Dermatol* 1988;**19**:1045–52.

12. Marks R, Staples M, Giles G. Trends in non-melanocytic skin cancer treated in Australia: the Second National Survey. *Int J Cancer* 1993;**53**:585–90.

13. Schwartz R. Therapeutic perspectives in actinic and other keratoses. *Int J Dermatol* 1996;**35**:533–8.

14. Preston D, Stern R. Nonmelanoma cancers of the skin. *N Engl J Med* 1992;**327**:1649–62.

15. Sanchez Yus E, de Diego V, Urrutia S. Large cell acanthoma: a cytologic variant of Bowen's disease. *Am J Dermatopath* 1988;**10**:197–208.

16. Reizner G, Chuang T, Elpern D, Stone J, Farmer E. Bowen's diseae (squamous cell carcinoma *in situ*) in Kauai, Hawaii. A population-based incidence report. *J Am Acad Dermatol* 1994;**31**:596–600.

17. Fiertz U. Catamnestic investigations of the side effects of therapy of skin diseases with inorganic arsenic. *Dermatologica* 1965;**131**:41–58.

18. Yeh S. Skin cancer in chronic arsenism. *Hum Pathol* 1967;**4**:469–85.

19. Yeh S, How S, Lin C. Arsenical cancer of the skin. Histologic study with special reference to Bowen's disease. *Cancer* 1968;**21**:312–39.

20. Shannon R, Strayer D. Arsenic-induced skin toxicity. *Hum Toxicol* 1989;**8**:99–104.

21. Cox N, Eedy D, Morton C. Guidelines for management of Bowen's disease. *Br J Dermatol* 1999;**141**:633–41.

22. Kettler A, Rutledge M, Tschen JG. Detection of human papillomavirus in nongenital Bowen's disease by *in situ* DNA hybridization. *Arch Dermatol* 1990;**126**:777–81.

23. Collina G, Rossie E, Betelli S. Detection of human papillomavirus in extragenital Bowen's disease using in situ hybridization and polymerase chain reaction. *Am J Dermatopath* 1995;**17**:326–41.

24. Czarnecki D, Staples M, Mar A, Giles G, Meehan C. Metastases from squamous cell carcinoma of the skin in southern Australia. *Dermatology* 1994;**189**:52.

25. Boddie AJ Jr, Fischer EP, Byers RM. Squamous carcinoma of the lower lip in patients under 40 years of age. *South Med J* 1977;**70**:711.

26. Glogau R. The risk of progression to invasive disease. *J Am Acad Dermatol* 2000;**42**:S23–S24.

27. Dodson J, DeSpain J, Hewett JE *et al.* Malignant potential of actinic keratoses and the controversy over treatments. A patient oriented perspective. *Arch Dermatol* 1991;**127**: 1029–31.

28. Frost C, Williams G, Green A. High incidence and regression rates of solar keratoses in a Queensland community. *J Invest Dermatol* 2000;**115**:273–7.

29. Jacobs D. Sebaceous carcinoma arising from Bowen's disease of the vulva. *Arch Dermatol* 1926;**122**:1191–3.

30. Saida T, Okabe Y, Uhara H. Bowen's disease with invasive carcinoma showing sweat gland differentiation. *J Cutan Pathol* 1989;**16**:222–6.

31. Kao G. Carcinoma arising in Bowen's disease. *Arch Dermatol* 1986;**122**:1124–6.

32. Beerman H. Tumors of the skin. *Am J Med Sci* 1946;**211**:480–504.

33. Graham J, Helwig E. Bowen's disease and its relationship to systemic cancer. *Arch Dermatol* 1959;**80**:133–159.

34. Epstein E. Association of Bowen's disease with visceral cancer. *Arch Dermatol* 1960;**82**:349–51.

35. Callen J, Headington J. Bowen's and non-Bowen's squamous intraepidermal neoplasia of the skin: relationship to internal malignancy. *Arch Dermatol* 1980;**116**:422–6.

36. Lycka B. Bowen's disease and internal malignancy. A meta-analysis. *Int J Dermatol* 1989;**28**:531–3.

37. Cox NH, Eedy DJ, Morton CA. Guidelines for management of Bowen's disease. British Association of Dermatologists. *Br J Dermatol* 1999;**141**:633–41.

38. Stevens A, Raftery, J. Health Care Needs Assessment. In: Williams HC, ed. *Dermatology*. Oxford: Radcliffe Medical Press 1997:261–341.

39. Pierre P, Weil E, Chen S. Cryotherapy versus topical 5-fluorouracil therapy of actinic keratoses: a systematic review. *Allergologie* 2001;**24**:204–5.

40. Lubritz R, Smolewski S. Cryosurgery cure rate of actinic keratoses. *J Am Acad Dermatol* 1982;**7**:631–2.

41. Dinehart S. The treatment of actinic keratoses. *J Am Acad Dermatol* 2000;**42**:S25–S28.

42. Ahmed I, Berth-Jones J, Charles-Holmes S, Callaghan C, Ilchyshyn A. Comparison of cryotherapy with curettage in the treatment of Bowen's disease: a prospective study. *Br J Dermatol* 2000;**143**:759–66.

43. Cox N, Dyson P. Wound healing on the lower leg after radiotherapy or cryotherapy of Bowen's disease and other malignant skin lesions. *Br J Dermatol* 1995;**133**:60–5.

44. Drnovsek-Olup B, Vedlin B. Use of Er:YAG laser for benign skin disorders. *Lasers Surg Med* 1997;**21**:13–19.

45. Jiang SB, Levine VJ, Nehal KS, Baldassano M, Kamino H, Ashinoff RA. Er:YAG laser for the treatment of actinic keratoses. *Dermatol Surg* 2000;**26**:437–40.

46. Gordon K, Garden J, Robinson J. Bowen's disease of the distal digit. *Dermatol Surg* 1996;**22**:723–8.

47. Tantikun N. Treatment of Bowen's disease of the digit with carbon dioxide laser. *J Am Acad Dermatol* 2000;**43**:1080–3.

48. Barta U, Grafe T, Wollina U. Radiation therapy for extensive actinic keratosis. *J Eur Acad Dermatol Venereol* 1999;**14**:293–5.

49. Stevens D, Kopf A, Gladstein A, Bart R. Treatment of Bowen's disease with grenz rays. *Int J Dermatol* 1977;**16**:329–39.

50. Caccialanza M, Piccinno R, Beretta M, Sopelana N. Radiotherapy of Bowen's disease. *Skin Cancer* 1993;**8**:115–18.

51. Umebayashi Y, Uyeno K, Tsujii H, Otsuka F. Proton radiotherapy of skin carcinoma. *Br J Dermatol* 1994;**130**:88–91.

52. Chung Y, Lee J, Bang D, Lee J, Kyung B, Lee M. Treatment of Bowen's disease with a specially designed radioactive skin patch. *Eur J Nucl Med* 2000;**27**:842–6.

53. Humphreys TR, Werth V, Dzubow L, Kligman A. Treatment of photodamaged skin with trichloroacetic acid and topical tretinoin. *J Am Acad Dermatol* 1996;**133**:638–44.

54. Lawrence N, Cox SE, Cockerell CJ, Freeman RG, Ponciano DC, Jr. A comparison of the efficacy and safety of Jessner's solution and 35% trichloroacetic acid v 5% fluorouracil in the treatment of widespread facial actinic keratoses. *Arch Dermatol* 1995;**131**:176–81.

55. Witheiler DD, Lawrence N, Cox SE, Cruz C, Cockerell CJ, Freeman RG. Long-term efficacy and safety of Jessner's solution and 35% trichloroacetic acid v 5% fluorouracil in the treatment of widespread facial actinic keratoses. *Dermatol Surg* 1997;**23**:191–6.

56. Spira M, Frreman R, Arfai P, Gerow F, Hardy S. A comparison of chemical peeling, dermabrasion, and 5-fluorouracil in cancer prophylaxis. *J Surg Oncol* 1971;**3**:367–8.

57. Winton GB, Salasche SJ. Dermabrasion of the scalp as a treatment for actinic damage. *J Am Acad Dermatol* 1986;**14**:661–8.

58. Sturm H. Bowen's disease and 5-fluorouracil. *J Am Acad Dermatol* 1979;**1**:513–22.

59. Hiruma M, Kawada A. Hyperthermic treatment of Bowen's disease with disposable chemical pocket warmers: a report of 8 cases. *J Am Acad Dermatol* 2000;**43**:1070–5.

60. Misiewicz J, Sendagorta E, Golebiowska A, Lorenc B, Czarnetzki B, Jablonska S. Topical treatment of mulitple actinic keratoses of the face with arotinoid methyl sulfone (Ro 14-9706) cream versus tretinoin cream: A double-blind, comparative study. *J Am Acad Dermatol* 1991;**24**:448–51.

61. Alirezai M, Dupuy P, Amblard P *et al.* Clinical evaluation of topical isotretinoin in the treatment of actinic keratoses. *J Am Acad Dermatol* 1994;**30**:447–51.

62. Kulp-Shorten CL, Konnikov N, Callen JP. Comparative evaluation of the efficacy and safety of masoprocol and 5-fluorouracil cream for the treatment of multiple actinic keratoses of the head and neck. *J Geriatr Dermatol* 1993;**1**:161–8.

63. Breza T, Taylor R, Eaglstein W. Noninflammatory destruction of actinic keratoses by fluorouracil. *Arch Dermatol* 1976;**112**:1256–8.

64. Carter V, Smith K, Noojin R. Xeroderma pigmentosum. Treatment with topically applied fluorouracil. *Arch Dermatol* 1968;**98**:526–7.

65. Simmonds W. Topical management of actinic keratoses with 5-fluorouracil: results of a 6-year follow-up study. *Cutis* 1972;**10**:737–41.

66. Neldner K. Prevention of skin cancer with topical 5-Fluorouracil. *Rocky Mountain Med J* 1966;**Nov**:74–8.

67. Epstein E. Treatment of lip keratoses (actinic cheilitis) with topical fluorouracil. *Arch Dermatol* 1977;**113**:906–8.

68. Marrero G, Katz B. The new fluor-hydroxy pulse peel. A combination of 5-fluorouracil and glycolic acid. *Dermatol Surg* 1998;**24**:973–8.

69. Klein E, Stoll H, Milgrom H, Helm F, Walker M. Tumors of the Skin. XII. Topical 5-fluorouracil for epidermal neoplasms. *J Surg Oncol* 1971;**3**:331–49.

70. Schultz E, Falkson G. Benign and malignant skin diseases response to topical 5-fluorouracil. *Med Proc* 1970;**Feb**:41–6.

71. Dogliotti M. Actinic keratoses in Bantu Albinos: Clinical experiences with the topical use of 5-fluorouracil. *S Afr Med J* 1973;**47**:2169–72.

72. Dillaha C, Jansen G, Honeycutt W, Holt G. Further studies with topical 5-fluorouracil. *Arch Dermatol* 1965;**92**:410–13.

73. Ott F, Eichenberger-De Beer H, Storck H. The local treatment of precancerous skin conmdition with 5-Fluorouracil ointment. *Dermatologica* 1970;**140**:109–13.

74. Robinson T, Kligman A. Treatment of solar keratoses of the extremities with retinoic acid and 5-Fluorouracil. *Br J Dermatol* 1975;**92**:703–6.

75. Bercovitch L. Topical chemotherapy of actinic keratoses of upper extremities with tretinoin and 5-fluorouracil: a double-blind controlled study. *Br J Dermatol* 1987;**116**:549–52.

76. Goncalves J. Treatment of solar keratoses with a 5-fluorouracil and salicylic acid varnish. *Br J Dermatol* 1975;**92**:85–8.

77. Dillaha C, Jansen G, Honeycutt WM *et al.* Selective cytotoxic effect of topical 5-fluorouracil. *Arch Dermatol* 1963;**88**:247–56.

78. Shuttleworth D, Marks R. A comparison of the effects of intralesional interferon alpha-2b and topical 5% 5-fluorouracil cream in the treatment of solar keratoses and Bowen's disease. *J Dermatol Treat* 1989;**1**:65–8.

79. Welch M, Grabski W, McCollough M, Skelton H, Smith K, Menon P. 5-fluorouracil iontophoretic therapy for Bowen's disease. *J Am Acad Dermatol* 1997;**36**:956–8.

80. Bell H, Rhodes L. Bowen's disease-a retrospective review of clinical management. *Clin Exp Dermatol* 1999;**24**:336–9.

81. Stone N, Burge S. Bowen's disease of the leg treated with weekly pulses of 5% fluorouracil cream. *Br J Dermatol* 1999;**140**:963–91.

82. Dillaha C, Jansen G, Honeycutt W. Topical therapy with fluorouracil. *Prog Dermatol* 1966;**1**:1–2.

83. Jansen G, Dillaha C, Honeycutt W. Bowenoid conditions of the skin: treatment with topical 5-fluorouracil. *Southern Med J* 1967;**60**:185–8.

84. Unis M. Short-term intensive 5-fluorouracil treatment of actinic keratoses [see comments]. *Dermatol Surg* 1995;**21**:162–3.

85. Pearlman D. Weekly pulse dosing: effective and comfortable topical 5-fluorouracil treatment of multiple facial actinic keratoses. *J Am Acad Dermatol* 1991;**25**:665–7.

86. Epstein E. Does intermittent "pulse" topical 5-fluorouracil therapy allow destruction of actinic keratoses without significant inflammation? *J Am Acad Dermatol* 1998;**38**:77–80.

87. Stockfleth E, Meyer T, Benninghoff B, Christophers E. Successful treatment of actinic keratosis with imiquimod cream 5%: a report of six cases. *Br J Dermatol* 2001;**144**:1050–3.

88. Mackenzie-Wood A, Kossard S, de Launey J, Wilkinson B, Owens M. Imiquimod 5% cream in the treatment of Bowen's disease. *J Am Acad Dermatol* 2001;**44**: 462–70.

89. Smith K, Germain M, Sketon H. Bowen's disease (squamous cell carcinoma in situ) in immunosuppressed patients treated with imiquimod 5% cream and a COX inhibitor, sulindac: potential applications for this combination of immunotherapy. *Dermatol Surg* 2001;**27**: 143–6.

90. Jeffes EW, McCullough JL, Weinstein GD *et al.* Photodynamic therapy of actinic keratosis with topical 5-aminolevulinic acid: a pilot dose-ranging study. *Arch Dermatol* 1997;**133**:727–32.

91. Ormrod D, Jarvis B. Topical aminolevulinic acid HCl photodynamic therapy. *Am J Clin Dermatol* 2000;**1**: 133–9.

92. Kurwa HA, Yong-Gee SA, Seed PT, Markey AC, Barlow RJ. A randomized paired comparison of photodynamic therapy and topical 5-fluorouracil in the treatment of actinic keratoses. *J Am Acad Dermatol* 1999;**41**: 414–18.

93. Morton C, Whitehurst C, Moore J, Mackie R. Comparison of red and green light in the treatment of Bowen's disease by photodynamic therapy. *Br J Dermatol* 2000;**143**: 767–72.

94. Morton C, Whitehurst C, Moseley H, McColl J, Moore J, Mackie R. Comparison of photodynamic therapy with cryotherapy in the treatment of Bowen's disease. *Br J Dermatol* 1996;**135**:766–71.

95. Jones C, Mang T, Cooper M, Wilson B, Stoll H. Photodynamic therapy in the treatment of Bowen's disease. *J Am Acad Dermatol* 1992;**27**:979–82.

96. Svanberg K, Anderson T, Killander D, Wang I, Sternam U, Andersson-Engels S. Photodynamic therapy of non-melanoma malignant tumours of the skin using topical alpha-amino levulinic acid sensitization and laser irradiation. *Br J Dermatol* 1994;**130**:743–51.

97. Wong T, Sheu H, Lee Y, Fletcher R. Photodynamic therapy for Bowen's disease (squamous cell carcinoma in situ) of the digit. *Dermatol Surg* 2001;**27**:452–5.

98. Stables G, Stringer M, Robinson D, Ash D. Large patches of Bowen's disease treated by topical aminolaevulinic acid photodynamic therapy. *Br J Dermatol* 1997;**136**:957–60.

99. Fijan S, Honigsmann H, Ortel B. Photodynamic therapy of epithelial skin tumours using delta-aminolaevulinic acid and desferrioxamine. *Br J Dermatol* 1995;**133**:282–8.

100. Olsen EA, Abernethy ML, Kulp-Shorten C *et al.* A double-blind, vehicle-controlled study evaluating masoprocol cream in the treatment of actinic keratoses on the head and neck. *J Am Acad Dermatol* 1991;**24**(5 Pt 1):738–43.

101. Epstein E. Warning! Masoprocol is a potent sensitizer. *J Am Acad Dermatol* 1994;**31**(2 Pt 1):295–7.

102. McEwan LE, Smith JG. Topical diclofenac/hyaluronic acid gel in the treatment of solar keratoses. *Australas J Dermatol* 1997;**38**:187–9.

103. Rivers JK, McLean DI. An open study to assess the efficacy and safety of topical 3% diclofenac in a 2·5% hyaluronic acid gel for the treatment of actinic keratoses. *Arch Dermatol* 1997;**133**:1239–42.

104. Burgess GH, Bloch A, Stoll H, Milgrom H, Helm F, Klein E. Effect of topical tubercidin on basal cell carcinomas and actinic keratoses. *Cancer* 1974;**34**:250–3.

105. Cham BE, Daunter B, Evans RA. Topical treatment of malignant and premalignant skin lesions by very low concentrations of a standard mixture (BEC) of solasodine glycosides. *Cancer Lett* 1991;**59**:183–92.

106. Moriarty M, Dunn J, Darragh A, Lambe R, Brick I. Etretinate in treatment of actinic keratosis. *Lancet* 1982;**i**(**8268**):364–5.

107. Watson AB. Preventative effect of etretinate therapy on multiple actinic keratoses. *Cancer Detect Prev* 1986;**9**:161–5.

108. Thianprasit M. Chronic cutaneous arsenism treated with aromatic retinoid. *J Med Assoc Thailand* 1984;**67**: 93–100.

109. Edwards L, Levine N, Weidner M, Piepkorn M, Smiles K. Effect of intralesional a2-interferon on actinic keratoses. *Arch Dermatol* 1986;**122**:779–82.

110. Edwards L, Levine N, Smiles K. The effect of topical interferon Alpha2b on actinic keratoses. *J Dermatol Surg Oncol* 1990;**16**:446–9.

111. Dyall-Smith D. Intralesional bleomycin. *Australas J Dermatol* 1998;**39**:123–4.

112. Weinstock MA, Bingham SF, Cole GW *et al.* Reliability of counting actinic keratoses before and after brief consensus discussion: the VA topical tretinoin chemoprevention (VATTC) trial. *Arch Dermatol* 2001;**137**:1055–8.

29
Kaposi's sarcoma

Imogen Locke and Margaret F Spittle

Background
Definition

Kaposi's sarcoma (KS), described by Moritz Kaposi in 1872, is a multifocal vascular tumour. It is characterised histologically by a proliferation of spindle-shaped tumour cells surrounding abnormal slit-like vascular channels with extravasated erythrocytes. It may present with cutaneous or mucosal lesions (mouth, gastrointestinal, bronchial), visceral lesions or lymphadenopathy.

There are four clinical variants of KS which appear in specific populations but have identical histological features:

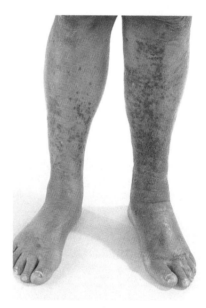

Figure 29.2 Endemic (African) Kaposi's sarcoma

1.   Classical Kaposi's sarcoma

Classical KS (Figure 29.1) typically affects elderly men of Mediterranean or Jewish descent. It presents with purple–blue ulcerated plaques on the lower legs, which progress over a period of years.

2.   Endemic (African) Kaposi's sarcoma

Endemic (or African) KS (Figure 29.2) is common in Sub-saharan Africa. In its nodular form it may run an indolent course similar to classical KS, with oedema of the lower legs. A more aggressive lymphadenopathic form of disseminated endemic KS is seen in children

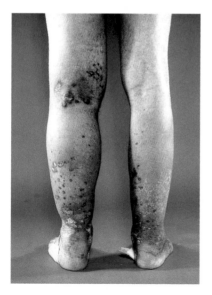

Figure 29.1 Classic Kaposi's sarcoma with oedema of the left leg

and young adults. Florid and infiltrative types of endemic KS affect adults and are locally aggressive.

3. Transplant/immunosuppression-related Kaposi's sarcoma

Transplant recipients and patients receiving immunosuppressive therapy are another group in which KS occurs. The same ethnic groups in which classical KS is seen are at higher risk but the disease tends to run a more aggressive course.

4. AIDS-related Kaposi's sarcoma

In 1981, Friedman-Kien *et al.* reported a cluster of young homosexual men with aggressive KS involving lymph nodes and viscera, in association with a syndrome of opportunistic infections and a defect in cell-mediated immunity, subsequently named the acquired immune deficiency syndrome (AIDS).[1] This aggressive form of KS (Figures 29.3 and 29.4) was seen up to 20 times more frequently in homosexual men with AIDS than in haemophiliac men with AIDS. KS is now an AIDS-defining illness in the Center for Disease Control guidelines.

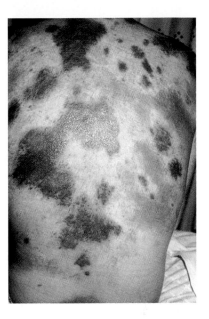

Figure 29.4   Extensive AIDS-related Kaposi's sarcoma

Incidence/prevalence

Classical KS is rare; it is much more common in men than in women, with a ratio of up to 15:1. The peak age of onset is 50–70 years. Endemic (African KS) is a common tumour in equatorial Africa and in 1971 comprised up to 9% of all cancers seen in Uganda.[2] Since the beginning of the AIDS epidemic, KS has become the most frequently occurring tumour in central Africa, in human immunodeficiency virus (HIV)-negative and HIV-positive men, accounting for up to 50% in some countries.[3] Since the introduction of highly active antiretroviral therapy (HAART), the proportion of patients with AIDS-related KS is decreasing but it remains the most common AIDS-associated malignancy, affecting 20–40% of homosexual men who are HIV positive.[4] In published series of organ transplant recipients, between 0·5% and 5·3% have developed KS; in one study the mean period between transplantation and development of KS was 12·5 months (range 1–37 months).[5–7]

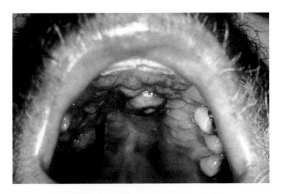

Figure 29.3   Kaposi's sarcoma affecting the hard palate in a patient with AIDS

Table 29.1   AIDS Clinical Trials Group (ACTG) staging classification

	Good risk (0) (all of the following)	Poor risk (1) (any of the following)
Tumour (T)	Confined to skin and/or lymph nodes and/or minimal oral disease[a]	Tumour-associated oedema or ulceration Extensive oral KS Gastrointestinal KS KS in other non-nodal viscera
Immune system (I)	CD4 count $\geq 200 \times 10^6$/litre	CD4 count $< 200 \times 10^6$/litre
Systemic illness (S)	No history of opportunistic infections or thrush No "B" symptoms[b] Performance status $\geq 70\%$ (Karnofsky)	History of opportunistic infections and/or thrush "B" symptoms present Performance status $<70\%$ Other HIV-related illness (for example neurological disease, lymphoma)

[a]Minimal oral disease is non-nodular KS confined to the palate.

[b]"B" symptoms are unexplained fever, night sweats, >10% involuntary weight loss or diarrhoea persisting for more than 2 weeks.

Aetiology

The unusual geographical distribution of KS has long suggested an infective cause. Epidemiological evidence, including the 20 times greater frequency of AIDS-related KS in homosexual men compared with haemophiliacs, suggested a sexually transmitted cofactor. In 1994, Chang *et al.* described the identification of fragments of a novel herpes virus in a biopsy of an AIDS-related KS lesion.[8] KS-associated herpes virus (KSHV), also known as human herpes virus 8 (HHV8), can be identified in virtually all KS specimens regardless of subtype, but is absent from uninvolved skin. The KSHV genome encodes proteins that are homologous to human oncoproteins and have the potential to induce cellular proliferation and inhibit apoptosis. The presence of KSHV seems to be necessary for the development of KS but the role of cofactors such as host immunosuppression, cytokines and HIV is unclear.

Prognosis

Classical KS typically runs an indolent course over years or decades, with gradual development of new lesions and complications such as lower-limb lymphoedema. An increased risk of developing a second malignancy, usually non-Hodgkin's lymphoma, has been reported. Endemic (African) KS may run an indolent course similar to classical KS, with nodules and plaques in association with lower limb oedema. The lymphadenopathic form of African KS in children has an aggressive course and carries a poor prognosis. Epidemic AIDS-related KS may be a disseminated and fulminant disease. The prognosis is determined by the extent of tumour, severity of immunodeficiency and the presence or absence of systemic illness. Each of these variables is independently associated with survival and has resulted in the prospectively validated tumour, immunodeficiency and systemic illness (TIS) staging classification (see Table 29.1).[9] Immune status is the most important prognostic factor, and patients with a CD4 count greater than 200×10^6 cells/litre have a better prognosis. Opportunistic infections are often the cause of death in this group of patients. However, with the advent of HAART and better prophylaxis of opportunistic infections, the prognosis of AIDS-associated KS may be improving although newer therapies specifically for KS have not been shown to improve overall survival.

Aims of treatment

In the UK and North America, AIDS-related KS is the most common variant. In this group, where overall prognosis is often determined by other complications such as opportunistic infections, treatment aims to improve the cosmetic appearance of cutaneous disease and palliate symptoms associated with lymph node or visceral disease (such as oedema, bleeding and shortness of breath), with minimal toxicity. However, the introduction of HAART and more effective prophylaxis of opportunistic infections is modifying the natural history of HIV infection and delaying progression to AIDS. Other endpoints such as time to treatment failure and overall survival may become more important in the future in this group of patients with KS.

Relevant outcomes

Response rate in terms of the number and size of lesions, flattening, and degree of pigmentation, is an important endpoint for systemic therapies in the treatment of cutaneous disease. One of the problems in comparing studies of systemic therapy in KS is the subjective nature of the assessment of response. Recent randomised studies of systemic therapies in AIDS-related KS have adopted the AIDS Clinical Trials Group (ACTG) criteria for assessment of response (Table 29.2).[10] The overall cosmetic effect is also an important endpoint, particularly for local therapies such as radiotherapy which have long-term effects on the normal skin surrounding lesions. Consider, for example, the young homosexual man with telltale purple nodular HIV-associated KS lesions on a highly visible area such as the face. Local radiotherapy to this area, with a wide margin of normal skin, may leave him with an equally unsightly area of residual brown discoloration and a contrasting "halo" of depigmentation. Palliation of associated symptoms such as tumour-associated oedema is another endpoint for which assessment is highly subjective.

Methods of search

We searched Medline from 1966 to 2001. We first performed a highly sensitive search using the truncated term "Kaposi*", which generated over 8400 abstracts. We then performed a more specific Medline search using "sarcoma, Kaposi" [MeSH terms] or "Kaposi's sarcoma" [text word] combined with the following interventions AND [surgery, laser*, photodynamic therapy, cryotherapy, cryosurgery, intralesional therapy, intralesional vincristine or vinblastine, radiotherapy, interferon, chemotherapy, anthracycline, bleomycin, vinca-alkaloid, vincristine, vinblastine, taxane, paclitaxel, liposomal therapy, gemcitabine, navelbine, thalidomide, antiangiogenic agent, retinoids, retinoic acid, antiretroviral therapy, zidovudine, ganciclovir, cidofovir or foscarnet].

We also searched the Cochrane Central Register of Controlled Trials and Database of Systematic Reviews using the search terms "Kaposi" and "Kaposi's sarcoma".

QUESTIONS

> **What are the effects of local therapies in Kaposi's sarcoma (surgical excision, cryotherapy, photodynamic therapy and intralesional chemotherapy)?**

We found no systematic reviews or randomised controlled trials of local therapies in KS. There were a relatively small number of uncontrolled phase II studies of each of the above interventions.

Surgical excision

We found no clinical trials.

Cryotherapy

One uncontrolled phase II study of 20 patients with cutaneous AIDS-related KS, treated with

Table 29.2   AIDS Clinical Trials Group (ACTG) response criteria

Complete response (CR) Clinical complete response (CCR)	The absence of any detectable residual disease, including tumour-associated oedema, persisting for at least 4 weeks. In patients in whom pigmented (brown or tan) macular skin lesions persist after apparent CR, biopsy of at least one representative lesion is required to document the absence of malignant cells. In patients known to have had visceral disease, an attempt at restaging with appropriate endoscopic or radiographic procedures should be made. If such procedures are medically contraindicated, the patient may be classified as having CCR.
Partial response (PR)	The absence of new cutaneous or oral lesions, new visceral sites of involvement, or the appearance or worsening of tumour-associated oedema or effusions in addition to at least one of the following: • A 50% or greater decrease in the number of all previously existing skin lesions (skin, oral, measurable or evaluable visceral disease) • A 50% decrease in the size of lesions (includes a 50% decrease in the sum of the products of the largest perpendicular diameters of bi-dimensionally measurable marker lesions and/or complete flattening of at least 50% of the lesions (i.e. 50% of previously nodular or plaque-like lesions become macules). • In those patients with predominantly nodular lesions, flattening to an indurated plaque of 75% or more of the nodules. • Patients with residual tumour-associated oedema or effusion who otherwise meet the criteria for CR.
Stable disease (SD)	Any response not meeting the criteria for progression or PR.
Progressive disease (PD)	An increase of 25% or more in the size of previously existing lesions and/or the appearance of new lesions or new sites of disease and/or a change in the character of 25% or more of the skin or oral lesions from macular to plaque-like or nodular. The development of new or increasing tumour-associated oedema or effusion is also considered to represent disease progression.

liquid-nitrogen cryotherapy, reported a complete response rate of 80% lasting a minimum of 6 weeks.[11] On average, each lesion required three treatments at three-weekly intervals and the main side-effects were blistering and local discomfort. Another uncontrolled study of patients with AIDS-related facial KS found cryosurgery to be effective for small lesions measuring less than 1 cm.[12]

Photodynamic therapy

In one uncontrolled phase I/II study of 348 AIDS-related KS lesions in 25 patients treated with

Photofrin photodynamic therapy, the maximum tolerated 630 nm light dose was determined to be 300 J/cm^2 if given with Photofrin, 1·0 mg/kg, 48 hours beforehand.[13] Of 289 evaluable lesions, 33% had a complete clinical response and 63% had a partial response. At light doses of 400 J/cm^2, full-field necrosis and scabbing occurred whereas at doses of 250 J/cm^2 side-effects were erythema and oedema within the treatment field. In another uncontrolled phase II study, Photofrin, 2 mg/kg, with 70–120 J/cm^2 of 630 nm light therapy for the treatment of 83 evaluable lesions in eight homosexual men with AIDS-related cutaneous KS resulted in high overall response rates (83–100%). However, acute toxicity was unacceptable and the long-term cosmetic result was poor, with scarring and hyperpigmentation.[14] A further small uncontrolled phase II study treated 30 AIDS-associated KS lesions with indocyanine green, 2×2 mg/kg intravenously, followed immediately by 850 nm light therapy, 100 J/cm^2.[15] Nineteen lesions resolved completely, leaving an atrophic scar, with no recurrences in 2 years.

Intralesional chemotherapy

Two uncontrolled phase II studies have examined the effect of treating intraoral, oropharyngeal and laryngeal AIDS-related KS by intralesional injection of vinblastine.[16,17] One obtained a 62% complete response rate (16/26 lesions) in 24 patients with AIDS-associated oropharyngeal or laryngeal KS.[16] Lesions were injected with vinblastine, 0·1–0·2 mg/ml repeated "every 4 to 5 weeks" until complete response or stable disease. Side-effects included self-limiting pain, and ulceration. In 11 of 24 patients the pain was not relieved by paracetamol. A similarly high complete response rate was found in another uncontrolled phase II study of intralesional vinblastine as a local treatment for oral-cavity AIDS-associated KS.[17] A total of 144 lesions in 50 patients were treated, and the complete response rate was 74%. The most common site of intraoral KS is the hard palate. Intralesional chemotherapy (vinblastine, vincristine or bleomycin) has also been used to treat cutaneous KS lesions, with overall response rates (complete response plus partial response) in small uncontrolled studies of 88–100%.[18,19]

Comment

In the absence of randomised controlled studies, the comparative efficacy of local therapies in the treatment of KS cannot be assessed. High response rates have been described in uncontrolled case series for cryotherapy,

photodynamic therapy and intralesional chemotherapy, but at the expense of troublesome local side-effects.

Is radiotherapy an effective local treatment for cutaneous Kaposi's sarcoma?

No systematic reviews were found. Two randomised trials in AIDS-related KS have compared different radiotherapy dose-fractionation schedules.[20,21] There have also been many case series typically using total doses of radiotherapy ranging from 8 Gy to 40 Gy. However, the dose each lesion received in these series was individualised depending on both patient and lesion factors. Conclusions cannot be drawn from such non-randomised studies as to the optimum dose-fractionation schedule in AIDS-related KS.

No randomised studies of radiotherapy in classical KS, endemic KS or immunosuppression-related KS were found. Many retrospective case series of radiotherapy as a local therapy for classical KS have been reported suggesting it is a radiosensitive disease, but often criteria for assessment of response are not stated and vary between studies.

Efficacy
AIDS-related KS

We found one randomised trial of radiotherapy in 71 cutaneous AIDS-associated KS lesions comparing three different dose-fractionation regimens: 8 Gy in a single fraction, 20 Gy in 10 fractions over 2 weeks and 40 Gy in 20 fractions over 4 weeks.[20] Lesions were treated using 6 MeV electrons with 0·5 cm skin bolus allowing a 2 cm margin around palpable tumour. An objective response was defined as at least a 50% decrease in palpable tumour area, which was taken as the product of the perpendicular dimensions. Complete response was defined as resolution of all palpable tumour, with or without residual pigmentation. More complete responses were achieved with 40 Gy in 20 fractions (83%) and 20 Gy in 10 fractions (79%) than with an 8 Gy single fraction (50%). A greater proportion of complete responses were without residual purple pigmentation in the group that received 40 Gy (53%) than in the groups that received 20 Gy or 8 Gy (11% and 17%, respectively).[20] The median time to treatment failure (defined as measurable growth in tumour area) for the 40 Gy, 20 Gy and 8 Gy groups were 43, 26 and 13 weeks, respectively.[20]

Another prospective randomised trial compared 8 Gy in a single fraction with 16 Gy in four fractions over 4 days for the treatment of cutaneous AIDS-related KS.[21] A total of 596 lesions in 57 patients were treated, of which 172 lesions in 27 patients were treated in a randomised fashion. The method of randomisation was not reported. A total of 424 lesions in 49 patients were treated in a concurrent non-randomised prospective trial where the radiotherapy regimen was given according to patient preference. Lesions were treated using 75 or 100 kV superficial radiotherapy with a margin of 3–5 mm.

The overall response rate for the randomised and non-randomised lesions was 79% (465/590), which included complete responses and pigmented complete responses. The overall response rate for lesions treated with a single 8 Gy fraction was 78% (305/392), and 81% (160/198) for the lesions that received 16 Gy in four fractions. The overall response rates for the 172 lesions treated as part of the randomised trial were 71% (57/80) and 82% (75/92) for the 8 Gy and 16 Gy groups, respectively. The two response rates do not differ significantly (0·25>P>0·1). The response rate was highest in facial lesions. The response rates for the lesions treated non-randomly were 79% (248/313) for those that received 8 Gy and 80% (85/106) for those in the 16 Gy arm.[21]

A large retrospective case series of 643 patients with AIDS-related KS treated over a 10-year period (June 1986–December 1996) reported an objective response rate of 92% in 621 evaluable patients.[22] The radiotherapy was delivered as a split course, with 20 Gy given in 2·5 Gy fractions over 2 weeks treating four times per week followed by 10 Gy in 1 week after a 2-week rest period. Extended cutaneous fields were treated with 4 MeV or 8 MeV electrons. Localised fields were treated with 45–100 KV superficial x rays.[22]

Another large series of AIDS-related KS lesions treated with radiotherapy retrospectively reviewed 375 lesions in 187 patients, of which 266 sites were cutaneous.[23] The lesions were treated in a non-randomised fashion with total doses of 2–40 Gy in fractions of 1·5–8 Gy. Of the 266 cutaneous lesions, 111 received an 8 Gy single fraction and 155 received a more protracted fractionation regimen. In this study a response was defined as complete flattening of a lesion or a decrease in size to at least 50% of its pretreatment size, with reduced pigmentation. In total, 93% of the cutaneous lesions that received an 8 Gy single fraction responded, compared with 96% of the lesions that received a fractionated course of radiotherapy. The response or time to relapse did not differ between the two groups.[23] Many smaller case series have used a variety of dose-fractionation schedules and have shown similarly high response rates of cutaneous KS to radiotherapy; however, criteria used to assess response vary.

Classical and endemic (African) Kaposi's sarcoma

We found no randomised studies of radiotherapy in endemic (African) or classical KS. A case series of 82 patients with classical KS treated with radiotherapy between 1972 and 1985 reported a complete response rate of more than 50% with doses ranging from 6·5 Gy in a single fraction to 35 Gy in 10 fractions.[24] Long-term control was greater with doses of 27·5 Gy or more delivered in 10 fractions over a 2-week period.[24] Brenner et al. reported a similar complete response rate for radiotherapy in classical KS of 58%.[25] Another case series of 60 patients with classical KS treated with radiotherapy reported an overall response rate of 93%. In this study a variety of radiotherapy techniques were used, including megavoltage electrons, megavoltage photons, a combination of both, and total skin electron beam therapy.[26]

One retrospective case series of 28 men with endemic (African) KS treated with radiotherapy between 1978 and 1990 reported a complete response rate of 32% and a partial response rate of 54%, but the criteria used to assess response were not stated.[27] The radiotherapy dose ranged from an 8–10 Gy single fraction to 14–24 Gy fractionated over 1–3 weeks using orthovoltage, cobalt[60] or 6–8 MeV electrons.

Drawbacks
In the randomised trial of Stelzer and Griffin, toxicity was graded using the Radiation Therapy Oncology Group scoring system.[20] Grade 1 acute toxicity (skin erythema, dry desquamation or alopecia) was seen in 3/24 (12%) of the patients who received 8 Gy, 11/24 (46%) of patients who received 20 Gy and 22/23 (96%) patients who received 40 Gy. No acute toxicity greater than grade 1 was seen. Late toxicity occurred only in the 40 Gy group (6/23 patients) but did not exceed grade 1 (slight hyperpigmentation or alopecia). In a large retrospective case series of 621 evaluable patients the frequency of grade 1, grade 2 and grade 3 skin reactions was 7%, 69% and 23·4%, respectively.[22]

Harrison et al. developed a subjective four-point grading system to assess pigmentation in the normal skin surrounding lesions following irradiation as part of overall cosmesis.[21] The

scoring system graded cosmesis from grade 0 (no evidence of pigmentation) to grade 3 (severe skin pigmentation or telangiectasia). Of the 172 randomised lesions, cosmesis grade 0 or 1 was found in 87% of those who received a single fraction and 90% of those who received four fractions, a non-significant difference.

Comment
Radiotherapy gives high response rates in the treatment of cutaneous KS and is an effective local palliative therapy. In the absence of any placebo group, it is difficult to state with certainty that the responses are due solely to the treatment, but inclusion of a placebo or sham radiotherapy group would be ethically unjustifiable. The rates of complete response and duration of lesion control are higher with increasing total doses of radiotherapy in AIDS-related KS.[20] However, in this group of patients prognosis is that of the underlying AIDS diagnosis. In the study of Harrison et al., for example, participating patients survived for only a median of 17 months. With the advent of HAART, however, prognosis for patients with AIDS may be improving.[21] Treatment is given with palliative intent and cosmesis is an important endpoint.

Difficulties in comparing trials of radiotherapy in cutaneous KS are variation in the definitions of response and the subjective nature of assessment, particularly of lesion colour and nodularity. A lesion may flatten or reduce in size with treatment but haemosiderin within the skin may leave residual brown pigmentation, influencing the overall cosmetic outcome. Uniform criteria of response in future trials should include assessment of lesion flatness, size, residual pigmentation and tumour-associated oedema after therapy. Evaluation of the effect of radiotherapy on the surrounding skin is also important in the overall cosmetic outcome following treatment. Patients should be warned that radiotherapy might lead to depigmentation of the surrounding normal skin, producing a "halo" effect.

Implications for clinical practice

Radiotherapy can improve the appearance of cutaneous KS lesions and provide temporary local control. In the population with AIDS-related cutaneous KS, a single 8 Gy fraction of radiotherapy with superficial *x* rays or electrons gives a high response rate. Some good evidence indicates that higher response rates and a greater duration of local control are seen with fractionated radiotherapy courses to a higher total dose. However, fractionated regimens more often cause acute toxicity and require more visits to hospital. This matters particularly in a group whose prognosis depends on the course of the underlying AIDS, although with more effective antiretroviral therapy longer term local control may become increasingly important.

> **Is interferon alfa an effective systemic treatment for AIDS-related Kaposi's sarcoma alone or in combination with zidovudine?**

Interferons have multiple effects on immune function and cell proliferation, and may act synergistically in the treatment of AIDS-related KS with antiretroviral therapy. We found no systematic reviews of the use of interferon in AIDS-related KS. Early phase II trials demonstrated activity of interferon as monotherapy for AIDS-related KS before the advent of nucleoside reverse transcriptase inhibitors. One small randomised trial compared two doses of interferon alfa as monotherapy in AIDS-related KS.[28] On the basis of *in vitro* studies suggesting synergy between interferon alfa and antiretroviral drugs, multiple subsequent phase II trials have examined the combination of interferon alfa and zidovudine in the treatment of AIDS-related KS. We found one randomised comparative trial of 108 patients with AIDS-related KS using zidovudine antiretroviral

therapy combined with one of two different doses of interferon alfa.[29] We found no placebo-controlled trials.

Interferon alfa alone
Efficacy

One small prospective randomised trial of interferon as monotherapy in AIDS-related KS tested the efficacy of high-dose versus low-dose interferon alfa in AIDS-associated KS.[28] Twenty patients were randomised between high-dose intravenous interferon (50 MU/m^2 for 5 days on alternate weeks) and low-dose subcutaneous interferon (1 MU/m^2 for 5 days on alternate weeks). The objective response rate was 40% in the high-dose arm and 20% in the low-dose arm.[28] Many uncontrolled phase II studies have been conducted and these have reported higher response rates for patients with CD4 lymphocyte counts >200 × 10^6 cells/litre, higher doses of interferon (>20 MU/day) and in the absence of previous opportunistic infections. However, most of these individual studies are small, and the use of a wide variety of interferon doses and schedules makes comparisons difficult. These trials often compare two different doses or preparations of interferon and we found no placebo-controlled randomised trials of interferon in the treatment of KS. In one larger series of 273 patients with AIDS-related KS, CD4 counts >400 × 10^6 cells/litre were associated with response rates of 45% whereas the response rate for patients with CD4 counts <200 × 10^6 cells/litre was only 7%.[30] Another series of uncontrolled phase II trials with a total of 114 patients given interferon alfa-2b demonstrated higher response rates with high-dose (50 MU/m^2 intravenously) than low-dose interferon (1 MU/m^2 subcutaneously).[31] Patients with early stage disease and without "B" symptoms were more likely to respond.[31]

Drawbacks

Almost all patients experienced flu-like symptoms with interferon alfa, and in the study of Volberding *et al.* 6% of patients discontinued therapy because of adverse reactions.[31] In addition to flu-like symptoms, adverse events include haematological toxicity and abnormalities in liver function tests. In the randomised study of Groopman *et al.*, mild haematological and hepatic toxicity were seen at both high and low doses of interferon alfa.[28]

Interferon alfa plus zidovudine
Efficacy
We found one randomised study comparing two doses of interferon alfa combined with zidovudine. In this study of 108 patients with AIDS-related KS, patients received zidovudine 500mg/day and were randomised to either a low (1 MU/day) or intermediate dose (8 MU/day) of subcutaneous interferon alfa.[29] Response rates for the 54 patients randomised to 8 MU/day were significantly greater than for the 53 patients who received 1 MU/day: 31% and 8%, respectively $(P = 0.001)$.[29] Time to progression was longer for intermediate-dose interferon (18 weeks) than for low-dose interferon (13 weeks) $(P = 0.002)$. Response rates were higher for patients who had a CD4 count $>150 \times 10^6$ cells/litre.[29]

Other phase I/II trials in AIDS-related KS using doses of interferon alfa ranging from 4.5 to 27 MU/day combined with zidovudine, 500–1200 mg/day, have achieved objective response rates of 5–47%.[32–38]

Drawbacks
In the above randomised study comparing two doses of interferon alfa combined with zidovudine in the treatment of AIDS-related KS, both haematological and non-haematological toxicities were higher for 8 MU daily than 1 MU daily, necessitating dose

reductions in 50 of the 54 patients receiving the higher dose.[29]

Interferon versus bleomycin
A small randomised study compared interferon alfa-2a plus zidovudine with bleomycin plus zidovudine in 26 patients with AIDS-related KS, of which 22 were evaluable for response.[39] Two of 10 (20%) assessable patients, who received bleomycin, 15 mg every 2 weeks, plus zidovudine, 250 mg twice daily, had an objective response to treatment after 5.3 months on treatment, compared with one of 12 (8%) evaluable patients who received interferon alfa-2a, 9 MU/day, plus zidovudine, 250 mg twice daily, after 4.7 months on treatment.[39]

Interferon combined with cytotoxic chemotherapy
One small uncontrolled study of 24 patients with AIDS-related KS treated with interferon alfa-2b and etoposide found an objective response rate of 38% (8/21 evaluable patients).[40] Another small study combined intermediate-dose interferon alfa with actinomycin D, vinblastine and bleomycin in 13 patients with AIDS-related KS. There was one complete response and four partial responses but four patients required hospital admission for febrile neutropenia.[41]

Comment
Zidovudine alone is no longer standard therapy for HIV infection, and the advent of HAART has changed the clinical course of AIDS-related KS. The effectiveness of interferon combined with HAART is unknown. No randomised trials have compared liposomal anthracyclines with interferon in early AIDS-related KS. The effectiveness of interferon combined with cytotoxic chemotherapy is unknown. All of the above trials compared two or more actives or different doses of interferon and therefore may

be comparing several ineffective treatments. None of these trials was placebo controlled.

Implications for practice

Patients with early stage disease, CD4 counts >200 cells × 10⁶/litre, no "B" symptoms and no previous opportunistic infections are most likely to respond to interferon alfa. Response rates are greater with higher doses of interferon, whether given alone or in combination with zidovudine. A disadvantage of interferon in the treatment of KS is the need for frequent subcutaneous injections. The development of pegylated interferon which requires less frequent administration may be an advantage.

> What are the effects of systemic chemotherapy in KS and do liposomal anthracyclines produce higher response rates (by ACTG criteria), with less toxicity, than conventional combination chemotherapy in advanced AIDS-related Kaposi's sarcoma?

We found no systematic reviews of chemotherapy in KS. The majority of the randomised evidence is in the treatment of advanced AIDS-related KS. We found three small randomised trials of chemotherapy in African KS. Several drugs have been found active as single agents in uncontrolled phase II studies, the most active of which include paclitaxel, liposomal anthracyclines, vinca alkaloids and bleomycin. Two commonly used combination cytotoxic regimens in the treatment of AIDS-related KS are bleomycin plus vincristine (BV), and doxorubicin, bleomycin and vincristine (ABV), which have been compared in randomised studies with single-agent chemotherapy, including newer drugs such as liposomal anthracyclines. We found no randomised placebo-controlled trials and all the trials compared two or more actives, apart from a small randomised crossover comparison of liposomal daunorubicin versus observation for early KS.

Single-agent chemotherapy
Bleomycin

We found three small uncontrolled phase II trials of bleomycin as single-agent therapy in the treatment of AIDS-related KS and one small non-randomised study comparing single-agent bleomycin with combination ABV chemotherapy.[42–45] In one non-randomised phase II study of single-agent bleomycin, 30 patients received intramuscular bleomycin, 5 mg/day for 3 days every 14–21 days, and another 30 patients received bleomycin by infusion, 6 mg/m²/day for 4 days every 28 days.[42] The overall partial response rate for the combined groups was 48% (29/60), and the response rates in the intramuscular group and the continuous infusion groups were similar (although the groups were not randomly assigned).[42] Mean duration of bleomycin therapy was 5 months. Nineteen patients died during the treatment and four patients after withdrawal of bleomycin. Opportunistic infections were the cause of death in 18 of the 23 patients who died.[42] In another small uncontrolled study, 17 patients with AIDS-related KS were treated with infusional bleomycin at 20 mg/m²/day for 3 days every 21 days and the partial response rate by ACTG criteria (see Table 29.2) was 65%.[43] Three of five previously treated patients also had a partial response. Median survival was 7 months.[43] In a third uncontrolled phase II study, 70 patients with AIDS-related mucocutaneous KS were given intramuscular bleomycin 5 mg/day for 3 days every 2 weeks. Two patients had a complete response and 50 patients had a partial response, giving an overall response rate of 74%.[44] The median time to relapse was 10 weeks.

In a small non-randomised study comparing bleomycin with ABV combination chemotherapy in 24 patients with extensive AIDS-related KS, there were no complete or partial responses in 12 patients who received bleomycin alone. Four of 12 patients who received ABV chemotherapy had a partial response.[45]

Vinca alkaloids

We found one randomised study comparing oral etoposide with vinblastine in the treatment of classical KS in elderly Mediterranean patients.[46] We found no randomised evidence for the use of single-agent vinca alkaloids in AIDS-related KS. Several uncontrolled phase II studies used single-agent vinblastine in the treatment of both classical and AIDS-related KS.[25,47–52]

In one study, 65 elderly patients with classical KS were randomised between oral etoposide and intravenous vinblastine.[46] Etoposide was given every 3 weeks at a dose of 60 mg/m^2 on days 1–3 for the first cycle, days 1–4 for the second cycle and days 1–5 for the third cycle. Vinblastine was given intravenously at a dose of 3 mg/m^2 weekly for the first 3 weeks then 6 mg/m^2 every 3 weeks. The overall response rate was 73% for etoposide and 58% for vinblastine ($P = 0.3$). An uncontrolled phase II study of single-agent vinblastine in 38 patients with AIDS-related KS reported an overall response rate of 26% with weekly vinblastine, 4–8 mg/week titrated against white blood cell count.[49] Reported response rates to vinblastine in small uncontrolled studies are higher for classical KS than for AIDS-related KS.

Etoposide

We found one randomised study comparing oral etoposide with intravenous vinblastine in classical KS, described above.[46] We also found one small uncontrolled phase II study of oral etoposide in the treatment of 17 evaluable patients with classical KS, which reported a response rate of 76% to 100 mg daily for 3–5 days every 3 weeks.[53] We found five small phase II trials of etoposide and one of teniposide in AIDS-related KS.[54–59] In four small uncontrolled phase II studies of oral etoposide in AIDS-related KS, with between 14 and 41 evaluable patients, the objective response rate varied from 0 to 83%.[54–56,58] In one study of infused etoposide in nine patients there was an overall partial response rate of only 22%, with one death resulting from drug toxicity.[57] An uncontrolled study of 25 patients with AIDS-related KS treated with teniposide, 360 mg/m^2 infused over 60 minutes, every 3 weeks, produced a partial response rate of 40%, which lasted a median of 9 weeks.[59]

Liposomal anthracyclines

Doxorubicin and daunorubicin have been produced in encapsulated forms in which the anthracycline drug is trapped within phospholipid spheres known as liposomes. These liposomal preparations have a prolonged circulatory half-life and are associated with enhanced delivery of active drug to KS lesions. They have been compared with standard combination chemotherapy in large randomised trials.[60–62] A randomised crossover study of 29 patients with early AIDS-related KS (<20 cutaneous lesions, no visceral involvement and a CD4 count >400 × 10^6/litre) randomised patients between initial liposomal daunorubicin and observation for 12 weeks.[63] Fifteen patients received liposomal daunorubicin, 40 mg/m^2 every 2 weeks for six cycles, and 14 patients were observed. ACTG criteria were used to assess response and patients crossed over after 12 weeks or on disease progression. There was a 40% initial response rate in the liposomal daunorubicin arm. Forty per cent of these patients developed progressive disease, compared with 72% in the observation arm.

Paclitaxel

We found no randomised studies. Three uncontrolled phase II studies of paclitaxel in advanced AIDS-related KS were found. Overall response rates in these three phase II studies were between 59% and 71%.[64–66] In each study the most frequent dose-limiting toxicity was neutropenia, and in one study grade 3 or 4 neutropenia occurred in 61% of patients.[65]

Newer cytotoxic drugs

There have been no phase III studies of newer agents such as vinorelbine and gemcitabine in KS. Vinorelbine has been used in an uncontrolled phase II study of 35 evaluable patients with AIDS-related KS who had progressed on one or more previous systemic chemotherapies. An overall response rate of 43% was found.[67]

One phase II study of gemcitabine in 11 evaluable patients with recurrent classical KS after previous chemotherapy reported 10/11 partial responses and one complete response.[68] Gemcitabine was given at 1·2 g/week for 2 weeks followed by a 1-week gap, and was continued until maximum response was achieved.[68]

Anti-angiogenic agents

Thalidomide is an anti-angiogenic agent that has been investigated in uncontrolled phase II trials in the treatment of AIDS-related KS. One such study of 20 patients, of whom 17 were assessable for response, reported a 40% (8/20) partial response rate with oral thalidomide, 200 mg/day, increased fortnightly to a maximum of 1000 mg/day.[69] Response lasted for a median of 7·1 months and the median thalidomide dose at the time of maximum response was 500 mg/day. Nine of 20 patients experienced drowsiness and seven patients experienced depression. Five patients withdrew from the study because of toxicity.[69] In another uncontrolled study, 17 patients with AIDS-related KS were given oral thalidomide, 100 mg at night for 8 weeks; 35% patients (6/17) had a partial response but six patients withdrew early because of toxicity.[70] The highly vascular nature of KS has produced interest in other anti-angiogenic agents such as matrix metalloproteinase inhibitors, which are being investigated in phase I studies.

Combination chemotherapy in endemic (African) Kaposi's sarcoma

We found a series of three small randomised comparative studies of chemotherapy in Ugandan patients with endemic (African) KS.[71–73] Chemotherapy is an important modality of treatment for endemic KS in developing countries without adequate access to radiotherapy facilities. On the basis of a previous small randomised study which found a higher response rate for actinomycin D than cyclophosphamide in patients with endemic (African) KS, a second randomised study compared actinomycin D with a combination of actinomycin D plus vincristine.[71,72] Twelve patients received actinomycin D alone, 0·42 mg/m^2/day for 5 days every 3–4 weeks, and 14 received this with vincristine, 1·4 mg/m^2/week until the end of the second course of actinomycin D then on days 1 and 5 of each subsequent course.[72] Twenty-four patients were evaluable for response. Two of the 12 patients who received actinomycin D alone died during the first cycle of chemotherapy (Gram-negative sepsis and adrenal failure). A further patient in the combination group developed sepsis after cycle three and died. Complete response was defined as the complete disappearance of all visible/measurable disease, and a partial response as >50% regression of disease. After 4–6 courses of chemotherapy, 13 of 14 patients who received actinomycin D plus vincristine had a complete or partial response, compared with nine of 12 patients randomised to receive actinomycin D alone. However the number of patients in this study is very small and more patients in the combination group had florid type KS or bone lesions.

A further randomised study compared actinomycin D plus vincristine (same schedule as above) with or without the addition of DTIC (dacarbazine), 250 mg/m^2 for 5 days with alternate courses of actinomycin D.[73]

Randomisation was achieved using random cards. The overall response rate for the 40 patients randomised to the two-drug arm was 88%. Of 32 patients randomised to receive the three-drug combination, 30 patients had a complete response (94%), with a further patient having a partial response (overall response rate 97%). Time to best response was quicker for the three-drug combination than the two-drug combination (2 courses versus 5–6 courses).

Combination chemotherapy in AIDS-related Kaposi's sarcoma
ABV chemotherapy versus doxorubicin

We found one small randomised study of 61 patients with extensive mucocutaneous or visceral AIDS-related KS, comparing ABV combination chemotherapy with doxorubicin alone.[74] The overall response rate was 88% for 30 patients who received ABV combination chemotherapy and 48% for the 31 patients who received doxorubicin, 20 mg/m^2, alone. The response rates differed significantly. Toxicity was similar in both arms, but neutropenia ($<1000 \times 10^6$ cells/litre) was more frequent with ABV (52%) than with doxorubicin alone (34%). Median survival was 9 months for both groups.[74]

ABV or BV chemotherapy versus liposomal anthracyclines

Three large randomised controlled trials have compared liposomal anthracyclines (either doxorubicin or daunorubicin) with standard ABV or BV combination chemotherapy. We found one randomised study comparing liposomal daunorubicin (DaunoXome) with ABV and two randomised trials comparing liposomal doxorubicin with standard combination chemotherapy (either ABV or BV).[60–62] All three trials assessed response using modified ACTG response criteria and graded toxicity according to standard criteria. Concurrent antiretroviral

therapy was allowed in all three trials. Table 29.3 summarises the results of these trials.

A further randomised controlled trial compared pegylated liposomal doxorubicin (PLD), 20 mg/m^2, alone with the combination PLD + bleomycin + vincristine (PLD, 20 mg/m^2, bleomycin, 10 IU/m^2, vincristine, 1 mg) given every two weeks.[75]

Efficacy
Liposomal daunorubicin versus ABV chemotherapy

One randomised trial comparing liposomal daunorubicin with ABV chemotherapy (doxorubicin, 10 mg/m^2, bleomycin, 15 IU, and vincristine, 1 mg every 2 weeks) in 227 patients with advanced AIDS-related KS reported equivalent overall response rates of 25% and 28%.[60] Median survival was similar in both groups (369 days versus 342 days), as was the median time to treatment failure.

The method of randomisation was not stated but patients were stratified at randomisation using a permuted-block design for the following prognostic factors: baseline CD4 count <100 cells $\times 10^6$/litre, visceral involvement, zidovudine-containing antiretroviral therapy, and Karnofsky performance status below 80%. Responses were assessed using modified ACTG criteria. In patients with persistent pigmented macular skin lesions after a clinically complete response, a biopsy of at least one representative skin lesion was required for complete response by ACTG criteria.

Liposomal daunorubicin was given at 40 mg/m^2 every 2 weeks until complete response, progressive disease or unacceptable toxicity. Patients who responded completely were given a further two cycles of chemotherapy and then observed on study. No prior chemotherapy was permitted but concurrent antiretroviral therapy was allowed. Alopecia and peripheral neuropathy were significantly more frequent with

Table 29.3 Randomised trials comparing liposomal anthracyclines and standard combination chemotherapy in AIDS-related Kaposi's sarcoma

Reference	Study type	Study population	No. of patients treated	Interventions compared (n = number of patients)	Co-treatments permitted	Overall percentage response rate (ORR)	Selected adverse events
60	Prospective randomised comparative study	Biopsy-proven AIDS-related KS with at least 25 mucocutaneous lesions, symptomatic visceral involvement or tumour-associated oedema	227	Liposomal daunorubicin (DaunoXome) 40 mg/m^2 every 2 weeks (n=116) OR ABV (doxorubicin 10 mg/m^2, bleomycin 15 IU and vincristine 1 mg) every 2 weeks (n = 111)	G-CSF if absolute neutrophil count <0·75 × 10^9 cells/litre Concurrent antiretroviral therapy	Responses assessed using modified ACTG criteria ORR: DaunoXome 25% ABV 27·9% Not significant	SWOG toxicity scoring system DaunoXome v ABV: Grade 1/2 alopecia 8% v 36% Grade 1/2 neuropathy 12% v 38% Grade 4 neutropenia 15% v 5%
61	Prospective randomised comparative study	Biopsy-proven AIDS-related KS with at least 25 mucocutaneous lesions or at least 10 new lesions in the preceding month or documented visceral disease	258	PLD 20 mg/m^2 every 2 weeks for 6 cycles (n = 133) OR ABV (doxorubicin 20 mg/m^2, bleomycin 10 mg/m^2 and vincristine 1 mg) every 2 weeks for 6 cycles (n = 125). Either treatment continued until complete response, progressive disease or unacceptable toxicity	CSF at the discretion of the investigators Concurrent antiretroviral therapy	Responses assessed using modified ACTG criteria ORR: PLD 45·9% ABV 24·8% P<0·001	World Health Organization criteria PLD v ABV: Grade 3/4 alopecia 1% v 19% Grade 3/4 peripheral neuropathy 6% v 14% Grade 3/4 leucopenia 36% v 42%
62	Prospective randomised comparative study	Biopsy-proven AIDS-related KS with at least 15 mucocutaneous lesions or more	241	PLD 20 mg/m^2 every 3 weeks	Concurrent antiretroviral therapy Maintenance ganciclovir therapy	Responses assessed using modified ACTG criteria	National Cancer Institute common toxicity criteria

(Continued)

Table 29.3 (*Continued*)

Reference Study type	Study population	Total number of patients treated	Interventions compared n = number of patients	Co-treatments permitted	Overall percentage response rate (ORR)	Selected adverse events
	than five new cutaneous lesions in the preceding month or documented visceral KS with at least five assessable cutaneous lesions		for 6 cycles (n=121) OR BV (bleomycin 15 IU/m^2 and vincristine 2 mg) every 3 weeks for 6 cycles (n =120)	Foscarnet for active cytomegalovirus infection (CSF not permitted)	ORR: PLD 58·7% BV 23·3% P <0·001	Adverse events seen in 10% or more patients for PLD v BV: Alopecia 3·3% v 8·3% Paraesthesia 3·3% v 14·2% Leucopenia 71·9% v 50·8% Constipation 1·7% v 10·8% Cardiotoxicity 1·7% v 0·8%

ACTG, AIDS Clinical Trials Group; CSF, colony stimulating factor; G-CSF, granulocyte-colony stimulating factor; PLD, pegylated liposomal doxorubicin; SWOG, Southwest Oncology Group

ABV than with liposomal daunorubicin ($P<0.0001$), but grade 4 neutropenia was more frequent with the liposomal drug ($P = 0.021$).

Liposomal doxorubicin versus ABV or BV chemotherapy

Two randomised trials have compared PLD and ABV or BV combination chemotherapy and reported significantly higher overall response rates with the liposomal drug.[61,62] Northfelt et al. studied 258 patients with AIDS-related KS and reported a 46% overall response rate for PLD, 20 mg/m^2, compared with 25% for ABV chemotherapy (doxorubicin, 20 mg/m^2 + bleomycin, 10 mg/m^2 + vincristine, 1 mg), given every 2 weeks for six cycles. The difference in overall response rates was statistically significant ($P<0.001$).[61] Time to treatment failure did not differ significantly between the groups. The method of randomisation for this study is not stated. Modified ACTG criteria were used to assess response, and standard World Health Organization criteria were used to grade toxicity. Prior anthracycline chemotherapy was an exclusion criterion but concurrent antiretroviral therapy was permitted. Significantly more grade 3 nausea and vomiting, alopecia and peripheral neuropathy occurred with ABV than with PLD, and the dropout rate due to adverse events was higher with ABV (37% versus 11%). The two regimens did not differ significantly in the frequency of grade 3 or greater leucopenia, anaemia or thrombocytopenia. PLD was found to be more effective than combination chemotherapy with standard ABV in the treatment of AIDS-related cutaneous KS and caused less toxicity.

The second randomised trial (Stewart et al.) compared PLD, 20 mg/m^2, with BV chemotherapy (bleomycin, 15 IU/m^2 + vincristine, 2 mg) every 3 weeks for six cycles in patients with AIDS-related KS.[62] The 241 patients were randomised to the alternative treatments using a table of random numbers, blocked by investigation site, which was achieved by faxing the patient's age, risk factors and staging criteria to a central office. Concurrent antiretroviral therapy and antimicrobial prophylaxis was permitted during the study – 49% of the PLD group and 57% of the BV group were taking antiretrovirals. Modified ACTG criteria were used to assess response. Lesions without any detectable residual disease but persistent pigmented macules (brown) were described as a clinical complete response, rather than a complete response by ACTG criteria, because they were not re-biopsied. Adverse events were graded according to the National Cancer Institute common toxicity criteria. The overall response rate was significantly higher for PLD (59%) than BV chemotherapy (23%) ($P <0.001$). Peripheral neuropathy occurred significantly more frequently in the BV group ($P <0.001$) but neutropenia was more frequent in the PLD group ($P <0.001$).

Liposomal doxorubicin versus liposomal doxorubicin + bleomycin + vincristine

We found one randomised comparison of PLD alone with PLD + bleomycin + vincristine.[75] The overall response rates were 79% for 62 patients who received PLD alone and 80% for 64 patients who received the combination. Median times to progression were similar for both groups. However, the addition of bleomycin and vincristine to PLD caused a more rapid fall in quality of life indices and a shorter median time to first grade 3 toxicity.

We found no randomised trials comparing liposomal daunorubicin and PLD in the treatment of cutaneous KS although response rates in studies tend to be higher for PLD.

Drawbacks

In two randomised controlled trials the early dropout rate due to adverse events was higher with standard combination chemotherapy than with PLD. One RCT comparing PLD with ABV chemotherapy reported early dropout rates due to adverse events of 37% for the ABV arm and 11% for PLD.[61] Similarly early withdrawal because of chemotherapy-related toxicity was higher in the BV arm (27%) than the PLD arm (11%) in the second comparative RCT.[62]

Neutropenia

The incidence of grade 3 neutropenia in a randomised study comparing liposomal daunorubicin and ABV chemotherapy was similar in both groups (36% versus 35% respectively).[60] However, grade 4 neutropenia was more frequent as an adverse effect of liposomal daunorubicin than of ABV chemotherapy in the same randomised trial (15% versus 5%, $P = 0.021$).[60]

The most common adverse event in both arms of an RCT comparing PLD with ABV chemotherapy was leucopenia, affecting 36% of 133 patients who received PLD and 42% of 125 patients in the ABV group.[61] No episodes of febrile neutropenia (neutrophils $<500 \times 10^6$ cells/litre) occurred in the PLD group but 37% developed opportunistic infections and 6% experienced episodes of sepsis.[61] In a further RCT 29% of 121 patients who received PLD developed grade 3 leucopenia compared with 12% in the comparative BV chemotherapy arm.[62]

Cardiotoxicity

Of 24 patients who received a cumulative dose of >500 mg/m^2 of liposomal anthracycline in one randomised study, none were found to have a 20% or greater decline in their left ventricular ejection fraction (LVEF).[60] Liposomal daunorubicin was discontinued in one patient whose LVEF fell from 47% to 33%. An angiogram then showed that this patient had had a complete occlusion of the left anterior descending artery. In one RCT of

liposomal doxorubicin versus ABV, pre- and post-treatment estimations of LVEF were available for 47 patients who received PLD. Of these, two patients were found to have had a >20% fall in LVEF.[61] One death attributable to cardiomyopathy occurred in 133 patients treated with PLD.[61] It seems that, unlike conventional anthracyclines, liposomal anthracyclines are not associated with significant cumulative cardiotoxicity.

Nausea and vomiting

Of the patients receiving liposomal daunorubicin, 51% experienced mild nausea.[60] Grade 3 nausea and vomiting was significantly more frequent with ABV than with PLD (34% versus 15%, $P<0.001$).[61]

Alopecia

In the randomised trial reported by Gill et al. alopecia occurred more frequently amongst the patients who received ABV chemotherapy than among those receiving liposomal daunorubicin.[60] Of the ABV group, 36% experienced grade 1–2 alopecia, compared with 8% in the liposomal daunorubicin group ($P < 0.0001$). In another RCT comparing PLD with ABV chemotherapy, grade 3 alopecia was also more frequent in the ABV group than in those receiving a liposomal anthracycline (19% versus 1%, $P<0.001$).[61]

Peripheral neuropathy

Peripheral neuropathy was seen in 41% of patients treated with ABV and 13% of those given liposomal daunorubicin ($P<0.0001$) in the study of Gill et al.[60] In another randomised study, peripheral neuropathy was also less common with liposomal doxorubicin than with ABV chemotherapy (6% versus 14%, $P = 0.002$).[61]

Acute infusion reactions

In the only large phase III study of liposomal daunorubicin, the incidence of acute infusion reactions was 2% (2/116 patients). In an RCT of PLD, six of 133 patients (5%) experienced an acute infusion-related reaction presenting as flushing, chest pain, hypotension and back pain. Five of the six patients needed premedication for subsequent cycles but could continue on the study.[61] In another study the frequency of acute infusion reactions with PLD was similar, affecting five of 121 patients (4%), but a severe anaphylactic reaction occurred in one patient.[62]

Mortality
In the RCT of Stewart et al., five of 121 patients in the PLD arm died during the study. The cause of death for four of these patients was progression of AIDS, and the remaining patient died from progression of KS. The investigators attributed none of the deaths to the liposomal drug.[62]

In another RCT 24/133 patients who received PLD died, mostly as a result of complications of HIV infection, with one death resulting from cardiomyopathy.[61] There was no significant difference in the death rates compared with the ABV arm of the study.[61] In an RCT comparing liposomal daunorubicin with ABV chemotherapy, five of 117 patients who received PLD and five of 115 patients who received ABV chemotherapy died because of complications of HIV infection.[60] Median survival in the two groups did not differ.[60]

Palmar-plantar erythrodysaesthesia
A 2% (3/133 patients) incidence of palmar-plantar erythrodysaesthesia (cutaneous toxicity resulting in dry peeling red hands and feet) was reported in one trial of liposomal doxorubicin.[61]

Comment
Many uncontrolled trials, particularly in AIDS-related KS, have suggested a response rate, in terms of reduction in number and/or size of lesions, to a variety of cytotoxic agents including bleomycin, vinca alkaloids, etoposide and paclitaxel. Evaluation of earlier studies is made difficult by variation in the definitions used to stage disease and to assess response to therapy. The adoption of standardised ACTG criteria for staging and assessing response to treatment has made it easier to compare studies and should be used in future therapeutic trials.[10]

One small RCT suggested that combination chemotherapy with ABV chemotherapy is more effective than single-agent standard doxorubicin. Subsequently, three large RCTs have provided good evidence, using ACTG criteria to assess response, that liposomal anthracyclines are at least as effective in AIDS-related cutaneous KS as standard ABV or BV combination chemotherapy.[60–62] The two RCTs that specifically compared PLD with ABV or BV chemotherapy provide good evidence that PLD is more effective than standard combination chemotherapy.[61,62] The better toxicity profiles found in all three studies, associated with less frequent early termination of therapy because of adverse events, also favours the use of liposomal chemotherapy over standard combination chemotherapy. The addition of bleomycin and vincristine to liposomal doxorubicin is unlikely to be of benefit.

Although overall response rates to PLD are higher than for ABV or BV chemotherapy, the median duration of response is similar. In the RCT comparing PLD with ABV chemotherapy, the median duration of response was 90 days and 92 days, respectively.[61] In the RCT comparing PLD with BV chemotherapy, the median duration of response was 142 days and 123 days, respectively, but the difference was not statistically significant.[62]

Although we found no RCTs directly comparing the two liposomal drugs, the response rates for patients with advanced AIDS-related KS appear to be higher with liposomal doxorubicin than with daunorubicin. There have been no studies of sequential chemotherapy. Newer single-agent cytotoxic therapies such as paclitaxel, vinorelbine and gemcitabine should be compared with liposomal anthracyclines in large phase III studies.

Implications for practice

There is good evidence that liposomal doxorubicin is likely to be beneficial for the palliative treatment of advanced AIDS-related KS. In view of its better toxicity profile than conventional chemotherapy, liposomal doxorubicin should be used as first-line systemic therapy for patients with advanced AIDS-related KS who have poor immune function and significant mucocutaneous disease or visceral disease. However the liposomal anthracyclines are expensive and not readily available in the developing countries where most HIV-related disease occurs.

There have been no recent RCTs of chemotherapy in the other less common types of KS. However, previous uncontrolled studies and case series have suggested that patients with classical KS or African KS are at least as chemosensitive as those with AIDS-related KS without the underlying immune suppression.

> What are the effects of topical and systemic retinoids in the treatment of Kaposi's sarcoma?

Retinoids are a group of natural and synthetic vitamin A derivatives. They are active against KS cells *in vitro* and are used topically in the treatment of hyperkeratotic skin conditions.[76,77] We found two RCTs of the use of topical retinoids in the treatment of cutaneous AIDS-related KS.[78,79] No placebo-controlled clinical trials of the use of oral retinoids in the treatment of any of the clinical variants of KS were found.

Topical alitretinoin gel
Efficacy

We found two randomised double-blind, vehicle-controlled trials of the use of alitretinoin (9-*cis*-retinoic acid) gel in the topical treatment of AIDS-related KS.[78,79] The larger one, a multicentre randomised double-blind trial involving 268 patients with AIDS-related cutaneous KS, compared 0.1% alitretinoin gel with vehicle gel, applied twice daily for 12 weeks.[79] Concurrent antiretroviral therapy was allowed. Six index lesions were used to assess response to therapy using ACTG criteria applied to topical therapy. The overall response rate (complete and partial responses) was 35% (45/134) in the alitretinoin group compared with 18% (24/134) for the vehicle group. Following the blinded phase of the study, 184 of the patients were then treated with alitretinoin gel on an open-label basis and the overall response rate was 49% (90/184).[79]

In another randomised double-blind vehicle-controlled study, patients were randomised between 0·1% alitretinoin gel and vehicle gel, applied twice daily for 12 weeks.[78]. The overall response rate, assessed by ACTG criteria applied to topical therapy, for 62 patients treated with alitretinoin was 37% compared with 7% for 72 patients who received vehicle gel ($P = 0.00003$).

Alitretinoin was superior to vehicle gel in both the above studies when multiple variables, including number of lesions, CD4 count, performance status and number of concurrent antiretroviral therapies, were adjusted for.

Drawbacks

The most common adverse event resulting from treatment with alitretinoin gel was irritation at the application site, usually mild to moderate and reversible on cessation of treatment. In one study 7% of patients discontinued alitretinoin therapy because of treatment-related adverse events.[79]

Comment

These two randomised double-blind vehicle-controlled trials provide good evidence for the superiority of 0·1% alitretinoin gel over vehicle gel in the treatment of cutaneous AIDS-related KS. The overall response rate, using standard ACTG criteria, for 0·1% alitretinoin gel (applied twice daily for 12 weeks) was between 35% and 37%. Response rates in the vehicle-only groups were between 7% and 18%, suggesting that KS can undergo some degree of spontaneous remission or that the application of a vehicle alone may be of some benefit. This observation underlines the need to consider including suitable placebo groups in further trials.

What are the effects of antiretrovirals in the treatment of AIDS-related Kaposi's sarcoma?

We found no systematic reviews or large RCTs of antiretroviral therapy as a systemic treatment for AIDS-related KS. One small RCT of oral zidovudine, intravenous zidovudine or oral placebo in AIDS-related KS was identified but zidovudine monotherapy is no longer standard treatment for HIV infection.[80] A small prospective cohort study and one larger retrospective cohort study examining the effect of HAART were found.[81,82]

Efficacy

Antiretroviral therapy has been shown to increase survival and delay progression to AIDS in HIV-positive patients. Population-based studies have shown that HAART (which includes two nucleoside reverse transcriptase inhibitors with either a non-nucleoside reverse transcriptase inhibitor or one or two protease inhibitors) decreases the incidence of KS as an AIDS-defining diagnosis.[83–85] In a multicentre cohort of 30 000 patients from centres in the US the incidence of KS fell from 4·8 per 100 person-years in 1990 to 1·5 per 100 person-years in

1997 during 54 000 person-years of follow up between 1990 and 1997.[85] The relative risk of developing KS was 0·41 (95% CI 0·2–0·8) for patients on triple antiretroviral therapy.

Reconstitution of the immune system following treatment with HAART may also affect established KS and prolong time to disease progression. Small uncontrolled studies and case reports have documented reduction of KS lesions after initiation of HAART.[86–88]

One small RCT of 37 evaluable patients with a high risk of developing AIDS-related KS (CD4 count >200 cells × 10^6/litre, no "B" symptoms and no history of opportunistic infections) randomised patients to 4-hourly treatment with one of the following: oral placebo, oral zidovudine, 250 mg, intravenous zidovudine, 0·5 mg/kg, or intravenous zidovudine, 2·5 mg/kg.[80] At 6 weeks, four of nine patients receiving oral placebo and 10 of 28 patients receiving oral or intravenous zidovudine had progressive KS. After 12 weeks, only five patients receiving zidovudine had a minor response (defined as the absence of new KS lesions and a 25–50% regression in at least 25% of existing lesions). In this study zidovudine was not an effective treatment for KS in terms of response rate or delay of progression. However, the number of patients in each of the four treatment arms was small, and monotherapy with zidovudine has been superseded by HAART as standard therapy in the treatment of HIV infection.

A small prospective cohort study of 39 patients with AIDS-related KS commenced on HAART found that 10 of 19 patients, who received no other systemic therapy for KS, achieved a complete response by ACTG criteria.[81] Patients were more likely to respond if their CD4 count was >150 cells × 10^6/litre. A retrospective cohort study identified 101 patients who received local or systemic therapy for KS and were subsequently commenced on HAART.[82]

Thirty-three patients were excluded because new anti-KS therapy was instituted at the same time as commencement of HAART. For the remaining 78 patients, the median time to treatment failure before starting HAART was 0·5 years (defined as the time between the final and penultimate anti-KS therapy before HAART). After the start of HAART, median time to treatment failure was 1·7 years (defined as time between start of HAART and next anti-KS therapy).[82] No correlation was demonstrated between CD4 count response and control of KS but a statistically significant correlation between progression of KS and virological failure of HAART (defined as viral load >5000 copies/ml) was found. However, five of 24 patients (21%) on HAART did not have virological failure (viral load <200 copies/ml) at the time of KS progression. Immune reconstitution has been postulated as the mechanism of response of KS to antiretroviral therapy but response to HAART and the relationship to CD4 count response is unpredictable.

Drawbacks

The side-effects of combination HAART depend on the profile of individual drugs used and interactions with other drugs. More frequent side-effects include nausea and vomiting, lethargy, diarrhoea, peripheral neuropathy, headache, deranged liver function, hypersensitivity reactions, myelosuppression, lactic acidosis and pancreatitis.

Implications for practice

HAART may delay the onset of KS as an AIDS-defining diagnosis in patients with HIV infection. HAART may also induce responses in AIDS-related KS via immune reconstitution but the response to therapy is unpredictable. Patients with high viral loads, low CD4 counts or with other HIV-related symptoms require antiretroviral therapy for control of HIV infection. HAART alone

in these patients is a reasonable initial therapy for KS, which may be combined later with other local or systemic treatments. However, immune reconstitution takes several weeks and patients with poor prognosis KS may require additional therapy in the interim.

> **What is the role of anti-herpes virus therapy in the prevention and treatment of AIDS-related Kaposi's sarcoma?**

The discovery of KSHV (also known as HHV8) has provided another potential target for the prevention and treatment of AIDS-related KS. KSHV replication is inhibited *in vitro* by cidofovir, ganciclovir and foscarnet, but not by aciclovir.[89,90] Cohort studies have reported a decreased risk of developing KS for HIV-positive patients treated with ganciclovir or foscarnet for cytomegalovirus (CMV) infection and there have been occasional case reports of patients with AIDS-related KS having prolonged responses to antiherpetic therapy.[91–95] One cohort study of 3688 HIV-positive patients followed up for a median of 4·2 years, during which time 16% (598 patients) developed KS, found a statistically significant reduction in the relative hazard of developing KS for those who received foscarnet or ganciclovir. The relative hazard for foscarnet was 0·38 (95% CI 0·15–0·95; $P = 0.038$) and for ganciclovir 0·39 (95% CI 0·19–0·84; $P = 0.015$).

A randomised study of the treatment of CMV retinitis with ganciclovir in patients with AIDS, found a reduced risk of developing KS with oral or intravenous ganciclovir treatment.[96] The 377 patients with AIDS and unilateral CMV retinitis were randomised to receive a ganciclovir implant and oral ganciclovir, 4·5 g daily, ganciclovir implant and oral placebo, or intravenous ganciclovir alone. The primary outcome was the development of new CMV disease but treatment with oral or intravenous ganciclovir was also found to reduce the risk of developing KS by 75% ($P = 0.008$) and 93% ($P<0.001$), respectively, compared with oral placebo.[96]

Implications for practice

Whilst there is some evidence that antiherpetic agents reduced the risk of developing AIDS-related KS, these agents are not currently used in routine practice as prophylaxis. RCTs evaluating these drugs for other outcomes such as CMV infections suggest important benefit. This observation needs to be followed up by well-designed studies with KS as the main outcome.

Key points

Local therapy

- Evidence is insufficient to make any firm recommendations as to the value of surgical excision, cryotherapy, photodynamic therapy and intralesional chemotherapy.
- In people with AIDS-related KS, an 8 Gy single fraction of radiotherapy is highly likely to improve the cosmetic outcome of individual cutaneous lesions, with minimal harm. Fractionated radiotherapy to a higher total dose causes greater skin toxicity but provides a longer duration of lesion control and therefore may be more appropriate for more indolent disease seen with classical KS and some forms of endemic (African) KS. However the optimum dose fractionation schedule in these conditions is yet to be determined.
- Topical 0.1% alitretinoin gel as a local treatment for AIDS-related KS is more effective than vehicle gel and has a response rate of approximately 35%.

Systemic therapy

- Interferon alfa is likely to be a beneficial systemic treatment for good prognosis AIDS-related KS. Interferon can be safely combined with antiretroviral therapy and is most suitable as first-line therapy for patients with CD4 counts $>200 \times 10^6$ cells/litre, no "B" symptoms and no history of prior opportunistic infection.
- We found good evidence that liposomal doxorubicin is more effective in AIDS-related KS than standard combination chemotherapy containing bleomycin + vincristine, with or without an anthracycline. Unlike conventional anthracyclines, liposomal anthracyclines do not appear to be associated with significant cardiotoxicity.
- Newer single-agent cytotoxic therapies such as paclitaxel, vinorelbine and gemcitabine have shown activity in AIDS-related KS in uncontrolled phase II trials. Future RCTs comparing these agents with the liposomal anthracyclines are required.
- Classical KS and endemic (African) are likely to be at least as chemosensitive as AIDS-related KS but are less common variants which have not been the subject of large randomised phase III studies.
- Antiretroviral therapy is reasonable initial therapy for minimally symptomatic cutaneous AIDS-related KS, although the response to therapy is unpredictable. It may be combined with other systemic therapies.
- Antiherpetic therapy for CMV disease is associated with a reduced risk of developing KS in HIV-positive patients. There is insufficient evidence to assess the value of cidofovir, ganciclovir or foscarnet as treatment for established AIDS-related KS.

References

1. Friedman-Kien AE, Laubenstein L, Marmor M et al. Kaposi's sarcoma and Pneumocystis pneumonia among homosexual men – New York City and California. MMWR Morb Mortal Wkly Rep 1981;**30**:305–8.

2. Taylor JF, Templeton AC, Vogel CL et al. Kaposi's sarcoma in Uganda: a clinico-pathological study. Int J Cancer 1971;**8**:122–35.

3. Wabinga HR, Parkin DM, Wabwire-Mangen F, Mugerwa JW. Cancer in Kampala, Uganda, in 1989–1991: changes in incidence in the AIDS era. Int J Cancer 1993;**54**:26–36.

4. Biggar RJ, Rabkin CS. The epidemiology of AIDS-related neoplasms. *Haematol Oncol Clin North Am* 1996;**10**: 997–1010.

5. Farge D. Kaposi's sarcoma in organ transplant recipients. *Eur J Med* 1993;**2**:339–43.

6. Shepherd FA, Maher E, Cardella C *et al.* Treatment of Kaposi's sarcoma after solid organ transplantation. *J Clin Oncol* 1997;**15**:2371–7.

7. Qunibi W, Akhtar M, Sheth K *et al.* Kaposi's sarcoma: the most common tumor after renal transplantation in Saudi Arabia. *Am J Med* 1988;**84**:225–32.

8. Chang Y, Cesarman E, Pessin MS *et al.* Identification of herpesvirus-like DNA sequences in AIDS-associated Kaposi's sarcoma. *Science* 1994;**266**:1865–9.

9. Krown SE, Testa MA, Huang J *et al.* for the AIDS Clinical Trials Group Oncology Committee: AIDS-related Kaposi's sarcoma: prospective validation of the AIDS Clinical Trials Group staging classification. *J Clin Oncol* 1997,**15**: 3085–92.

10. Krown SE, Metroka C, Wernz JC. Kaposi's sarcoma in the acquired immune deficiency syndrome: a proposal for uniform evaluation, response, and staging criteria. *J Clin Oncol* 1989;**7**:1201–7.

11. Tappero JW, Berger TG, Kaplan LD *et al.* Cryotherapy for cutaneous Kaposi's sarcoma (KS) associated with acquired immune deficiency syndrome (AIDS) a phase II trial. *J Acquir Immune Defic Syndr* 1991;**4**:839–46.

12. Schofer H, Ochsendorf FR, Hochscheid I, Milbradt R. Facial kaposi's sarcoma. Palliative treatment with cryotherapy, intralesional chemotherapy, low-dose roentgen therapy and camouflage. *Hautarzt* 1991;**42**:492–8.

13. Bernstein ZP, Wilson BD, Oseroff AR *et al.* Photofrin photodynamic therapy for treatment of AIDS-related cutaneous Kaposi's sarcoma. *AIDS* 1999;**13**:1697–704.

14. Hebada KM, Huizing MT, Brouwer PA *et al.* Photodynamic therapy in AIDS-related cutaneous Kaposi's sarcoma. *J Acquir Immune Defic Syndr Hum Retrovirol* 1995;**10**:61–70.

15. Szeimes RM, Lorenzen T, Karrer S *et al.* Photochemotherapy of cutaneous AIDS-associated Kaposi's sarcoma with indocyanine green and laser light. *Hautarzt* 2001;**52**:322–6.

16. Friedman M, Venkakesan TK, Caldanelli DD. Intralesional vinblastine for treating AIDS-associated Kaposi's sarcoma of the oropharynx and larynx. *Ann Otol Rhinol Laryngol* 1996;**105**:272–4.

17. Flaitz CM, Nichols CM, Hicks MJ. Role of intralesional vinblastine administration in treatment of intraoral Kaposi's sarcoma in AIDS. *Eur J Cancer B Oral Oncol* 1995;**31B**:280–5.

18. Boudreaux AA, Smith LL, Cosby CD *et al.* Intralesional vinblastine for cutaneous Kaposi's sarcoma associated with acquired immunodeficiency syndrome. A clinical trial to evaluate efficacy and discomfort associated with injection. *J Am Acad Dermatol* 1993;**28**.61–5.

19. Brambilla L, Boneschi V, Beretta G, Finzi AF. Intralesional chemotherapy for Kaposi's sarcoma. *Dermatologica* 1984;**169**:150–5.

20. Stelzer KJ, Griffin TW. A randomized prospective trial of radiation therapy for AIDS-associated Kaposi's sarcoma. *Int J Radiat Oncol Biol Phys* 1993;**27**:1057–61.

21. Harrison M, Harrington KJ, Tomlinson DR, Stewart JS. Response and cosmetic outcome of two fractionation regimens for AIDS-related Kaposi's sarcoma. *Radiother Oncol* 1998;**46**:23–8.

22. Belmbaogo E, Kirova Y, Frikha H *et al.* (Radiotherapy of epidemic Kaposi's sarcoma: the experience of Henri-Mondor Hospital (643 patients)). *Cancer Radiother* 1999;**2**:49–52.

23. Berson AM, Quivey JM, Harris JW, Wara WM. Radiation therapy for AIDS-related Kaposi's Sarcoma. *Int J Radiat Oncol Biol Phys* 1990;**19**:569–75.

24. Cooper JS. The influence of dose on the long-term control of Classic (non–AIDS associated) Kaposi's sarcoma by radiotherapy. *Int J Radiat Oncol Biol Phys* 1988;**15**: 1141–6.

25. Brenner B, Rakowsky E, Katz A *et al.* Tailoring treatment for classical Kaposi's sarcoma: Comprehensive clinical guidelines. *Int J Oncol* 1999;**14**:1097–102.

26. Nisce LZ, Safai B, Poussin-Rosillo H. Once weekly total and subtotal skin electron beam therapy for Kaposi's sarcoma. *Cancer* 1981;**47**:640–4.

27. Stein ME, Lakier R, Kuten A *et al.* Radiation therapy in endemic (African) Kaposi's sarcoma. *Int J Radiat Oncol Biol Phys* 1993;**27**:1181–4.

28. Groopman JE, Gottlieb MS, Goodman J *et al.* Recombinant alpha-2 interferon therapy for Kaposi's sarcoma associated with the acquired immunodeficiency syndrome. *Ann Intern Med* 1984;**100**:671–6.

29. Shepherd FA, Beaulieu R, Gelmon K *et al.* Prospective randomized trial of two dose levels of interferon with zidovudine for the treatment of Kaposi's sarcoma associated with human immunodeficiency virus infection: a Canadian HIV Clinical Trials Network study. *J Clin Oncol* 1998;**16**:1736–42.

30. Evans LM, Itri LM, Campion M *et al.* Interferon-alpha 2a in the treatment of acquired immunodeficiency syndrome-related Kaposi's sarcoma. *J Immunother* 1991;**10**:39–50.

31. Volberding PA, Mitsuyasu RT, Golando JP, Spiegel RJ. Treatment of Kaposi's sarcoma with interferon alfa-2b (Intron A). *Cancer* 1987;**59**(Suppl):620–5.

32. Krown SE, Gold JW, Niedzwiecki D *et al.* Interferon-alpha with zidovudine: safety, tolerance, and clinical and virologic effects in patients with Kaposi sarcoma associated with acquired immunodeficiency syndrome (AIDS). *Ann Intern Med* 1990;**112**:812–21.

33. Fischl MA, Uttamchandani RB, Resnick L *et al.* A phase I study of recombinant human interferon-alpha 2a or human lymphoblastoid interferon-alpha n1 and concomitant zidovudine in patients with AIDS-related Kaposi's sarcoma. *J Acquir Immune Defic Syndr* 1991;**4**:1–10.

34. de Wit R, Danner SA, Bakker PJ *et al.* Combined zidovudine and interferon-alpha treatment in patients with AIDS-associated Kaposi's sarcoma. *J Intern Med* 1991;**229**:35–40.

35. Baumann R, Tauber MG, Opravil M *et al.* Combined treatment with zidovudine and lymphoblast interferon alpha in patients with HIV-related Kaposi's sarcoma. *Klin Wochenschr* 1991;**69**:360–7.

36. Podzamczer D, Bolao F, Clotet B *et al.* Low-dose interferon alpha combined with zidovudine in patients with AIDS-associated Kaposi's sarcoma. *J Intern Med* 1993;**233**:247–53.

37. Fischl MA, Finkelstein DM, He W *et al.* A phase II study of recombinant human interferon-alpha 2a and zidovudine in patients with AIDS-related Kaposi's sarcoma. *J Acquir Immune Defic Syndr Hum Retrovirol* 1996;**11**:379–84.

38. Stadler R, Bratzke B, Schaart F, Orfanos CE. Long-term combined rIFN-alpha-2a and zidovudine therapy for HIV-associated Kaposi's sarcoma: clinical consequences and side effects. *J Invest Dermatol* 1990;**95**(Suppl):170–5.

39. Opravil M, Hirschel B, Bucher HC, Luthy R. A randomised trial of interferon-alpha2a and zidovudine versus bleomycin and zidovudine for AIDS-related Kaposi's sarcoma. Swiss HIV Cohort Study. *Int J STD AIDS* 1999;**10**:369–75.

40. Krigel RL, Slywotzky CM, Lonberg M *et al.* Treatment of epidemic Kaposi's sarcoma with a combination of interferon-alpha 2b and etoposide. *J Biol Response Mod* 1988;**7**:359–64.

41. Shepherd FA, Evans WK, Garvey B *et al.* Combination chemotherapy and alpha-interferon in the treatment of Kaposi's sarcoma associated with acquired immune deficiency syndrome. *Can Med Assoc J* 1988;**139**:635–9.

42. Lassoued K, Clauvel JP, Katlama C *et al.* Treatment of the acquired immune deficiency syndrome-related Kaposi's sarcoma with bleomycin as a single agent. *Cancer* 1990;**66**:1869–72.

43. Remick SC, Reddy M, Herman D *et al.* Continous infusion bleomycin in AIDS-related Kaposi's sarcoma. *J Clin Oncol* 1994;**12**:1130–6.

44. Caumes E, Guermonprez G, Katlama C *et al.* AIDS-associated mucocutaneous Kaposi's sarcoma treated with bleomycin. *AIDS* 1992;**6**:1483–7.

45. Hernandez DE, Perez JR. Advanced epidemic Kaposi's sarcoma: treatment with bleomycin or combination of doxorubicin, bleomycin and vincristine. *Int J Dermatol* 1996;**35**:831–3.

46. Brambilla L, Labianca R, Boreschi V *et al.* Mediterranean Kaposi's sarcoma in the elderly. A randomised study of oral etoposide versus vinblastine. *Cancer* 1994;**74**:2873–8.

47. Zidan J, Robenstein W, Abzah A *et al.* Treatment of Kaposi's sarcoma with vinblastine in patients with disseminated dermal disease. *Isr Med Assoc J* 2001;**3**:251–3.

48. Kaplan L, Abrams D, Volberding P. Treatment of Kaposi's sarcoma in acquired immunodeficiency syndrome with an alternating vincristine-vinblastine regime. *Cancer Treat Rep* 1986;**70**:1121–2.

49. Volberding PA, Abrams DI, Conant M *et al.* Vinblastine therapy for Kaposi's sarcoma in the acquired immunodeficiency syndrome. *Ann Intern Med* 1985;**103**:335–8.

50. Solan AJ, Greenwald ES, Silvay O. Long-term complete remissions of Kaposi's sarcoma with vinblastine therapy. *Cancer* 1981;**47**:637–9.

51. Klein E, Schwartz RA, Laor Y *et al.* Treatment of Kaposi's sarcoma with vinblastine. *Cancer* 1980;**45**:427–31.

52. Tucker SB, Wintelmann RK. Treatment of Kaposi's sarcoma with vinblastine. *Arch Dermatol* 1976;**112**:958–61.

53. Brambilla L, Boneschi V, Fossati S *et al.* Oral etoposide for Kaposi's Mediterranean sarcoma. *Dermatologica* 1988;**177**:365–9.

54. Laubenstein LJ, Krigel RL, Odajnyk CM *et al.* Treatment of epidemic Kaposi's sarcoma with etoposide or a combination of doxorubicin, bleomycin and vinblastine. *J Clin Oncol* 1984;**2**:1115–20.

55. Sprinz E, Caldas AP, Mans DR *et al.* Fractionated doses of oral etoposide in the treatment of patients with *AIDS*-related Kaposi's sarcoma: clinical and pharmocologic study to improve therapeutic index. *J Clin Oncol* 2001;**24**:177–84.

56. Schwartsmann G, Sprinz E, Kromfield M *et al.* Clinical and pharmacokinetic study of oral etoposide in patients with AIDS-related Kaposi's sarcoma with no prior exposure to cytotoxic therapy. *J Clin Oncol* 1997;**15**:2118–24.

57. Remick SC, Reddy M, Ekman K *et al.* Continuous infusion etoposide in advanced AIDS-related Kaposi sarcoma. *J Infus Chemother* 1996;**6**:92–6.

58. Bakker PJ, Danner SA, Lange JM *et al.* Etoposide for epidemic Kaposi's sarcoma: a phase II study. *Eur J Cancer Clin Oncol* 1988;**24**:1047–8.

59. Schwartsmann G, Sprinz E, Kronfeld M *et al.* Phase II study of teniposide in patients with AIDS-related Kaposi's sarcoma. *Eur J Cancer* 1991;**27**:1637–9.

60. Gill PS, Wernz J, Scadden DT *et al.* Randomized phase III trial of liposomal daunorubicin versus doxorubicin, bleomycin, and vincristine in AIDS-related Kaposi's sarcoma. *J Clin Oncol* 1996;**14**:2353–64.

61. Northfelt DW, Dezube BJ, Thommes JA *et al.* Pegylated-liposomal doxorubicin versus doxorubicin, bleomycin and vincristine in the treatment of AIDS-related Kaposi's sarcoma: results of a randomized phase III clinical trial. *J Clin Oncol* 1998;**16**:2445–51.

62. Stewart S, Jablonowski H, Goebel FD *et al.* Randomized comparative trial of pegylated liposomal doxorubicin versus bleomycin and vincristine in the treatment of AIDS-related Kaposi's sarcoma. *J Clin Oncol* 1998;**16**:683–91.

63. Uthayakumar S, Bower M, Money-Kyrle J *et al.* Randomized cross-over comparison of liposomal daunorubicin versus observation for early Kaposi's sarcoma. *AIDS* 1996;**10**:515–19.

64. Gill PS, Tulpule A, Espina BM *et al.* Paclitaxel is safe and effective in the treatment of advanced AIDS-related Kaposi's sarcoma. *J Clin Oncol* 1999;**17**:1876–83.

65. Welles L, Saville MW, Lietzau J *et al.* Phase II trial with dose titration of paclitaxel for the therapy of human immunodeficiency virus-associated Kaposi's sarcoma. *J Clin Oncol* 1998;**16**:1112–21.

66. Saville MW, Lietzau J, Pluda JM *et al.* Treatment of HIV-associated Kaposi's sarcoma with paclitaxel. *Lancet* 1995;**346**:26–8.

67. Nasti G, Errante D, Talamini R *et al.* Vinorelbine is an effective and safe drug for AIDS-related Kaposi's sarcoma: results of a phase II study. *J Clin Oncol* 2000;**18**:1550–7.

68. Brambilla L, Labianca R, Ferrucci SM *et al.* Treatment of classical Kaposi's sarcoma with gemcitabine. *Dermatology* 2001;**202**.119–22.

69. Little RF, Wyvill KM, Pluda JM *et al.* Activity of thalidomide in AIDS-related Kaposi's sarcoma. *J Clin Oncol* 2000;**18**:2593–602.

70. Fife K, Howard MR, Gracie F *et al.* Activity of thalidomide in AIDS-related Kaposi's sarcoma and correlation with HHV8 titre. *Int J STD AIDS* 1998;**9**:751–5.

71. Vogel CL, Templeton CJ, Templeton AC *et al.* Treatment of Kaposi's sarcoma with actinomycin-D and cyclophosphamide: a randomized clinical trial. *Int J Cancer* 1971;**8**:136–43.

72. Vogel CL, Primack A, Dhru D *et al.* Treatment of Kaposi's sarcoma with a combination of actinomycin D and vincristine: a randomized clinical trial. *Cancer* 1973;**31**:1382–91.

73. Olweny CL, Toya T, Mbidde EK, Lwanga SK. Treatment of Kaposi's sarcoma by combination of actinomycin-D, vincristine and carboxamide (nsc-45388): results of a randomized clinical trial. *Int J Cancer* 1974;**14**:649–56.

74. Gill PS, Rarick M, McCutchan JA *et al.* Systemic treatment of AIDS-related Kaposi's sarcoma: results of a randomized trial. *Am J Med* 1991;**90**:427–33.

75. Mitsuyasu R, von Roenn J, Krown S *et al.* Comparison study of liposomal doxorubicin alone or with bleomycin and vincristine for treatment of advanced AIDS-associated Kaposi's sarcoma: AIDS Clinical Trial Group protocol 286. *Proc Annu Meet Am Soc Clin Oncol.* May 1997; abstract 191.

76. Guo WX, Gill PS, Antakly T. Inhibition of AIDS-Kaposi's sarcoma cell proliferation following retinoic acid receptor activation. *Cancer Res* 1995;**55**:823–9.

77. Corbeil J, Rapaport E, Richmann DD, Looney DJ. Antiproliferative effect of retinoid compounds on Kaposi's sarcoma cells. *J Clin Invest* 1994;**93**:1981–6.

78. Bodsworth NJ, Bloch M, Bower M *et al.* Phase III vehicle-controlled, multi-centred study of topical alitretinoin gel 0.1% in cutaneous AIDS-related Kaposi's sarcoma. *Am J Clin Dermatol* 2001;**2**:77–87.

79. Walmsley S, Northfelt DW, Melosky B *et al.* Treatment of AIDS-related cutaneous Kaposi's sarcoma with alitretinoin (9-cis-retinoic acid) gel. Panretin Gel North American Study Group. *J Acquir Immune Defic Syndr* 1999;**22**: 235–46.

80. Lane HC, Falloon J, Walter RE *et al.* Zidovudine in patients with human immunodeficiency virus (HIV) infection and Kaposi's sarcoma. A phase II randomised placebo-controlled trial. *Ann Intern Med* 1989;**111**:41–50.

81. Dupont C, Vasseur E, Beauchet A *et al.* Long-term efficacy on Kaposi's sarcoma of highly active antiretroviral therapy in a cohort of HIV-positive patients. CISIH 92. Centre d'information et de soins de l'immunodeficience humaine. *AIDS* 2000;**14**:987–93.

82. Bower M, Fox P, Fife K *et al.* Highly active anti-retroviral therapy (HAART) prolongs time to treatment failure in Kaposi's sarcoma. *AIDS* 1999;**13**:2105–11.

83. Grulian AE, Li Y, McDonald AM *et al.* Decreasing rates of Kaposi's sarcoma and non-Hodgkins lymphoma in the era of potent combination anti-retroviral therapy. *AIDS* 2001;**15**:629–33.

84. Pezzotti P, Serraino D, Rezza G *et al.* The spectrum of AIDS-defining diseases: temporal trends in Italy prior to the use of highly active anti-retroviral therapies, 1982–1996. *Int J Epidemiol* 1999;**28**:975–81.

85. Jones J, Hanson DL, Dworkin MS *et al.* Effect of antiretroviral and other antiviral therapies on the incidence of Kaposi's sarcoma and trends in Kaposi's sarcoma. Proc 12th World AIDS conference. *J Acquir Immune Defic Syndr* 2000;**24**:270–4.

86. Wit FW, Sol CJ, Renwick N *et al.* Regression of AIDS-related Kaposi's sarcoma associated with clearance of human herpesvirus-8 from peripheral blood mononuclear cells following initiation of antiretroviral therapy. *AIDS* 1998;**12**:218–19.

87. Volm MD, Wenz J. Patients with advanced AIDS-related Kaposi's sarcoma (EKS) no longer require systemic therapy after introduction of effective antiretroviral therapy (abstract). *Proc Am Soc Clin Oncol* 1997; **16**:469.

88. Tavio M, Nash G, Spina M *et al.* Highly active antiretroviral therapy in HIV-related Kaposi's sarcoma. *Ann Oncol* 1998;**9**:923.

89. Medveczky MM, Horvath E, Lund T, Medveczky PG. In vitro antiviral drug sensitivity of the Kaposi's sarcoma-associated herpesvirus. *AIDS* 1997;**11**:1327–32.

90. Kedes DH, Ganem D. Sensitivity of Kaposi's sarcoma-associated herpesvirus replication to antiviral drugs. Implications for potential therapy. *J Clin Invest* 1997;**99**:2082–6.

91. Mocroft A, Youle M, Gazzard B *et al.* Anti-herpesvirus treatment and risk of Kaposi's sarcoma in HIV infection. Royal Free/Chelsea and Westminster Hospitals Collaborative Group. *AIDS* 1996;**10**:1101–5.

92. Glesby MJ, Hoover DR, Weng S *et al.* Use of antiherpes drugs and the risk of Kaposi's sarcoma: data from the Multicenter AIDS Cohort Study. *J Infect Dis* 1996;**173**: 1477–80.

93. Robles R, Lugo D, Gee L, Jacobson MA. Effect of antiviral drugs used to treat cytomegalovirus end-organ disease on subsequent course of previously diagnosed Kaposi's sarcoma in patients with AIDS. *J Acquir Immune Defic Syndr Hum Retrovirol* 1999;**20**:34–8.

94. Jones JL, Hanson DL, Dworkin MS, Jaffe HW. Incidence and trends in Kaposi's sarcoma in the era of effective antiretroviral therapy. *J Acquir Immune Defic Syndr* 2000;**24**:270–4.

95. Morfeldt L, Torssander J. Long-term remission of Kaposi's sarcoma following foscarnet treatment in HIV infected patients. *Scand J Infect Dis* 1994;**26**:749–52.

96. Martin DF, Kuppermann BD, Wolitz RA *et al.* Oral ganciclovir for patients with cytomegalovirus retinitis treated with a ganciclovir implant. Roche Ganciclovir Study Group. *N Engl J Med* 1999;**340**:1063–70.

Part 3: The evidence

Section C: Infective skin diseases

Editors: Thomas Diepgen and Hywel Williams

30
Local treatments for cutaneous warts

Sam Gibbs

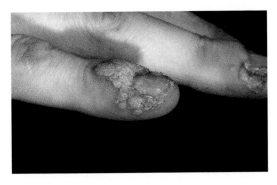

Figure 30.1   Ordinary viral warts on the fingers

Background
Definition

Viral warts are extremely common, benign and usually self-limiting. Infection of epidermal cells with the human papillomavirus (HPV) results in cell proliferation and a thickened, warty papule on the skin. The most common sites involved are the hands and feet but any area of skin can be infected.

Incidence/prevalence

There are few reliable, population-based data on the incidence and prevalence of common warts. Prevalence probably varies widely between different age groups, populations and periods of time. Two large population-based studies found prevalence rates of 0·84% and 12·9%, respectively.[1,2] Prevalence rates are highest in children and young adults; studies in school populations have shown prevalence rates of 12% in 4–6 year olds[3] and 24% in 16–18 year olds.[4]

Aetiology and risk factors

Warts are caused by HPV, of which there are over 70 different types. Viral warts are most common at sites of trauma such as the hands and feet, and lesions probably result from inoculation of virus into minimally damaged areas of epithelium. Plantar warts are often acquired from common bare-foot areas[5] and severe hand warts are an occupational risk for butchers and meat handlers.[6] Genital warts are also common and are frequently sexually transmitted; they are not discussed in this chapter.

Prognosis

Extragenital warts in immunocompetent people are harmless and usually resolve spontaneously as a result of natural immunity within months or years. The rate of resolution is highly variable and probably depends on a number of factors, including host immunity, age, HPV type and site of infection. One frequently cited study of an institutionalised population showed that two-thirds of warts resolved within a 2-year period.[7] Evaluation of control group clearance rates within randomised controlled trials (RCTs) may also give some indication of natural clearance rates, although a non-specific benefit of vehicle bases may make interpretation difficult. Seventeen of the RCTs discussed in more depth later in this chapter included a placebo group and used participants rather than warts as the unit of analysis. The average cure rate with placebo preparations in these trials was 30% (range 0–73%) after an average period of 10 weeks (range 4–24 weeks).

Diagnostic tests

Simple warts are nearly always diagnosed clinically. Microscopic examination of warts removed surgically can confirm the diagnosis if there is doubt. HPV typing is used in research laboratories and occasionally in medicolegal cases investigating child abuse.

Aims of treatment

To clear warts completely and permanently.

Relevant outcomes

- Total clearance
- Non-recurrence
- Adverse reactions such as pain and blistering

Methods of search

For a systematic review[8] we searched for all RCTs of local treatments for extragenital warts in immunocompetent people in the Cochrane Central Register of Controlled Trials, Medline, Embase and a number of other electronic databases using standardised search strategies. The bibliographies of all identified trials and key review articles were searched manually. All relevant pharmaceutical companies were contacted and a search for unpublished trials was carried out by contacting a number of clinicians and researchers worldwide. The most recent searches were completed in September 2001.

QUESTIONS

How effective are the various available local treatments for clearing warts and what are the side-effects of these treatments?

Topical treatments containing salicylic acid (SA)

Efficacy

Reported cure rates in 13 RCTs ranged from 0% to 84%.[8]

SA versus placebo

Six RCTs[9–14] (376 adults and children) compared SA with placebo. SA preparations gave higher cure rates: 75% versus 48%; odds ratio (OR) 3·91 (95% confidence interval (CI) 2·40–6·36); number needed to treat (NNT) 3·67 (CI 2·72–5·60).

SA versus cryotherapy

Two RCTs[15,16] compared SA with cryotherapy (272 adults and children). Cure rates ranged between 60% and 70% and did not differ significantly between the two treatments; OR 1·15 (CI 0·72–1·82).

Other comparisons

Seven other RCTs[15,17–20] compared different products containing SA or compared SA with other topical treatments such as glutaraldehyde and dithranol. The limited evidence provided by these different trials showed no convincing advantage of any particular delivery system for SA, or of the other topical treatments.

Drawbacks

In one RCT that compared a mixture of monochloroacetic acid and 60% SA with placebo,[13] one of the 29 patients in the active treatment group developed cellulitis. Minor skin irritation was noted occasionally in some of the other trials but generally topical SA was reported to have no significant harmful effects.

Comment

There is some reservation about the validity of pooled data from the different RCTs because of the generally low quality of trials and the heterogeneity of their design and methodology. For instance, different RCTs used slightly different topical SA products and while some RCTs included patients with refractory warts, others excluded them. Despite this we feel there is good evidence for a modest but definite beneficial clinical effect of SA in treating ordinary warts.

Implications for practice

Topical preparations containing SA are generally effective and safe for treating warts.

Cryotherapy with liquid nitrogen

Reported cure rates in 16 RCTs were highly variable, ranging from 9% to 87%.[8]

Efficacy
Cryotherapy versus placebo or no treatment

Two small RCTs[21,22] involving 69 adults compared cryotherapy with either placebo cream[21] or no treatment.[22] The pooled data did not demonstrate a significant difference in cure rates: 35% v 34%; OR 0·82 (CI 0·16–4·24). One trial[21] had a very low cure rate for cryotherapy (1/11) and the other[22] had a very high cure rate in its placebo group (8/20).

Cryotherapy versus SA

Two RCTs[15,16] compared SA with cryotherapy in 320 adults and children. There was no significant difference in cure rates between the two treatments: 65% v 62%; OR 1·15 (CI 0·72–1·82).

Length of freeze

Four RCTs[23-26] compared aggressive and gentle cryotherapy in 592 adults and children; however, definitions of aggressive and gentle differed and some studies included refractory warts whereas others did not. Overall, cure was achieved in 52% with aggressive cryotherapy and 31% with gentle cryotherapy; OR 3·69 (CI 1·45–9·41).

Interval between freezes

Three RCTs[15,27,28] showed no significant difference in cure rates between 2- 3- and 4-week intervals. Cure was generally achieved more quickly with shorter treatment intervals.

Optimum number of freezes

Only one RCT[29] examined this question in 115 adults and children not cured after 3 months of three-weekly cryotherapy and showed no benefit of prolonging cryotherapy for a further 3 months. Cure rates were 43% and 38% in the treated and non-treated groups, respectively (no data available to calculate OR).

Drawbacks

Only two RCTs had precise data on adverse events. Pain or blistering was reported by 64/100 (64%) of participants treated with an "aggressive" (10-second) regimen compared with 44/100 (44%) of those treated with a "gentle" (brief freeze) regimen (OR 2·26 (CI 1·28–3·99)). Five participants withdrew from the aggressive group and one from the gentle group because of pain and blistering[23]. Pain and/or blistering was reported in 29%, 7% and 0% of those treated at 1-, 2- and 3-week intervals, respectively (no available data for OR).[27] The rate of reported adverse affects was higher with a shorter interval between treatments but this is likely to be a reporting artefact because these participants were seen sooner after each treatment.

Comment

The evidence from available RCTs for the absolute and relative effectiveness of cryotherapy for warts is both limited and contradictory. Moreover, as with the RCTs on topical SA, heterogeneity of study design and methods and the likely heterogeneity of the populations being studied make it impossible to synthesise data and draw firm conclusions. For instance, some trials included all types of warts on the hands and feet in all age groups whereas others were more selective and simply looked at hand warts or excluded certain groups such as mosaic plantar warts or refractory warts. Of particular note is the likelihood that wart clinic "populations" used for these studies may have had very different characteristics in different periods of time. For instance, studies done in the 1970s in the UK would have included a higher proportion of participants with incident warts and a greater chance of cure and/or spontaneous resolution. In the 1980s and 1990s, more people with warts were treated in primary care; thus, hospital wart clinics would have had a more selected population with a higher proportion of refractory warts and correspondingly lower cure rates.

Implications for practice

- The available, rather limited, evidence shows that cryotherapy is probably of equivalent efficacy to topical treatments containing SA.
- Aggressive cryotherapy (defined by longer freezing times) is more effective than gentle cryotherapy.
- Harmful effects such as pain and blistering are probably more frequent with aggressive cryotherapy.
- There is no significant difference in cure rates between 2-, 3- and 4-week-interval regimens.
- There is no significant benefit of prolonging 3-weekly cryotherapy beyond 3 months.

Contact immunotherapy with dinitrochlorobenzene (DNCB)
Efficacy

Two small RCTs.[22,30] of DNCB in 80 children and adults achieved a cure rate of 80% (32/40) compared with 38% (15/40) in the placebo/no treatment groups (OR 6·67 (CI 2·44–18·23)).

Drawbacks

No precise data on adverse effects were reported in either of these trials. Rosado-Cancino et al.[30] commented that 6 of 20 participants treated with 2% DNCB were sensitised only after the second application. All of them subsequently experienced significant local irritation with or without blistering when they were treated with 1% DNCB. None withdrew from the study.

Comment

DNCB, a potent contact allergen, can cause significant local irritation and dermatitis, which probably precludes its use outside specialist centres.

Implications for practice

Contact immunotherapy with DNCB appears to be a promising treatment but is probably best reserved for highly refractory warts.

Photodynamic therapy (PDT)
Efficacy

Four RCTs[31-34] of different types of PDT reported varying success. Cure rates ranged from 8% (of patients) to 73% (of warts).

PDT versus placebo

One trial[31] in 52 adults and children using a left–right design (randomising active and placebo treatments to warts on the left and right side of the body) showed resolution of warts in 40% of participants. In all those that responded to treatment, the warts on the placebo-treated side also resolved. In another trial in 40 adults,[32] aminolaevulenic acid (ALA) PDT achieved a cure rate of 56% of warts compared with 42% of warts in the placebo PDT group. Topical SA was also used for all participants.

PDT versus SA

One RCT[33] in 120 adults and children compared methylene blue/DMSO PDT with a mixture of SA and creosote. The cure rates achieved were 8% and 15%, respectively.

PDT versus cryotherapy

One RCT[34] in 28 adults with refractory warts compared four different types of light source for PDT with cryotherapy. PDT was administered three times and cryotherapy four times. The cure rates ranged from 28% to 73% of warts with the different types of PDT; 20% of warts were cured with cryotherapy. Topical SA was also used for all patients.

Drawbacks

Two trials[31,32] provided no data on adverse effects. Burning and itching during treatment and mild discomfort afterwards was reported universally with ALA PDT.[34] All participants with plantar warts were able to walk after treatment. In another study,[32] severe or unbearable pain during treatment was reported for an average of 17% of warts with active treatment and an average of 4% of warts with placebo PDT.[32]

Comment

Methodological heterogeneity makes it difficult to draw conclusions from these different trials. One used a left–right design, two others used warts as the unit of analysis and each trial used different types of PDT.

Implications for clinical practice

PDT seems to offer no particular advantage in terms of higher cure rates or fewer adverse effects than other simpler and cheaper local treatments available.

Intralesional bleomycin
Efficacy

Conflicting results were reported in five RCTs of intralesional bleomycin. Cure rates ranged from 16% to 94%. Two trials[35,36] showed higher cure rates with bleomycin than with placebo, one[37] showed placebo to achieve higher cure rates than bleomycin and one[38] showed no significant difference between bleomycin and placebo. One other trial found no significant difference in cure rates between three different concentrations of bleomycin injections.[39]

Bleomycin versus placebo

One RCT[35] using a left–right design in 24 adults showed cure rates of 58% and 10% of warts with 0·1% bleomycin and saline (placebo) injections, respectively. Another RCT[36] in 16 adults and children showed cure rates of 82% and 35% of warts with 0·1% bleomycin and saline injections, respectively. Yet another RCT[37] in 62 adults achieved cure rates of 16% and 44% with 1% bleomycin in oil or saline, and oil or saline placebo injections, respectively. A further RCT[38] in 31 adults and children showed cure rates of 94% and 73% of participants with 0·1% bleomycin and saline injections respectively.

Different concentrations of bleomycin

One RCT[39] in 26 adults comparing 0·25, 0·5 and 1·0 units/ml bleomycin showed cure rates of 73%, 88% and 90% of warts, respectively; differences were not statistically significant.

Drawbacks

No precise data on adverse effects were provided in any of the RCTs. Munkvad et al.[37] reported "adverse events" in 19/62 (31%) participants but the nature of the adverse events and the proportions in the active treatment and placebo groups were not specified. Three of the other four trials[35,36,39] reported that most participants experienced pain. In two[36,38] of the five trials local anaesthetic was used routinely before the injection of bleomycin. Hayes et al.[39] reported pain in most participants, irrespective of dose. In the trial by Bunney et al.,[35] of the 24 participants, all of whom received bleomycin, one withdrew because of the pain of the injections and another one withdrew because of pain in the period after injection.

Comment

Again, methodological and statistical heterogeneity (different outcomes, trial periods, units of analysis, numbers of injections, vehicles and concentrations) make it impossible to synthesise the data from these trials.

Implications for clinical practice

There is no compelling evidence for the efficacy of intralesional bleomycin.

Other local treatments for warts

One trial of the pulsed dye laser[40] involving 40 patients showed no significant difference in cure rates between four pulsed dye laser treatments at monthly intervals and "conventional treatment" with either cryotherapy or cantharidin.

5-Fluorouracil and intralesional interferons as treatments for warts are more of historical interest. Four[41-44] and six[45-50] trials, respectively, were found for these treatments, most dating from the 1970s and 1980s. Evidence provided by all the trials was severely limited by heterogeneity of methodology and design and overall did not suggest any striking efficacy of either treatment.

No RCTs were identified that studied the efficacy of the following treatments: carbon dioxide laser, surgical excision, curettage and cautery, formaldehyde, podophyllin and podophyllotoxin.

Key points

- Topical preparations containing SA are generally effective and safe for treating warts.
- The available, rather limited, evidence shows that cryotherapy is probably of equivalent efficacy to topical treatments containing SA.
- Contact immunotherapy with DNCB appears to be a promising treatment but is probably best reserved for highly refractory warts.
- PDT and pulsed dye laser therapy do not appear to have any particular advantage in terms of higher cure rates or fewer adverse effects than the other simpler and cheaper local treatments available.
- There is no compelling evidence for the efficacy of intralesional bleomycin.

References

1. Johnson ML, Roberts J. Skin conditions and related need for medical care among persons 1–74 years. US Department of Health Education and Welfare Publication 1978;**1660**:1–26.

2. Beliaeva TL. The population incidence of warts. Vestn Dermatol Venerol 1990;**2**:55–8.

3. Williams HC, Pottier A, Strachan D. The descriptive epidemiology of warts in British schoolchildren. Br J Dermatol 1993;**128**:504–11.

4. Kilkenny M, Merlin K, Young R, Marks R. The prevalence of common skin conditions in Australian school students: 1. Common, plane and plantar viral warts. Br J Dermatol 1998;**138**:840–5.

5. Johnson LW. Communal showers and the risk of plantar warts. J Fam Pract 1995;**40**:136–8.

6. Keefe M, al-Ghamdi A, Coggon D et al. Cutaneous warts in butchers. Br J Dermatol 1995;**132**:166–7.

7. Massing AM, Epstein WL. Natural history of warts. Arch Dermatol 1963;**87**:303–10.

8. Gibbs S, Harvey I, Sterling J, Stark R. Local treatments for cutaneous warts. In: Cochrane Collaboration. Cochrane Library. Issue 2. Oxford: Update Software, 2001.

9. Abou-Auda H, Soutor C, Neveaux JL. Treatment of verruca infections (warts) with a new transcutaneous controlled release system. *Curr Ther Res Clin Exp* 1987;**41**:552–6.

10. Bart BJ, Biglow J, Vance JC, Neveaux JL. Salicylic acid in karaya gum patch as a treatment for verruca vulgaris. *J Am Acad Dermatol* 1989;**20**:74–6.

11. Felt BT, Hall H, Olness K *et al*. Wart regression in children: comparison of relaxation imagery to topical treatment and equal time interventions. *Am J Clin Hypn* 1998;**41**:130–7.

12. Spanos NP, Williams V, Gwynn MI. Effects of hypnotic, placebo, and salicylic acid treatments on wart regression. *Psychosom Med* 1990;**52**:109–14.

13. Steele K, Shirodaria P, O'Hare M *et al*. Monochloroacetic acid and 60% salicylic acid as a treatment for simple plantar warts: effectiveness and mode of action. *Br J Dermatol* 1988;**118**:537–43.

14. Bunney MH, Hunter JA, Ogilvie MM, Williams DA. The treatment of plantar warts in the home. A critical appraisal of a new preparation. *Practitioner* 1971;**207**:197–204.

15. Bunney MH, Nolan MW, Williams DA. An assessment of methods of treating viral warts by comparative treatment trials based on a standard design. *Br J Dermatol* 1976;**94**:667–79.

16. Steele K, Irwin WG. Liquid nitrogen and salicylic/lactic acid paint in the treatment of cutaneous warts in general practice. *J R Coll Gen Pract* 1988;**38**:256–8.

17. Auken G, Gade M, Pilgaard CE. Treatment of warts of the hands and feet with Verucid. *Ugeskr Laeger* 1975;**137**:3036–8.

18. Flindt-Hansen H, Tikjob G, Brandrup F. Wart treatment with anthralin. *Acta Derm Venereol* 1984;**64**:177–9.

19. Parton AM, Sommerville RG. The treatment of plantar verrucae by triggering cell-mediated immunity. *Br J Pod Med* 1994;**131**:883–6.

20. Veien NK, Madsen SM, Avrach W, Hammershoy O, Lindskov R, Niordson A-MMSD. The treatment of plantar warts with a keratolytic agent and occlusion. *J Dermatol Treat* 1991;**2**:59–61.

21. Gibson JR, Harvey SG, Barth J, Darley CR, Reshad H, Burke CA. A comparison of acyclovir cream versus placebo cream versus liquid nitrogen in the treatment of viral plantar warts. *Dermatologica* 1984;**168**:178–81.

22. Wilson P. Immunotherapy v cryotherapy for hand warts; a controlled trial (abstract). *Scottish Med J* 1983;**28**:191.

23. Connolly M, Basmi K, O'Connell M, Lyons JF, Bourke JF. Efficacy of cryotherapy is related to severity of freeze (abstract). *Br J Dermatol* 1999;**141**(S55):31.

24. Sonnex TS, Camp RDR. The treatment of recalcitrant viral warts with high dose cryosurgery under local anaesthesia (abstract). *Br J Dermatol* 1988;**119**(S33):38–9.

25. Berth-Jones J, Bourke J, Eglitis H *et al*. Value of a second freeze-thaw cycle in cryotherapy of common warts. *Br J Dermatol* 1994;**131**:883–6.

26. Hansen JG, Schmidt H. Plantar warts. Occurrence and cryosurgical treatment. *Ugeskr Laeger* 1986;**148**:173–4.

27. Bourke JF, Berth-Jones J, Hutchinson PE. Cryotherapy of common viral warts at intervals of 1, 2 and 3 weeks. *Br J Dermatol* 1995;**132**:433–6.

28. Larsen PO, Laurberg G. Cryotherapy of viral warts. *J Dermatol Treat* 1996;**7**:29–31.

29. Berth-Jones J, Hutchinson PE. Modern treatment of warts: cure rates at 3 and 6 months. *Br J Dermatol* 1992;**127**:262–5.

30. Rosado-Cancino MA, Ruiz-Maldonado R, Tamayo L, Laterza AM. Treatment of multiple and stubborn warts in children with 1-chloro-2,4-dinitrobenzene (DNCB) and placebo. *Dermatol Rev Mex* 1989;**33**:245–52.

31. Veien NK, Genner J, Brodthagen H, Wettermark G. Photodynamic inactivation of verrucae vulgares. II. *Acta Derm Venereol* 1977;**57**:445–7.

32. Stender IM, Na R, Fogh H, Gluud C, Wulf HC. Photodynamic therapy with 5-aminolaevulinic acid or placebo for recalcitrant foot and hand warts: randomised double-blind trial. *Lancet* 2000;**355**:963–6.

33. Stahl D, Veien NK, Wulf HC. Photodynamic inactivation of virus warts: a controlled clinical trial. *Clin Exp Dermatol* 1979;**4**:81–5.

34. Stender IM, Lock-Anderson J, Wulf HC. Recalcitrant hand and foot warts successfully treated with photodynamic therapy with topical 5-aminolaevulinic acid: a pilot study. *Clin Exp Dermatol* 1999;**24**:154–9.

35. Bunney MH, Nolan MW, Buxton PK, Going SM, Prescott RJ. The treatment of resistant warts with intralesional bleomycin: a controlled clinical trial. *Br J Dermatol* 1984;**111**:197–207.

36. Rossi E, Soto JH, Battan J, Villalba L. Intralesional bleomycin in verruca vulgaris. Double-blind study. *Dermatol Rev Mex* 1981;**25**:158–65.

37. Munkvad M, Genner J, Staberg B, Kongsholm H. Locally injected bleomycin in the treatment of warts. *Dermatologica* 1983;**167**:86–9.

38. Perez Alfonzo R, Weiss E, Piquero Martin J. Hypertonic saline solution *v* intralesional bleomycin in the treatment of common warts. *Dermatol Venez* 1992;**30**:176–8.

39. Hayes ME, O'Keefe EJ. Reduced dose of bleomycin in the treatment of recalcitrant warts. *J Am Acad Dermatol* 1986;**15**(5 Pt 1):1002–6.

40. Robson KJ, Cunningham NM, Kruzan KL. Pulsed dye laser versus conventional therapy for the treatment of warts: a prospective randomized trial. *J Am Acad Dermatol* 2000;**43**:275–80.

41. Artese O, Cazzato C, Cucchiarelli S, Iezzi D, Palazzi P, Ametetti M. Controlled study: medical therapy (5-fluorouracil, salicylic acid) *v* physical therapy (DTC) of warts. *Dermatol Clinics* 1994;**14**:55–9.

42. Bunney MH. The treatment of plantar warts with 5-fluorouracil. *Br J Dermatol* 1973;**89**:96–7.

43. Hursthouse MW. A controlled trial on the use of topical 5-fluorouracil on viral warts. *Br J Dermatol* 1975;**92**:93–6.

44. Schmidt H,.Jacobsen FK. Double-blind randomized clinical study on treatment of warts with fluorouracil-containing topical preparation. *Z Hautkr* 1981;**56**:41–3.

45. Berman B, Davis-Reed L, Silverstein L, Jaliman D, France D, Lebwohl M. Treatment of verrucae vulgaris with alpha 2 interferon. *J Infect Dis* 1986;**154**:328–30.

46. Lee SW, Houh D, Kim HO, Kim CW, Kim TY. Clinical trials of interferon-gamma in treating warts. *Ann Dermatol* 1990;**2**:77–82.

47. Niimura M. Application of beta-interferon in virus-induced papillomas. *J Invest Dermatol* 1990;**95**:149S–51S.

48. Pazin GJ, Ho M, Haverkos HW *et al.* Effects of interferon-alpha on human warts. *J Interferon Res* 1982;**2**:235–43.

49. Vance JC, Bart BJ, Hansen RC *et al.* Intralesional recombinant alpha-2 interferon for the treatment of patients with condyloma acuminatum or verruca plantaris. *Arch Dermatol* 1986;**122**:272–7.

50. Varnavides CK, Henderson CA, Cunliffe WJ. Intralesional interferon: ineffective in common viral warts. *J Dermatol Treat* 1997;**8**:169–72.

Acknowledgements

Many thanks to my colleagues for their involvement in this systematic review of the literature: Professor Ian Harvey, School of Health Policy and Practice, University of East Anglia, Norwich, Dr Jane Sterling, Department of Dermatology, Addenbrooke's NHS Trust, Cambridge, and Rosemary Stark, Department of Service Development, Finance and Information, Norfolk Health Authority.

31
Impetigo

*Sander Koning, Lisette WA van Suijlekom-Smit
and Johannes C van der Wouden*

Background
Definition

Impetigo is a contagious superficial skin infection, characterised by superficial erosions covered with honey-coloured crusts, most often on the face. Bullous and non-bullous impetigo can be distinguished. Impetigo may be primary or secondary.

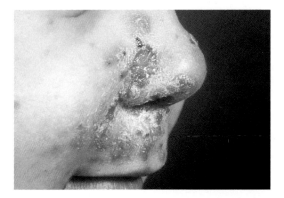

Figure 31.1   Child with impetigo. By kind permission of AP Oranje

Incidence

Impetigo is most frequent in children; incidence rates peak at 4–5 years of age. Population-based incidence rates are unknown. Impetigo is common in general practice, with incidence rates of around 20 episodes per 1000 children per year seen by the general practioner.[1–3]

Aetiology

In moderate climates, the primary pathogen in non-bullous impetigo is *Staphylococcus aureus*.

However, in warm and humid climates *Streptococcus pyogenes* or both *S. pyogenes* and *S. aureus* are more often isolated. The relative frequency of *S. aureus* infections has also changed with time. It was predominant in the 1940s and 1950s, then group-A streptococci became more prevalent. Recently *S. aureus* has become more common again.[4] Bullous impetigo is a staphylococcal disease.

Prognosis

Impetigo is believed to be self-limiting, taking several weeks to cure without intervention. However, no research is available to substantiate this statement. Prompt resolution usually occurs with adequate treatment. The course of the disease is usually mild, but sometimes general symptoms such as fever and lymphadenopathy occur.

Aims of treatment

Impetigo is treated to accelerate cure and to prevent spread of the infection.

Relevant outcomes

Clinical cure (clearance of crusts, blisters and redness) is the most relevant outcome. Criteria such as relief of pain, itching and soreness, and bacteriological cure can be considered as secondary outcomes.

Methods of search

We included randomised trials of all interventions for impetigo by using the following search terms in Medline (June 2001): impetigo

(MESH) or staphylococcal skin infections (MESH) or impetigo (in title or abstract) or pyoderma (in title or abstract).

QUESTIONS

What are the effects of treatments on the clearance of impetiginous lesions after 1 week?

Disinfecting treatments
Efficacy
We found one systematic review.[5]

Versus placebo
We found one randomised controlled trial (RCT) comparing hexachlorophene with placebo.[6] Scrubbing with hexachlorophene added no notable benefit to placebo treatment.

Versus topical antibiotic treatment
One multicentre RCT compared hydrogen peroxide cream with fusidic acid cream/gel.[7] There was no significant difference in treatment effect, but there was a tendency towards a better effect of fusidic acid cream/gel. There was no significant difference between hexachlorophene and bacitracin ointment in a small and ancient study.[6]

Versus oral antibiotic treatment
Hexachlorophene scrubbing was much less effective than oral treatment with penicillin.[6]

Drawbacks
Eleven per cent of the patients using hydrogen peroxide cream reported mild side-effects (non specified). No patient was withdrawn from the study because of side-effects.[7] No adverse effects of scrubbing with hexachlorophene were recorded.[6]

Comment
The disinfecting drugs, such as povidone-iodine and chlorhexidine, advised in some guidelines have not been compared with a placebo.

Hydrogen peroxide cream had a good treatment result in relatively large a trial. Blinding in this trial was not done correctly.

Implications for topical disinfectants in clinical practice
There is no good evidence for the value of disinfecting measures in the treatment of impetigo.

Topical antibiotics
Efficacy
We found one systematic review.[5]

Versus placebo
Mupirocin has been studied in two placebo-controlled trials, both of which found a better effect with mupirocin.[8,9] One other RCT showed that fusidic acid was much more effective than placebo (55% of patients cured versus 13%).[10]

Versus each other
Several topical antibiotics have been compared directly. Mupirocin and fusidic acid were compared in three studies,[11–13] none of which showed a significant difference in treatment effect. Three other studies compared several other antimicrobial preparations with each other and sometimes combined with a topical steroid. Hydrocortisone/potassium hydroxyquinoline sulphate was significantly better than hydrocortisone/miconazole at 2 weeks.[14] Sulconazole was better than miconazole (63% versus 50% cure) at 14 days of treatment.[15] No significant differences were found in a three-armed RCT between fusidic acid cream, tetracycline/ polymyxine ointment and neomycin/bacitracin ointment.[16]

Versus oral antibiotics
Three RCTs compared topical mupirocin with erythromycin,[4,17,18] two of which found a small but not significant difference favouring erythromycin.[17,18]

One trial of good quality (n = 102) showed a big difference in favour of mupirocine.[4] In a meta-analysis, mupirocin was significantly better than erythromycin.[5] In a small RCT (n = 32), cephalexin and mupirocin were both significantly more effective than bacitracin cream.[19]

Drawbacks

RCT reports usually note few, if any, side-effects with local antibiotics. The two studies comparing mupirocin with placebo reported none.[8,9] In studies comparing mupirocin with fusidic acid, the greasy nature of mupirocin was reported as a side-effect in 7·4% of patients versus 1·0%[11]; minor itching/burning occurred in 6/116 (5%) versus 2/50 (4%) respectively.[13] No side-effects were reported in Gilbert's study.[12] Studies comparing erythromycin versus mupirocin recorded gastrointestinal side-effects in 23% versus 8%,[4] none in either group,[18] and equal distribution between the two groups.[17] Hydrocortisone/potassium hydroxyquinoline caused two cases of mild staining in 65 patients.[14] Miconazole caused "mild burning" in one case.[15] In general, resistance rates against topical antibiotics such as fusidic acid and mupirocin will rise when an antibiotic is used excessively.

Comments

Many RCTs deal with a range of (skin) infections, including impetigo. Only trials that had separate results for the group of impetigo patients were included. The time of follow up and definition of "cure" and "improvement" differ and are often not clear, making comparison difficult. There is a lack of placebo-controlled studies.

Implications for topical antibiotics in clinical practice

Although traditionally considered less effective than oral therapy, there is some good evidence that local treatments are equal to or more effective than oral treatment. In general, oral antibiotics have more side-effects, especially gastrointestinal side-effects. Fusidic acid and mupirocin are equally effective. Most studies date back 10 years or more. Resistance patterns have changed since then. Contemporary and local characteristics and resistance patterns of the causative bacteria should always be taken into account when choosing treatment. When a large area is affected or when the patient has general symptoms such as fever, oral therapy seems more appropriate.

Systemic antibiotics
Efficacy

We found one systematic review.[5]

Versus placebo

No placebo-controlled trials of systemic antibiotics were found.

Versus topical antibiotics

Discussed under topical antibiotics above.

Versus each other

Two RCTs compared penicillin and erythromycin, both finding erythromycin to be more effective.[20,21] One very small study (n = 18) found no difference between azithromycin and cephalexin.[22] A larger study showed equally good results of erythromycin and dicloxacilin.[23] Amoxicillin plus clavulanic acid gave better results than amoxicillin alone, but without reaching significance in a small study.[24] No differences were found between cefdinir and cephalexin.[25] Cephalexin was equal to erythromycin in a small study.[20]

Drawbacks

Incidence of side-effects were:

- azithromycin: 16·5%, mainly mild gastrointestinal[22]
- cephalexin:10·9% mainly mild gastrointestinal,[22] 11% mainly diarrhoea,[25] no adverse effects in one study.[20]
- cefdinir: 16%, mainly diarrhoea.[25]

Comments

Many RCTs include a range of (skin) infections, with a subset of impetigo patients. Only trials reporting separate results for the group of impetigo patients were considered in this chapter. There is a lack of placebo-controlled studies. Resistance rates of the bacteria were determined in some studies, and differed from study to study. The time of follow up differs widely between the studies, making comparison difficult.

Implications for use of systemic antibiotics in clinical practice

There is some good evidence that local treatment is equal to or more effective than oral treatment. Macrolide antibiotics give better treatment results than penicillin. In general, oral antibiotics have more side-effects, especially gastrointestinal side-effects. Most studies date back 10 years or more. Resistance patterns have changed since then. Contemporary local characteristics and resistance patterns of the causative bacteria should always be taken into account when choosing treatment. When a large area is affected or when the patient has general symptoms such as fever, oral therapy seems preferable.

Key points

- The natural history of impetigo is not known.
- Few placebo-controlled studies have been done.
- Many different antibiotic treatments have been studied against each other, often in small studies showing no significant differences.
- There is no evidence supporting the value of disinfecting treatments.
- Macrolide and cephalosporine antibiotics are more effective than non-betalactamase-resistant pencillins.
- Topical antibiotics such as mupirocin and fusidic acid are equally effective as oral antibiotics such as erythromycin and have fewer side-effects.
- Resistance patterns in causative bacteria change over time and should be taken into account when choosing a therapy for impetigo.

References

1. Bruijnzeels MA, van Suijlekom-Smit LWA, van der Velden J, van der Wouden JC. *The child in general practice*. Rotterdam/Utrecht: Erasmus Universiteit/NIVEL, 1993.

2. van der Ven-Daane I, Bruijnzeels MA, van der Wouden JC, van Suijlekom-Smit LWA. Occurrence and treatment of impetigo vulgaris in children. *Huisarts Wet* 1993;**36**:291–3.

3. McCormick A, Fleming D, Charlton J. Morbidity statistics from general practice: fourth national study 1991–1992. London: Department of Health, Office of Population Censuses and Royal College of General Practitioners, 1995.

4. Dagan R, Bar-David Y. Double-blind study comparing erythromycin and mupirocin for treatment of impetigo in children: implications of a high prevalence of erythromycin-resistant *Staphylococcus aureus* strains. *Antimicrob Agents Chemother* 1992;**36**:287–90.

5. Van Amstel L, Koning S, van Suijlekom-Smit LWA, Oranje A, van der Wouden JC. The treatment of impetigo contagiosa, a systematic review. *Huisarts Wet* 2000;**43**:247–52.

6. Ruby RJ, Nelson JD. The influence of hexachlorophene scrubs on the response to placebo or penicillin therapy in impetigo. *Pediatrics* 1973;**52**:854–9.

7. Christensen OB, Anehus S. Hydrogen peroxyde cream: an alternative to topical antibiotics in the treatment of impetigo contagiosa. *Acta Derm Venerol* 1994;**74**:460–2.

8. Eells LD, Mertz PM, Piovanetti Y, Pekoe GM, Eaglstein WH. Topical antibiotic treatment of impetigo with mupirocin. *Arch Dermatol* 1986;**122**:1273–6.

9. Gould JC, Smith JH, Moncur H. Mupirocin in general practice: a placebo-controlled trial. *Royal Society of Medicine: international congress and symposium series* 1984;**80**:85–93.

10. Koning S, van Suijlekom-Smit LWA, Nouwen JL *et al.* Fusidic acid cream in the treatment of impetigo in general practice: double blind randomised placebo controlled trial. *BMJ* 2002;**324**:203–6.

11. Morley PAR, Munot LD. A comparison of sodium fusidate ointment and mupirocin ointment in superficial skin sepsis. *Curr Med Res Opin* 1988;**11**:142–8.

12. Gilbert M. Topical 2% mupirocin versus 2% fusidic acid ointment in the treatment of primary and secondary skin infections. *J Am Acad Dermatol* 1989;**20**:1083–7.

13. White DG, Collins PO, Rowsell RB. Topical antibiotics in the treatment of superficial skin infections in general

practice – a comparison of mupirocin with sodium fusidate. *J Infect* 1989;**18**:221–9.

14. Jaffe GV, Grimshaw JJ. A clinical trial of hydrocortisone/potassium hydroxyquinoline sulphate (Quinocort) in the treatment of infected eczema and impetigo in general practice. *Pharmatherapeutica* 1986;**4**:628–36.

15. Nolting S, Strauss WB. Treatment of impetigo and ecthyma. A comparison of sulconazole with miconazole. *Int J Derm* 1988;**27**:716–19.

16. Vainer G, Torbensen E. Behandling af impetigo i almen praksis. *Ugeskr laeger* 1986;**148**:1202–6.

17. Britton JW, Fajardo JE, Krafte-Jacobs B. Comparison of mupirocin and erythromycin in the treatment of impetigo. *J Pediatr* 1990;**117**:827–9.

18. Mertz PM, Marshall DA, Eaglstein WH, Piovanetti Y, Montalvo J. Topical mupirocin treatment of impetigo is equal to oral erythromycin therapy. *Arch Dermatol* 1989;**125**:1069–73.

19. Bass JW, Chan DS, Creamer KM *et al.* Comparison of oral cephalexin, topical mupirocin, and topical bacitracin for treatment of impetigo. *Pediatr Inf Dis J* 1997;**16**:708–9.

20. Demidovich CW, Wittler RR, Ruff ME, Bass JW, Browning WC. Impetigo: current etiology and comparison of penicillin, erythromycin, and cephalexin therapies. *Am J Dis Child* 1990;**144**:1313–15.

21. Barton LL, Friedman AD. Impetigo: A reassessment of etiology and therapy. *Pediatr Dermatol* 1987;**4**:185–8.

22. Kiani R, Double-blind, double-dummy comparison of azithromycin and cephalexin in the treatment of skin and skin structure infections. *Eur J Clin Microbiol Infect Dis* 1991;**10**:880–4.

23. Barton LL, Friedman AD, Portilla MG. Impetigo contagiosa: a comparison of erythromycin and dicloxacillin therapy. *Pediatr Dermatol* 1988;**5**:88–91.

24. Dagan R, Bar-David Y. Comparison of amoxicillin and clavulanic acid (Augmentin) for the treatment of nonbullous impetigo. *Am J Dis Child* 1989;**143**:916–18.

25. Tack KJ, Keyserling CH, McCarty J, Hedrick JA Study of use of cefdinir versus cephalexin for treatment of skin infections in pediatric patients. *Antimicrob Agents Chemother* 1997;**41**:739–42.

32
Athlete's foot

Fay Crawford

Background
Definition
Athlete's foot or tinea pedis is most frequently caused by dermatophyte (ringworm) invasion of the skin of the feet. It usually manifests in one of three ways: interdigital skin appears macerated (white) and soggy; patches of skin on the foot may be affected by recurrent vesicular eruptions which make the skin itchy and red; and finally the soles of the feet, including the sides and heels can appear dry and scaly.[1]

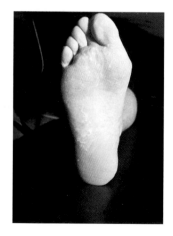

Figure 32.1   Athlete's foot

Incidence/prevalence
Tinea infections are common. It has been estimated that 15% of the general population have a fungal infection of the feet.[2] Gentles and Evans[3] found the prevalence of athlete's foot to be 21·5% in a sample of adult male swimmers, but the prevalence amongst adult females participating in the same survey was only 3·3%.

Aetiology
The dermatophytes most frequently reported in clinical trials to be present on patients' skin at trial entry are *Trichophyton rubrum, T. mentagrophytes, Epidermophyton floccosum* and *T. interdigitale*.[4]

Scaling, fissuring, pruritus and itching are some of the clinical features of fungal infections of the skin and it is these irritations that make the patient seek treatment. The natural history of the condition if untreated is a chronic, worsening infection which can lead to fissuring and breaks in the epidermis. Although the condition will not resolve spontaneously, some evidence from cure rates collected from people in the placebo arms of controlled trials suggests that improved foot hygiene alone may cure the infection in a proportion of people.[5,6]

Diagnosis
The use of laboratory tests to diagnose the presence of dermatophyte infection is very important because athlete's foot can be mistaken for other skin conditions. For example, interdigital maceration can look exactly like interdigital athlete's foot, and juvenile chronic dermatosis and bacterial infections such as erythrasma can also have a similar appearance to fungal infections on the skin of the feet.

Aims of treatment
Treatment aims to reduce the signs and symptoms such as itching and flaking of the skin, and ultimately to eradicate the infection.

The many creams available for the treatment of athlete's foot differ in cost and availability. The azoles (for example miconazole, clotrimazole) and allylamines (terbinafine, naftifine) are sold over the counter in pharmacies. Other creams (for example tolnaftate, undecenoic acid) are available in supermarkets. This last group is the cheapest of the topical preparations and the allylamine creams are the most expensive.

Oral drugs are sometimes used in the management of chronic manifestations of athlete's foot. Griseofulvin is the oldest and cheapest of the oral antifungal drugs but it must be taken for a long time. Newer azoles such as itraconazole, ketoconazole and fluconazole are effective in a much shorter time. The newest oral antifungal drugs are allylamines (terbinafine, naftifine). The allylamines (both topical and oral) are fungicidal whereas all other antifungal agents are fungistatic.

Relevant outcomes

The effects of treatment on these symptoms are measured in randomised controlled trials (RCTs) but microscopy and culture are usually the primary outcomes. Secondary outcomes are measured using a variety of signs and symptoms (redness, flaking, itching etc.). A reduction in symptoms may be achieved quite quickly but the tenacity of tinea infections often means that complete cure takes a long time.

Methods of search

Systematic reviews and RCTs were identified using a search strategy published elsewhere.[7] This was updated to September 2001 with a Medline and Embase search using the same strategy and supplemented by a search of the Cochrane Central Register of Controlled Trials (September 2001).

The inclusion criterion for study selection was the mycological confirmation of the presence of fungi in the trial populations. The search found two systematic reviews, one of topical treatments for skin infections[7] and the other of oral treatments for skin infections.[4] The search also identified three RCTs not included in the reviews, which compared topical allylamines with topical azoles.

Generic drug names are used in the effectiveness analyses below. Martindale[8] gives a complete list of brand names of antifungal drugs.

QUESTIONS

How effective are allylamine creams in the treatment of athlete's foot?

One systematic review[7] found 12 RCTs comparing allylamines (terbinafine 1% cream or naftifine 1% gel) with placebo controls, used for 4 weeks. The two active preparations were similarly effective. A pooled analysis of data from seven trials (n = 683) comparing either naftifine or terbinafine with placebo controls produced a relative risk (RR) of 3·69 (95% confidence intervals (CI) 2·41 to 5·66). The allylamine creams, used twice daily for 4 weeks, are highly effective in the management of athlete's foot.

How effective are azole creams in the treatment of athlete's foot?

One systematic review[7] found 14 RCTs comparing 4–6 weeks treatment with azole creams (1% clotrimazole, 1% tioconazole, 1% bifonazole, 1% econazole, 2% miconazole nitrate with placebo controls. They were similarly effective.

Treatment with 6 weeks of clotrimazole or tioconazole applied twice daily was evaluated in four trials (n = 434) (RR 1·85, CI 1·27 to 2·69). Shorter treatment times (4 weeks) with bifonazole, econazole nitrate or miconazole nitrate gave a RR of 2·25 (CI 1·44 to 3·52, n = 520). All the creams were similarly effective whether used for 4 or 6 weeks. Over-the-counter antifungal creams are very effective in the treatment of athlete's foot when compared with placebo controls.

How do allylamines creams compare with azole creams in curing athlete's foot?

One systematic review of topical treatments (search date December 1997) indicated slightly better mycological cure rates with the allylamines (terbinafine 1% and butenafine 1% creams) than with azoles (clotrimazole 1% and miconazole 1% creams) used for 4 weeks (RR 1·1·95% CI 0·99 to 1·23). This analysis was based on data from 11 RCTs (n = 1554).[7] The analysis showed the allylamines to cure 80% of cases of athlete's foot, compared with a cure rate of 72% achieved with azole creams.

The systematic review[7] included one RCT[9] which compared 1 week of terbinafine 1% cream with 4 weeks of clotrimazole 1% cream. There was no difference in the cure rates (n = 211) after 1 week of treatment but 6 weeks after the start of treatment the cure rate for terbinafine was significantly better than that of clotrimazole (RR 1·16, CI 1·06 to 1·27).

Patel et al.[10] found exactly the opposite effect in a smaller but similar trial (n = 104). They compared 1 week of terbinafine cream with 4 weeks of clotrimazole cream in people with interdigital tinea pedis. Terbinafine was found to more effective after 1 week (RR 1·51, CI 1·16 to 1·98) but there were no differences in effectiveness for outcomes assessed at later times.

In the smallest of the trials, comparing 1 week of 1% terbinafine with 4 weeks of 2% miconazole

(n = 48),[11] no difference in cure rate emerged at any time during the trial (RR at 1 week 0·99, CI 0·57 to 1·7). At 4 weeks there were 12/22 cures (54·6%) in the terbinafine group and 15/23 (65·2%) in the miconazole group (RR 0·83, CI 0·51 to 1·35).

Schopoff et al.[12] compared terbinafine cream used for 1 week with clotrimazole cream for 4 weeks in 429 people with interdigital tinea pedis and found no differences in the effectiveness at any time during the trial.

Pooling the data from all three trials (n = 792) comparing 1 week of terbinafine cream with either 2% miconazole or 1% clotrimazole found no statistical difference between these treatments (RR 1·15, CI 0·82 to 1·61).

How effectively do creams that can be bought in the supermarket cure athlete's foot?

A systematic review[7] found two three-arm trials comparing undecenoic acid with tolnaftate and placebo, another trial comparing undecenoic acid with placebo and no treatment, a fourth trial comparing undecenoic acid with placebo and a fifth trial comparing tolnaftate with tea-tree oil and placebo. Pooling the tolnaftate data from the arms of three trials that compared it with placebo indicates that tolnaftate is more effective than placebo against dermatophyte infections (RR 1·56; CI 1·05 to 2·31). Pooled data from four trials showed undecenoic acid to be more effective than placebo in the management of athlete's foot (RR 2·83, CI 1·91 to 4·19).

Two trials of ciclopirox olamine 1% (which is not available in the UK) found it effective in treating athlete's foot. In one placebo-controlled trial (n = 163) the RR was 6·85 (CI 3·10 to 15·15). A second small trial (n = 87) comparing ciclopirox olamine with clotrimazole found no statistical difference (RR 1·12, CI 0·90 to 1·38).

Are oral drugs more effective than topical compounds in the treatment of athlete's foot?

Only one small RCT (n = 137) has compared the efficacy of an oral drug with a cream in the management of interdigital athlete's foot.[13] Cure rates were similar in those treated for 1 week with oral terbinafine 250 mg/day and those using clotrimazole 1% cream twice daily for 4 weeks. The relapse rates among those who were cured differed significantly, however: 11/39 in the terbinafine group and 5/50 in the clotrimazole group relapsed after 3 months.

What are the most effective oral drugs in the treatment of athlete's foot?

One systematic review[4] found 10 RCTs that compared two antifungal drugs and two RCTs that compared oral antifungal drugs with placebos. The sample sizes in all trials were small (range 14–66).

The review found four trials comparing oral terbinafine 250 mg/day with itraconazole 100 mg/day. One trial (n = 117) compared 2 weeks of terbinafine with 2 weeks of itraconazole and found a significant difference in favour of terbinafine (RR 1·5, CI 1·23 to 2·02). Three trials (n = 339) comparing 2 weeks of terbinafine with 4 weeks of itraconazole found no statistical differences in cure rates (RR 1·17, CI 0·94 to 1·46).

The systematic review found two small trials that compared griseofulvin 500 mg/day with terbinafine 250 mg/day for 4 or 6 weeks. The pooled data from the two trials found terbinafine to be significantly more effective (RR 2·20, CI 1·45 to 3·32).

The systematic review[4] found similar low cure rates for ketoconazole 200 mg (53%) and griseofulvin 1000 mg (57%). The cure rates with fluconazole 50 mg did not differ significantly from those with itraconazole 100 mg or ketoconazole 200 mg, but in both trials the cure rates were high (89–100%). Treatments were taken for 6 weeks in these trials.

Drawbacks

Topical antifungal compounds are well tolerated and are not associated with high rates of adverse events. One systematic review[7] found that few trial reports gave details of adverse events and the few that were reported were not severe (for example itching, redness or burning).

The systematic review of oral treatments for fungal infections of the skin[4] noted that all 12 included trials reported side-effects. All drugs produced side-effects; the rate was lowest for fluconazole (11%) and highest for terbinafine (18%). Gastrointestinal effects and rashes were reported most frequently.

Comment

The evidence from one small trial[13] shows that oral treatments are no more effective in the management of interdigital athlete's foot than the creams. The same study also found higher relapse rates after oral treatments.

Implications for practice

All antifungal creams, whether over the counter or those available in supermarkets are effective in the treatment of athlete's foot.

Prescription-only antifungal creams produce slightly higher cure rates than all other creams. The available evidence indicates that the most cost-effective management strategy for athlete's foot is an over-the-counter cream twice daily for 4 weeks, with prescription only cream reserved for treatment failures.[14]

There appears to be no therapeutic advantage in using an allylamine cream (terbinafine or naftifine) for 1 week rather than an azole cream for 4 weeks. The hypothesis that higher compliance rates are likely to be associated with shorter treatment times is often quoted but has not been tested.[15]

If no advantage is gained from treating interdigital athlete's foot with oral antifungals, physicians should be cautious in prescribing oral drugs to manage moccasin type (infection over the sole of the foot). The belief that recalcitrant cases of athlete's foot are more effectively managed with oral drugs has not been extensively tested.

Key points

- Athlete's foot is common and can be hard to cure.
- Long-standing case of athlete's foot should be confirmed using microscopy and culture laboratory tests.
- All fungal creams are effective in treating athlete's foot. There is evidence that different antifungal creams are associated with different cure rates; creams containing allylamines are the most effective in producing a cure followed by the azoles and undecenoic acid and tolnaftate.
- There is some evidence to suggest that oral drugs (tablets) are no more effective than creams in producing a cure for athlete's foot.

References

1. Springett K, Merriman L. Assessment of the skin and its appendages. In: Merriman L, Tollafield D, eds. *Assessment of the Lower Limb*. Edinburgh: Churchill Livingstone, 1995.

2. Gupta AK, Saunder DN, Shear NH. Efficacy of antifungal agent Terbinafine in the treatment of superficial dermatophyte infections – an overview. *Today Ther Trends* 1995;**13**:9–20.

3. Gentles JC, Evans EGV. Foot infections in swimming baths. *BMJ* 1973;**3**:260–2.

4. Bell-Syer SEM, Hart R, Crawford F *et al.* A systematic review of oral treatments for fungal infections of the skin of the feet. *J Dermatol* 2001;**12**:69–74.

5. Smith EB, Graham JL, Ulrich JA. Topical clotrimazole in tinea pedis. *South Med J* 1977;**70**:47–8.

6. Evans EGV, James IGV, Joshipura RC. Two week treatment of tinea pedis with terbinafine a placebo controlled study. *J Dermatol Treat* 1991;**2**:95–7.

7. Crawford F, Bell Syer S, Hart R, Torgerson D, Young P, Russell I. Topical treatments for fungal infections of skin and nails of the foot. In: Cochrane Collaboration. *Cochrane Library*, Issue 1. Oxford: Update Software, 2002.

8. Martindales. *The Complete Drug Reference, 32nd ed.* London: Pharmaceutical Press, 1999.

9. Evans EGV, Dodman B, Williamson DM. Comparison of terbinafine and clotrimazole in treating tinea pedis. *BMJ* 1993;**307**:645–7.

10. Patel A, Brookman SD, Bullen MU *et al.* Topical treatment of interdigital tinea pedis: terbinafine compared with clotrimazole. *Australas J Dermatol* 1999;**40**:197–200.

11. Leenutaphong V, Tangwiwat S, Muanprasat C, Niumpradit N, Spitaveesuawan R. Double-blind study of the efficacy of one week topical terbinafine cream compared to 4 weeks miconazole cream in patients with Tinea pedis. *J Med Assoc Thailand* 1999;**82**:1006–9.

12. Schopof R, Hettler O, Brautigam M *et al.* Efficacy and tolerability of 1% topical solution used for 1 week compared with 4 weeks clotrimazole 1% topical solution in the treatment of interdigital tinea pedis: a randomised controlled clinical trial. *Mycoses* 1999;**42**:415–20.

13. Barnetson R St, Marley J, Bullen M *et al.* Comparison of one week of oral terbinafine (250 mg/per day) with four weeks of treatment with clotrimazole 1% cream in interdigital tinea pedis. *Br J Dermatol* 1998;**139**:675–8.

14. Hart R, Bell-Syer S, Crawford F, Torgerson D, Young P, Russell I. Systematic review of topical treatments for fungal infections of the skin and nails of the feet. *BMJ* 1999;**319**:79–82.

15. Williams H. Pragmatic clinical trial is now needed. [Letters] *BMJ* 1999;**319**:1070.

33
Onychomycosis

Aditya K Gupta, Jennifer Ryder and Robyn Bluhm

Background
Definition
Onychomycosis is a fungal infection of the nail, caused predominantly by anthropophilic dermatophytes, less commonly by yeast (*Candida* spp.), and by non-dermatophyte mould infections.[1-3] Onychomycosis may present with hyperkeratosis, subungual debris, thickening or discoloration of the nail plate. Total nail dystrophy may also result with advanced onychomycosis.[3]

Incidence/prevalence
Onychomycosis is the most common nail disorder in adults. It accounts for approximately 50% of all nail diseases[4,5] and the incidence has increased over the past 80 years.[3] In North American centres, the prevalence of onychomycosis is between approximately 6·5% and 13·8%.[4,6-8] Onychomycosis affects predominantly toenails rather than fingernails; in some reports the ratio of toenail:fingernail onychomycosis ranges from 4:1 to 19:1.[4,7,9,10]

Aetiology/risk factors
Predisposing factors for onychomycosis include tinea pedis, positive family history, increasing age, male sex, trauma, immunosuppression, diabetes mellitus, poor peripheral circulation and smoking.[3,4,6,7,11-17] In addition, for fingernails persistent exposure to water, the use of artificial nails and trauma induced by pushing back the cuticles and aggressive manicuring may also be predisposing factors.

Prognosis
Onychomycosis may be effectively treated with systemic and/or topical antifungal agents. Traditional systemic agents used to treat onychomycosis include griseofulvin and ketoconazole. The newer oral agents used to treat onychomycosis are terbinafine, itraconazole and fluconazole.[18-25] Recent available data suggests that ravuconazole, a triazole, is effective for this indication.[26] Topical treatments include ciclopirox and amorolfine nail lacquers.[27,28] Only ciclopirox 8% nail lacquer has been approved in the US for the treatment of onychomycosis.[29]

Relapse of onychomycosis, especially of toenails, is not uncommon, particularly in predisposed individuals. Fingernail onychomycosis may respond better to treatment than toenail disease because perfusion of the upper extremity is generally better than of the lower extremity, which may result in improved drug delivery to the fingers compared with the toes. Also, fingernails have a faster rate of outgrowth compared with toenails (3 mm/month compared with 1 mm/month),[30] resulting in the infected fingernail growing out faster than its lower extremity counterpart.

Aims of treatment
Onychomycosis may be a cosmetic problem, especially when fingernails are infected.[31] The treatment objectives are to reduce the fungal burden within the nail, ultimately curing the fungal infection, and to promote healthy regrowth of

affected nails. In instances where onychomycosis is associated with a degree of morbidity, for example, pain, discomfort and soft tissue infection, timely treatment may help to eliminate symptoms and prevent complications that could be associated with more severe consequences.[32]

Relevant outcomes

The most commonly reported therapeutic measure of efficacy is mycological cure, which is defined, by most, as negative light microscopic examination and negative culture. Clinical improvement has been reported in several ways. Some studies have used the parameter of clinical success, which is defined as cleared or markedly improved (90–100% clear nail).[33] Others have defined clinical success as cure or improvement sufficient to reduce the involved area of the target nail to less than 25% at the end of therapy.[34] Another term used is clinical effectiveness, which is taken to be mycological cure and at least 5 mm of new clear toenail growth.[35] Clinical cure refers to the nail after therapy appearing completely cured to the naked eye. Complete cure rate is the combined results of mycological and clinical cure.

Search methods

To identify studies where oral treatments – itraconazole (continuous and pulse), fluconazole, terbinafine (continuous and pulse) and griseofulvin – were used to treat adults with toenail or fingernail onychomycosis caused by dermatophytes, we searched Medline (1966–2002) for randomised controlled trials (RCTs). The reference sections of the published reports were also examined for potential studies not listed in the database.

Some of the studies were completely[26,27,36–135] or partially[33,34,136–145] excluded for the following reasons.

Open trials, studies conducted in a special population (for example diabetics, patients with Down's syndrome, transplant recipients) and reports where we were unable to extract the relevant data, double publications, non-English language studies, and retrospective studies were excluded.

The use of nail lacquers such as ciclopirox and amorolfine to treat onychomycosis is not considered. There are many anecdotal reports of various topical agents being effective for the management of onychomycosis; however, published reports of the efficacy of topical agents in onychomycosis in the indexed, peer-reviewed literature are far fewer. Other clinical trials have included tioconazole 28% solution, bifonazole with urea, fungoid tincture, miconazole, and tea tree oil.

Also excluded were studies that used non-standard treatment dosage or duration for toenails (for example terbinafine therapy for less than 3 months or more than 4 months; continuous itraconazole therapy for less than 3 months or more than 4 months and less than 200 mg/day; itraconazole pulse therapy for fewer than three pulses or more than four pulses; fluconazole dosage other than 150 mg/week; griseofulvin therapy for less than 3 months), fingernails (terbinafine therapy for more than 6 weeks, continuous itraconazole therapy for more than 6 weeks, pulse itraconazole for more than two pulses, fluconazole dosage other than 150 mg/week), or other non-standard regimens, such as sequential or combination therapy.

We have not considered trials where ketoconazole was used to treat onychomycosis, given the potential of this agent to cause hepatotoxicity and the availability of alternative agents.

The use of ravuconazole for the management of onychomycosis has not been considered further because information currently available in a published format is restricted to abstracts.[26]

This chapter discusses the distal and lateral presentation of onychomycosis, which is the most common type; treatment of the other types of onychomycosis is not considered.[3,146] Onychomycosis caused by *Candida* spp. and non-dermatophyte moulds is less common and is not considered in this chapter.

Evidence was graded using the quality of evidence scale system employed by Cox and colleagues[147] (Box 33.1).

Box 33.1 The quality of evidence scale system employed by Cox and colleagues[147]

I   Evidence obtained from at least one properly designed randomised control trial

II-i Evidence obtained from well-designed controlled trials without randomisation

II-ii Evidence obtained from well-designed cohort or case-control analytic studies, preferably from more than one centre or research group

II-iii Evidence obtained from multiple time series with or without the intervention. Dramatic results in uncontrolled experiments could also be included

III Options of respected authorities based on clinical experience, descriptive studies or reports of expert committees

IV Evidence inadequate owing to problems of methodology (for example sample size, length of comprehensiveness of follow up or conflicts in evidence)

QUESTIONS

What is the role of oral antifungal therapy in the management of dermatophyte onychomycosis in adults?

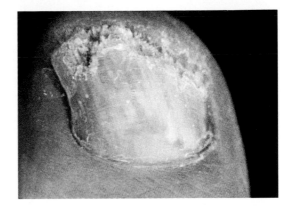

Figure 33.1   This patient is a 47-year-old non-diabetic male exhibiting an infection of the left great toenail with no other health problems. He gave a history of approximately 15-year duration of nail abnormality that may be related to previous nail trauma. The thickened nail had large areas of yellowish–white discoloration typical of fungal nail infection. Culture revealed infection with the dermatophyte fungus, *Trichophyton rubrum*.

Griseofulvin was the first significant oral antifungal agent available for the management of dermatomycoses. Although its use in the treatment of onychomycosis has decreased over the years, it is still widely used for the treatment of tinea capitis.[148] Ketoconazole, an oral imidazole, is no longer recommended for the treatment of onychomycosis, which requires a long duration of therapy, because of the potential for hepatotoxicity.[148] The introduction of the new oral antifungal agents, terbinafine, itraconazole and fluconazole has led to improved efficacy, decreased treatment duration and fewer adverse events.

What are the effects of systemic treatments on fingernail and toenail onychomycosis?

Griseofulvin

The regimen for treating onychomycosis is continuous therapy using 500–1000 mg/day, typically administered for 6–12 months for fingernail onychomycosis and for 9–18 months for toenail disease.

Fingernail onychomycosis

Quality of evidence – I

One double-blind RCT compared griseofulvin, 500 mg/day for 12 weeks, with terbinafine in the treatment of onychomycosis (Table 33.1).[141] The mycological cure rate and complete cure rate were 63% and 39%, respectively.

Toenail onychomycosis
Quality of evidence – I

Three double-blind RCTs[140,144,149] and one open RCT[142] compared griseofulvin with continuous terbinafine or itraconazole in the treatment of onychomycosis (Table 33.2).

Effectiveness
In the RCTs, griseofulvin, 500 mg/day or 1 g/day, was administered to treat onychomycosis. In the double-blind RCTs the mycological cure rate ranged from 46% to 69% and complete cure occurred in 2–56% of patients. In the open RCT, 6% of patients were completely cured.

Drawbacks
The use of griseofulvin may be associated with adverse events such as gastrointestinal upset, nausea, diarrhoea, headache, central nervous system symptoms and urticaria.[150] Few drug interactions are associated with griseofulvin therapy and no drugs are contraindicated.

Comment
Griseofulvin was the first systemic agent used to treat onychomycosis on a widespread basis. The newer oral agents (itraconazole, terbinafine and fluconazole) have been found to be more effective than griseofulvin and the duration of active therapy is also shorter with the more recently introduced antimycotics.[151,152] Moreover, when griseofulvin is used to treat dermatophyte toenail onychomycosis, relapse rates may be higher (40–60%)[129] than with the newer oral antifungal agents.[33,153–156]

Continuous terbinafine
The regimen for fingernail and toenail onychomycosis is 250 mg/day, administered for 6 and 12 weeks, respectively.

Fingernail onychomycosis
Quality of evidence – I

Two double-blind RCTs evaluated subjects with fingernail onychomycosis only (see Table 33.1). One study administered terbinafine for 12 weeks and therefore was not included in this analysis.[141]

Effectiveness
The double-blind randomised placebo-controlled study used terbinafine, 250 mg/day for 6 weeks, to treat fingernail onychomycosis (Table 33.1).[156] Mycological cure was achieved in 79% of patients and complete cure in 59%.

Toenail onychomycosis
Quality of evidence – I

The majority of studies were double-blind RCTs (Table 33.3). Terbinafine was administered at a dose of 250 mg/day for 3–4 months.

Effectiveness
Six double-blind RCTs compared terbinafine with placebo.[33,145,156–159] Each study reported terbinafine, 250 mg/day, to be significantly more effective than placebo in treating onychomycosis.

Ten double-blind RCTs compared continuous terbinafine with other drugs.[35,149,160–167] Mycological cure rates ranged from 67% to 95% and the corresponding clinical response rates from 66% to 97% with a follow up of no more than 72 weeks.

Four open RCTs reported the efficacy of continuous terbinafine for 3 or 4 months.[168–171]

Table 33.1 Treatment of dermatophyte fingernail onychomycosis

Year	Authors	Treatment	Study type	No. of evaluable patients	Regimen	Treatment duration	Follow up (post-treatment)	Efficacy measure (%)		
								MC	CR	CC
2001	Itraconazole package insert (US)[155]	Continuous itraconazole	Double-blind, randomised, placebo-controlled	37	200 mg/day	2 months		(61)	*	(47)
2001	Terbinafine package insert (US)[156]	Continuous terbinafine	Double-blind, randomised, placebo-controlled	Not stated	250 mg/day	6 wks	24 wks	(79)	*	(59)
1997	Odom et al.[179]	Pulse itraconazole	Double-blind, randomised, multicentre, placebo-controlled	37	400 mg/day 1 wk/month	2 months	Up to 19 wks	16/22 (73)	17/22 (77)	15/22 (68)
1998	Drake et al.[137]	Fluconazole	Double-blind, randomised, parallel, multicentre, placebo-controlled	78	150 mg/wk	Up to 9 months	6 months	70/78 (90)*	69/78 (88)	61/78 (78)*
1998	Haneke[141]	Griseofulvin	Double-blind, randomised, comparative (continuous terbinafine)	92	500 mg/day	12 wks, followed by 12 wks placebo	6 months	45/72 (63)		(39)

Mycological cure (MC) is defined as negative microscopy and culture unless indicated otherwise; clinical response (CR) is defined as cured or markedly improved unless indicated otherwise; Complete cure (CC) is defined as mycological and clinical cure or improvement unless indicated otherwise; *not defined; ‡CC defined as clinical cure and negative mycological culture; ‡‡‡CC defined as MC and continuous growth of unaffected nail; ^CR variable definitions; ⊥⊥ MC defined as negative microscopy

Table 33.2 Treatment of dermatophyte toenail onychomycosis using griseofulvin therapy

Year	Authors	Study type	No. of evaluable patients	Regimen	Treatment duration	Follow up (post-treatment)	Efficacy measure (%) MC	CR	CC
1997	Baran et al.[144]	Double-blind, randomised, parallel, multicentre, comparative (continuous terbinafine)	58	1 g/day	Up to 12 months		(69)		(44)
1995	Faergemann et al.[149]	Double-blind, randomised, parallel, comparative (continuous terbinafine)	41	500 mg/day	13 months		19/41 (46)*	*	1/41 (2)‡‡
1995	Hofmann et al.[140]	Double-blind, randomised, comparative (continuous terbinafine)	88	1000 mg/day	48 wks	24 wks	42/68 (62)		49/88 (56)‡‡‡
1993	Korting et al.[142]	Open, randomised, comparative (continuous itraconazole)	36	660 mg/day	Up to 18 months			*	2/36 (6)
			36	990 mg/day				*	2/36 (6)

See Table 33.1 for abbreviations.

(Continued)

Table 33.3 Treatment of dermatophyte toenail onychomycosis using terbinafine continuous therapy

Year	Authors	Study type	No. of evaluable patients	Regimen	Treatment duration	Follow up (from baseline)	Efficacy measure (%) MC	CR	CC
2002	Heikkila et al.[160]	Double-blind, double dummy, randomised multicentre, comparative (pulse itraconazole)	23	250 mg/day	12 wks	72 wks	Negative microscopy: 21/23 (91)	*	11/23 (48)*
			18		16 wks		Negative culture: 20/23 (87)		
							Negative microscopy: 18/18 (100)	*	9/18 (50)*
							Negative culture: 7/18 (94)		
2002	Sigurgeirsson et al.[161]	Double-blind, double dummy, randomised comparative (pulse itraconazole)	74	250 mg/day	12 or 16 wks	Up to 5 years	34/74 (46)	*	26/74 (35)
2001	TER Package Insert (US)[156]	Double-blind, randomised, placebo-controlled	Not Stated	250 mg/day	12 wks	48 wks	(70)	*	(38)
2000	Havu et al.[162]	Double-blind; double-placebo, randomised multicentre, comparative (fluconazole)	46	250 mg/day	12 wks	60 wks	41/46 (89)	39/46 (85)^	*
1999	Evans et al.[35]	Double-blind, double dummy, randomised parallel, multicentre, comparative (pulse itraconazole)	110	250 mg/day	12 wks	72 wks	81/107 (76)	67/102 (66)^	49/107 (46)
			99		16 wks		80/99 (81)	67/95 (71)^	54/98 (55)
1999	Degreef et al.[165]	Double-blind, randomised parallel, multicentre, comparative (continuous itraconazole)	144	250 mg/day	12 wks	48 months	(67)	(87)	*
1999	Billstein et al.[157]	Double-blind, randomised parallel, multicentre, placebo-controlled	29	250 mg/day	12 wks	72 wks	18/21 (86)	*	*
			27		16 wks		13/16 (81)	*	*

Table 33.3 *(Continued)*

Year	Authors	Study type	No. of evaluable patients	Regimen	Treatment duration	Follow up (from baseline)	Efficacy measure (%)		
							MC	CR	CC
1998	De Backer et al.[163]	Double-blind, randomised parallel, multicentre, comparative (continuous itraconazole)	186	250 mg/day	12 wks	48 wks	119/163 (73)	(76) *	(38)
1997	Drake et al.[33]	Double-blind, randomised multicentre, placebo-controlled	142	250 mg/day	12 wks	48 wks	(70)	58/71 (82)	*
1997	Sveigaard et al.[158]	Double-blind, randomised multicentre, placebo-controlled	48	250 mg/day	3 months	9 or 12 months	19/48 (40)	*	18/48 (38)
1997	Honeyman et al.[164]	Double-blind, double dummy, randomised parallel, multicentre, comparative (continuous itraconazole)	64	250 mg/day	4 months	48 wks	61/64 (95)⊥⊥	62/64 (97)	61/64 (95)
1997	Tausch et al.[139]	Double-blind, randomised multicentre, duration finding	56	250 mg/day	12 wks	48 wks	46/56 (82)	33/56 (59)^	33/56 (59)
1995	Brautigam et al.[166]	Double-blind, randomised parallel, multicentre, comparative (continuous itraconazole)	86	250 mg/day	12 wks	52 wks	70/86 (81)	69/86 (80)*	*
1995	Faergemann et al.[149]	Double-blind, randomised parallel, comparative (griseofulvin)	43	250 mg/day	4 months		36/43 (84)*	*	18/43 (42)‡‡
1995	Watson et al.[159]	Double-blind, randomised, placebo-controlled	56	250 mg/day	12 wks	24 wks	33/56 (59)	*	*
1994	De Backer et al.[167]	Double-blind, randomised parallel, comparative (continuous terbinafine)	49	250 mg/day	4 months	48 wks	41/49 (84)	44/49 (90)	*
			51	500 mg/day			46/51 (90)	45/51 (88)	*

(Continued)

Table 33.3 (Continued)

Year	Authors	Study type	No. of evaluable patients	Regimen	Treatment duration	Follow up (from baseline)	Efficacy measure (%)		
							MC	CR	CC
1992	van der Schroeff[143]	Double-blind, randomised, duration-finding	30	250 mg/day	6 wks	48 wks	12/29 (41)	*	12/30 (40)
			34		12 wks		24/34 (71)		24/34 (71)
			34		24 wks		28/34 (82)	*	27/34 (79)
1992	Goodfield et al.[145]	Double-blind, randomised parallel, multicentre, placebo-controlled	45	250 mg/day	12 wks	48 wks	37/45 (82)	*	*
2002	Arca et al.[168]	Open, randomised comparative (pulse itraconazole, fluconazole)	16	250 mg/day	3 months	6 months	12/16 (75)	*	10/16 (63)
1996	Alpsoy et al.[170]	Open, randomised comparative (pulse terbinafine)	24	250 mg/day	3 months	12 months	*	*	19/24 (79)
1999	Kejda[171]	Open, randomised parallel, comparative (pulse itraconazole)	25	250 mg/day	3 months	12 months	(76)	17/25 (68)	*
1996	Tosti et al.[169]	Open, randomised, comparative (pulse itraconazole, pulse terbinafine)	19	250 mg/day	4 months	10 months	16/17 (94)	*	13/17 (76)

See Table 33.1 for abbreviations

Mycological cure ranged between 75% and 94%. In one study, clinical response was reported to be 68%.[171] Complete cure ranged from 63% to 79%.

Drawbacks

Treatment of onychomycosis with continuous terbinafine is associated with a low frequency of adverse events.[151,172] These adverse events are generally mild to moderate in severity and are reversible. The more common adverse events involve the gastrointestinal tract, skin and central nervous system. Only a small proportion of patients discontinue treatment with terbinafine. Few drug interactions have been reported and some of these may arise because the allylamine inhibits the hepatic cytochrome P450 CYP2D6.[173,174] In the US and Canada, the package inserts[156,175] state that pretreatment serum transaminase tests (alanine transaminase and aspartate transaminase) tests should be considered before initiating terbinafine therapy.

Comments

Terbinafine is effective and safe for the treatment of onychomycosis. Terbinafine is an allylamine, which inhibits squalene epoxidase, resulting in an accumulation of squalene and a deficiency of ergosterol. The accumulation of squalene may be associated with fungicidal action.[176] In one study the clinical relapse rate was recorded in 11% of patients when followed up for up to 96 weeks from the start of therapy.[33] A substantial number of high-quality studies demonstrate the effectiveness of continuous terbinafine in the treatment of toenail onychomycosis, some of which have stated that this may be the most effective agent available for this indication.[177,178]

Pulse terbinafine

In pulse regimens, terbinafine is administered at 250 mg twice a day for 1 week, followed by 3 weeks with no treatment between successive pulses. Typically, two pulses are required to treat fingernail onychomycosis and three or four pulses for toenail disease.

Toenail onychomycosis

Quality of evidence – I

Three randomised comparator studies have reported the use of intermittent terbinafine therapy in the treatment of onychomycosis (Table 33.4). Two were open studies[169,170] and one was single-blind.[136] The duration of follow up was 10–18 months.

Effectiveness

One single-blind randomised study[136] compared terbinafine pulse with sequential treatment in which two itraconazole pulses were followed by terbinafine pulse (see Table 33.4). The mycological cure rate in the terbinafine group was 49%, and therapy was effective (mycological cure plus at least 5 mm of new nail growth) in 46% of patients, with 32% of patients completely cured (n = 90).

In the two open randomised comparative studies,[169,170] intermittent terbinafine therapy was associated with complete cure rates of 50% (n = 20)[169] and 74% (n = 23).[170] Furthermore, in the study by Tosti et al.[169] the mycological cure rate was 80% (n = 20).

Drawbacks

Intermittent terbinafine therapy has been associated with few adverse events. Adverse events are generally mild to moderate and are reversible. The spectrum of adverse effects is similar to that seen with the continuous terbinafine regimen. The pulse terbinafine regimen is not indicated for the treatment of onychomycosis, and therefore there are no monitoring guidelines in the US.

Table 33.4 Treatment of dermatophyte toenail onychomycosis using terbinafine pulse therapy

Year	Authors	Study type	No. of evaluable patients	Regimen	Treatment duration	Follow up (post-treatment)	Efficacy measure (%)		
							MC	CR	CC
2001	Gupta et al.[136]	Single-blind, randomised parallel, comparative (pulse itraconazole + pulse terbinafine)	90	500 mg/day 1 wk/month	3 months	18 months	44/90 (49)	41/90 (46)^	29/90 (32)
1996	Alpsoy et al.[170]	Open, randomised comparative (continuous terbinafine)	23	500 mg/day 1 wk/month	3 months	12 months	*	*	17/23 (74)
1996	Tosti et al.[169]	Open, randomised comparative (pulse itraconazole, continuous terbinafine)	20	500 mg/day 1 wk/month	4 months	10 months	16/20 (80)	*	10/20 (50)

See Table 33.1 for abbreviations

Comment

The preferred regimen for the treatment of onychomycosis using terbinafine is continuous rather than pulse therapy. Compared with the continuous regimen, which has been well studied, there are relatively less data available on the efficacy and safety of the pulse regimen.

Pulse itraconazole

In a pulse regimen, itraconazole is taken 200 mg twice a day for 1 week, followed by 3 weeks without treatment between successive pulses. Typically two pulses are administered for fingernail onychomycosis and three or four pulses for toenail disease.

Fingernail onychomycosis

Quality of evidence – I

One double-blind placebo-controlled trial investigated the efficacy of pulse itraconazole in fingernail onychomycosis (see Table 33.1).[179] The mycological cure and clinical response rates were 73% and 77%, respectively.

Toenail onychomycosis

Quality of evidence – I

Eleven RCTs, five of which were double blind, evaluated pulse itraconazole in the treatment of toenail onychomycosis (Table 33.5).

Effectiveness

One double-blind RCT compared three pulses of itraconazole with placebo.[180] The mycological cure rate was 62% with itraconazole, which was significantly higher than that in the placebo group ($P<0.0001$). There was also a significant difference between the clinical response rate in the active treatment (65%) compared with the placebo group ($P<0.001$).

Four double-blind randomised comparative studies evaluated itraconazole pulse treatment, three compared with continuous terbinafine treatment,[35,160,161] and one compared with continuous itraconazole treatment.[181] The mycological cure rates for the itraconazole pulse groups, with a follow up of no more than 72 weeks, ranged from 38% to 69%. The corresponding range for clinical response rates were 28–81%.

Five open randomised comparative studies[168,169,171,183,184] reported mycological cure rates with itraconazole of 61–75%, and clinical response rates of 77–88%. One randomised study[182] compared three-pulse therapy with four pulses; however, since the number of treatment cycles had little effect on cure rates, a combined mycological cure rate of 77% was reported; hence this study was not included in the table.

Drawbacks

Pulse itraconazole therapy is approved for fingernail, but not toenail, onychomycosis in the US. Adverse events occur with a low frequency and are generally mild to moderate in severity and are reversible. These events include gastrointestinal upset, cutaneous eruption and headache.[185] Studies report a low discontinuation rate because of adverse events. Itraconazole may interact with several drugs, some of which are contraindicated with this triazole.[155,173,174,186] In some cases the drug interaction may be explained by inhibition of cytochrome P450 CYP3A4 by itraconazole. Itraconazole is contraindicated in North America (USA and Canada) in patients with evidence of ventricular dysfunction, for example, congestive heart failure or a history of heart failure.[155,187] Hepatic enzymes should be monitored in patients with pre-existing hepatic function abnormalities or those who have experienced liver toxicity with other medications. Hepatic enzymes should be monitored periodically in all patients receiving continuous treatment for more than 1 month, or at any time a patient develops signs or symptoms suggestive of liver dysfunction.[155,187]

Comment

Itraconazole pulse therapy is effective and safe in onychomycosis. The pulse regimen used to

Table 33.5 Treatment of dermatophyte toenail onychomycosis using itraconazole pulse therapy

Year	Reference	Study type	No. of evaluable patients	Regimen	Treatment duration	Follow up period (from baseline)	Efficacy measure (%) MC	CR^	CC
2002	Heikkila et al.[160]	Double-blind, double dummy, randomised, multicentre, comparative (continuous terbinafine)	18	400 mg/day 1 wk/month	12 wks	72 wks	Negative microscopy: 11/18 (61) Negative culture: 12/18 (67)	*	6/18 (33)*
			17		16 wks		Negative microscopy: 11/17 (65) Negative culture: 13/17 (76)	*	3/17 (18)*
2002	Sigurgeirsson et al.[161]	Double-blind, double dummy, randomised, comparative (continuous terbinafine)	77	400 mg/day 1 wk/month	12 or 16 wks	Up to 5 years	10/77 (13)	*	11/77 (14)
2000	Gupta et al.[180]	Double-blind, randomised, placebo-controlled	78	400 mg/day 1 wk/month	3 months	48 wks	48/78 (62)	51/78 (65)	*
1999	Evans et al.[35]	Double-blind, double dummy, randomised, parallel, multicentre, comparative (continuous terbinafine)	107	400 mg/day 1 wk/month	12 wks	72 wks	41/107 (38)	29/102 (28)^	25/107 (23)
			109		16 wks		53/108 (49)	35/104 (34)^	28/108 (26)
1997	Havu et al.[181]	Double-blind, randomised, parallel, multicentre, comparative (continuous itraconazole)	59	400 mg/day 1 wk/month	3 months	12 months	41/59 (69)	48/59 (81)	*
2002	Arca et al.[168]	Open, randomised, comparative (continuous terbinafine, fluconazole)	18	400 mg/day 1 wk/month	3 months	6 months	11/18 (61)	*	11/18 (61)

(Continued)

Table 33.5 (Continued)

Year	Reference	Study type	No. of evaluable patients	Regimen	Treatment duration	Follow up period (from baseline)	Efficacy measure (%)		
							MC	CR	CC
1999	Shemer et al.[183]	Open, randomised, comparative (continuous itraconazole)	Minimum of 16 patients in each group	400 mg/day 1 wk/month	3 months 4 months	48 wks	* *	* *	(50) (65)
1999	Kedja[171]	Open, randomised, parallel, comparative (continuous terbinafine)	26	400 mg/day 1 wk/month	3 months	12 months	(75)	20/26 (77)	*
1996	Tosti et al.[169]	Open, randomised, comparative (continuous v pulse terbinafine)	21	400 mg/day 1 wk/month	4 months	10 months	15/20 (75)	*	8/21 (38)
1996	De Doncker et al.[184]	Open, randomised, comparative (pulse itraconazole)	25 25	400 mg/day 1 wk/month	3 months 4 months	Up to 1 yr	16/25 (64) 18/25 (72)	22/25 (88) 21/25 (84)	* *

See Table 33.1 for abbreviations.

treat toenail onychomycosis decreases the itraconazole required by one-half compared with the continuous regimen with this triazole. This may result in monetary saving, increased compliance and may reduce the frequency of adverse events.[180,185,188–190] In fact, the pulse regimen is the preferred mode of drug delivery when using itraconazole. No significant difference was found between three- and four-pulse regimens of itraconazole for the primary efficacy parameters in the treatment of toenail onychomycosis.[184] In one report, after the use of three pulses for the treatment of toenail onychomycosis, the relapse rate at follow up 12 months after the start of therapy was 10·4%.[190] Two pulses of itraconazole should be effective and safe in fingernail onychomycosis.

Continuous itraconazole

The regimen for fingernail and toenail onychomycosis is 200 mg/day administered for 6 and 12 weeks, respectively.

Fingernail onychomycosis

Quality of evidence – I

One double-blind RCT compared continuous itraconazole with placebo in the treatment of fingernails only (see Table 33.1).[155] The mycological cure rate was 61% and the corresponding complete cure rate was 47%.

Toenail onychomycosis

Quality of evidence – I

The majority of reported studies were double-blind RCTs (Table 33.6).

Effectiveness

In the four double-blind RCTs that compared continuous itraconazole with placebo, significantly more patients receiving active treatment achieved mycological cure and clinical response ($P<0·01$).[155,191–193] The mycological cure rates for the RCTs treating patients with continuous itraconazole ranged from 46% to 84%; the corresponding range for clinical response rates was 58–83%.

Drawbacks

Adverse events associated with the use of continuous itraconazole for the treatment of onychomycosis are not common, and those experienced are generally mild to moderate in severity. Adverse events include gastrointestinal disorders (for example nausea, abdominal pain), rashes, and central nervous system effects (for example headache).[181,185,188–190] Only a small proportion of patients discontinue treatment with the triazole. A number of drugs are contraindicated with itraconazole (see section on itraconazole pulse therapy above). In addition, the triazole has several drug interactions (see section above). Itraconazole is contraindicated in North America in patients with evidence of ventricular dysfunction, for example, congestive heart failure or a history of heart failure. The US package insert suggests that liver function tests be performed in patients receiving continuous therapy for more than 1 month or at any time a patient develops signs and symptoms suggestive of liver disease.[155]

Comment

Continuous itraconazole therapy is an effective and well-tolerated treatment for onychomycosis. Historically, treatment of onychomycosis with itraconazole was with the continuous regimen; later work done by de Doncker et al.[184,190] resulted in the widespread adaptation of pulse therapy for this indication. When patients with toenail onychomycosis were treated with continuous itraconazole therapy, 21% of the overall success group had a relapse (worsening of the global

Table 33.6 Treatment of dermatophyte toenail onychomycosis using itraconazole continuous therapy

Year	Reference	Study type	No. of evaluable patients	Regimen	Treatment duration	Follow up period (from baseline)	Efficacy measure (%)		
							MC	CR	CC
2001	Itraconazole package insert (US)[155]	Double-blind, randomised, placebo-controlled	110	200 mg/day	12 wks		(54)	*	(14)
1999	Degreef et al.[165]	Double-blind, randomised, parallel, multicentre, comparative (continuous terbinafine)	145	200 mg/day	12 wks	48 wks	(61)	(82)	*
1998	Haneke et al.[138]	Double-blind, randomised, parallel, multicentre, comparative (continuous itraconazole + pulse itraconazole, miconazole)	479	200 mg/day	3 months	12 months	354/479 (74)	395/479 (82)	*
1998	De Backer et al.[163]	Double-blind, randomised, parallel, multicentre, comparative (continuous terbinafine)	186	200 mg/day	12 wks	48 wks	77/168 (46)	(58) *	(23)*
1997	Elewski et al.[191]	Double-blind, randomised, multicentre, placebo-controlled	109	200 mg/day	12 wks	48 wks	59/109 (54)	71/109 (65)	
1997	Havu et al.[181]	Double-blind, randomised, multicentre, parallel, comparative (pulse itraconazole)	62	200 mg/day	3 months	12 months	41/62 (66)	43/62 (69)	*
1997	Honeyman et al.[164]	Double-blind, double dummy, randomised, parallel, multicentre, comparative (continuous terbinafine)	70	200 mg/day	4 months	12 months	59/70 (84) ⊥⊥	58/70 (83)^	53/70 (76)

(Continued)

Table 33.6 (Continued)

Year	Reference	Study type	No. of evaluable patients	Regimen	Treatment duration	Follow up period (from baseline)	Efficacy measure (%)		
							MC	CR	CC
1995	Brautigam et al.[166]	Double-blind, randomised, parallel, multicentre, comparative (continuous terbinafine)	84	200 mg/day	12 wks	52 wks	53/84 (63)	63/84 (75)*	*
1996	Jones et al.[192]	Double-blind, randomised, placebo-controlled	35	200 mg/day	12 wks		24/35 (69)*	27/35 (77)*	18/35 (51)*
1996	Odom et al.[193]	Double-blind, randomised, placebo-controlled	38	200 mg/day	12 wks	48 wks	18/38 (47)*	26/38 (68)	14/38 (37)
1999	Shemer et al.[183]	Open, randomised, comparative (pulse itraconazole)	Minimum of 16 patients in each group	200 mg/day	3 months 4 months	48 wks	* *	* *	(68) (65)

See Table 33.1 for abbreviations.

score or conversion of KOH (potassium hydroxide) or culture from negative to positive).[155]

Fluconazole

Fluconazole is given at 150 mg once weekly until the affected nail has grown out. Typically, the duration of therapy for fingernail and toenail disease has been 4–9 months and 9–15 months, respectively.[194]

Fingernail onychomycosis

Quality of evidence – I

One double-blind RCT assessed the efficacy of fluconazole in the treatment of fingernail onychomycosis,[137] comparing various regimens of fluconazole with each other and with placebo (see Table 33.1). Fluconazole 150 mg/week for up to 9 months resulted in a mycological cure rate of 90% and a clinical response rate of 88%.[137]

Toenail onychomycosis

Quality of evidence – I

Few double-blind RCTs have been reported (Table 33.7).[34,162]

Effectiveness

In one double-blind RCT,[34] mycological cure was 53%. The corresponding clinical response rate was 77%. In an open RCT, 31% of patients were mycologically cured.[168]

Drawbacks

Fluconazole is not approved for the treatment of onychomycosis in North America. The more common adverse effects observed with fluconazole affect the gastrointestinal tract, cutaneous system and central nervous system.[174,194] Adverse events do not commonly occur, and those experienced are usually of mild to moderate severity and are reversible. Only a small proportion of patients discontinue treatment with fluconazole. Cisapride and terfenadine are contraindicated with fluconazole. Some drug interactions may occur with the triazole; in certain cases, the drug interactions arise because fluconazole inhibits cytochrome P450 CYP2C9 and at higher doses the triazole may inhibit cytochrome P450 CYP3A4.[173,174]

Comment

Fluconazole is effective and safe for the treatment of onychomycosis. Compared with terbinafine and itraconazole, there are relatively few studies that have evaluated the efficacy of fluconazole in the treatment of toenail onychomycosis. The preferred regimen for fluconazole is once weekly therapy, typically 150 mg per week for several months until the abnormal-appearing nail plate has grown out. In the study reported by Scher et al.[34] the clinical relapse rate over a 6-month follow up was 4.4%.[153] Studies evaluating the use of once-weekly fluconazole at a higher doses such as 300 mg or 450 mg once weekly[34,137] or continuous fluconazole administration have not been discussed.

General comments

Several pharmacoeconomic analyses of the various oral treatments used in dermatophyte onychomycosis have been published. These studies calculate the cost-effectiveness of each therapy on the basis of the efficacy results of multiple clinical trials. The two most cost-effective regimens for the treatment of onychomycosis are continuous terbinafine and pulse itraconazole.[174,195–199]

In certain nail presentations, response to therapy may be improved by combining oral antifungal

Table 33.7 Treatment of dermatophyte toenail onychomycosis using fluconazole therapy

Year	Authors	Study type	No. of evaluable patients	Regimen	Treatment duration	Follow up (post-treatment)	Efficacy measure (%) MC	CR	CC
2000	Havu et al.[162]	Double-blind, double-placebo, randomised multicentre, comparative (continuous terbinafine)	43		12 wks		22/43 (51)	10/43 (23)t	*
			41	150 mg/wk	24 wks	60 wks	20/41 (49)	18/41 (44)t	*
1998	Scher et al.[34]	Double-blind, randomised parallel, multicentre, placebo-controlled	73	150 mg/wk	Up to 12 months	6 months (only those patients that were clinically cured or improved)	38/72 (53)	56/73 (77)	*
2002	Arca et al.[168]	Open, randomised comparative (pulse itraconazole, continuous terbinafine)	16	150 mg/wk	3 months	6 months	5/16 (31)	*	5/16 (31)

See Table 33.1 for abbreviations

therapy with either an effective topical therapy or mechanical/chemical measures (for example mechanical avulsion, debridement or chemical avulsion). For example, when there is lateral onychomycosis, a dermatophytoma, severe onycholysis, a thickened nail or severe onychomycosis, it may be advantageous to consider a combination approach.[42,59,68,200–202]

Key points

- The main oral antifungal agents used to treat onychomycosis are terbinafine, itraconazole and fluconazole. Griseofulvin and ketoconazole are the traditional antifungal agents, but their use has decreased substantially since the introduction of the newer oral antifungal agents. In addition, the use of ketoconazole for onychomycosis, where long duration therapy is required, has diminished markedly given the potential for hepatotoxicity.
- The preferred regimens with the new oral antifungal agents are continuous terbinafine, pulse itraconazole and once-weekly fluconazole. The duration of therapy with these agents for fingernail onychomycosis is typically 6 weeks with continuous terbinafine, two pulses of itraconazole and 6–9 months of once-weekly fluconazole. The corresponding durations of therapy with these antifungal agents for toenail onychomycosis are 12 or 16 weeks, three or four pulses, and 9–15 months, respectively.
- RCTs have demonstrated that griseofulvin, continuous terbinafine, itraconazole (pulse and continuous) and fluconazole are effective and safe for treatment of dermatophyte fingernail onychomycosis.
- RCTs have demonstrated that continuous terbinafine, itraconazole (pulse and continuous) and fluconazole are effective and safe for treatment of dermatophyte toenail onychomycosis.
- Several factors need to be considered when deciding which agent to prescribe for onychomycosis. These include, efficacy, causative organism, regimen preference (for example continuous versus pulse versus once weekly, and expected duration of therapy), safety of antifungal agent, medical status of patient, potential for drug interactions, relapse rates and cost of therapy.
- None of the newer oral antifungal agents have been approved for the treatment of onychomycosis in children, where the disease occurs much less frequently than in adults.

References

1. Roberts DT. Onychomycosis: current treatment and future challenges. *Br J Dermatol* 1999;**141**(Suppl. 56):1–4.

2. Zaias N. Onychomycosis. *Arch Dermatol* 1972;**105**: 263–74.

3. Hay RJ, Baran R, Haneke E. Fungal (onychomycosis) and other infections involving the nail apparatus. In: Baran R, Dawber RPR, eds. *Diseases of the nails and their management*, 2nd ed. Oxford: Blackwell Scientific Publications,1994;97–134.

4. Gupta AK, Jain HC, Lynde CW *et al.* Prevalence and epidemiology of onychomycosis in patients visiting physicians' offices: a multicenter Canadian survey of 15,000 patients. *J Am Acad Dermatol* 2000;**43**:244–8.

5. Gupta AK, Scher RK. Management of onychomycosis: a North American perspective. *Dermatol Ther* 1997;**3**: 58–65.

6. Ghannoum MA, Hajjeh RA, Scher R *et al.* A large-scale North American study of fungal isolates from nails: the frequency of onychomycosis, fungal distribution, and antifungal susceptibility patterns. *J Am Acad Dermatol* 2000;**43**:641–8.

7. Gupta AK, Jain HC, Lynde CW *et al.* Prevalence and epidemiology of unsuspected onychomycosis in patients visiting dermatologists' offices in Ontario, Canada – a multicenter survey of 2001 patients. *Int J Dermatol* 1997;**36**:783–7.

8. Elewski BE, Charif MA. Prevalence of onychomycosis in patients attending a dermatology clinic in northeastern Ohio for other conditions. *Arch Dermatol* 1997;**133**:1172–3.

9. Sais G, Jucgla A, Peyri J. Prevalence of dermatophyte onychomycosis in Spain: a cross-sectional study. *Br J Dermatol* 1995;**132**:758–61.

10. Williams HC. The epidemiology of onychomycosis in Britain. *Br J Dermatol* 1993;**129**:101–9.

11. Gupta AK, Gupta MA, Summerbell RC *et al*. The epidemiology of onychomycosis: possible role of smoking and peripheral arterial disease. *J Eur Acad Dermatol Venereol* 2000;**14**:466–9.

12. Del Mar M, De Ocariz S, Arenas R *et al*. Frequency of toenail onychomycosis in patients with cutaneous manifestations of chronic venous insufficiency. *Int J Dermatol* 2001;**40**:18–25.

13. Gupta AK, Taborda P, Taborda V *et al*. Epidemiology and prevalence of onychomycosis in HIV-positive individuals. *Int J Dermatol* 2000;**39**:746–53.

14. Gupta AK, Humke S. The prevalence and management of onychomycosis in diabetic patients. *Eur J Dermatol* 2000;**10**:379–84.

15. Gupta AK, Konnikov N, MacDonald P *et al*. Prevalence and epidemiology of toenail onychomycosis in diabetic subjects: a multicentre survey. *Br J Dermatol* 1998;**139**: 665–71.

16. Gupta AK, Lynde CW, Jain HC *et al*. A higher prevalence of onychomycosis in psoriatics compared with non- psoriatics: a multicentre study. *Br J Dermatol* 1997;**136**:786–9.

17. Zaias N, Rebell G. Chronic dermatophytosis caused by *Trichophyton rubrum*. *J Am Acad Dermatol* 1996;**35**: S17–20.

18. Gupta AK. Onychomycosis in the elderly. *Drugs Aging* 2000;**16**:397–407.

19. Gupta AK, Shear NH. A risk-benefit assessment of the newer oral antifungal agents used to treat onychomycosis. *Drug Saf* 2000;**22**:33–52.

20. Hart R, Bell-Syer SE, Crawford F *et al*. Systematic review of topical treatments for fungal infections of the skin and nails of the feet. *BMJ* 1999;**319**:79–82.

21. Scher RK. Onychomycosis: therapeutic update. *J Am Acad Dermatol* 1999;**40**:S21–6.

22. Elewski BE. Onychomycosis: pathogenesis, diagnosis, and management. *Clin Microbiol Rev* 1998;**11**:415–29.

23. Gupta AK, Scher RK, De Doncker P. Current management of onychomycosis. An overview. *Dermatol Clin* 1997;**15**:121–35.

24. Hay RJ. Onychomycosis. Agents of choice. *Dermatol Clin* 1993;**11**:161–9.

25. Haneke E. Fungal infections of the nail. *Semin Dermatol* 1991;**10**:41–53.

26. Gupta AK, Leonardi C, Stolz R *et al*. Evaluation of ravuconazole for the treatment of toenail onychomycosis (abstract). *Ann Dermatol Venereol* 2002;**129**:1S607–842.

27. Gupta AK, Fleckman P, Baran R. Ciclopirox nail lacquer topical solution 8% in the treatment of toenail onychomycosis. *J Am Acad Dermatol* 2000;**43**:S70–80.

28. Haria M, Bryson HM. Amorolfine. A review of its pharmacological properties and therapeutic potential in the treatment of onychomycosis and other superficial fungal infections. *Drugs* 1995;**49**:103–20.

29. Dermik Laboratories Inc. Ciclopirox topical solution 8% nail lacquer. Berwyn, PA, USA: Dermik Laboratories Inc., 2000.

30. Dawber RPR, De Berker D, Baran R. Science of the nail apparatus. In: Baran R, Dawber RPR, eds. *Diseases of the nails and their management*, 2nd ed. Oxford: Blackwell Scientific Publications,1994;1–34.

31. Scher RK. Onychomycosis is more than a cosmetic problem. *Br J Dermatol* 1994;**130**(Suppl. 43):15.

32. Drake LA, Patrick DL, Fleckman P *et al*. The impact of onychomycosis on quality of life: development of an international onychomycosis-specific questionnaire to measure patient quality of life. *J Am Acad Dermatol* 1999;**41**:189–96.

33. Drake LA, Shear NH, Arlette JP *et al*. Oral terbinafine in the treatment of toenail onychomycosis: North American multicenter trial. *J Am Acad Dermatol* 1997;**37**:740–5.

34. Scher RK, Breneman D, Rich P *et al*. Once-weekly fluconazole (150, 300, or 450 mg) in the treatment of distal subungual onychomycosis of the toenail. *J Am Acad Dermatol* 1998;**38**:S77–86.

35. Evans EG, Sigurgeirsson B. Double blind, randomised study of continuous terbinafine compared with intermittent itraconazole in treatment of toenail onychomycosis. The LION Study Group. *BMJ* 1999;**318**:1031–5.

36. Albanese G, Di Cintio R, Martini C, Nicoletti A. Short therapy for tinea unguium with terbinafine: four different courses of treatment. *Mycoses* 1995;**38**:211–14.

37. Andre J, De Doncker P, Laporte M *et al*. Onychomycosis caused by *Microsporum canis*: treatment with itraconazole. *J Am Acad Dermatol* 1995;**32**:1052–3.

38. Arenas R, Fernandez G, Dominguez L. Onychomycosis treated with itraconazole or griseofulvin alone with and without a topical antimycotic or keratolytic agent. *Int J Dermatol* 1991;**30**:586–9.

39. Arenas R, Dominguez-Cherit J, Fernandez LM. Open randomized comparison of itraconazole versus terbinafine in onychomycosis. *Int J Dermatol* 1995;**34**:138–43.

40. Assaf RR, Elewski BE. Intermittent fluconazole dosing in patients with onychomycosis: results of a pilot study. *J Am Acad Dermatol* 1996;**35**:216–19.

41. Bahadir S, Inaloz HS, Alpay K *et al.* Continuous terbinafine or pulse itraconazole: a comparative study on onychomycosis. *J Eur Acad Dermatol Venereol* 2000;**14**:422–3.

42. Baran R, Feuilhade M, Combernale P *et al.* A randomized trial of amorolfine 5% solution nail lacquer combined with oral terbinafine compared with terbinafine alone in the treatment of dermatophytic toenail onychomycoses affecting the matrix region. *Br J Dermatol* 2000;**142**:1177–83.

43. Baran R, Tosti A, Piraccini BM. Uncommon clinical patterns of *Fusarium* nail infection: report of three cases. *Br J Dermatol* 1997;**136**:424–7.

44. Baudraz-Rosselet F, Rakosi T, Wili PB, Kenzelmann R. Treatment of onychomycosis with terbinafine. *Br J Dermatol* 1992;**126**(Suppl. 39):40–6.

45. Bentley-Phillips B. The treatment of onychomycosis with miconazole tincture. *S Afr Med J* 1982;**62**:57–8.

46. Bohn M, Kraemer KT. Dermatopharmacology of ciclopirox nail lacquer topical solution 8% in the treatment of onychomycosis. *J Am Acad Dermatol* 2000;**43**:S57–69.

47. Bonifaz A, Carrasco-Gerard E, Saul A. Itraconazole in onychomycosis: intermittent dose schedule. *Int J Dermatol* 1997;**36**:70–2.

48. Brandrup F, Larsen PO. Long-term follow-up of toe-nail onychomycosis treated with terbinafine. *Acta Derm Venereol* 1997;**77**:238.

49. Brautigam M. Terbinafine versus itraconazole: a controlled clinical comparison in onychomycosis of the toenails. *J Am Acad Dermatol* 1998;**38**:S53–6.

50. Buck DS, Nidorf DM, Addino JG. Comparison of two topical preparations for the treatment of onychomycosis: *Melaleuca alternifolia* (tea tree) oil and clotrimazole. *J Fam Pract* 1994;**38**:601–5.

51. Campbell CK, Johnson EM, Warnock DW. Nail infection caused by *Onychocola canadensis*: report of the first four British cases. *J Med Vet Mycol* 1997;**35**:423–5.

52. Chen J, Liao W, Wen H *et al.* A comparison among four regimens of itraconazole treatment in onychomycosis. *Mycoses* 1999;**42**:93–6.

53. Coldiron B. Recalcitrant onychomycosis of the toenails successfully treated with fluconazole. *Arch Dermatol* 1992;**128**:909–10.

54. Cribier B, Grosshans E. [Efficacy and tolerance of terbinafine (Lamisil) in a series of 50 cases of dermatophyte onychomycoses]. *Ann Dermatol Venereol* 1994;**121**:15–20.

55. De Backer M, De Keyser P, De Vroey C, Lesaffre E. A 12-week treatment for dermatophyte toe onychomycosis: terbinafine 250 mg/day *v.* itraconazole 200 mg/day – a double-blind comparative trial. *Br J Dermatol* 1996;**134** (Suppl. 46):16–17.

56. De Cuyper C. Long-term evaluation of terbinafine 250 and 500 mg daily in a 16-week oral treatment for toenail onychomycosis. *Br J Dermatol* 1996;**135**:156–7.

57. De Doncker P, Van Lint J, Dockx P, Roseeuw D. Pulse therapy with one-week itraconazole monthly for three or four months in the treatment of onychomycosis. *Cutis* 1995;**56**:180–3.

58. DiSalvo AF, Fickling AM. A case of nondermatophytic toe onychomycosis caused by *Fusarium oxysporum*. *Arch Dermatol* 1980;**116**:699–700.

59. Dominguez-Cherit J, Teixeira F, Arenas R. Combined surgical and systemic treatment of onychomycosis. *Br J Dermatol* 1999;**140**:778–80.

60. Downs AM, Lear JT, Archer CB. *Scytalidium hyalinum* onychomycosis successfully treated with 5% amorolfine nail lacquer. *Br J Dermatol* 1999;**140**:555.

61. Eastcott DF. Terbinafine and onychomycosis. *N Z Med J* 1991;**104**:17.

62. Effendy I, Kolczak H, Ossowski B, Hohler T. [Topical therapy of onychomycoses with 8% ciclopirox laquer. An open, non-comparative study]. *Fortschr Med* 1993;**111**: 205–8.

63. Elewski BE. Onychomycosis caused by *Scytalidium dimidiatum*. *J Am Acad Dermatol* 1996;**35**:336–8.

64. Galimberti R, Kowalczuk A, Flores V, Squiquera L. Onychomycosis treated with a short course of oral terbinafine. *Int J Dermatol* 1996;**35**:374–5.

65. Galitz J. Successful treatment of onychomycosis with ciclopirox nail lacquer: a case report. *Cutis* 2001; **68**:23–4.

66. Gianni C, Cerri A, Crosti C. Unusual clinical features of fingernail infection by *Fusarium oxysporum*. *Mycoses* 1997;**40**:455–9.

67. Gianni C, Cerri A, Crosti C. Non-dermatophytic onychomycosis. An understimated entity? A study of 51 cases. *Mycoses* 2000;**43**:29–33.

68. Goodfield MJ, Evans EG. Combined treatment with surgery and short duration oral antifungal therapy in patients with limited dermatophyte toenail infection. *J Dermatol Treat* 2000;**11**:259–62.

69. Goodfield MJ, Rowell NR, Forster RA *et al*. Treatment of dermatophyte infection of the finger- and toe-nails with terbinafine (SF 86-327, Lamisil), an orally active fungicidal agent. *Br J Dermatol* 1989;**121**:753–7.

70. Goodfield MJ, Evans EG. Treatment of superficial white onychomycosis with topical terbinafine cream. *Br J Dermatol* 1999;**141**:604–5.

71. Gupta AK, Gregurek-Novak T, Konnikov N *et al*. Itraconazole and terbinafine treatment of some nondermatophyte molds causing onychomycosis of the toes and a review of the literature. *J Cutan Med Surg* 2001;**5**:206–10.

72. Gupta AK, Horgan-Bell CB, Summerbell RC. Onychomycosis associated with *Onychocola canadensis*: ten case reports and a review of the literature. *J Am Acad Dermatol* 1998;**39**:410–17.

73. Gupta AK, De Doncker P, Haneke E. Itraconazole pulse therapy for the treatment of *Candida* onychomycosis. *J Eur Acad Dermatol Venereol* 2000;**15**:112–15.

74. Hay RJ, Mackie RM, Clayton YM. Tioconazole nail solution – an open study of its efficacy in onychomycosis. *Clin Exp Dermatol* 1985;**10**:111–15.

75. Hay RJ, Clayton YM, Moore MK. A comparison of tioconazole 28% nail solution versus base as an adjunct to oral griseofulvin in patients with onychomycosis. *Clin Exp Dermatol* 1987;**12**:175–7.

76. Hiruma M, Matsushita A, Kobayashi M, Ogawa H. One week pulse therapy with itraconazole (200 mg day-1) for onychomycosis. Evaluation of treatment results according to patient background. *Mycoses* 2001;**44**:87–93.

77. Kirshbaum BA. Itraconazole therapy for onychomycosis: case reports. *Cutis* 1996;**58**:371–4.

78. Koenig H, Ball C, de Bievre C. First European cases of onychomycosis caused by *Onychocola canadensis*. *J Med Vet Mycol* 1997;**35**:71–2.

79. Lauharanta J. Comparative efficacy and safety of amorolfine nail lacquer 2% versus 5% once weekly. *Clin Exp Dermatol* 1992;**17**(Suppl. 1):41–3.

80. Lebwohl MG, Daniel CR, Leyden J *et al*. Efficacy and safety of terbinafine for nondermatophyte and mixed nondermatophyte and dermatophyte toenail onychomycosis. *Int J Dermatol* 2001;**40**:358–60.

81. Lecha M. Amorolfine and itraconazole combination for severe toenail onychomycosis; results of an open randomized trial in Spain. *Br J Dermatol* 2001;**145**(Suppl. 60):21–6.

82. Lee KH, Kim YS, Kim MS *et al*. Study of the efficacy and tolerability of oral terbinafine in the treatment of onychomycosis in renal transplant patients. *Transplant Proc* 1996;**28**:1488–9.

83. Ling MR, Swinyer LJ, Jarratt MT *et al*. Once-weekly fluconazole (450 mg) for 4, 6, or 9 months of treatment for distal subungual onychomycosis of the toenail. *J Am Acad Dermatol* 1998;**38**:S95–102.

84. Mahgoub ES. Clinical trial with clotrimazole cream (Bay b 5097) in dermatophytosis and onychomycosis. *Mycopathologia* 1975;**56**:149–52.

85. Mensing H, Polak-Wyss A, Splanemann V. Determination of the subungual antifungal activity of amorolfine after 1 month's treatment in patients with onychomycosis: comparison of two nail lacquer formulations. *Clin Exp Dermatol* 1992;**17**(Suppl. 1):29–32.

86. Meyerson MS, Scher RK, Hochman LG *et al*. Open-label study of the safety and efficacy of Fungoid tincture in patients with distal subungual onychomycosis of the toes. *Cutis* 1992;**49**:359–62.

87. Meyerson MS, Scher RK, Hochman LG *et al*. Open-label study of the safety and efficacy of naftifine hydrochloride 1 percent gel in patients with distal subungual onychomycosis of the fingers. *Cutis* 1993;**51**:205–7.

88. Molin L, Tarstedt M, Engman C. Oral terbinafine treatment for toenail onychomycosis: follow-up after 5– 6 years. *Br J Dermatol* 2000;**143**:682–3.

89. Moncada B, Loredo CE, Isordia E. Treatment of onychomycosis with ketoconazole and nonsurgical avulsion of the affected nail. *Cutis* 1983;**31**:438–40.

90. Montana JB, Scher RK. A double-blind, vehicle-controlled study of the safety and efficacy of Fungoid Tincture in patients with distal subungual onychomycosis of the toes. *Cutis* 1994;**53**:313–16.

91. Montero-Gei F, Robles-Soto ME, Schlager H. Fluconazole in the treatment of severe onychomycosis. *Int J Dermatol* 1996;**35**:587–8.

92. Nahass GT, Sisto M. Onychomycosis: successful treatment with once-weekly fluconazole. *Dermatology* 1993;**186**:59–61.

93. Ninomiya J, Yamazaki K, Ito Y *et al*. [Evaluation of the efficacy of small-dose itraconazole pulse therapy (200 mg/day) for tinea unguium]. *Nippon Ishinkin Gakkai Zasshi* 1999;**40**:35–7.

94. Nolting S, Brautigam M, Weidinger G. Terbinafine in onychomycosis with involvement by non-dermatophytic fungi. *Br J Dermatol* 1994;**130**(Suppl. 43):16–21.

95. Onsberg P, Stahl D, Veien NK. Onychomycosis caused by *Aspergillus terreus*. *Sabouraudia* 1978;**16**:39–46.

96. Onsberg P, Stahl D. *Scopulariopsis* onychomycosis treated with natamycin. *Dermatologica* 1980;**160**:57–61.

97. Piepponen T, Blomqvist K, Brandt H *et al*. Efficacy and safety of itraconazole in the long-term treatment of onychomycosis. *J Antimicrob Chemother* 1992;**29**: 195–205.

98. Piraccini BM, Morelli R, Stinchi C, Tosti A. Proximal subungual onychomycosis due to *Microsporum canis*. *Br J Dermatol* 1996;**134**:175–7.

99. Pittrof F, Gerhards J, Erni W, Klecak G. Loceryl nail lacquer – realization of a new galenical approach to onychomycosis therapy. *Clin Exp Dermatol* 1992; **17**(Suppl 1):26–8.

100. Pollak R, Billstein SA. Efficacy of terbinafine for toenail onychomycosis. A multicenter trial of various treatment durations. *J Am Podiatr Med Assoc* 2001;**91**:127–31.

101. Ramos-e-Silva, Marques SA, Gontijo B *et al*. Efficacy and safety of itraconazole pulse therapy: Brazilian multicentric study on toenail onychomycosis caused by dermatophytes. *J Eur Acad Dermatol Venereol* 1998;**11**:109–16.

102. Reinel D, Clarke C. Comparative efficacy and safety of amorolfine nail lacquer 5% in onychomycosis, once-weekly versus twice-weekly. *Clin Exp Dermatol* 1992;**17**(Suppl. 1):44–9.

103. Reinel D. Topical treatment of onychomycosis with amorolfine 5% nail lacquer: comparative efficacy and tolerability of once and twice weekly use. *Dermatology* 1992;**184**(Suppl. 1):21–4.

104. Rollman O. Treatment of onychomycosis by partial nail avulsion and topical miconazole. *Dermatologica* 1982;**165**:54–61.

105. Rollman O, Johansson S. *Hendersonula toruloidea* infection: successful response of onychomycosis to nail avulsion and topical ciclopiroxolamine. *Acta Derm Venereol* 1987;**67**:506–10.

106. Romano C, Miracco C, Difonzo EM. Skin and nail infections due to *Fusarium oxysporum* in Tuscany, Italy. *Mycoses* 1998;**41**:433–7.

107. Romano C, Paccagnini E, Difonzo EM. Onychomycosis caused by *Alternaria* spp. in Tuscany, Italy from 1985 to 1999. *Mycoses* 2001;**44**:73–6.

108. Rosenthal SA, Stritzler R, Vilafane J. Onychomycosis caused by *Aspergillus fumigatus*. Report of a case. *Arch Dermatol* 1968;**97**:685–7.

109. Savin RC, Atton AV. Terbinafine in onychomycosis – a mini study. *Int J Dermatol* 1993;**32**:918–19.

110. Scher RK, Barnett JM. Successful treatment of *Aspergillus flavus* onychomycosis with oral itraconazole. *J Am Acad Dermatol* 1990;**23**:749–50.

111. Seebacher C, Nietsch KH, Ulbricht HM. A multicenter, open-label study of the efficacy and safety of ciclopirox nail lacquer solution 8% for the treatment of onychomycosis in patients with diabetes. *Cutis* 2001;**68**:17–22.

112. Segal R, Kritzman A, Cividalli L *et al*. Treatment of *Candida* nail infection with terbinafine. *J Am Acad Dermatol* 1996;**35**:958–61.

113. Shemer A, Bergman R, Cohen A, Friedman-Birnbaum R. [Treatment of onychomycosis using 40% urea with 1% bifonazole]. *Harefuah* 1992;**122**:159–60.

114. Shuster S, Munro CS. Single dose treatment of fungal nail disease. *Lancet* 1992;**339**:1066.

115. Sigler L, Congly H. Toenail infection caused by *Onychocola canadensis* gen. et sp. nov. *J Med Vet Mycol* 1990;**28**:405–17.

116. Sigler L, Abbott SP, Woodgyer AJ. New records of nail and skin infection due to *Onychocola canadensis* and description of its teleomorph *Arachnomyces nodosetosus* sp. nov. *J Med Vet Mycol* 1994;**32**:275–85.

117. Smith SW, Sealy DP, Schneider E, Lackland D. An evaluation of the safety and efficacy of fluconazole in the treatment of onychomycosis. *South Med J* 1995; **88**:1217–20.

118. Syed TA, Ahmadpour OA, Ahmad SA, Shamsi S. Management of toenail onychomycosis with 2%

butenafine and 20% urea cream: a placebo-controlled, double-blind study. *J Dermatol* 1998;**25**:648–52.

119. Syed TA, Qureshi ZA, Ali SM *et al.* Treatment of toenail onychomycosis with 2% butenafine and 5% *Melaleuca alternifolia* (tea tree) oil in cream. Trop *Med Int Health* 1999;**4**:284–7.

120. Tang WY, Chong LY, Leung CY *et al.* Intermittent pulse therapy with itraconazole for onychomycosis. Experience in Hong Kong Chinese. *Mycoses* 2000;**43**:35–9.

121. Torok I, Simon G, Dobozy A *et al.* Long-term post-treatment follow-up of onychomycosis treated with terbinafine: a multicentre trial. *Mycoses* 1998;**41**:63–5.

122. Tosti A, Piraccini BM, Stinchi C, Lorenzi S. Onychomycosis due to *Scopulariopsis brevicaulis*: clinical features and response to systemic antifungals. *Br J Dermatol* 1996;**135**:799–802.

123. Tosti A, Piraccini RM Proximal subungual onychomycosis due to *Aspergillus niger*: report of two cases. *Br J Dermatol* 1998;**139**:156–7.

124. Tosti A, Piraccini BM, Lorenzi S. Onychomycosis caused by nondermatophytic molds: clinical features and response to treatment of 59 cases. *J Am Acad Dermatol* 2000;**42**:217–24.

125. Tseng SS, Longley BJ, Scher RK, Treiber RK. *Fusarium* fingernail infection responsive to fluconazole intermittent therapy. *Cutis* 2000;**65**:352–4.

126. Tsuboi H, Unno K, Komatsuzaki H *et al.* [Topical treatment of onychomycosis by occlusive dressing using bifonazole cream containing 40% urea]. *Nippon Ishinkin Gakkai Zasshi* 1998;**39**:11–16.

127. Tulli A, Ruffilli MP, De Simone C. The treatment of onychomycosis with a new form of tioconazole. *Chemioterapia* 1988;**7**:160–3.

128. Ulbricht H, Worz K. [Therapy with ciclopirox lacquer of onychomycoses caused by molds]. *Mycoses* 1994;**37**(Suppl. 1):97–100.

129. Villars VV, Jones TC. Special features of the clinical use of oral terbinafine in the treatment of fungal diseases. *Br J Dermatol* 1992;**126**(Suppl. 39):61–9.

130. Walsoe I, Stangerup M, Svejgaard E. Itraconazole in onychomycosis. Open and double-blind studies. *Acta Derm Venereol* 1990;**70**:137–40.

131. Warshaw EM, Carver SM, Zielke GR, Ahmed DD. Intermittent terbinafine for toenail onychomycosis: is it

effective? Results of a randomized pilot trial. *Arch Dermatol* 2001;**137**:1253.

132. Wong CK, Cho YL. Very short duration therapy with oral terbinafine for fingernail onychomycosis. *Br J Dermatol* 1995;**133**:329–31.

133. Wu J, Wen H, Liao W. Small-dose itraconazole pulse therapy in the treatment of onychomycosis. *Mycoses* 1997;**40**:397–400.

134. Zaias N, Serrano L. The successful treatment of finger *Trichophyton rubrum* onychomycosis with oral terbinafine. *Clin Exp Dermatol* 1989;**14**:120–3.

135. Zaias N, Rebell G, Zaiac MN, Glick B. Onychomycosis treated until the nail is replaced by normal growth or there is failure. *Arch Dermatol* 2000;**136**:940.

136. Gupta AK, Lynde CW, Konnikov N. Single-blind, randomized, prospective study of sequential itraconazole and terbinafine pulse compared with terbinafine pulse for the treatment of toenail onychomycosis. *J Am Acad Dermatol* 2001;**44**:485–91.

137. Drake L, Babel D, Stewart DM *et al.* Once-weekly fluconazole (150, 300, or 450 mg) in the treatment of distal subungual onychomycosis of the fingernail. *J Am Acad Dermatol* 1998;**38**:S87–94.

138. Haneke E, Tajerbashi M, De Doncker P, Heremans A. Itraconazole in the treatment of onychomycosis: a double-blind comparison with miconazole. *Dermatology* 1998;**196**:323–9.

139. Tausch I, Brautigam M, Weidinger G, Jones TC. Evaluation of 6 weeks treatment of terbinafine in tinea unguium in a double-blind trial comparing 6 and 12 weeks therapy. The Lagos V Study Group. *Br J Dermatol* 1997;**136**:737–42.

140. Hofmann H, Brautigam M, Weidinger G, Zaun H. Treatment of toenail onychomycosis. A randomized, double-blind study with terbinafine and griseofulvin. LAGOS II Study Group. *Arch Dermatol* 1995;**131**: 919–22.

141. Haneke E, Tausch I, Brautigam M et al. Short-duration treatment of fingernail dermatophytosis: a randomized, double-blind study with terbinafine and griseofulvin. LAGOS III Study Group. *J Am Acad Dermatol* 1995;**32**:72–7.

142. Korting HC, Schafer-Korting M, Zienicke H *et al.* Treatment of tinea unguium with medium and high doses

of ultramicrosize griseofulvin compared with that with itraconazole. *Antimicrob Agents Chemother* 1993;**37**: 2064–8.

143. van der Schroeff JG, Cirkel PK, Crijns MB *et al.* A randomized treatment duration-finding study of terbinafine in onychomycosis. *Br J Dermatol* 1992;**126**(Suppl. 39):36–9.

144. Baran R, Belaich S, Beylot C *et al.* Comparative multicentre double-blind study of terbinafine (250 mg per day) versus griseofulvin (1 g per day) in the treatment of dermatophyte onychomycosis. *J Dermatol* 1997;**8**:93–7.

145. Goodfield MJ. Short-duration therapy with terbinafine for dermatophyte onychomycosis: a multicentre trial. *Br J Dermatol* 1992;**126**(Suppl. 39):33–5.

146. Baran R, Hay RJ, Tosti A, Haneke E. A new classification of onychomycosis. *Br J Dermatol* 1998;**139**:567–71.

147. Cox NH, Eedy DJ, Morton CA. Guidelines for management of Bowen's disease. *Br J Dermatol* 1999;**141**:633–41.

148. Gupta AK. Systemic antifungal agents. In: Wolverton SE, ed. *Comprehensive Dermatologic Drug Therapy.* Philadelphia: WB Saunders, 2001;55–84.

149. Faergemann J, Anderson C, Hersle K *et al.* Double-blind, parallel-group comparison of terbinafine and griseofulvin in the treatment of toenail onychomycosis. *J Am Acad Dermatol* 1995;**32**:750–3.

150. Gupta AK, Sauder DN, Shear N. Antifungal agents: an overview. Part I. *J Am Acad Dermatol* 1994;**30**:677–8.

151. Gupta AK, Shear NH. The new oral antifungal agents for onychomycosis of the toenails. *J Eur Acad Dermatol Venereol* 1999;**13**:1–13.

152. Gupta AK, Sauder DN, Shear NH. Antifungal agents: an overview. Part II. *J Am Acad Dermatol* 1994;**30**:911–33.

153. Elewski BE. Once-weekly fluconazole in the treatment of onychomycosis: introduction. *J Am Acad Dermatol* 1998;**38**:S73–6.

154. De Doncker PR, Scher RK, Baran RL *et al.* Itraconazole therapy is effective for pedal onychomycosis caused by some nondermatophyte molds and in mixed infection with dermatophytes and molds: a multicenter study with 36 patients. *J Am Acad Dermatol* 1997;**36**:173–7.

155. Janssen Pharmaceutica Products LP. Itraconazole package insert (United States). Titusville, New Jersey, USA: Janssen Pharmaceutica, 2002.

156. Novartis Pharmaceutical Corporation. Terbinafine package insert (United States). East Hanover, New Jersey, USA: 2001.

157. Billstein S, Kianifard F, Justice A. Terbinafine *v.* placebo for onychomycosis in black patients. *Int J Dermatol* 1999;**38**:377–9.

158. Svejgaard EL, Brandrup F, Kragballe K *et al.* Oral terbinafine in toenail dermatophytosis. A double-blind, placebo-controlled multicenter study with 12 months' follow-up. *Acta Derm Venereol* 1997;**77**:66–9.

159. Watson A, Marley J, Ellis D, Williams T. Terbinafine in onychomycosis of the toenail: a novel treatment protocol. *J Am Acad Dermatol* 1995;**33**:775–9.

160. Heikkila H, Stubb S. Long-term results in patients with onychomycosis treated with terbinafine or itraconazole. *Br J Dermatol* 2002;**146**:250–3.

161. Sigurgeirsson B, Olafsson JH, Steinsson JB *et al.* Long-term effectiveness of treatment with terbinafine *v* itraconazole in onychomycosis: a 5–year blinded prospective follow-up study. *Arch Dermatol* 2002;**138**:353–7.

162. Havu V, Heikkila H, Kuokkanen K *et al.* A double-blind, randomized study to compare the efficacy and safety of terbinafine (Lamisil) with fluconazole (Diflucan) in the treatment of onychomycosis. *Br J Dermatol* 2000; **142**:97–102.

163. De Backer M, De Vroey C, Lesaffre E *et al.* Twelve weeks of continuous oral therapy for toenail onychomycosis caused by dermatophytes: a double-blind comparative trial of terbinafine 250 mg/day versus itraconazole 200 mg/day. *J Am Acad Dermatol* 1998;**38**:S57–63.

164. Honeyman JF, Talarico FS, Arruda LHF *et al.* Itraconazole versus terbinafine (LAMISIL): which is better for the treatment of onychomycosis? *J Eur Acad Dermatol Venereol* 1997;**9**:215–21.

165. Degreef H, del Palacio A, Mygind S *et al.* Randomized double-blind comparison of short-term itraconazole and terbinafine therapy for toenail onychomycosis. *Acta Derm Venereol* 1999;**79**:221–3.

166. Brautigam M, Nolting S, Schopf RE, Weidinger G. Randomised double blind comparison of terbinafine and itraconazole for treatment of toenail tinea infection. Seventh Lamisil German Onychomycosis Study Group. *BMJ* 1995;**311**:919–22.

167. De Backer M, De Keyser P, Massart DL, Westelinck KJ. Terbinafine (Lamisil) 250 mg/day and 500 mg/day are

equally effective in a 16 week oral treatment of toenail onychomycosis. A double-blind multicentre trial. In: Hay RJ, ed. *International Perspective on Lamisil. London: CCT Healthcare Communications*,1994;39–43.

168. Arca E, Tastan HB, Akar A *et al*. An open, randomized, comparative study of oral fluconazole, itraconazole and terbinafine therapy in onychomycosis. *J Dermatol Treat* 2002;**13**:3–9.

169. Tosti A, Piraccini BM, Stinchi C *et al*. Treatment of dermatophyte nail infections: an open randomized study comparing intermittent terbinafine therapy with continuous terbinafine treatment and intermittent itraconazole therapy. *J Am Acad Dermatol* 1996;**34**: 595–600.

170. Alpsoy E, Yilmaz E, Basaran E. Intermittent therapy with terbinafine for dermatophyte toe-onychomycosis: a new approach. *J Dermatol* 1996;**23**:259–62.

171. Kejda J. Itraconazole pulse therapy *v* continuous terbinafine dosing for toenail onychomycosis. *Postgrad Med* 1999;**Spec no.**:12–15.

172. Gupta AK, Shear NH. Safety review of the oral antifungal agents used to treat superficial mycoses. *Int J Dermatol* 1999;**38**(Suppl. 2):40–52.

173. Katz HI, Gupta AK. Oral antifungal drug interactions. *Dermatol Clin* 1997;**15**:535–44.

174. Gupta AK, Katz HI, Shear N. Drug interactions with itraconazole, fluconazole and terbinafine and their management. *Int J Dermatol* 1999;**41**(2 Pt 1):237–49.

175. Novartis Pharmaceuticals Canada. Terbinafine package insert (Canada). Dorval, Quebec: Novartis Pharmaceuticals Canada, 2001.

176. Ryder NS. Terbinafine: mode of action and properties of the squalene epoxidase inhibition. *Br J Dermatol* 1992;**126**(Suppl. 39):2–7.

177. Haugh M, Helou S, Boissel JP, Cribier BJ. Terbinafine in fungal infections of the nails: a meta-analysis of randomized clinical trials. *Br J Dermatol* 2002;**147**: 118–21.

178. Crawford F, Young P, Godfrey C *et al*. Oral treatments for toenail onychomycosis: a systematic review. *Arch Dermatol* 2002;**138**:811–16.

179. Odom RB, Aly R, Scher RK *et al*. A multicenter, placebo-controlled, double-blind study of intermittent therapy with itraconazole for the treatment of onychomycosis of the fingernail. *J Am Acad Dermatol* 1997;**36**:231–5.

180. Gupta AK, Maddin S, Arlette J *et al*. Itraconazole pulse therapy is effective in dermatophyte onychomycosis of the toenail: a double-blind placebo-controlled study. *J Dermatol Treat* 2000;**11**:33–7.

181. Havu V, Brandt H, Heikkila H *et al*. A double-blind, randomized study comparing itraconazole pulse therapy with continuous dosing for the treatment of toe-nail onychomycosis. *Br J Dermatol* 1997;**136**:230–4.

182. Ginter G, De Doncker P. An intermittent itraconazole 1–week dosing regimen for the treatment of toenail onychomycosis in dermatological practice. *Mycoses* 1998;**41**:235–8.

183. Shemer A, Nathansohn N, Kaplan B *et al*. Open randomized comparison of different itraconazole regimens for the treatment of onychomycosis. *J Dermatol Treat* 1999;**10**:245–9.

184. De Doncker P, Decroix J, Pierard GE *et al*. Antifungal pulse therapy for onychomycosis. A pharmacokinetic and pharmacodynamic investigation of monthly cycles of 1–week pulse therapy with itraconazole. *Arch Dermatol* 1996;**132**:34–41.

185. Gupta AK, De Doncker P, Scher RK *et al*. Itraconazole for the treatment of onychomycosis. *Int J Dermatol* 1998;**37**:303–8.

186. Gupta AK, Albreski D, Del Rosso JQ, Konnikov N. The use of the new oral antifungal agents, itraconazole, terbinafine, and fluconazole to treat onychomycosis and other dermatomycoses. *Curr Prob Dermatol* 2001;**13**:213–48.

187. Janssen Pharmaceutica. Itraconazole package insert (Canada). Toronto, Canada: Janssen Pharmaceutica, 2001.

188. De Doncker P, Gupta AK, Cel Rosso JQ *et al*. Safety of itraconazole pulse therapy for onychomycosis. An update. *Postgrad Med J* 1999;**Spec no.**:17–25.

189. De Doncker P, Gupta AK. Itraconazole and terbinafine in perspective. From petri dish to patient. *Postgrad Med J* 1999;**Spec no.**:6–11.

190. De Doncker P, Gupta AK, Marynissen G *et al*. Itraconazole pulse therapy for onychomycosis and dermatomycoses: an overview. *J Am Acad Dermatol* 1997;**37**:969–74.

191. Elewski BE, Scher RK, Aly R *et al*. Double-blind, randomized comparison of itraconazole capsules *v*. placebo in the treatment of toenail onychomycosis. *Cutis* 1997;**59**:217–20.

192. Jones HE, Zaias N. Double-blind, randomized comparison of itraconazole capsules and placebo in onychomycosis of toenail. *Int J Dermatol* 1996;**35**: 589–90.

193. Odom R, Daniel CR, Aly R. A double-blind, randomized comparison of itraconazole capsules and placebo in the treatment of onychomycosis of the toenail. *J Am Acad Dermatol* 1996;**35**:110–11.

194. Gupta AK, Scher RK, Rich P. Fluconazole for the treatment of onychomycosis: an update. *Int J Dermatol* 1998;**37**:815–20.

195. Jansen R, Redekop WK, Rutten FF. Cost effectiveness of continuous terbinafine compared with intermittent itraconazole in the treatment of dermatophyte toenail onychomycosis: an analysis of based on results from the L.I.ON. study. Lamisil versus Itraconazole in Onychomycosis. *Pharmacoeconomics* 2001;**19**:401–10.

196. Gupta AK. Pharmacoeconomic analysis of oral antifungal therapies used to treat dermatophyte onychomycosis of the toenails. A US analysis. *Pharmacoeconomics* 1998;**13**:243–56.

197. Marchetti A, Piech CT, McGhan WF *et al.* Pharmacoeconomic analysis of oral therapies for onychomycosis: a US model. *Clin Ther* 1996;**18**:757–77.

198. Arikian SR, Einarson TR, Kobelt-Nguyen G, Schubert F. A multinational pharmacoeconomic analysis of oral therapies for onychomycosis. The Onychomycosis Study Group. *Br J Dermatol* 1994;**130**(Suppl. 43): 35–44.

199. Einarson TR, Arikian SR, Shear NH. Cost-effectiveness analysis for onychomycosis therapy in Canada from a government perspective. *Br J Dermatol* 1994;**130**(Suppl. 43):32–4.

200. Gupta AK, Baran R. Ciclopirox nail lacquer solution 8% in the 21st century. *J Am Acad Dermatol* 2000;**43**: S96–102.

201. Roberts DT, Evans EG. Subungual dermatophytoma complicating dermatophyte onychomycosis. *Br J Dermatol* 1998;**138**:189–90.

202. Gupta AK. Are boosters or supplementation of antifungal drugs of any use for treating onychomycosis? *J Drugs Dermatol* 2002;**1**:35–41.

34
Tinea capitis

Urbà González

Background
Definition

Tinea capitis (scalp ringworm) is an infection of the scalp skin and hair caused by fungi (dermatophyte) mainly of the genera *Trichophyton* and *Microsporum*. The clinical hallmark is single or multiple patches of hair loss, sometimes with a "black dot" pattern (Figure 34.1), which may be accompanied by signs of inflammation such as scaling, pustules and itching.[1,2]

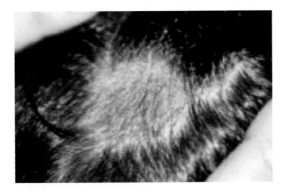

Figure 34.1   Tinea capitis

Incidence/prevalence[3,4]

Tinea capitis is uncommon in adults and it is seen predominantly in prepubertal children. It has affected mainly disadvantaged communities in both developing and industrialised nations. During the past 30 years some significant changes have occurred in the reported incidences of tinea capitis. Travel and migration have led to changes in the epidemiology of the species of dermatophyte causing tinea capitis.

Aetiology[5,6]

Tinea capitis is contagious. It can be acquired through contact with people, animals or objects carrying the fungus. The presence of fungi within the scalp may not be sufficient to result in tinea capitis (carrier state). Approximately eight dermatophyte species are characteristically associated with tinea capitis. Infections due to *Trichophyton tonsurans* predominate from Central America to the United States and in parts of Western Europe. *Microsporum canis* infections are mainly seen in South America, Southern and Eastern Europe, Africa and the Middle East. Reported cases of kerion (inflammatory tinea capitis) are rare outside Africa.

Prognosis

Tinea capitis is not life threatening in people with normal immunity. Untreated cases cause persistent symptoms and in some types of tinea capitis, mainly the inflammatory type or kerion, may lead to scarring alopecia.

Diagnostic tests[7–9]

The clinical diagnosis should be confirmed by mycological examination. The main methods of collecting samples for microbiological diagnosis involve either scraping or brushing the scalp. Microscopy provides the most rapid means of diagnosis and allows treatment to commence, but is not always positive. Culture allows accurate identification of the organism involved and may be positive even when microscopy is negative but may take up to 4 weeks. Wood's light or filtered ultraviolet light can be used to identify infections that fluoresce under this type of light such as *M. canis* and *M. audounii*, but not *T. tonsurans*.

Aims of treatment[10–15]

The first aim of treatment is to achieve complete clinical and mycological cure as quickly as possible, with no or minimal adverse effects. Effective short-course therapy is especially desirable in children, because prolonged therapy increases the risk of adverse effects as well as non-compliance. Another goal is prevention of spread to other children from objects, infected animals or children and from asymptomatic carriers.

Relevant outcomes

Outcomes are based on resolution of clinical signs (redness, scaling, oedema and hair loss) and symptoms (itch), and negative mycological data including microscopy and culture. Complete cure (clinical and mycological cure), cure (clinical or mycological cure), improvement (clinical) and failure (ineffective therapy or worsening) are the most widely used outcomes.

Methods of search

Controlled clinical trials and other relevant information were located by searching the *Cochrane Library* (March 2001), Medline (1966–2001) and Embase (1988–2001). I included all randomised controlled trials (RCTs) that met quality criteria but because of the limited studies available for some questions; studies with shortcomings in the methods were also included, which I mention in the text.

Systemic antifungal therapy for tinea capitis in children

Griseofulvin has been the most widely used and the most prescribed treatment for tinea capitis and has served as a standard for the evaluation of any newer agent to be considered for this infection. New drugs being used against other fungal infections in adults, such as ketoconazole, itraconazole, terbinafine and fluconazole, are being considered more frequently for the treatment of tinea capitis. Sufficient pharmacological and pharmaceutical data exist on these five antifungal drugs to make them suitable for treating tinea capitis in children.[16,17]

QUESTIONS

In children with tinea capitis, which oral antifungal drug leads to high rates of cure with the fewest adverse events?

Griseofulvin

There is moderate RCT evidence that griseofulvin at doses of 125–500 mg/day (according to patient's weight) for 6–8 weeks is effective and safe for the treatment of tinea capitis caused by *T. tonsurans*, *T. violaceum* and *M. canis*.

Efficacy

I found no systematic review. I found nine RCTs comparing griseofulvin with other oral antifungals in tinea capitis (Table 34.1).

Versus ketoconazole

I found four RCTs. In two RCTs[18,19] where *T. tonsurans* was the most commonly isolated organism, griseofulvin at doses of 10–20 mg/kg/day[18] and 250–500 mg/day[19] were compared with ketoconazole 3·3–6·6 mg/kg/day[18] and 200 mg/day,[19] for 12 and 6 weeks, respectively. There were no statistically significant differences between the mycological cure rate of the two drugs. Cure rates in the griseofulvin groups at the end of treatment were 96%[18] and 57·1%.[19] A small RCT[20] of 47 children compared griseofulvin 350 mg/day for 6 weeks with ketoconazole 100 mg/day for 6 weeks in inflammatory tinea capitis (*T. mentagrophytes* and *M. canis*). At the end of treatment, 80% and 100% of children respectively had improved clinically, but no mycological data were reported. An RCT of unknown blinding[21] done in 63 children where *Trichophyton* spp. predominated, compared griseofulvin 15 mg/kg/day with ketoconazole 5 mg/kg/day, each given as a single daily dose, and treatment stopped when there was complete cure or after 6 months. After 8 weeks' therapy 92% of the patients given griseofulvin had complete cure of their infection compared with only 59% of ketoconazole-treated patients. After 12 weeks 96% of griseofulvin patients were mycologically cured compared with 74% of the ketoconazole-treated group. Hair sample cultures took significantly longer to become sterile in ketoconazole-treated (median 8 weeks) than in griseofulvin-treated (4 weeks) patients.

Versus itraconazole

I found one RCT[22] done in 34 children where the majority of fungal organisms were *M. canis*, comparing 6 weeks of ultramicrosized griseofulvin 500 mg/day and itraconazole 100 mg/day and a follow up of 14 weeks that showed a complete cure rate of 88% for the two drugs.

Versus terbinafine

I found four RCTs. A double-blind RCT[23] compared 140 children from Pakistan, of whom 87 had *T. violaceum* tinea capitis. They were treated with either terbinafine (by weight) for 4 weeks or with griseofulvin 6–12 mg/kg/day for 8 weeks. After 12 weeks, 93% of the terbinafine

group were completely cured compared with 80% of the griseofulvin group; not a significant difference. A double-blind RCT[24] evaluated 50 children from Peru, 74% of whom had *T. tonsurans* infections. Half were treated with terbinafine according to weight, for 4 weeks plus 4 weeks with placebo; the other half received microsized griseofulvin according to weight for 8 weeks. After 8 weeks of treatment, complete cure was noted in 76% of the griseofulvin group and in 72% of terbinafine group, but 4 weeks later the complete cure rate increased to 76% in the terbinafine group but in the griseofulvin group it had fallen to 44%, a statistically significant difference. In a large RCT,[25] *T. tonsurans* accounted for 77% of the terbinafine group and 88% of the griseofulvin group; *Microsporum* spp. accounted for 14% of both groups. The RCT compared 8 weeks of griseofulvin suspension 10 mg/kg/day with 4 weeks of terbinafine. Complete cure rates at week 24 were 64% with terbinafine and 67% with griseofulvin – no significant difference. However, there was a trend to better responses in *Microsporum* spp. infections with 8 weeks of griseofulvin than with 4 weeks of terbinafine. In another RCT[26] the complete cure rate at the final follow up visit (week 12) was 74% in the group treated with 8 weeks' ultramicrosized griseofulvin, compared with 78% of the group treated with 4 weeks' terbinafine, with no significant differences between *M. canis* and *Trichophyton* spp. infections.

Drawbacks

Two patients had nausea and intense stomach ache with severe vomiting at weeks 2 and 4 of treatment and required discontinuation of therapy.[22] One griseofulvin-treated patient showed a two fold increase in serum alanine aminotransferase and aspartate aminotransferase after 3 weeks of treatment but values returned to normal at the following weekly clinic visit.[20]

The following adverse events have been described as of uncertain relationship with the study drug: skin infections, skin infestations, raised hepatic enzymes, raised triglycerides, raised uric acid, anaemia, eosinophilia, leucocytosis and granulocytopenia.[26,27] In the largest RCT,[25] a total of 52 adverse events were detected in 27 patients in the griseofulvin group and including abdominal discomfort and vomiting. None was rated as severe but one patient was withdrawn from the study because of abdominal pain, headaches and vomiting. In other studies no, or no significant, adverse effects were reported.[18,19,21,23,24]

Comment

A study published as an RCT[28] was excluded because it was still in progress and the codes about concealment of randomisation had not yet been broken. Another study described as an RCT[29] was excluded because it gave no separate clinical and mycological data for each group. I found two RCTs[27,30] that were duplicate publications of other studies.[23,24] I think that all the other studies included are relevant in showing the efficacy of griseofulvin for tinea capitis, even though the definition of cure varies from study to study, and some investigators carefully follow microbiological findings, whereas others place greater emphasis on clinical response. The high patient dropout rate in most of the studies may have masked the improvement in griseofulvin groups as those who achieve cure may have less incentive to attend follow up visits. It will also have reduced the power to detect a difference between the groups, indicating that griseofulvin may be even more effective. Duration of follow up varies from study to study (6–24 weeks) and only RCTs with long-term follow up can show the relapse rates, which are very important in determining therapeutic efficacy. Five of nine studies were supported by the pharmaceutical industry.[18–20,22,25]

Ketoconazole versus griseofulvin

Data from some RCTs.[18,21] indicate that ketoconazole may require a longer course of therapy than griseofulvin and it had no better cure rates. However, while ketoconazole is associated with rare but important hepatic and endocrine adverse events, none of these were noted in the paediatric studies described. Because oral itraconazole now exists and the safety of long-term use of oral ketoconazole is uncertain, I have not considered the latter further as a treatment of choice in children with tinea capitis. Three[18–20] of the four RCTs with ketoconazole described in Table 34.1 were supported by companies producing this drug.

Implications for practice

There is good evidence to support the use of griseofulvin to treat tinea capitis caused by *T. tonsurans*, *M. canis*, *T. mentagrophytes* and *T. violaceum*. Overall, griseofulvin is considered to be safe in children. On the basis of the RCTs described, the recommended dosage regimen for children is continuous therapy with tablets or suspension, adjusted according to patient weight (10–20 kg: 125 mg/day; 20–40 kg: 250 mg/day; >40 kg: 500 mg/day) for 6–8 weeks, including microsized and ultramicrosized preparations. Other advantages of griseofulvin are that it is inexpensive and that the suspension allows accurate dosage in children. As far as I know it is licensed for tinea capitis in most countries.[30]

Terbinafine

Moderate RCT evidence indicates that terbinafine at doses of 62·5–250 mg/day (according to body weight) for 2 weeks in *T. violaceum* infections and for 4 weeks in *T. tonsurans* infections, is effective and safe for the treatment of *Trichophyton* spp. tinea capitis. A few RCTs (limited evidence) suggest that longer therapeutic regimens of 6 weeks may be necessary to treat *Microsporum* spp. infections.

Efficacy

I found no systematic reviews but five RCTs comparing terbinafine with other oral antifungals in tinea capitis (Table 34.1).

Versus griseofulvin

I found four RCTs. A double-blind RCT[23,27] compared 140 children from Pakistan, 87% of whom had *T. violaceum* infection. They were treated with either terbinafine 62·5–250 mg/day by weight for 4 weeks, or with griseofulvin, 125–500 mg/day according to patient's weight, for 8 weeks. Four weeks after the conclusion of the study 93% of the terbinafine group were completely cured, compared with 80% in the griseofulvin group, a statistically non-significant difference. A double-blind RCT study[24,30] evaluated 50 children from Lima, Peru, 74% of whom had *T. tonsurans* infection. Half received terbinafine, 62·5–250 mg/day for 4 weeks, the other half griseofulvin, 125–500 mg/day for 8 weeks; dosage was according to body weight. At the end of week 8, 76% of the terbinafine group and 80% of the griseofulvin group showed complete cure. However, 4 weeks later the 76% cure rate in the terbinafine group was sustained, whereas in the griseofulvin group the cure rate had decreased to 44%. An RCT[26] compared ultramicrosized griseofulvin for 8 weeks with terbinafine for 4 weeks, both dosed according to body weight. At the final follow up visit at week 12, 88% of the terbinafine-treated group was mycologically cured, compared with 91% of the griseofulvin-treated group; complete cure was reported in 78% and 74% of patients, respectively. *Trichophyton* spp. and *M. canis* responded similarly to terbinafine. A large RCT[25] compared griseofulvin suspension 10 mg/kg/day for 8 weeks with terbinafine for 4 weeks. *T. tonsurans* infection accounted for 65% of the

terbinafine group and 73% of the griseofulvin group; 14% of each group had *Microsporum* spp. infection. At week 24, 4 weeks of terbinafine (complete cure rate: 64%) was at least as effective as 8 weeks of griseofulvin (complete cure rate: 67%). However, the *Microsporum* spp. infections tended to do better with 8 weeks of griseofulvin than with 4 weeks of terbinafine.

Versus itraconazole

One RCT[32] compared 2-week courses of terbinafine, 62·5–250 mg, and itraconazole, 50–200 mg (both according to weight). Twelve weeks after the start of treatment, 78% and 86% patients were completely cured in the terbinafine and itraconazole groups, respectively. *T. violaceum* was the major pathogen in both groups, and there were no *Microsporum* spp. infections.

Different terbinafine regimens compared

I found four RCTs (Table 34.1). One RCT[33] compared 1, 2 and 4 weeks of terbinafine therapy, 62·5–250 mg according to weight. The cure rate was 74% after 1 week of therapy, 80% after 2 weeks and 86% after 4 weeks. However, this study included no griseofulvin control group; 71% of patients had *T. violaceum* infections. A second RCT[34] compared 1, 2 and 4 weeks of terbinafine, 62·5–250 mg according to weight, in 79 children and three adults with *T. tonsurans* and *M. ferruginieum* tinea capitis. At week 12, the complete cure rate was 33·3% in the 1-week therapy group, 42·9% in the 2-week therapy group and 63% in the 4-week group. An RCT[35] published in two additional abstracts,[36,37] compared 1 and 2 weeks of terbinafine, 62·5–250 mg according to weight. At week 12 of follow up, in *Trichophyton* spp. infections the complete cure rate was 56% with 1 week of therapy and 86% with 2 weeks, but acceptable cure rates in *M. canis* infection were achieved only after an additional 4 weeks of treatment. An

Table 34.1 Data from all RCTs found comparing oral antifungals or differents doses of the same antifungal in tinea capitis

Study	Trial design, sample size, study population and types of fungus isolated	Interventions	Time of follow up, quality of reporting, dropouts and comments	Outcome measures Adverse effects
Tanz *et al.* 1985[19] USA (Chicago)	Double-blind, randomised. 22 children 2–16 years old **Griseofulvin group:** *T. tonsurans* 57·8% (7/12). **Ketoconazole group:** *T. tonsurans* 40% (4/10); *Penicillium* spp. 10% (1/10); *Scopulariopsis* spp 10% (1/10); unidentified fungus 10% (1/10)	**Griseofulvin** tablet, 500 mg/day, plus "ketoconazole" placebo tablet (patients <40 kg: half tablet) for **6 weeks** n = 12 **Ketoconazole** tablet, 200 mg/day, plus "griseofulvin" placebo tablet (patients weighting <40 kg: half tablet) for **6 weeks** n = 10 Co-treatment: antiseborrhoeic shampoo	**Follow up: 6 weeks** Described as randomised Some description of method of blinding, no ITT analysis **Dropouts:** 5 in griseofulvin group and 3 in ketoconazole group did not complete the study Compliance assessed Supported by Janssen (ketoconazole)	**Mycological cure rates:** griseofulvin group: 57·1% (4/7); ketoconazole group: 57·1% (4/7) **Clinical cure:** In both groups, total severity score decreased similarly during the course of the study **Complete cure:** not reported **Adverse effects:** 0 in griseofulvin group; ketoconazole group: 2 mild abdominal pain, 1 urticaria (concomitantly receiving penicillin)
Gan *et al.* 1987[21] USA (Dallas)	Unknown blinding, randomised 80 children 2·1–11 years old *T. tonsurans* 70% (42/60); *M. canis* 11·6% (7/60); *T. mentagrophytes* 1·6% (1/60); *T. violaceum* 1·6% (1/60); uncertain classification 15% (9/60)	**Griseofulvin** tablet or suspension, 15 mg/kg/day, single daily dose; **2–6 weeks** depending on the patient's clinical response to therapy n = 40 **Ketoconazole** tablet or crushed tablets suspended in sucrose syrup, 5 mg/kg/day, single daily dose **2–6 weeks** depending on the patient's clinical response to therapy n = 40 No co-treatment	**Follow up: 26 weeks** Method of randomisation: table of random numbers No mention of blinding No ITT analysis **Dropouts:** 11 of griseofulvin group and 6 of ketoconazole group failed to keep follow up visits Compliance assessed No mention of industry funding	**Mycological cure rates at week 12:** griseofulvin group: 96%; 1 reversion to negative between 12 and 26 weeks; ketoconazole group: 74%; 6 reversions to negative between 12 and 26 weeks **Clinical cure:** not reported **Complete cure rates at week 8:** 92% in griseofulvin group; 59% in ketoconazole group **None reported**

(Continued)

Table 34.1 (*Continued*)

Study	Trial design, sample size, study population and types of fungus isolated	Interventions	Time of follow up, quality of reporting, dropouts and comments	Outcome measures Adverse effects
Tanz et al. 1988[18] USA (Chicago)	Double-blind, randomised 48 children 2–16 years old T. tonsurans (64%) M. canis (12%)	**Griseofulvin** (micros ze) 250 mg tablet (10–20 mg/kg/ day) plus "ketoconazole" placebo tablet, single daily dose, for **12 weeks** n = 26 **Ketoconazole** 200 mg tablet (3.3–6.6 mg/kg/day) plus "griseofulvin" placebo tablet in a single daily dose for **12 weeks** n = 22 Co-treatment: antiseborrhoeic shampoos	**Follow up:** 12 weeks Method of randomisation: coded list, clear description of method of blinding No ITT analysis **Dropouts:** 7 of ketoconazole group; 16 of griseofulvin group failed to return for follow up visit Compliance not assessed Supported by Janssen (ketoconazole)	**Mycological cure rates at week 12:** griseofulvin group: 96%; ketoconazole group: 89% **Clinical cure at week 12:** Patients in both treatment groups showed significan: improvement in their severity score with no statistically significant differences **Complete cure rates at weeks 12:** griseofulvin group: 95.15%; ketoconazole group: 72·72% **Adverse effects:** griseofulvin group: none reported ; ketoconazole group: 1 with nausea
Martinez-Roig et al. 1988[20] Spain (Barcelona)	Double-blind, randomised 47 children 2–16 years old with tinea but only 13 affected by tinea capitis, all with the inflammatory type **Ketoconazole group:** T. mentagrophytes, M. canis, E. floccossum (no distinction between tinea capitis and tinea corporis) **Griseofulvin group:** T. mentagrophytes, M. canis, M. gypseum (no distinction between tinea capitis and tinea corporis)	**Griseofulvin** tablet, 350 mg/day, at 12-hourly intervals for **6 weeks** n = 5 **Ketoconazole** tablet, 100 mg/day at 12-hourly intervals for **6 weeks** n = 8 Co-treatment: manual depilation in cases of inflammatory tinea capitis	**Follow up:** 6 weeks Method of randomisation: computer-generated random number table Described as double blind No ITT analysis **Dropouts:** none in patients with tinea capitis Compliance assessed Supported by Laboratorios Dr Esteve (ketoconazole)	**Mycological cure rates:** not reported **Clinical cure rates at week 6:** griseofulvin group: 80% (4/5) improved; 20% (1/5) deteriorated; ketoconazole group: 100% (8/8) improved **Other outcomes:** Mean time to clinical cure (weeks): griseofulvin group: 5; ketoconazole group: 4·2; mean time to negative culture (weeks): griseofulvin group 4·7; ketoconazole group 3·6 **Complete cure:** not reported **Adverse effects:** griseofulvin group: one patient with reversible two fold increase in serum alanine aminotransferase and aspartate aminotransferase after 3 weeks' treatment; ketoconazole group: none reported

(Continued)

Table 34.1 (Continued)

Study	Trial design, sample size, study population and types of fungus isolated	Interventions	Time of follow up, quality of reporting, dropouts and comments	Outcome measures Adverse effects
Alvi et al. 1993[23] Pakistan (Karachi, Lahore)	Double-blind, randomised 140 subjects 2–65 years (90% children <12 years old)	Griseofulvin capsules, 10–20 kg: 125 mg/day; 20–40 kg: 250 mg/day; >40 kg: 500 mg/day) once daily for 8 weeks n = 68	Follow up: 12 weeks. Described as randomised Described as double blind No ITT analysis Dropouts: 16 patients from the	**Mycological cure rates at weeks 12:** griseofulvin group: 87·75% (43/49); terbinafine group: 92·86% (52/56) **Clinical cure scores at week 12:** griseofulvin group: 0·76; terbinafine group: 0·46 (where 0 = absent; 1 = mild; 2 = moderate; 3 = severe)
Duplicate publication Haroon et al. 1995[27] Pakistan (Lahore, Karachi)	**Griseofulvin group:** T. violaceum 89·8% (44/49); T. verrucosum 8·2% (4/49); T. tonsurans 2% (1/49) **Terbinafine group:** T. violaceum 86% (48/56); T. verrucosum 5·3% (3/56); T. tonsurans 5·3% (3/56); T. rubrum 5·3% (1/5); M. audouinii 5·3% (1/56)	**Terbinafine** capsules, 10–20 kg: 62·5 mg/day; 20–40 kg: 125 mg/day; >40 kg: 250 mg/day) once daily for 4 weeks plus 4 weeks of placebo n = 72 No co-treatment	terbinafine group and 19 patients from griseofulvin group withdrawn because of irregularities in follow up No mention of compliance assessments. Supported by Sandoz (terbinafine)	**Complete cure rates at week 12:** griseofulvin group: 79·59% (39/49); terbinafine group: 92·86% (52/56) **Adverse effects:** mostly of uncertain relationship and/or of no relationship to drugs: griseofulvin group: 1 cutaneous infection; 1 cutaneous infestation; 1 raised hepatic enzymes; 5 raised triglycerides; 1 raised uric acid; 1 eosinophilia; 1 leucocytosis; 1 granulocytopenia; terbinafine group: 1 tonsillitis; 1 cutaneous infestation; 2 raised hepatic enzymes; 1 raised triglycerides; 3 eosinophilia
Memişoğlu et al. 1999[26] Turkey (Adana. Izmir, Ankara)	Double-blind, randomised, parallel group 78 children 2–13 years old **Griseofulvin group:** T. violaceum 11·4% (4/35); T. rubrum 22·8% (8/35); M. canis 48·5% (17/35); T. tonsurans 5·7% (2/35); T. mentagrophytes 5·7% (2/35); T. verrucosum 5·7% (2/35) **Terbinafine group:** T. violaceum 15·6% (5/32); T. rubrum 15·6% (5/32); M. canis 46·8% (15/32);	Griseofulvin (ultramicrosized), 10–20 kg: 125 mg/day; 20–40 kg: 250 mg/day; >40 kg: 500 mg/day) for 8 weeks n = 39 **Terbinafine,** 10–20 kg: 62·5 mg/day; 20–40 kg: 125 mg/day; >40 kg: 250 mg/day) for 4 weeks plus 4 weeks of placebo n = 39 No co-treatment	Follow up: 12 weeks Described as randomised Described as double blind No ITT analysis Dropouts: 7 in terbinafine group and 4 in griseofulvin group No mention of compliance assessment No mention of industry support	**Mycological cure rates at week 12:** griseofulvin group: 91·4% (32/35); terbinafine group: 87·5% (28/32) **Clinical cure scores at week 12:** griseofulvin group: 1·2; terbinafine group: 1·2; clinical signs and symptoms, including erythema, oedema, pruritus, hair loss and desquamation scored on a scale where 0 = none, 1 = mild, 2 = moderate, 3 = severe **Complete cure rates at week 12:** griseofulvin group: M. canis 71% (12/17); Trichophyton spp. 78% (14/18); terbinafine group: M. canis 87% (13/15); Trichophyton spp. 73% (11/15) **Adverse effects:** griseofulvin group: 1 elevated aspartate aminotransferase; 1 elevated triglycerides; 2 anaemia (of uncertain drug relationship): terbinafine group: 1 mild elevated triglycerides (of uncertain drug relationship)

(Continued)

Table 34.1 (Continued)

Study	Trial design, sample size, study population and types of fungus isolated	Interventions	Time of follow up, quality of reporting, dropouts and comments	Outcome measures / Adverse effects
	T. tonsurans 6·25% (2/32); *T. mentagrophytes* 3·1% (1/32); *T. verrucosum* 3·1% (1/32); *M. audouinii* 3·1% (1/32); unidentified 6·25% (2/32)			
Cáceres-Rios *et al.* 2000[24] Peru (Lima) See abstract[30]	Double-blind, randomised 50 children 1–14 years old with non-inflammatory tinea capitis **Griseofulvin group:** *T. tonsurans* 84% (21/25); *M. canis* 16% (4/25) **Terbinafine group:** *T. tonsurans* 64% (16/25); *M. canis* 36% (9/25)	**Griseofulvin** (microsized) tablet, 10–20kg; 125 mg/day; 20–40kg: 250 mg/day; >40 kg:500 mg/day, once a day for **8 weeks** *n* = 25 **Terbinafine** tablet, 10–20 kg: 62·5 mg/day; 20–40 kg: 125 mg/day; >40 kg: 250 mg/day) once a day for **4 weeks plus 4 weeks of placebo** n = 25 No co-treatment	**Follow up:** 12 weeks Described as "alternately randomised" Described as double blind No ITT analysis **Dropouts:** one patient withdrew with viral hepatitis (group not mentioned) No mention of compliance assessment No mention of industry support	**Mycological cure rates at week 12:** griseofulvin group: 44%; terbinafine group: 76% **Clinical cure at week 12:** Statistically significant differences between treatment groups at end of week 12 **Complete cure rates at week 12:** griseofulvin group: 44%; terbinafine group: 76% **Adverse effects:** minimal side-effects such as gastric upset and nausea reported in both groups in 4% of patients, but it was not necessary to discontinue therapy
Fuller *et al.* 2001[25] UK (London)	Open, randomised, parallel group 210 children 2–16 years old **Griseofulvin group** *T. tonsurans* 73%, other *Trichophyton* spp. 10%, *Microsporum* spp. 14%	**Griseofulvin** suspension, 10 mg/kg/day, for **8 weeks** n = 107 **Terbinafine** tablet, <20 kg: 62·5 mg/day; 20–40 kg: 125 mg/day; >40kg: 250 mg/ day) for **4 weeks** n = 103	**Follow up:** 24 weeks Method of randomisation: computer-generated; patients randomised in blocks of four Described as open ITT analysis **Dropouts:** 26 patients from	**Mycological cure rates at week 24:** griseofulvin group: 72%; terbinafine group: 70% *Clinical cure rates:* No statistically significant difference in clinical response between treatment groups at weeks 4, 8, 12 and 24 **Complete cure rates at week 24:** griseofulvin group: 67%; terbinafire group: 34%

(Continued)

Table 34.1 (Continued)

Study	Trial design, sample size, study population and types of fungus isolated	Interventions	Time of follow up, quality of reporting, dropouts and comments	Outcome measures / Adverse effects
	Terbinafine group: T. tonsurans 65%, other Trichophyton spp. 19.5%, Microsporum spp. 14%	Co-treatment: selenium sulphide shampoo, twice weekly for the first 2 weeks of treatment	terbinafine group: 37 from griseofulvin group excluded from ITT analysis. Compliance assessed by direct questioning. Supported by Novartis (terbinafine)	**Adverse effects:** griseofulvin group: 52 adverse events in 27 patients: abdominal discomfort and vomiting; 1 withdrawn (abdominal pain, headaches and vomiting); terbinafine group 57 adverse events in 36 patients: pruritus, urticaria and skin scaling; 4 withdrawn (vomiting, dizziness, urticaria and weight loss)
López-Gómez, et al. 1994[22] Spain (Madrid)	Double-blind, randomised; 34 children <12 years; 1 adult. Itraconazole group: M. canis 88.8% (16/18); T. mentagrophytes 5.5% (1/18); T. tonsurans 5.5% (1/18); Griseofulvin group: M. canis 94.1% (16/17); T. violaceum 5.9% (1/17)	Itraconazole 100 mg/day for 6 weeks n = 18; Griseofulvin (ultramicrosized) 500 mg/day for **6 weeks** n = 17; No co-treatment	**Follow up:** 14 weeks; Described as randomised; Described as double blind; No ITT analysis; **Dropouts:** 1 in itraconazole group; 2 patients in griseofulvin group because of adverse events; No mention of compliance assessment; Supported by Janssen (Itraconazole)	**Mycological cure rates at week 14:** itraconazole group: 76·47% (13/17);griseofulvin group: 78·57% (11/14); **Clinical cure at week 14:** Total combined symptom severity score decreased by 9% in the itraconazole group and by 7% in the griseofulvin group; **Complete cure rates at week 14:** itraconazole group: 88·23% (15/17); griseofulvin group: 88·23% (15/17); **Adverse effects:** griseofulvin group: nausea; intense stomach ache with severe vomiting; itraconazole group: none reported
Jahangir et al. 1998[32] Pakistan (Lahore)	Double-blind, randomised; 60 children any age: >10 kg. Itraconazole group: T. violaceum 82·1% (23/28); T. tonsurans 7·1% (2/28); T. mentagrophytes 7·1% (2/28); T. verrucosum 3·6% (1/28)	Itraconazole, <20 kg: 50 mg; 20–40 kg: 100 mg; >40 kg: 200 mg – supposed daily – for **2 weeks** n = 30; Terbinafine, <20 kg: 62·5 mg; 20–40 kg: 125 mg; >40 kg: 200–250 mg – supposed	**Follow up:** 12 weeks; Described as randomised; Described as double blind; No ITT analysis; **Dropouts:** 2 in itraconazole group; 3 in terbinafine group because of irregular follow up	**Mycological cure rates at week 12:** itraconazole group: 85·7%; terbinafine group: 77·8%; **Clinical cure at week 12:** mean sum score of clinical signs reduced by 83·7% in the itroconazole group and by 84·9% in the terbinafine group; **Complete cure rates at week 12:** itraconazole group: 85·7%; all failures (n = 4) had T. violaceum tinea capitis; terbinafine

(Continued)

Table 34.1 (Continued)

Study	Trial design, sample size, study population and types of fungus isolated	Interventions	Time of follow up, quality of reporting, dropouts and comments	Outcome measures Adverse effects
	Terbinafine group: T. violaceum 88·8% (24/27); T. tonsurans 3·7% (1/27); T. mentagrophytes 3·7% (1/27); T. verrucosum 3·7% (1/27)	daily – for **2 weeks** n = 30 No co-treatment	unrelated to therapy No mention of compliance assessment No mention of industry support	group: 77·8% all failures (n = 6) has T violaceum tinea capitis **Adverse effects:** itraconazole group: 2 urticaria; terbinafine group: 2 fever, body aches and vertigo
Haroon et al. 1996[33] Pakistan (Lahore, Karachi)	Double-blind, randomised 161 patients; 156 (96·3%) were children <12 years old T. violaceum 71·4% (115/161); T. tonsurans 14·9% (24/161); T. verrucosum 4·3% (7/161); M. audouinii 4·3% (7/161); M. canis 2·5% (4/161); T. schoenleinii 1·8% (3/161); T. mentagrophytes 0·6% (1/161)	**Terbinafine**, 10–20 kg: 62·5 mg/day; 20–40 kg: 125 mg/day; >40 kg: 250 mg/day) once daily **for 1 week** plus 3 weeks of placebo n = 53 **for 2 weeks** plus 2 weeks of placebo n = 51 **for 4 weeks** n = 57 No co-treatment	**Follow up:** 12 weeks Described as randomised. Described as double blind No ITT analysis **Dropouts:** no mention of withdrawals or dropouts No mention of compliance assessment. Supported by Sandoz (terbinafine)	**Mycological cure rates at week 12:** 1-week terbinafine: 49·1%; 2-week terbinafine: 19·6%; 4-week group 19·3% **Clinical improvement at week 12:** 1-week group: 83%; 2-week group: 85%; 4-week group: 86% **Complete cure rates at week 12:** 1-week group: 49·1% (26/53); 2-week group: 60·8% (31/51); 4-week group: 66·7% (38/57) **Adverse effects:** 1-week group: 1 headache; 5 raised hepatic enzymes; 3 raised triglycerides; 1 eosinophilia, 1 leucocytosis; 2-week group: 2 raised hepatic enzymes; 1 eosinophilia; 4-week group: 2 raised hepatic enzymes; 2 raised triglycerides; 3 eosinophilia and 1 leucocytosis
Kullavanijaya et al. 1997[34] Thailand (Bangkok)	Single-blind, randomised 86 children ≥7 years old; 3 adults T. tonsurans, M. ferruginosum, 7 patients (of the three groups) had kerion, among these patients, 3 had M. ferrugineum infection, 3 had mixed infection and 1 had T. tonsurans infection	**Terbinafine** 62·5–250 mg according to body weight – supposed once daily – **for 1 week** n = 27 (completed the study) **for 2 weeks** n = 28 (completed the study) **for 4 weeks** n = 27 (completed the study)	**Follow up:** 20 weeks. Described as randomised. Described as single blind but no mention of which one (patients or observers) No ITT analysis **Dropouts:** 7 children were lost to follow up and excluded No mention of compliance	**Overall** cure rates (**complete cure** and **mycological cure**) at week 12: 44·4% in the 1-week group; 57·1% in the 2-week group; 77·8% in the 4-week group; no further improvement in the cure rates noted at week 20 (data not shown) **Clinical cure:** not reported **Adverse effects:** none reported

(Continued)

Table 34.1   (Continued)

Study	Trial design, sample size, study population and types of fungus isolated	Interventions	Time of follow up, quality of reporting, dropouts and comments	Outcome measures Adverse effects
			assessment. Supported by Sandoz (terbinafine)	
		No co-treatment		
Talarico Filho et al. 1998[38] Brazil (São Paulo, Paraná)	Single-blind, randomised 132 children 1–14 years old 1-week group: M. canis 77·1% (27/35); T. rubrum 8·6% (3/35); T. tonsurans 88·6% (3/35); T. mentagrophytes 2·8% (1/35); T. schoenleinii 2·8% (1/35) 2-week group: M. canis 73·3% (28/38); T. rubrum 7·9% (3/38); T. tonsurans 18·5% (7/38) 4-week group: M. canis 55·9% 19/34; T. rubrum 5·9% (2/34); T. tonsurans 26·5% (9/34); T. mentagrophytes 5·9% (2/34); T. schoenleinii 2·9% (1/34); M. gypseum 2·9% (1/34)	Terbinafine 10–20 kg: 62·5 mg/day; 20–40 kg: 125 mg/day; >40 kg: 250 mg/day once daily for 1 week plus 3 weeks of placebo n = 42 for 2 weeks plus 2 weeks of placebo n = 44 for 4 weeks n = 46 No co-treatment	Follow up: 12 weeks. Described as randomised. Patients blinding (single blind). No ITT analysis. Dropouts: only 107 patients completed the study (no mention in which group). No mention of compliance assessment. Supported by Sandoz (terbinafine)	Mycological cure rates at week 12: 1-week group: 48·6%; 2-week group: 60·5%; 4-week group: 69·7% Clinical cure rates at week 12: 1-week group: 54·3%; 2-week group: 60·5%; 4-week group: 84·8% Complete cure rates at week 12: 1-week group: 45·7%; 2-week group: 52·63%; 4-week group: 78·78% Adverse effects: 1-week group: 1 mild pruritus, 1 mild constipation; 2-week group: 1 mild headache, 2 moderate nausea; 4-week group: 1 mild urticaria, 1 labial oedema, 1 mild constipation , 1 moderate loss of appetite, 1 mild diarrhoea, 1 mild nausea, 1 moderate partial loss of taste (recovery within 8 weeks)
Hamm et al. 1999[35] and abstracts[36,37] Germany (Würzburg, Nürnberg)	Double-blind, randomised 35 children; mean age 9·3 years 1-week group: M. canis 43·7% (7/16); T. tonsurans 37·5% (6/16); T. violaceum 6·25% (1/16); T. mentagrophytes 12·5% (2/16)	Terbinafine 10–20 kg: 62·5 mg/day; 20–40 kg: 125 mg/day; >40 kg: 250 mg/day once daily for 1 week n = 16 for 2 weeks n = 19 No co-treatment	Follow up: 12 weeks. No description of randomisation process. Described as double blind but no description of blinding between 1and 2 weeks groups No ITT analysis	Mycologycal cure rates: 86·9% (20/23) Trichophyton spp. infections treated successfully with 1 or 2 weeks' terbinafine; 8·3% (1/12) patients with M. canis with short-course treatment Clinical cure scores: symptoms score decreased from 12·9 to 3·8 in Trichophyton infections and from 12·1 to 8·0 in Microsporum infections in the 1-week group; from 11·3 to 0·6 in Trichophyton infections and from 15·2 to 11·4 in Microsporum infections in the 2-week group

(Continued)

Table 34.1 (Continued)

Study	Trial design, sample size, study population and types of fungus isolated	Interventions	Time of follow up, quality of reporting, dropouts and comments	Outcome measures Adverse effects
	2-week group: *M. canis* 26·3% (5/19); *T. tonsurans* 31·5% (6/19); *T. violaceum* 26·3% (5/19); *T. mentagrophytes* 5·3% (1/19); *T. soudanense* 5·3% (1/19); *T. verrucosum* 5·3% (1/19)		**Dropouts:** no mention of withdrawals or dropouts. No mention of compliance assessment. Supported by Novartis (terbinafine)	**Complete cure rates:** 1-week group: *Trichophyton* spp. 44·4% (4/9); *Microsporum* spp. 0% (0/5); 2-week group: *Trichophyton* spp. 64 28% (9/14); *Microsporum* spp. 0% (0/7); additional 4 weeks treatment: *Trichophyton* spp. 33·3% (1/3); *Microsporum* spp. 33·3% (2/6) **Adverse effects:** 1-week group: 1 abdominal pain (mild to moderate), 1 abdominal pain and epistaxis (mild to moderate), 1 lack of appetite, headache and facial oedema (severe); 1 coughing and fever (mild to moderate); 2-week group: 1 abdominal pain, 1 abdominal pain and fatigue, 1 nausea, dyspepsia and headache, 1 fever; 4-week group: 1 lack of appetite and gastroenteritis
Solomon *et al.* 1997[49] USA (New York)	Open, randomised 41 children 2–15 years old Non-inflammatory, *T. tonsurans* 100%	**Fluconazole** tablets or suspension: 1·5 mg/kg/day for **20 days** n = 8 (completed the study) 3 mg/kg/day for **20 days** n = 10 (completed the study) 6 mg/kg/day for **20 days** n = 9 (completed the study) No co-treatment	**Follow up:** 4 months Described as randomised Described as open-label study No intention-to-treat analysis **Dropouts:** 14 patients were lost to follow up No mention of compliance assessment. No mention as supported by industry	**Mycological cure rates at month 4:** 25% in the 1·5 mg/kg/day group; 60% in the 3 mg/kg/day group; 89% in the 6 mg/kg/day group **Clinical cure:** Clinical improvement noted on average by the 17th day n the 1·5 mg/kg/day group, the 16th day in the 3 mg/kg/day group and the 12th day in the 6 mg/kg/day group **Complete cure rates:** not reported **Adverse effects:** none reported

ITT = intention-to-tract

RCT[38] of 107 children with mainly *M. canis* tinea capitis compared 1, 2 and 4 weeks of terbinafine, 125–250 mg/day according to weight. At week 12, the mycological cure rate was 49% with only 1 week of therapy, 61% with 2 weeks and 70% with 4 weeks.

Drawbacks

In the RCT comparing itraconazole with terbinafine,[32] fever, body aches and vertigo occurred in one patient in the terbinafine group, but no patient showed any significant haematological or biochemical change. In some RCTs tolerability was reported as good, or as no or few adverse events of uncertain relationship or of no relationship.[23,24,27,30,36] Cases of tonsillitis, cutaneous infestations, raised hepatic enzymes, raised triglycerides and eosinophilia,[23,27] and mild elevated triglycerides of uncertain drug relationship[26] have been reported. Fifty-seven adverse events (pruritus, urticaria, skin scaling) were reported by 36 patients and four patients were withdrawn from a study because of adverse events (vomiting, dizziness, urticaria and weight loss).[25] The following adverse events were reported in an RCT comparing different regimens of terbinafine[23]: headache, raised hepatic enzymes, raised triglycerides, eosinophilia and leucocytosis in the 1-week terbinafine group; raised hepatic enzymes and eosinophilia in the 2-week terbinafine group; raised hepatic enzymes, raised triglycerides, eosinophilia and leucocytosis in the 4-week terbinafine group. The following adverse events were reported in another RCT comparing different regimens of terbinafine[38]: mild pruritus and mild constipation in the 1-week terbinafine group; mild headache and nausea in the 2-week terbinafine group; mild urticaria, labial oedema, mild constipation; moderate loss of appetite, mild diarrhoea, mild nausea and moderate/ partial loss of taste (recovered within 8 weeks) in the 4-week terbinafine group. Other RCTs comparing different regimens of terbinafine reported[35–37]: abdominal pain (mild to moderate), epistaxis (mild to moderate), lack of appetite, headache and facial oedema (severe), coughing and fever (mild to moderate) in the 1-week terbinafine group; abdominal pain, fatigue, nausea, dyspepsia, headache and fever in the 2-week terbinafine group. One additional patient reported lack of appetite and gastroenteritis only during the additional 4-week treatment period.

Comment

I excluded one study that was still in progress.[28] Another[29] was excluded because it gave no separate clinical and mycological data for each study group. I found a study reported as an RCT[29] in a group of New Zealand patients with mainly *M. canis* infections. The authors concluded that 4 weeks of terbinafine was as efficacious as 8 weeks of griseofulvin treatment, using topical econazole cream and ketoconazole shampoo as adjunct therapy. However, complete clinical and mycological data for study end and follow up time points were not provided. One RCT[27] was presented as a duplicate publication.[23] The manufacturer of terbinafine has been involved in most of the RCTs. Some uncontrolled studies have found oral terbinafine at higher doses or over 6–8 weeks to be effective in the treatment of *M. canis* tinea capitis and well tolerated.[13] Definition of cure varies from study to study: some investigators follow microbiological findings, others place greater emphasis on clinical response. High dropout rates in some studies may artificially decrease the response rate, as those who are cured may be lost to follow up.

Implications for practice

Good evidence supports the use of terbinafine for treating *T. tonsurans* tinea capitis in children, and fair evidence supports its use in *M. canis* tinea capitis. Terbinafine has the advantage over griseofulvin of producing good results in a shorter time, making patient compliance less a problem. An important disadvantage is that it is available only in tablet form – there is no suspension. According to RCTs, the recommended regimen in children with tinea capitis is continuous therapy once daily for 4 weeks with dosage according to body weight: 62·5 mg/day for children weighing 10–20 kg; 125 mg/day for 20–40 kg; 250 mg/day for those weighing over 40 kg. *M. canis* infections may require treatment for 6–8 weeks. Terbinafine is not licensed for this indication in children in some countries.

Itraconazole

Limited RCT evidence shows that oral itraconazole at doses according to the patient's weight (<20 kg: 50 mg/day; >20 kg: 100 mg/day) for 2–6 weeks is effective and safe for tinea capitis caused by *T. violaceum* (2 weeks of treatment) and *M. canis* (6 weeks of treatment). Only observational data suggest that itraconazole may be effective against *T. tonsurans* infections.

Efficacy

Two RCTs have compared itraconazole with other oral antifungals (Table 34.1).

Versus griseofulvin

A double-blind RCT of 35 patients mostly infected with *M. canis*, compared 6 weeks' itraconazole, 100 mg/day, with 6 weeks' griseofulvin, 500 mg/day.[22] At the 14-week follow up they showed the same complete cure rate – 88%.

Versus terbinafine

A double-blind RCT of 60 patients with predominantly *T. violaceum* tinea capitis compared 2 weeks' itraconazole with 2 weeks' terbinafine.[32] After 2 weeks the complete cure rates in the two groups differed little: 86% in the itraconazole group versus 78% in the terbinafine group.

A non-randomised trial[39] compared 15 children (9 with *M. canis* and 6 with *T. violaceum* infections) treated with 50 mg itraconazole versus 56 children (38 with *M. canis*, 18 with other *Trichophyton* and *Microsporum* spp. infections) treated with 100 mg itraconazole orally, as capsules, once daily for a minimum of 4 and a maximum of 8 weeks. Two months after the final dose the mycological cure rates were 60% in the of 50 mg group and 89% in the 100 mg group.

I found nine uncontrolled studies, with more than 10 patients, conducted with different therapeutic regimens of itraconazole.[40–48] Some studies used continuous treatment (50–100 mg/day or 5 mg/kg/day for 3–11 weeks) with capsules[40,42, 46–48] or oral solution[41] and others used pulse therapy (3–5 mg/kg/day for 1 week a month with a maximum of 3–5 pulses) with capsules[43,45] or oral solution.[44] Complete cure rates ranged from 81% to 100%; causative fungi were *T. tonsurans* and *M. canis*. One study[46] found a complete cure rate of only 40% in children infected with *T. tonsurans*.

Drawbacks

Transient gastrointestinal side-effects are the most frequently reported and rarely a reversible increase in serum aminotransferase. In the RCT comparing itraconazole with griseofulvin[22] two patients on griseofulvin stopped therapy prematurely because of nausea and intense stomach ache with severe vomiting that occurred in weeks 2 and 4 of treatment and subsided after the withdrawal of griseofulvin. In the RCT comparing itraconazole with terbinafine,[32] two patients in the itraconazole group reported with urticaria. Other studies have noted: a papular skin eruption not clearly related to treatment with itraconazole,[39] minor gastrointestinal disturbances,[41,44,46,47] headache,[46] epistaxis and seizure (not drug related),[46] and "tired legs".[48]

Comment

The methods of randomisation and blinding were not clearly described in either RCT.[22,32] No intention-to-treat analysis was done in these studies but the dropout rates were 3/35[22] and 5/60.[32] One of the RCTs[22] was funded by the manufacturer of itraconazole. In one uncontrolled study[46] that reported a complete cure rate of 40%, the high dropout rate of 54% may have artificially decreased the response rate because those who are cured may be less likely to return for follow up. I found much information from uncontrolled studies but additional RCTs comparing itraconazole with other antifungals are clearly needed.

Implications for practice

Fair but still limited evidence supports the use of itraconazole for the treatment of tinea capitis in children caused by *M. canis*, *T. violaceum* and *T. tonsurans*. On the basis of limited evidence, the recommended dosage for itraconazole for tinea capitis in children is 100 mg/day or dose adjusted to body weight, for 6 weeks in *M. canis* and for 2 weeks in *T. violaceum* infections. Uncontrolled studies suggest that shorter or pulse regimens may also be useful.

Fluconazole

Limited evidence (mostly observational) suggests that fluconazole continuously at 6–8 mg/kg/day for 3 weeks or intermittently at 6–8 mg/kg/week for 4–8 weeks is effective and safe for treating *T. tonsurans* and *M. canis* tinea capitis in children.

Efficacy

I found no RCTs comparing fluconazole with griseofulvin or other systemic antifungals for tinea capitis. A small RCT[49] comparing various doses of fluconazole (1·5, 3·0 and 6 mg/kg/day) for 20 days in the treatment of *T. tonsurans* tinea capitis showed a complete cure rate of 25% in the 1.5 mg group, 60% in the 3 mg group and 89% in the 6 mg group (Table 34.1). I found three uncontrolled studies of fluconazole in at least 20 patients[50–52]; *M. canis* and *T. tonsurans* were the main causative fungi. Mycological cure rates ranged from 88% to 100%. These studies used intermittent therapy: 6 mg/kg/day for 2 weeks followed after 4 weeks and if indicated by an extra week of treatment at the same dose[50]; 6–8 mg/kg/week for 4–8 weeks[52] and 8 mg/kg/week for 8–12 weeks.[51]

Drawbacks

Only mild reversible gastrointestinal complaints and asymptomatic and reversible elevated liver function tests were noted.[51]

Comment

Studies are needed to compare fluconazole with other antifungals and to determine proper dosing and duration of therapy. The only RCT I found was very small.[49] Two studies were supported in part by the manufacturer.[50,51]

Implications for practice

There is no good evidence to recommend a dosage regimen with fluconazole for tinea capitis in children. Observational studies suggest that continuous 6 mg/kg/day for 3 weeks or intermittent 6–8 mg/kg/week for 4–8 weeks may be effective. Fluconazole is not licensed for this indication in children in some countries.

> ### What are the effects of topical treatment of tinea capitis in adults and children?

Adjunctive topical therapy has been used together with oral antifungal treatment to eradicate the fungi from the infected site, decrease spread to other people and to speed the cure. Various topical agents are available for adjunctive therapy.[53]

Shampoos

There is moderate RCT evidence that the addition of biweekly shampooing with selenium sulphide substantially reduces the period of active shedding. However, some evidence indicates that topical treatment is not useful to treat tinea capitis.

Efficacy

An RCT[54] reported that 75% of griseofulvin-treated patients with uncomplicated *T. tonsurans* tinea capitis had sterile hair sample cultures 4 weeks after initiation of griseofulvin. By contrast, 94% of patients who received griseofulvin together with biweekly selenium sulphide shampoos had sterile hair cultures at 4 weeks. Another RCT[55] of 54 patients receiving griseofulvin 15 mg/kg/day for *T. tonsurans* tinea capitis, compared selenium sulphide 2·5% lotion or 1% shampoo with a bland non-medicated shampoo. Patients were observed every 2 weeks until they were clinically and mycologically cured. The selenium sulphide products were statistically superior to the non-medicated shampoo for time required to eliminate shedding and viable fungi. However, no difference was noted between the two selenium products.

I found an RCT[56] performed in a very depressed area of Africa where griseofulvin is not generally available. It compared 6 weeks of miconazole cream with 6 weeks of Whitfield's ointment (6% benzoic acid plus 3% salicylic acid) in *T. violaceum* and *M. audouinii* tinea capitis and found no significant cure rates. A small open study[57] of children with *T. tonsurans* tinea capitis treated solely with 2% ketoconazole shampoo daily for 8 weeks reported a clinical cure in 93%

but at 6-month follow up only 33% showed a mycological cure and remained cured during the 1 year follow up.

Drawbacks

No adverse events were reported.

Comment

RCTs of adjunctive therapy were described as randomised, but did not adequately describe the method and were not blinded.[54,55] One of the studies was supported by Janssen, the manufacturer of the ketoconazole shampoo.[57]

Implications for practice

Some evidence supports the use of adjunctive topical therapy of tinea capitis with antifungal shampoos (for example 1% selenium sulphide shampoo) for reducing the time of cure and for decreasing spread of infectious fungi to other persons.

> In children with inflammatory tinea capitis (kerion) does an oral antifungal plus a corticosteroid lead to faster cure and complete hair regrowth than an oral antifungal alone?

Corticosteroids

Moderate RCT evidence indicates that the use of oral or intralesional corticosteroids as adjunctive therapy with griseofulvin for inflammatory tinea capitis (kerion) does not lead to additional or faster improvement.

Efficacy

Three RCTs showed no evidence that the use of oral[58,59] or intralesional[60] corticosteroids as adjunctive therapy with oral griseofulvin in inflammatory tinea capitis (kerion) results in additional or faster improvement of kerion. One RCT[60] of 30 children with *T. tonsurans* tinea capitis showed that intralesional injection of corticosteroid combined with oral griseofulvin is no better than griseofulvin alone for treatment of kerion and found no significant differences in the time to negative culture, time of onset of new hair growth, complete regrowth of hair or time to scalp clearing. In this study all patients were instructed to shampoo their hair with 1% selenium sulphide twice weekly for 3 weeks. Two RCTs[58,59] using oral corticosteroids showed no additional benefit in terms of improvement, reduction in the severity of clinical signs or pathogen eradication.

Drawbacks

No adverse events were noted. In particular no patient had post-therapy alopecia, permanent scarring or biochemical evidence of hepatic dysfunction.[60]

Comment

One RCT[60] described the method of randomisation using a table of random numbers, but was not blinded. Triamcinolone acetonide, 2·5 mg, was used in this study, but whether larger doses of steroid might be effective remains unknown. The other two RCTs[58,59] were described as randomised but only one[59] was double blind). In this latter RCT, scaling and pruritus were eliminated more quickly in the group that used erythromycin and prednisone in addition to griseofulvin but the authors think this may have been due to the smaller volume of the kerions in this group rather than the effects of therapy, so that the patients became symptom free sooner.

Implications for practice

Addition of corticosteroids to oral antifungals is unlikely to be useful. Fair evidence supports the rejection of the use of oral or intralesional corticosteroids as adjunctive therapy for inflammatory tinea capitis (kerion).

> **What strategies are best for reducing spreading and re-infection in tinea capitis in adults and children?**

Carrier state is defined as the individuals with no signs or symptoms of tinea capitis but from whom scalp positive cultures can be isolated.[1] Strategies for management of the carrier state include: preventive treatments such as fungicidal shampoos, decontamination of objects that come into contact with the scalp, education programmes for children to avoid sharing of objects that can spread tinea capitis to others (such as caps, combs and toys) and shaving of hair.

There is no RCT evidence for optimal management of symptom-free carriers.

Efficacy

I found no systematic reviews and no RCTs about the impact of the strategies for management of the asymptomatic carrier state. A non-randomised study[61] compared different shampoos in carriers and found that povidone-iodine shampoo produced a cure rate of 94%, compared with 47% with econazole shampoo, 50% with selenium sulphide 2·5% shampoo and 50% with a control shampoo.

Drawbacks

None were reported.

Implications for practice

The effectiveness is unknown. Although it is agreed that decontamination of objects that come into contact with scalp, education programmes for children and avoidance of sharing of objects can reduce the spread of fungal infections,[1] I found no good evidence to support this. Limited evidence supports the regular use of antifungal shampoos in controlling the carrier state of populations at risk. Povidone-iodine shampoo may be the most suitable for prophylaxis.

Key points

Systemic antifungal therapy for tinea capitis in children

- RCT evidence suggests that griseofulvin for 6–8 weeks is effective and safe for tinea capitis.
- The best evidence available also suggests that terbinafine, itraconazole and fluconazole can cure most patients with tinea capitis with a shorter course of therapy.
- All these drugs have good safety profiles in children.
- Regional as well as dermatophyte species variation may play an important role in the response rate, and may determine what dosage regimens are recommended.
- RCT evidence indicates that terbinafine for 4 weeks is effective and safe for treating *Trichophyton* spp. tinea capitis.
- Some RCTs suggest that longer ferbinafine therapeutic regimens of 6 weeks are necessary to treat *Microsporum* spp. infections.
- Some RCT evidence suggests that oral itraconazole for 2–6 weeks is effective and safe to treat tinea capitis in children.
- Limited, mostly observational, evidence suggests that fluconazole for 3–6 weeks is effective and safe for treating tinea capitis in children.

Adjunctive therapy for tinea capitis in adults and children

- Some RCT evidence suggests that antifungal shampoos can reduce the period of active shedding in patients treated with oral antifungals.
- Existing RCT evidence indicates that corticosteroids used with griseofulvin for inflammatory tinea capitis (kerion) give no additional or faster improvement.

Strategies to reduce spreading and re-infection in tinea capitis

- No RCT evidence exists for optimal management of symptom-free carriers. I found insufficient evidence suggesting that antiseptic shampoos can reduce

References

1. Eleweski BE. Tinea capitis: a current perspective. *J Am Acad Dermatol* 2000;**42**:1–24.
2. Čeburkovas O, Schwartz RA, Janniger CK. Tinea capitis: current concepts. *J Dermatol* 2000;**27**:144–8.
3. Aly R. Ecology, epidemiology and diagnosis of tinea capitis. *Pediatr Infect Dis J* 1999;**18**:180–5.
4. Figueroa JI, Hay RJ. Skin infections II: Fungi. In: Williams HC, Strachan DP, eds. *The challenge of dermato-epidemiology*. Boca Raton: CRC Press, Inc,1997;257–9.
5. Al Sogair S. Fungal infections in children: tinea capitis. *Clinics Dermatol* 2000;**18**:679–85.
6. Hay RJ, Moore M. Mycology. In: Champion RH, Burton JL, Burns DA *et al.*, eds. *Textbook of Dermatology, 6th ed.* Oxford: Blackwell Science, 1998;1303–6.
7. Friedlander SF, Pickering B, Cunningham B *et al.* Use of the cotton swap method in diagnosing tinea capitis. *Am Acad Pediatrics* 199;**104**:276–9.
8. Hubbard TW, Triquet JM. Brush-culture method for diagnosing tinea capitis. *Pediatrics* 1992;**90**:416–18.
9. Drake LA, Dinehart CSM, Farmer ER *et al.* Guidelines of care for superficial mycotic infections of the skin: tinea capitis and tinea barbae. *J Am Acad Dermatol* 1996;**34**:290–4.
10. Temple ME, Nahata MC, Koranyi KI. Pharmacotherapy of tinea capitis. *J Am Board Fam Pract* 1999;**12**:236–42.
11. Eleweski BE. Treatment of tinea capitis: beyond griseofulvin. *J Am Acad Dermatol* 1999;**40**:S27–30.
12. Abdel-Rahman SM, Nahata MC. Treatment of tinea capitis. *Ann Pharmacother* 1997;**31**:338–48.
13. Gupta AK, Hofstader SLR, Adam P *et al.* Tinea capitis: an overview with emphasis on management. *Pediatr Dermatol* 1999;**16**:171–89.
14. McMichael AJ. Effective management of tinea capitis in the pediatric population. *Today Ther Trends* 2001;**19**:93–104.

15. Nesbitt LT Jr. Treatment of tinea capitis. *Int J Dermatol* 2000;**39**:261–2.

16. Blumer JL. Pharmacologic basis for the treatment of tinea capitis. *Pediatr Infect Dis J* 1999;**18**:191–9.

17. Friedlander SF. The evolving role of itraconazole, fluconazole and terbinafine in the treatment of tinea capitis. *Pediatr Infect Dis J* 1999;**18**:205–10.

18. Tanz RR, Hebert AA, Esterly BN. Treating tinea capitis: should ketoconazole replace griseofulvin? *J Pediatr* 1988;**112**:987–91.

19. Tanz RR, Stagl S, Esterly BN. Comparison of ketoconazole and griseofulvin for treatment of tinea capitis in childhood: A preliminary study. *Pediatr Emerg Care* 1985;**1**:16–18.

20. Martínez-Roig A, Torres-Rodriguez JM, Bartlett-Coma A. Double blind study of ketoconazole and griseofulvin in dermatophytoses. *Pediatr Infect Dis J* 1988;**7**:37–40.

21. Gan VN, Petruska M, Ginsburg CM. Epidemiology and treatment of tinea capitis: ketokonazole *v.* griseofulvin. *Pediatr Infect Dis J* 1987;**6**:46–9.

22. López-Gómez S, Del Palacio A, Cutsem JV *et al.* Itroconazole versus griseofulvin in the treatment of tinea capitis: a double-blind randomized study in children. *Int J Dermatol* 1994;**33**:743–7.

23. Alvi KH, Iqbal N, Khan KA *et al.* A randomized, double-blind trial of the efficacy and tolerability of terbinafine once daily compared to griseofulvin once daily in the treatment of tinea capitis. In. Shuster S, Jafary MH, eds. Terbinafine in the treatment of superficial fungal infections. Royal Society of Medicine Services International Congress and Symposium Series No. 205. London: Royal Society of Medicine Services,1993:35–40.

24. Cáceres-Rios H, Rueda M, Ballona R *et al.* Comparison of terbinafine and griseofulvin in the treatment of tinea capitis. *J Am Acad Dermatol* 2000;**42**:80–4.

25. Fuller LC, Smith CH, Cerio R *et al.* A randomized comparison of 4 weeks of terbinafine *v.* 8 weeks of griseofulvin for the treatment of tinea capitis. *Br J Dermatol* 2001;**144**:321–7.

26. Memisoğlu HR, Erboz S, Akkaya S *et al.* Comparative study of the efficacy and tolerability of 4 weeks of terbinafine therapy with 8 weeks of griseofulvin therapy in children with tinea capitis. *J Dermatol Treat* 1999;**10**:189–93.

27. Haroon TS, Hussain I, Aman S *et al.* A randomized double-blind comparative study of terbinafine and griseofulvine in tinea capitis. *J Dermatol Treat* 1995;**6**:167–9.

28. Haroon TS, Hussain I, Aman S *et al.* A randomized, double-blind, comparative study of terbinafine *v* griseofulvine in tinea capitis. *J Dermatol Treat* 1992;**3**(Suppl. 1):25–7.

29. Rademaker M, Havill S. Griseofulvin and terbinafine in the treatment of tinea capitis in children. *N Z Med J* 1998;**111**:55–7.

30. Cáceres H, Rueda M, Ballona R *et al.* Comparison of terbinafine and griseofulvin in the treatment of tinea capitis. *Ann Dermatol Venereol* 1998;**125**(Suppl. 1):1S21.

31. Higgins EM, Fuller LC, Smith CH. Guidelines for the management of tinea capitis. *Br J Dermatol* 2000;**143**:53–8.

32. Jahangir M, Hussain M, Hassan M *et al.* A double-blind, randomized, comparative trial of itraconazole versus terbinafine for 2 weeks in tinea capitis. *Br J Dermatol* 1998;**139**:672–4.

33. Haroon TS, Hussain I, Aman S *et al.* A randomized double-blind comparative study of terbinafine for 1, 2 and 4 weeks in tinea capitis. *Br J Dermatol* 1996;**135**:86–8.

34. Kullavanijaya P, Reangchainam S, Ungpakorn R. Randomized single-blind study of efficacy and tolerability of terbinafine in the treatment of tinea capitis. *J Am Acad Dermatol* 1997;**37**:272–3.

35. Hamm H, Schwinn A, Bräutigam M *et al.* Short duration treatment with terbinafine for tinea capitis caused by *Trichophyton* or *Microsporum* species. *Br J Dermatol* 1999;**140**:480–2.

36. Schwinn A, Hamm H, Bräutigam M *et al.* What is the best approach to tinea capitis with terbinafine? *J Eur Acad Dermatol Venereol* 1998;**11**(Suppl. 2):S232 (abstract P199).

37. Schwinn A, Hamm H, Bräutigam M *et al.* What is the best approach to tinea capitis with terbinafine?. *Ann Dermatol Venereol* 1998;**125**(Suppl. 1):1S133–4 (abstract P147).

38. Talarico Filho S, Cucé LC, Foss NT *et al.* Efficacy, safety and tolerability of terbinafine for tinea capitis in children: Brazilian multicentric study with daily oral tablets for 1, 2 and 4 weeks. *J Eur Acad Dermatol Venereol* 1998;**11**:141–6.

39. Degreef H. Itraconazole in the treatment of tinea capitis. *Cutis* 1996;**58**:90–3.

40. Greer DL. Treatment of tinea capitis with itraconazole. *J Am Acad Dermatol* 1996;**35**:637–8.

41. Ginter G. *Microsporum canis* infections in children: results of a new oral antifungal therapy. *Mycoses* 1996;**39**:265–9.

42. Elewski BE. Treatment of tinea capitis with itraconazole. *Int J Dermatol* 1997;**36**:539–41.

43. Gupta AK, Alexis ME, Raboobee N *et al*. Itraconazole pulse therapy is effective in the treatment of tinea capitis in children: an open multicentre study. *Br J Dermatol* 1997;**137**:251–4.

44. Gupta AK, Solomon R, Adam P. Itraconazole oral solution for the treatment of tinea capitis. *Br J Dermatol* 1998;**139**:104–6.

45. Gupta AK, Hofstader SL, Summerbell RC *et al*. Treatment of tinea capitis with itraconazole capsule pulse therapy. *J Am Acad Dermatol* 1998;**39**:216–19.

46. Abdel-Rahmen SM, Powell DA, Nahata MC. Efficacy of itraconazole with *Trichophyton tonsurans* tinea capitis. *J Am Acad Dermatol* 1998;**38**:443–6.

47. Möhrenschlager M, Schnopp C, Fesq H *et al*. Optimizing the therapeutic approach in tinea capitis of childhood with itraconazole. *Br J Dermatol* 2000;**143**:1011–15.

48. Legendre R, Escola-Macre J. Itraconazole in the treatment of tinea capitis. *J Am Acad Dermatol* 1990;**23**:559–60.

49. Solomon BA, Collins R, Sharma R *et al*. Fluconazole for the treatment of tinea capitis in children. *J Am Acad Dermatol* 1997;**37**:274–5.

50. Gupta AK, Adam P, Hofstader SLR *et al*. Intermittent short duration therapy with fluconazole is effective for tinea capitis. *Br J Dermatol* 1999;**141**:304–6.

51. Gupta AK, Dlova N, Taborda P *et al*. Once weekly fluconazole is effective in children in the treatment of tinea capitis: a prospective, multicentre study. *Br J Dermatol* 2000;**142**:965–8.

52. Montero-Gei F. Fluconazole in the treatment of tinea capitis. *Int J Dermatol* 1998;**37**:870–3.

53. Bettoli V, Tosti A. Antifungals. In: Katsambas AD, Lotti TM, eds. *European Handbook of Dermatological Treatments*. Berlin Heilderberg: Springer-Verlag, 2000:748–55.

54. Allen HB, Honig PJ, Leyden JJ *et al*. Selenium sulfide: adjunctive therapy for tinea capitis. *Pediatrics* 1982;**69**:81–3.

55. Givens TG, Murray MM, Baker RC. Comparison of 1% and 2·5% selenium sulfide in the treatment of tinea capitis. *Arch Pediatr Adolesc Med* 1995;**149**:808–11.

56. Wright S, Robertson VJ. An institutional survey of tinea capitis in Harare, Zimbabwe and a trial of miconazole cream versus Whitefield's ointment in its treatment. *Clin Exp Dermatol* 1986;**2**:371–7.

57. Greer DL. Successful treatment of tinea capitis with 2% ketoconazole shampoo. *Int J Dermatol* 2000;**39**:302–4.

58. Hussain I, Muzaffar F, Rashid T *et al*. A randomized, comparative trial of treatment of kerion celsi with griseofulvin plus oral prednisolone *v*. griseofulvin alone. *Med Mycol* 1999;**37**:97–9.

59. Honig PJ, Caputo GL, Leyden JJ *et al*. Treatment of kerions. *Pediatr Dermatol* 1994;**11**:169–71.

60. Ginsburg CM, Gan VN, Petruska M. Randomized controlled trial of intralesional corticosteroid and griseofulvin *v*. griseofulvin alone for treatment of Kerion. *Pediatr Infect Dis J* 1987;**6**:1084–7.

61. Neil G, Hanslo D. Control of the carrier state of scalp dermatophytes. *Pediatr Infect Dis J* 1990;**9**:57–8.

35
Candidiasis

Peter von den Driesch

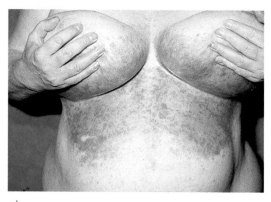

a)

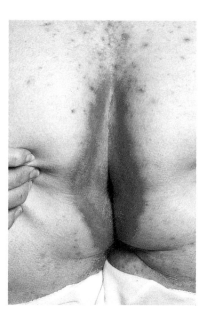

b)

Figure 35.1 Characteristic intertriginous *Candida* infections of the skin

Background
Definition

The term candidiasis or candidosis covers a number of clinical diseases caused by infection with the yeast *Candida albicans* or, on occasion, by other yeasts of the genus *Candida*. Infections most often affect the intertriginous areas of the skin as well as the mouth and gut, although under certain circumstances may become systemic and involve internal organs.

Incidence/prevalence

The gut is the major reservoir for *Candida* yeasts, without causing clinical disease. Newborn babies are normally not colonised. Follow up studies showed that the most important and rapid route of colonisation is from mother to child.[1] Among the elderly, 36–78% are colonised with *Candida*; denture wearing, smoking and poor oral hygiene are risk factors for the presence of the yeasts.[2] The incidence and prevalence of cutaneous *Candida* infections in the general population is unknown, nor is the frequency of clinically manifest oral or genital candidiasis.

Aetiology

It is generally believed that yeast colonisation of the mouth or the gut is not by itself a disease. Under certain circumstances, however, the aggressive potential of the yeast increases and defined diseases occur. Intensive chemotherapy, immunosuppressive drugs, HIV infection and other diseases that cause immunosuppression, for example diabetes mellitus, and being overweight contribute to this problem.[3]

The causative agent *C. albicans* and other less pathogenic yeasts of the genus *Candida* are a heterogeneous collection of yeast species that do not produce ascospores or teliospores. The morphological feature of this group of yeasts (with the exception of *C. glabrata*) is the capacity to form pseudomycelia. *C. albicans* alone is suggested to be the causative agent in 85–90% of clinically manifest infections.[4]

Candida infections of the skin most often affect the intertriginous folds of the genitocrural, as well as the submammary and subaxillary areas. These "intertrigos" have a erythematous moist appearance, sometimes with removable white smear, and characteristically with single erythematous satellite vesicopustules at the periphery. Interdigital *Candida* infections occur on the feet and, especially in workers with high exposure to humidity, on the hands. Nails can also be infected. *Candida* is one major cause of diaper dermatitis in infants.

Oral clinically manifest *Candida* infections may occur as pseudomembranous, atrophic or hyperplastic candidosis. Black hairy tongue and the so-called perleche of the lateral lips are other typical oral manifestations.

Other conditions such as seborrhoeic eczema as well as general weakness and other ill-defined symptoms, the so-called *Candida* hypersensitivity syndrome, have been associated with gut colonisation by yeasts. However, formal proof of the relevance of any of these conditions to colonisation by *Candida* is lacking.[5]

Diagnosis

Diagnosis of *Candida* infection can be rapidly confirmed by direct microscopic examination of smears or potassium-hydroxide-pretreated skin scrapings. Further confirmation can be achieved by a prompt inoculation on a Sabouraud's agar. Subspecies are subsequently identified by inoculation in selective agars such as rice agar.

Aims of treatment and relevant outcomes

Treatment normally aims at complete relief of any symptoms caused by the yeasts. On the skin, cultures should be negative for the presence of *Candida* yeasts after treatment. Apart from controlled studies, however, the latter is proved in only a minority of patients. Possible outcomes of any studies are therefore complete clearing of the clinical manifestations and/or (repeated) demonstration of the lack of *Candida* yeasts in the appropriate specimen.

QUESTIONS

> Does prophylactic therapy against yeasts make sense?

Very-low-birth-weight infants

One RCT investigated 103 babies weighing less than 1500 g treated with fluconazole, 6 mg/kg, and found candidal rectal colonisation from day 14 to day 56 after birth in 15% of the drug-treated and 46% of the placebo-treated babies. The treatment was safe and no fluconazole-resistant *Candida* strains occurred during the study.[6]

Haematological malignancies

In one randomised controlled trial (RCT) comparing different treatment modalities, itraconazole (oral solution) was compared with fluconazole for antifungal prophylaxis.[7] Adults with haematological malignancies receiving chemotherapy or bone marrow transplants were randomly allocated itraconazole solution, 5 mg/kg/day, or fluconazole suspension, 100 mg, from before the onset of neutropenia until neutrophil recovery or suspected fungal infection. More proven systemic fungal infections occurred with fluconazole (four *Aspergillus*, one *C. tropicalis* and *C. krusei*) than with itraconazole (one *C. albicans*) and more of these were fatal (four versus none). Significantly more cases of proven aspergillosis occurred with fluconazole than with itraconazole (six versus none).[7]

In a non-randomised Bulgarian study, 69 patients with haematological malignancies and neutrophil count below 1×10^9/litre received oral fluconazole, 150 mg every other day. The incidence of mycotic infections was lower in the patients on antifungal prophylaxis compared with patients who received no prophylaxis. Most of the clinically and/or microbiologically verified infections were superficial oropharyngeal (61%) or oesophageal infections (22%), or single cases of skin, genital or rectal infections. *C. albicans* was isolated in 85% of the cases.[8]

An RCT compared fluconazole, 400 mg/day, with placebo in patients after bone-marrow transplantation treated for up to 75 days. Systemic fungal infections were found in 10 (7%) of 152 fluconazole-treated patients and in 26 (18%) of 148 placebo-treated patients ($P = 0.004$). No *C. albicans* infections occurred in fluconazole recipients, compared with 18 in placebo recipients ($P<0.001$) and no significant increase in infection with *Candida* species other than *C. albicans*. Fluconazole also significantly reduced the incidence of superficial fungal infections ($P<0.001$), fungal colonisation ($P = 0.037$) and empiric amphotericin B use ($P = 0.005$). Fluconazole recipients were more likely to survive: 31 of them died up to day 110 after transplantation, compared with 52 among the placebo recipients ($P = 0.004$).[9] Fluconazole toxicity was well manageable.

Critically ill patients

In a study of 292 critically ill adult surgical and trauma patients, admitted to hospital for at least 48 hours, patients were randomised to no antimycotic therapy, clotrimazole, 10 mg three times a day, ketoconazole, 200 mg/day or nystatin, 2 000 000 units 6-hourly. In this group treatment with three or more antibiotics, APACHE II >10, and ventilatory support for more than 48 hours significantly predicted yeast colonisation and sepsis. The four groups did not differ significantly with regard to yeast colonisation (23%, 18%, 12% and 15%, respectively), yeast sepsis (3%, 1%, 2% and 7% respectively), or mortality (15%, 14%, 6% and 20% respectively).[10]

In another group of ill high-risk surgical patients, an RCT on 49 patients revealed candidiasis in two patients who received intravenous fluconazole 400 mg/day and in seven patients who received placebo ($P = 0.06$). Fluconazole was well tolerated, and adverse events occurred at similar frequencies in both treatment groups.[11]

An RCT addressed the safety and efficacy of fluconazole therapy in 143 liver-transplant recipients. Seventy-six patients received oral fluconazole, 100 mg/day, and 67 received nystatin 4×10^6 units/day) for the first 28 days after transplantation. *Candida* colonisation occurred in 25% and 53% of patients in the fluconazole and nystatin groups, respectively ($P = 0.04$), and 13% and 34% of patients respectively had *Candida* infections ($P = 0.022$). Of these patients, 10.5% in the fluconazole group and 25.3% in the nystatin group had superficial *Candida* infections ($P = 0.024$). Invasive candidiasis developed in two patients in the fluconazole group (2.6%) and six in the nystatin group (9.0%) ($P = 0.12$). No increased hepatotoxicity, ciclosporin interaction or emergence of clinically relevant resistant *Candida* strains was attributable to fluconazole.[12]

HIV infection

A randomised unblinded study compared clotrimazole troches with oral fluconazole in

92 patients with manifest HIV infection. One-year clinical cure rates were similar with fluconazole (96%) and clotrimazole (91%), but mycological cure was better with fluconazole (49%) than clotrimazole (27%). Fluconazole resistance in *C. albicans* occurred most often in patients who had low CD4 counts.[13]

In a placebo-controlled RCT of nystatin in the prevention of oral candidosis in 128 HIV-infected men, a multivariate proportional hazards model showed that four factors were significant (*P*<0·001) in predicting time to oral candidiasis: nystatin treatment (hazard ratio 0·59), history of oral candidiasis (3·58), *C. albicans* carriage (2·79), and CD4 count at randomisation (0·65). In this small group of patients, nystatin appeared to delay the onset of oral candidiasis. Patients with CD4 counts <200 who carried *C. albicans* and who had a history of oral candidiasis were most likely to benefit from antifungal prophylaxis. No severe side-effects were reported.[14]

Another study investigated 323 women with HIV infection and CD4+ cell counts of 300 cells/mm^3 or less. Patients received fluconazole, 200 mg/week, or placebo. Crossover to open-label fluconazole treatment was permitted after two episodes of infection. After a median follow up of 29 months, 72 of 162 patients receiving fluconazole and 93 of 161 patients receiving placebo had at least one episode of candidiasis (*P*<0·001). Weekly fluconazole was effective in preventing oropharyngeal and vaginal candidiasis but not oesophageal candidiasis. Fluconazole resistance occurred in less than 5% of patients in each group. No severe side-effects were reported.[15]

What is the best treatment for cutaneous candidosis?

Topical nystatin

Topical application of nystatin in zinc-containing emollients is widely regarded as the "standard" treatment for *Candida* infection of the skin. However, there are no new controlled randomised studies to underline this general opinion. In studies primarily investigating newer drugs, only one very small study compared the new drug with the "standard" nystatin. This RCT enrolled 20 patients (mean age 12 months; range 1–48 months) with moderate-to-severe diaper dermatitis who were treated with either mupirocin ointment or nystatin cream applied to the infected area 8 hourly or after every diaper change for 7 days. In both groups the yeasts were eliminated within 5 days in all subjects. The authors attributed their impression of a better clinical response to mupirocin to its broader antimicrobial effect.[16]

Azole drugs

A number of RCTs have investigated the effect of newer azolic drugs in different cutaneous candidiasis variants. One RCT compared sertaconazole 1% and 2% cream in 10 patients, who used each for 28 days. Clinical, microscopic and microbiological parameters were evaluated. The cure was total for 19 out of the 20 patients, demonstrating high efficacy. There were no relapses of infection in any of the cured patients. No local or general effects were recorded during this trial.[17]

Another RCT enrolled 60 patients with culturally proven dermatophytosis (47 patients) or cutaneous candidosis (13 patients) in a double-blind, randomised study to compare the efficacy and tolerability of flutrimazole 1% cream with ketoconazole 2% cream, applied once daily for 4 weeks. Both groups of patients and distribution of target lesions were similar. The clinical results at the end of treatment were similar in both groups. The proportion of patients with negative microscopy and culture after 4 weeks of treatment was 70% in the flutrimazole group and 53% in the ketoconazole group; seven ketoconazole-treated patients (23%) compared with two flutrimazole-treated patients (6·6%) remained asymptomatic carriers (clinically cured with positive cultures).[18]

A larger recent RCT included infants age 2–13 months with diaper rash who were treated with either 0·25% miconazole nitrate (101 patients) or ointment base (101 patients) for 7 days. Both treatment groups improved, but patients receiving miconazole had significantly fewer rash sites and lower mean total rash scores on days 5 and 7 (P<0·001). In the miconazole group, improvement was greatest among those with moderate or severe diaper dermatitis at baseline and among patients whose baseline rashes were positive for *C. albicans*. Treatment with miconazole was as safe as with ointment base alone.[19]

An experimental study using an *ex vivo* system to evaluate fungal growth on stratum corneum strippings found a good antifungal effect of itraconazole whereas terbinafine had only marginal activity on *Candida*.[20]

Oral treatment

Regarding oral antifungal therapy, Stengel *et al.* compared fluconazole, 150 mg once weekly, with ketoconazole, 200 mg daily, in an RCT of 158 patients who had different forms of dermatophytosis, including a few with cutaneous candidiasis. Cure rates were similar in the patients with cutaneous candidiasis (fluconazole three of three, ketoconazole two of three).[21]

In a similar design, fluconazole, 150 mg once weekly, was compared with 50 mg daily. The results for cutaneous candidiasis at one month were 100% (9/9) and 92% respectively. The overall intention-to-treat analysis for all kinds of treated fungal infections showed no significant differences for the two regimens.[22]

What is the best treatment for oropharyngeal candidosis?

A parallel, double-blind RCT evaluated the effectiveness of nystatin pastilles (200 000 and 400 000 units) with placebo. Twenty-four subjects were selected on the basis of clinical signs of denture stomatitis and culture isolation of *Candida*. Both dosages were found to be effective after 7 and 14 days' treatment, significantly reducing or eliminating *Candida* during active therapy, and 10 days after cessation of treatment. Data from the 10-day follow up, however, demonstrated reinfection with the organism in most subjects.[23]

Another RCT evaluated the effectiveness of an antifungal denture soaking solution (nystatin, 10 000 IU/ml) used as an adjunct to a nystatin vaginal lozenge (100 000 IU/g), three times daily for 7 days, compared with tap water in a group of older chronically ill adults. Although the clinical signs and symptoms of oral candidiasis were resolved in all subjects, the presence of *Candida* hyphae was detected in about 80% of tissue and/or dentures. When compared with tap water, the use of an antifungal denture soaking solution produced no detectable difference in the presence of *C. albicans* hyphae over a 3-month period, but it did reduce the rate of recurrence of clinical signs and symptoms.[24]

A multicentre RCT by Murray *et al.* compared the efficacy and safety of oral itraconazole solution, 200 mg once daily, and clotrimazole troches, 10 mg five times daily, in 162 (142 evaluable) immunocompromised patients, mostly with AIDS. At the end of treatment significantly more patients in the clotrimazole group had negative cultures and a clinical cure than in the itraconazole group (53% versus 30%). Both drugs were well tolerated.[25]

In another RCT a total of 167 HIV-infected patients with oropharyngeal candidiasis received 14 days' therapy with either fluconazole suspension, 100 mg once daily, or liquid nystatin, 500 000 units four times daily. At day 14, 87% of the fluconazole-treated patients were clinically cured, compared with 52% in the nystatin-treated group ($P<0.001$). Fluconazole eradicated Candida organisms from the oral flora in 60%, compared with a 6% eradication rate with nystatin ($P<0.001$). The fluconazole group had fewer relapses noted on day 28 (18% versus 44% in the nystatin group; $P<0.001$) but this difference in relapse rates was no longer evident by day 42.[26]

What is the best treatment for vulvovaginal candidosis?

Topical treatment

In an early study, three days' treatment with 2% butoconazole vaginal cream was compared with a 7-day regimen of 2% miconazole vaginal cream in 271 women. After 30 days, 78% of the butoconazole-treated patients and 80% of the miconazole-treated patients remained free of vulvovaginitis. No difference in clinical and mycological cure or safety was found.[27]

In an RCT of prophylactic treatment, 38 of 42 patients (90.4%) who had achieved clinical cure with clotrimazole, 500 mg vaginal suppositories, continued to receive either 500 mg suppositories once monthly or placebo. Only a modest effect of the prophylactic regimen was evident.[28]

In another early placebo-controlled study, a single-dose 500 mg clotrimazole vaginal suppository was compared with placebo. After 7–10 days, Candida was present in 21 (38%) of those treated with clotrimazole and in 30 (75%) in the placebo group ($P<0.05$). In questionnaires completed 4 weeks later, however, half the women in each group reported recurrence of vaginal symptoms.[29]

An interesting study investigated the relationship between female genital candidiasis and Candida colonisation of their partners. A total of 125 women experiencing an acute episode of recurrent candidal vaginitis were enrolled.[30] Oral, penile and ejaculate cultures were also prepared from their male sexual partners. The rates of oral and rectal colonisation with Candida species in the women were 36% (45/125) and 45% (56/125), respectively. The male partners' oral cavities were positive in 23% (29/125) the penile coronal sulcus in 16% (20/125) and seminal fluid in 14% (18/125), respectively. In a follow up of 1 year, the clinical and microbiologic cure rate in the study group was 72% (95/125). The rate of relapse was not influenced by the treatment of Candida colonisation of the female intestinal tract, but the recurrence rate in the group with treatment of the sexual partner was lower (16% versus 45%, $P = 0.0019$).[30] This is the first study to show that treatment of the partner had an effect whereas treatment of gut colonisation of the females did not.

No difference could be detected between 1% ciclopirox olamine and 0.8% terconazole vaginal cream in the treatment of genital candidiasis in 170 women in a multicentre RCT. Despite higher and not significantly different initial microbial and clinical cure rates in both arms, at the end of the follow up at day 42 the cure rates were only 32.5% for ciclopirox and 31.5% for terconazole.[31]

Newer studies have investigated the effect of topical sustained-release creams. Dellenbach et al. treated 183 women with a sertaconazole 300 mg suppository and 186 with an econazole 150 mg suppository in a multicentre, double-blind RCT. The two groups did not differ in the rate of clinical recovery (disappearance of signs and symptoms) or mycological recovery (negative culture) 1 month after the last application (65.3 and 62.0%, respectively).[32]

Del Palacio *et al.* enrolled 124 patients who were randomly allocated to receive single doses of 1%, 2% or 4% flutrimazole vaginal cream or placebo. The percentages of patients cured at 4 weeks were 60·6% 78·0% and 81·6% with 1%, 2% and 4% cream, and 48·4% with placebo. The differences in effectiveness between 2% and 4% flutrimazole and placebo were significant (*P* = 0·01 and *P* = 0·003, respectively).Treatment failure was significantly associated with isolation of *C. glabrata*.[33]

Oral treatment

An early RCT compared oral itraconazole, 200 mg/day, with topical clotrimazole, 200 mg/day for 6 days, and with placebo in 95 patients. One week after the end of treatment 96%, 100% and 77% of the women, respectively, were clinically cured. Mycological cultures were negative in 73%, 95% and 32%. At 4 weeks no differences were found between itraconazole and clotrimazole. Side-effects were moderate and manageable but, as expected, were more frequent with itraconazole (nausea, headache) than with the locally applied clotrimazole.[34]

In a similar study design, a single oral 200 mg dose of fluconazole was not superior to daily application of a terconazole 80 mg vaginal suppository for 3 days.[35] Another RCT compared a single oral 150 mg dose of fluconazole with 7 days' clotrimazole 100 mg vaginal suppository. At the 35-day evaluation, 75% of both groups remained clinically cured; 56% of the fluconazole and 52% of the clotrimazole group were considered therapeutic cures.[36]

In a more extended comparison in a recent RCT, 150 women with clinical and mycological vaginal candidiasis received oral itraconazole, 200 mg for 3 days, or a single oral 150 mg dose of fluconazole or intravaginal clotrimazole, 100 mg/day for 6 days. The rates of clinical

effectiveness were 88%, 76% and 58%, respectively, which was not statistically significant.

What is the best therapeutic option for *Candida* urinary tract infection?

Two newer RCTs deal with the problem of candiduria. Potasman *et al.*[37] compared the efficacy of oral fluconazole (100 mg first day, then 50 mg/day for 14 days) plus catheter replacement with the efficacy of catheter replacement alone. Fluconazole caused a more rapid and an almost complete eradication of funguria, but catheter replacement alone was also followed by an 87–93% clearance of urinary findings at follow up 8 weeks later.

Another RCT enrolled 316 consecutive candiduric (asymptomatic or minimally symptomatic) hospitalised patients treated with fluconazole, 200 mg, or placebo daily for 14 days. In an intention-to-treat analysis, candiduria cleared by day 14 in 79 (50%) of 159 patients receiving fluconazole and 46 (29%) of 157 receiving placebo (*P*<0·001). Fluconazole initially produced high eradication rates, but cultures at 2 weeks showed similar candiduria rates among treated and untreated patients.[38] Thus, catheter replacement, if applicable, is the primary choice in candiduria. Oral antifungal treatment is acceptably safe but seems justified only in symptomatic patients.

What is proved about treatment of blood and systemic *Candida* infections?

Three newer RCTs deal with the treatment of blood and systemic *Candida* infections. One compared amphotericin B, 0·5–0·6 mg/kg/day, with fluconazole, 400 mg/day, as treatment for candidaemia in 237 patients. The outcome was similar: of the 103 patients treated with amphotericin B, 79% were treated successfully, compared with 70% of the 103 patients treated with fluconazole. The number of deaths did not differ significantly. The species most commonly associated with treatment failure was *C. albicans*. Fluconazole caused less toxicity than amphotericin B.[39]

A similarly designed German study of 72 patients found equal overall treatment results, but less toxicity with fluconazole than with amphotericin B/5-flucytosine. The latter, however, was more efficient in the treatment of *Candida* peritonitis and mycological cure.[40]

Regarding the route of administration of amphotericin B in critically ill patients with *Candida* sepsis, one RCT found treatment with amphotericin B in a lipid emulsion to be safer and as effective as the conventional mode of administration.[41]

Does a *Candida* hypersensitivity syndrome exist?

Public discussion in recent years has focused on a syndrome including fatigue, premenstrual tension, gastrointestinal symptoms and depression. Dismukes *et al.*[5] conducted a 32-week randomised, double-blind, crossover study using four different combinations of nystatin or placebo given orally or vaginally in 42 premenopausal women who met current criteria for the syndrome and had a history of *Candida* vaginitis. The outcomes studied were the changes from baseline scores for vaginal, systemic and overall symptoms, and the results of standardised psychological tests. Both active drug and placebo significantly reduced the clinical symptoms. The active-treatment regimens were more effective than placebo in relieving vaginal symptoms. All regimens, however, produced similar reductions in psychological symptoms and global indexes of distress.[5]

Key points

Prevention

- There is no evidence in the literature for a so-called *Candida* hypersensitivity syndrome.
- There is no RCT that supports eradication in colonised subjects who do not have an associated disease.
- In certain medical situations, such as in critically ill patients, those undergoing cancer chemotherapy, or those with complication of HIV infection, the majority of studies give evidence for a benefit of prophylactic antifungal therapy, especially in patients who are colonised with yeasts.
- There is limited evidence for any major differences between the possible treatment modalities (for example nystatin, ketoconazole, or fluconazole). In general, side-effects of this treatment are easily managed.
- There is no evidence that long-term treatment is of benefit.

Treatment

- In cutaneous candidiasis there is only limited evidence from studies on the effectiveness of "standard" nystatin.
- There is no evidence that newer topical or oral azole drugs are superior to nystatin.
- In general, clinical cure rates in all studies dealing with cutaneous candidiasis were high. The easier applicability of, for example, once-weekly oral treatment must be weighed against the greater chance of side-effects.
- In diaper dermatitis, application of an antifungal drug was superior in those cases in which *Candida* was identified at the start.
- In oropharyngeal candidosis one RCT showed itraconazole to be better than clotrimazole and another showed fluconazole to be better than nystatin. The differences, however, are only short lasting and may not have been demonstrable at longer follow up.

- In vulvovaginal candidosis the majority of RCTs have failed to demonstrate higher efficacy for any therapy approach. Short-term remission rates are between 70% and 80%, but many patients relapse after the end of treatment. Oral treatment is no better than local treatment, especially regarding long-term results. One RCT suggests that eradication of *Candida* in the sexual partner may improve long-term prognosis.

Additional comments

In countries with western lifestyle and nutrition, the majority of the population carry *Candida* in the gut. This should be considered normal and there is no evidence that elimination of the yeast makes sense or is even possible. In certain medical situations, however, prophylactic antifungal treatment to prevent the occurrence of a defined organ or systemic outbreak has been shown to be of benefit.

Under normal circumstances skin manifestations of candidosis seem to be easily treated, but only very limited information is available from studies. In other organ manifestations RCTs often fail to show significant differences between the different regimens and the results of placebo treatments are often surprisingly good, demonstrating that many patients have effective defence systems against the yeasts. Nevertheless, recalcitrant manifestations of local candidosis are frequent and may be a therapeutic problem since many RCTs show good short-term symptom relief but evidence of frequent recurrence in the long term.

References

1. Reef SE, Lasker BA, Butcher DS *et al.* Nonperinatal nosocomial transmission of *Candida albicans* in a neonatal intensive care unit: prospective study. *J Clin Microbiol* 1998;**36**:1255–9.

2. Abu-Elteen KH, Abu-Alteen RM. The prevalence of *Candida albicans* populations in the mouths of complete denture wearers. *New Microbiol* 1998;**21**:41–8.

3. Garber G. An overview of fungal infections. *Drugs* 2001;**61**(Suppl. 1):1–12.

4. Martin AG, Kobayashi GS. Yeast infections: candidiasis, pityriasis (tinea) versicolor. In: Freedberg JM, Eisen AZ, Wolff K *et al.*, eds. *Fitzpatrick's Dermatology in General Medicine, 5th ed.* New York: McGraw Hill, 1999: 2358–70.

5. Dismukes WE, Wade JS, Lee JY, Dockery BK, Hain JD. A randomized, double-blind trial of nystatin therapy for the candidiasis hypersensitivity syndrome. *N Engl J Med* 1990;**323**:1717–23.

6. Kicklighter SD, Springer SC, Cox T, Hulsey TC, Turner RB. Fluconazole for prophylaxis against candidal rectal colonization in the very low birth weight infant. *Pediatrics* 2001;**107**:293–8.

7. Morgenstern GR, Prentice AG, Prentice HG, Ropner JE, Schey SA, Warnock DW. A randomized controlled trial of itraconazole versus fluconazole for the prevention of fungal infections in patients with haematological malignancies. UK Multicentre Antifungal Prophylaxis Study Group. *Br J Haematol* 1999;**105**:901–11.

8. Goranov S, Spasov E, Grudeva-Popova J, Vakrilov V. Antifungal prophylaxis with low doses fluconazole in patients with hematological malignancies. *Folia Med* (Plovdiv) 1999;**41**:68–72.

9. Slavin MA, Osborne B, Adams R *et al.* Efficacy and safety of fluconazole prophylaxis for fungal infections after marrow transplantation – a prospective, randomized, double-blind study. *J Infect Dis* 1995;**171**:1545–52.

10. Savino JA, Agarwal N, Wry P, Policastro A, Cerabona T, Austria L. Routine prophylactic antifungal agents (clotrimazole, ketoconazole, and nystatin) in nontransplant/nonburned critically ill surgical and trauma patients. *J Trauma* 1994;**36**:20–5.

11. Eggimann P, Francioli P, Bille J *et al.* Fluconazole prophylaxis prevents intra-abdominal candidiasis in high-risk surgical patients. *Crit Care Med* 1999;**27**:1066–72.

12. Lumbreras C, Cuervas-Mons V, Jara P *et al.* Randomized trial of fluconazole versus nystatin for the prophylaxis of *Candida* infection following liver transplantation. *J Infect Dis* 1996;**174**:583–8.

13. Sangeorzan JA, Bradley SF, He X *et al.* Epidemiology of oral candidiasis in HIV-infected patients: colonization, infection, treatment, and emergence of fluconazole resistance. *Am J Med* 1994;**97**:339–46.

14. MacPhail LA, Hilton JF, Dodd CL, Greenspan D. Prophylaxis with nystatin pastilles for HIV-associated oral candidiasis. *J Acquir Immune Defic Syndr Hum Retrovirol* 1996;**12**:470–6.

15. Schuman P, Capps L, Peng G *et al*. Weekly fluconazole for the prevention of mucosal candidiasis in women with HIV infection. A randomized, double-blind, placebo-controlled trial. Terry Beirn Community Programs for Clinical Research on AIDS. *Ann Intern Med* 1997;**126**: 689–96.

16. de Wet PM, Rode H, van Dyk A, Millar AJ. Perianal candidosis – a comparative study with mupirocin and nystatin. *Int J Dermatol* 1999;**38**:618–22.

17. Umbert P, Nasarre J, Bello A *et al*. Phase II study of the therapeutic efficacy and safety of the new antimycotic sertaconazole in the treatment of superficial mycoses caused by *Candida albicans*. *Arzneimittel Forschung* 1992;**42**:757–60.

18. del Palacio A, Cuetara S, Perez A, Garau M, Calvo T, Sanchez-Alor G. Topical treatment of dermatophytosis and cutaneous candidosis with flutrimazole 1% cream: double-blind, randomized comparative trial with ketoconazole 2% cream. *Mycoses* 1999;**42**:649–55.

19. Concannon P, Gisoldi E, Phillips S, Grossman R. Diaper dermatitis: a therapeutic dilemma. Results of a double-blind placebo controlled trial of miconazole nitrate 0·25%. *Pediatr Dermatol* 2001;**18**:149–55.

20. Pierard GE, Arrese JE, De Doncker P. Antifungal activity of itraconazole and terbinafine in human stratum corneum: a comparative study. *J Am Acad Dermatol* 1995;**32**:429–35.

21. Stengel F, Robles-Soto M, Galimberti R, Suchil P. Fluconazole versus ketoconazole in the treatment of dermatophytoses and cutaneous candidiasis. *Int J Dermatol* 1994;**33**:726–9.

22. Nozickova M, Koudelkova V, Kulikova Z, Malina L, Urbanowski S, Silny W. A comparison of the efficacy of oral fluconazole, 150 mg/week versus 50 mg/day, in the treatment of tinea corporis, tinea cruris, tinea pedis, and cutaneous candidosis. *Int J Dermatol* 1998;**37**:703–5.

23. Johnson GH, Taylor TD, Heid DW. Clinical evaluation of a nystatin pastille for treatment of denture- related oral candidiasis. *J Prosthet Dent* 1989;**61**:699–703.

24. Banting DW, Greenhorn PA, McMinn JG. Effectiveness of a topical antifungal regimen for the treatment of oral candidiasis in older, chronically ill, institutionalized, adults. *J Can Dent Assoc* 1995;**61**:199–205.

25. Murray PA, Koletar SL, Mallegol I, Wu J, Moskovitz BL. Itraconazole oral solution versus clotrimazole troches for the treatment of oropharyngeal candidiasis in immunocompromised patients. *Clin Ther* 1997;**19**:471–80.

26. Pons V, Greenspan D, Lozada-Nur F *et al*. Oropharyngeal candidiasis in patients with AIDS: randomized comparison of fluconazole versus nystatin oral suspensions. *Clin Infect Dis* 1997;**24**:1204–7.

27. Kaufman RH, Henzl MR, Brown D, Jr *et al*. Comparison of three-day butoconazole treatment with seven-day miconazole treatment for vulvovaginal candidiasis. *J Reprod Med* 1989;**34**:479–83.

28. Sobel JD, Schmitt C, Meriwether C. Clotrimazole treatment of recurrent and chronic candida vulvovaginitis. *Obstet Gynecol* 1989;**73**:330–4.

29. Bro F. Single-dose 500–mg clotrimazole vaginal tablets compared with placebo in the treatment of *Candida* vaginitis. *J Fam Pract* 1990;**31**:148–52.

30. Spinillo A, Carratta L, Pizzoli G *et al*. Recurrent vaginal candidiasis. Results of a cohort study of sexual transmission and intestinal reservoir. *J Reprod Med* 1992;**37**:343–7.

31. Garcia Figueroa RG, Sauceda L, Ramirez PD, Cruz TF, Romero CR. Effectiveness and safety of ciclopirox olamine 1% vaginal cream versus terconazole 0·8% vaginal cream in the treatment of genital candidiasis. *Gynecol Obstet Mex* 2000;**68**:154–9.

32. Dellenbach P, Thomas JL, Guerin V, Ochsenbein E, Contet-Audonneau N. Topical treatment of vaginal candidosis with sertaconazole and econazole sustained-release suppositories. *Int J Gynecol Obstet* 2000;**71**(Suppl. 1):S47–S52.

33. del Palacio A, Sanz F, Sanchez-Alor G *et al*. Double-blind randomized dose-finding study in acute vulvovaginal candidosis. Comparison of flutrimazole site-release cream (1, 2 and 4%) with placebo site-release vaginal cream. *Mycoses* 2000;**43**:355–65.

34. Stein GE, Mummaw N. Placebo-controlled trial of itraconazole for treatment of acute vaginal candidiasis. *Antimicrob Agents Chemother* 1993;**37**:89–92.

35. Slavin MB, Benrubi GI, Parker R, Griffin CR, Magee MJ. Single dose oral fluconazole *v* intravaginal terconazole in treatment of *Candida* vaginitis. Comparison and pilot study. *J Fla Med Assoc* 1992;**79**:693–6.

36. Sobel JD, Brooker D, Stein GE *et al.* Single oral dose fluconazole compared with conventional clotrimazole topical therapy of *Candida* vaginitis. Fluconazole Vaginitis Study Group. *Am J Obstet Gynecol* 1995;**172**: 1263–8.

37. Potasman I, Castin A, Moskovitz B, Srugo I, Nativ O. Oral fluconazole for *Candida* urinary tract infection. *Urol Int* 1997;**59**:252–6.

38. Sobel JD, Kauffman CA, McKinsey D *et al.* Candiduria: a randomized, double-blind study of treatment with fluconazole and placebo. The National Institute of Allergy and Infectious Diseases (NIAID) Mycoses Study Group. *Clin Infect Dis* 2000;**30**:19–24.

39. Rex JH, Bennett JE, Sugar AM *et al.* A randomized trial comparing fluconazole with amphotericin B for the treatment of candidemia in patients without neutropenia. Candidemia Study Group and the National Institute. *N Engl J Med* 1994;**331**:1325–30.

40. Abele-Horn M, Kopp A, Sternberg U *et al.* A randomized study comparing fluconazole with amphotericin B/5–flucytosine for the treatment of systemic *Candida* infections in intensive care patients. *Infection* 1996;**24**:426–32.

41. Sorkine P, Nagar H, Weinbroum A *et al.* Administration of amphotericin B in lipid emulsion decreases nephrotoxicity: results of a prospective, randomized, controlled study in critically ill patients. *Crit Care Med* 1996;**24**:1311–15.

36
Deep fungal infections

Roderick J Hay

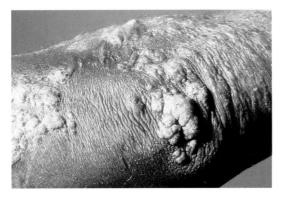

Figure 36.1 Chromoblastomycosis on the site of a traumatic injury

Introduction

Deep fungal infections or mycoses comprise a group of diseases which spread within the subcutaneous tissues (subcutaneous mycoses) or predominantly involve deeper structures including blood and bone marrow, along with other organs such as the lung and the liver (systemic mycoses). They include a number of different diseases, shown in Table 36.1.

Involvement of the skin in subcutaneous mycoses is usually secondary to direct spread from adjacent sites of infection, as in mycetoma where sinuses from deep abscesses reach the skin surface. The skin is usually breached in the process of infection and the organisms are often found in the environment with which the patient has contact.

In the case of the systemic mycoses, skin involvement is much less common but may occur through bloodstream spread where skin lesions are a consequence of dissemination and the formation of active infective foci in the dermis. The lung is usually the portal of entry in infections such as histoplasmosis, known as the endemic respiratory mycoses. Rarely the skin is the portal of entry in systemic fungal infections and the clinical course in such cases may be more benign, sometimes responding to minimal therapy. This pattern of infection, where there is local inoculation followed by local lesions and regional lymphadenopathy, is referred to as the cutaneous chancriform syndrome. By contrast, fully developed and widely disseminated disease spreading via fungaemia to affect the skin is often fatal. Infections with certain fungi such as *Penicillium marneffei* are more likely to result in skin lesions; in the latter infection over 70% of AIDS-associated cases present with skin lesions. An important subset of systemic mycoses is referred to as the opportunistic mycoses because there is always an underlying abnormality such as neutropenia or AIDS. Systemic candidosis and aspergillosis belong to this group. Skin involvement is rare and is usually the result of bloodstream spread.

This section is largely concerned with the subcutaneous mycoses. The systemic mycoses are, by definition, severe internal infections and a discussion of their management is beyond the

Table 36.1   The deep mycoses

Subcutaneous mycoses	
Mycetoma	*Madurella mycetomatis, M. grisea* (fungi)
	Nocardia spp, *Streptomyces somaliensis* (actinomycetes) and others
Chromoblastomycosis (chromomycosis)	*Fonsecaea pedrosoi, Cladophialophora carrionii* and others
Sporotrichosis	*Sporothrix schenckii*
Lobomycosis	*Loboa loboi*
Subcutaneous zygomycosis	*Basidiobolus* or *Conidiobolus* spp.
Systemic mycoses	
Endemic respiratory infections	
Histoplasmosis	*Histoplasma capsulatum* var. *capsulatum*
African histoplasmosis	*H. capsulatum* var. *duboisii*
Blastomycosis	*Blastomyces dermatitidis*
Coccidioidomycosis	*Coccidioides immitis*
Paracoccidioidomycosis	*Paracoccidioides brasiliensis*
Infections due to *Penicillium marneffei*	
Opportunistic infections	
Systemic candidosis	*Candida albicans, C. tropicalis, C. glabrata*
Aspergillosis	*Aspergillus fumigatus, A. flavus, A. niger*
Cryptococcosis	*Cryptococcus neoformans*
Mucormycosis (invasive zygomycosis)	Species of *Absidia, Rhizopus* and *Rhizomucor*
Others	
Infections due to *Fusarium, Trichosporon*	

scope of a dermatological work. In addition, there are no clinical studies directly relevant to the cutaneous manifestations of the systemic diseases, with the exception of a debate about the relevance of direct cutaneous invasion in their pathogenesis. Subcutaneous infections are rare and are generally confined to developing countries. There are few well-organised clinical studies in these infections and randomised double-blind controlled trials are exceedingly rare.

I have based the evidence search for this chapter on the Cochrane Central Register of Controlled Trials (version 2, 2002) and my own collection of studies and personal contacts in the field. Most drugs used for these infections have been developed to treat other mycotic infections and their application to deep mycoses is based on individual cases or case clusters. I will deal with each of the subcutaneous mycoses separately.

Mycetoma

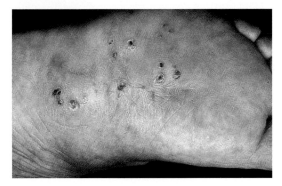

Figure 36.2   A eumycetoma infection

Definition

Mycetoma is a subcutaneous infection caused by either fungi (eumycetoma) or actinomycetes (actinomycetoma). The focus of infection is the subcutaneous tissue, including subcutaneous fat. The hallmark of the infection is that the microorganisms involved form into clusters of filaments called grains and these are surrounded by a dense neutrophil response, forming an abscess. These abscesses subsequently discharge onto the skin surface via draining sinuses but may affect underlying bone, resulting in osteomyelitis. Infective organisms are implanted into the skin, usually following a thorn injury.[1]

Incidence/prevalence

Mycetoma is an uncommon infection and there are no community-based data on prevalence. Information on worldwide incidence is based on an old study conducted by postal questionnaire in which interested departments (133) submitted data on numbers of cases occurring between 1940 and 1960. The results were published in 1963[2] and indicate that certain countries such as Sudan and Mexico had the highest numbers of cases. However, some countries such as India where the disease is endemic, did not

participate; so the data are only partially complete.

Aetiology and risk factors

Infections follow traumatic implantation of contaminated material from the environment. Because there are no known animal models, the method of infection is unknown. There are also no known risk factors apart from rural occupation. One report suggested that there was a higher incidence of diabetes mellitus in those with the disease but it did not include appropriate controls and this observation has not been substantiated elsewhere.[3]

Prognosis

There are no studies indicating prognosis of this infection. Most patients have been found to have some morbidity, usually resulting from limb deformity, but death has been known to occur where the infection affects the scalp or chest wall.

Treatment aims

The primary aim of treatment of mycetoma is to eradicate the infection and thereby halt the progression of deformity. This is possible in the case of actinomycetomas; however, there is insufficient evidence to support a particular regimen of treatment for eumycetomas, although individual responses have been recorded for ketoconazole, itraconazole and terbinafine and amphotericin B.[4] Generally, response rates amongst eumycetoma infections to chemotherapy are low and unpredictable. Therefore, in eumycetoma a secondary objective is to slow the course of the disease thus delaying the time when amputation is necessary. Amputation provides a radical cure.

Outcomes

Outcomes range from recovery to slowing of the disease progress. Mycetoma is rarely fatal and in even extensive disease the main problems are deformity and disability. In a few cases where the disease affects areas close to vital structures, such as the chest wall or cranium, the outcome is fatal.

The main approaches to management are therefore chemotherapy, combined in some cases of eumycetoma with surgery. Surgery itself may cause problems, particularly if this involves removing tissue from weight-bearing areas where the lack of support may result in pain and further disability.

QUESTION

Can mycetoma be treated successfully?

Efficacy

The usual treatments are chemotherapy for actinomycetomas and surgery and/or chemotherapy for eumycetomas. I have been unable to find any systematic reviews of treatment and there are no controlled clinical trials. Good responses to drugs such as sulphonamides and sulphones as well as co-trimoxazole have been reported in the management of actinomycetomas.[5,6] Treatment of eumycetoma with chemotherapy produces unpredictable results[4,6] and recovery is unusual. Radical surgery including limb amputation is curative in most cases.

Drawbacks

There are also no studies reporting side-effects of therapy in the specific case of mycetoma. The adverse events related to azoles such as ketoconazole and itraconazole are symptomatic hepatitis (rare with itraconazole), urticaria and drug interactions with some common medications such as terfenadine, astemazole, ciclosporin, tacrolimus, digoxin and statins, interaction with the latter resulting in rhabdomyolysis.

Comment

Mycetoma is a rare disease caused by more than ten different microorganisms distributed throughout much of the developing world. The likelihood of seeing a new generation of clinical trials on which to base an evidence-based review of treatment remains unlikely and one that can only be achieved by a coordinated multinational approach.

Implications for clinical practice

Treatment is likely to continue to be based on anecdotal evidence of the efficacy of different regimens.

Key points for mycetoma

- Treatment of actinomycetoma usually depends on two drugs such as co-trimoxazole plus rifampicin. The latter is given for up to 6 months while the other medication is continued until clinical recovery.
- Sulphonamides or sulphones can be used instead of co-trimoxazole and streptomycin instead of rifampicin.[4,6]
- Another proposed two-step regimen based on a small case series involves an intensive phase of therapy with penicillin, gentamicin and co-trimoxazole for 5–7 weeks, followed by maintenance therapy with amoxicillin and co-trimoxazole.[7]
- Successful outcome of treatment is less likely for eumycetomas. Therapy is therefore based on the premise of control of the infection by suppression of the disease, using fluconazole,[8] itraconazole[9,10] or terbinafine[11] plus amphotericin B.[4] Patients are followed over years.
- Where necessary, surgery is used to supplement the medical approach for slowing eumycetomas. Indications for amputation are advancing disease threatening the whole limb (for example involvement of the femur) and severe pain.
- Arterial perfusion with amphotericin B has also been tried for eumycetoma, with variable success rates.[12]

Sporotrichosis

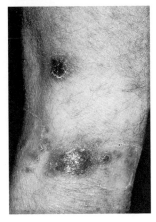

Figure 36.3 Lymphangitic sporotrichosis

Definition

Sporotrichosis is a subcutaneous and systemic infection caused by a single fungus species *Sporothrix schenckii,* a dimorphic fungal pathogen found in leaf and plant debris. The subcutaneous variety described here presents with solitary or lymphangitic nodules or ulcers on exposed cutaneous sites.

Incidence and prevalence

This is an uncommon infection and there are few data on prevalence. A problem in estimating exposure is that the frequency of subclinical infection is unknown. Using the crude antigen sporotrichin, it appears that many of the local unaffected population in endemic areas have positive reactions to the skin test (for example 22%)[13] but it is not clear if this is the result of exposure to *S. schenckii* or to cross-reactive fungal species.

By plotting the spread of cases, it appears that sporotrichosis is mainly seen in the tropics and subtropics and in parts of the US. Before the 1940s it was regularly seen in Europe, where it is now uncommon.

It is clear that cutaneous sporotrichosis may occur in the form of isolated cases or in case clusters associated with exposure to a common source of infection such as straw used in packing.[14] A major and continued outbreak was associated with contaminated pit props used in mines in South Africa. In addition, it appears that there are areas termed hyperendemic in parts of the world, for example Guatemala. Mexico and Peru. In the Peruvian focus, for instance, there has been an abnormally high frequency of cases in the vicinity of a single valley in the Andean foothills.[15] A key feature though is the absence of any obvious association between the infection and any local or geographical feature.

Aetiology and risk factors

Infections follow traumatic implantation of infected material from the environment, although it is not clear whether this is always followed by clinical disease. Risk factors include occupation: for example, miners, flower workers, those using plant material for packing and armadillo hunters have all been cited as at risk from exposure.

Prognosis

There are no studies to show if there is spontaneous resolution but this seems possible. There is clearly a wider spread of cutaneous lesions in patients with AIDS and there is a risk of internal dissemination from skin lesions in such cases. Rare cases of systemic sporotrichosis usually appear to have arisen independently of skin injury and are thought to have followed inhalation and subsequent dissemination from the lung.

Treatment aims

The aim of treatment is cure of the disease. Generally, full recovery is achievable.

QUESTION

What is the best treatment for sporotrichosis?

Efficacy

The classic treatment of sporotrichosis is a saturated solution of potassium iodide. It is started at a dose of 1 ml three time daily and the dose is increased dropwise until 4–6 ml is being administered three times daily.[16,17] The solution is often associated with side-effects such as nausea, vomiting and swelling of the salivary glands. However, recently terbinafine, itraconazole and fluconazole have been used with some success in this infection.[11,18-20]

Saturated potassium iodide is still widely used because it is cheap. One unblinded randomised comparative study of 57 people with culture-confirmed sporotrichosis showed that there was no advantage in splitting the dose of potassium iodide into three and that a single daily dose was as effective and no more toxic, with cure rates of around 89% in both groups after 45 days of follow up.[21] The alternative therapies are itraconazole, 200–600 mg daily and terbinafine, 250 mg daily. Itraconazole given for up to 36 months is recommended in a guideline for cutaneous sporotrichosis by the American Infectious Disease Society.[22] The efficacy of itraconazole is mainly supported by open studies[18,19] and there are fewer studies of terbinafine.[11] One study of fluconazole, 200–800 mg daily,[20] produced a cure in 10 of 14 patients (71%) with lymphocutaneous sporotrichosis.

Other proposed methods of treatment include liquid nitrogen as cryotherapy.[23] I have been unable to find any systematic reviews of treatment and there are no controlled clinical studies of oral antifungal agents.

Drawbacks

There are no studies reporting side-effects of therapy specific for sporotrichosis and readers are referred to references to itraconazole and terbinafine. Potassium iodide causes other specific side-effects such as sickness, vomiting, hypersalivation and salivary gland swelling. These side-effects are common (affecting around half of the trial participants in the one comparative study described above[21]) and usually mild.

Comment

There are opportunities for controlled studies of therapy in sporotrichosis, even though the disease is uncommon in many areas

Implications for clinical practice

Given the absence of randomised studies that evaluate different treatment approaches for sporotrichosis, current recommendations are based mainly on anecdotal experience. One study has suggested that there seems to be little advantage in giving potassium iodide three times as opposed to once daily in terms of cure rates.

Key points for treatment of sporotrichosis

- The main treatments in use are saturated potassium iodide solution and itraconazole.
- The disadvantage of potassium iodide is the high frequency of side-effects but the preparation is cheap.
- Fluconazole and terbinafine are alternatives, both of which show promise.
- Itraconazole appears to be effective but is used for similar long treatment periods to those used with potassium iodide. Comparative studies with terbinafine and fluconazole are needed.

Chromoblastomycosis
Definition

Chromoblastomycosis is a subcutaneous infection caused by a number of different fungi such as *Cladophialophora carrionii* and

Fonsecaea pedrosoi; a less common cause is *Phialophora dermatitidis.* The infection starts in the subcutaneous tissue or dermis and this is followed by progressive enlargement of cutaneous plaques that are usually either verrucose or plaque-like with central scarring. The organisms can be found in skin scrapings or biopsies as small pigmented cells often divided by a cross wall.

Incidence and prevalence

This is an uncommon infection and there are no data on prevalence. The disease is therefore known by clinical anecdote and reported cases. The endemic zone includes the tropics, particularly the humid zones; countries such as Costa Rica, Brazil and Madagascar probably have the largest number of cases.[24]

Aetiology and risk factors

Infection follows traumatic implantation of material from the environment. Fungi such as *Fonsecaea* species can be isolated from leaves and plant material. Although agricultural workers appear to be most at risk, there are no multicentre studies evaluating this issue.[24]

Prognosis

There are no studies indicating prognosis of this infection. However a small (5%) proportion of individuals may progress to squamous carcinoma of the skin in the affected area.

Treatment aims

The primary aim of treatment is complete recovery.[24] This is not always achievable in advanced disease. A secondary aim is prevention of complications such as squamous cell carcinoma.

Outcomes

As stated above, full recovery is not always achievable, although in early cases full recovery can be expected.

QUESTION

What is the best treatment for chromoblastomycosis?

Efficacy

The treatment of chromoblastomycosis is complex. I have not found controlled clinical studies of therapy. It is not clear though whether a single drug can cure extensive disease. Most of the treatment failures appear to occur where the infection covers a wide area.

The main treatments currently in use are itraconazole and terbinafine. Itraconazole has been used in doses of 100–200 mg daily with good results, particularly in early cases.[25] Terbinafine has been used in doses of 250 mg daily, also with good responses.[26,27] There is less experience with fluconazole, although it has been cited as an effective therapy.[28] There is no clear evidence that there are different responses to the two agents. In unresponsive cases, alternatives include combination therapy with amphotericin B and flucytosine,[29] or itraconazole and flucytosine.[30] Physical methods such as heat therapy and cryotherapy have also been used. Heat therapy involves application of heat-retaining materials to the lesions, repeated daily or less frequently over a number of weeks.[31] Itraconazole has also been used in a pulsed format[32] and in combination with other agents such as shaving, cryotherapy and 5-flucytosine.[33] One comparative trial of 12 patients with histologically confirmed chromoblastomycosis evaluated the benefit of cryotherapy in addition to itraconazole.[34] The authors suggested that itraconazole can be used initially to reduce the size of lesions, with cryotherapy being given to the residual lesion.

Drawbacks

The potential risks of treatment with terbinafine and itraconazole are discussed elsewhere in this volume. Flucytosine is an oral/intravenous drug. Potential side-effects include nausea, diarrhoea and headache, and dose-dependent bone marrow suppression. The latter occurs where plasma flucytosine levels exceed 100 mg/ml. The dose of flucytosine should be reduced in patients with renal impairment (there is a useful guide in the packet insert). Full blood and platelet counts should be followed during therapy; electrolyte and urea levels are also indicative of impending renal impairment. It is possible to monitor serum levels of flucytosine, reducing the dose if necessary. The optimum level is 40–60 mg/ml.

Comment and implications for clinical practice

The best approach to treatment in most cases is to give terbinafine or itraconazole. Where the disease is extensive, combination therapy with flucytosine plus itraconazole is of potential use.

Other subcutaneous mycoses

The other subcutaneous mycoses are even rarer and occur in remote areas. It is not possible to provide an evidence base for their diagnosis and treatment. They include the subcutaneous zygomycete infections due to *Conidiobolus* and *Basidiobolus* species, which cause woody swellings infiltrated by the strap-like fungi that cause the infections, fibroblasts and eosinophils.

Systemic mycoses

The systemic mycoses occasionally exhibit direct skin invasion following infiltration of organisms, or indirect skin manifestations such

> **Key points for chromoblastomycosis**
>
> - Chromoblastomycosis is caused by a number of different environmental fungi that are implanted through the skin.
> - Based on several case series, most infections probably respond to terbinafine or itraconazole.
> - Physical therapies such as cryotherapy and heat treatment have also been used and may confer additional benefit to drug therapy.
> - Flucytosine plus itraconazole may be of value in people who have extensive disease.

as erythema nodosum or multiforme, which are thought to develop following immune complex deposition. These are discussed briefly below.

The endemic mycoses

Skin involvement is seen as a consequence of one of three different mechanisms: direct penetration, bloodstream spread from a deep focus, and as an immunological reaction to primary, often respiratory, infection. In the latter instance the skin lesions most commonly seen are erythema nodosum or multiforme.

In the endemic mycoses the usually portal of entry is the lung. Direct entry via inoculation has been proposed in the case of some mycoses such as paracoccidioidomycosis caused by *Paracoccidioides brasiliensis* where mucocutaneous lesions are common (for example around the nose or mouth). The incidence of pulmonary disease in *P. brasiliensis* infection, even in the presence of skin lesions, is much higher in the endemic areas, suggesting that widespread subclinical exposure is most likely acquired through the airborne route. The demonstration of dissemination to mucocutaneous areas following fungaemia in animal models and the existence of subclinical pulmonary forms of disease support the view that skin lesions of paracoccidioidomycosis result from dissemination to skin from the lung. This is likely to be true of most cases of systemic endemic mycosis.

Opportunistic mycoses

The opportunistic mycoses include the infections due to *Candida, Aspergillus* and zygomycete fungi of the genera *Rhizopus, Rhizomucor* and *Absidia* amongst others. Infection affecting the skin is uncommon and these infections seldom present to a dermatologist; any skin involvement has to be set against the background of widespread and life-threatening disease. These infections often occur in patients with severe defects of either neutrophil numbers or function, such as recipients of stem cell transplants and cancer patients. *Candida* also affects seriously ill patients in intensive care or after abdominal surgery, neonates and after prolonged intravenous feeding. Isolated cases of cutaneous aspergillosis and zygomycosis have been recognised following abrasion at a specific site. Disseminated candidosis rarely affects the skin either in the neutropenic subject or the intravenous drug abuser. Systemic cryptococcus infection has been extensively evaluated in at least 13 randomised controlled trials in people with AIDS.

Patients with deep systemic mycoses rarely present directly to the dermatologist. However, there is an extensive literature on the treatment of disseminated fungal infection and through the involvement of organisations such as the Mycosis Study Group (USA) and the European Organisation for the Research and Treatment of Cancer (EORTC), a number of ground-breaking controlled clinical trials have been undertaken independently, but with the full cooperation, of the pharmaceutical industry. These have focused on various forms of treatment from prevention to specific therapy or empirical therapy.

One form of systemic mycosis that a dermatologist may be called to see is primary cutaneous cryptococcosis. Proving the existence of genuine isolated cutaneous forms of disseminated fungal disease following local trauma and possible direct inoculation compared with localised lesions following bloodstream spread has been difficult, but the concept is important as it has implications for treatment (for example the use of smaller doses that might be effective in localised forms of infection). The problem is well encapsulated by consideration of primary cutaneous cryptococcosis.

Cases of primary cutaneous cryptococcosis are rarely reported and the evidence for direct entry through the skin is often poorly substantiated and generally anecdotal. There are no clinical signs that are likely to provide an accurate indicator that the infection has developed as a result of cutaneous inoculation.[35] The evidence for its occurrence therefore can be summarised as follows:

- The first sign of infection is the development of an isolated skin lesion.
- There are no other signs or symptoms of disease, apart from regional lymphadenopathy.
- There is no circulating cryptococcal antigen or antigen in the cerebrospinal fluid measured by conventional tests such as cryptococcal latex antigen test or enzyme-linked immunoabsorbent assay.
- Oral antifungal therapy with fluconazole or itraconazole is effective.

An alternative interpretation for the development of cryptococcal skin lesions was described some time ago by Noble and Fajado[36] and was based on the subsequent identification of another focus of infection (for example lung, prostate) and evidence of positive serology in blood or cerebrospinal fluid.[37,38] This suggests that many cases of cutaneous cryptococcosis are not primary skin lesions at all but result from fungamia.[39,40] In some cases this process produces only a single skin lesion.

Examination of the literature shows that there are some patients who meet the criteria for primary cutaneous cryptococcosis.[35] These are generally elderly individuals who do not have any underlying condition known to predispose to cryptococcosis (AIDS, sarcoidosis, T cell lymphoma or chronic oral steroid therapy). Often they give a history of local skin injury, sometimes even associated with a peck of a bird that might be carrying *Cryptococcus*. Often strains isolated from such lesions belong to *C. neoformans* serotype D.[41] In AIDS patients, cutaneous cryptococcal infections may also be superimposed on some other process such as Kaposi's sarcoma[42] and are really part of a disseminated infection.

It is important to emphasise that these are observed criteria and have not, by virtue of the rarity of cutaneous cryptococcosis, been subjected to analysis of sufficient scientific rigour. However, the implications for therapy are sufficiently important that it is recommended that patients who meet the broad criteria for cutaneous cryptococcosis receive treatment with an oral azole antifungal agent, such as fluconazole (at least 200 mg daily) or itraconazole (at least 200 mg daily) until the lesions have resolved, treatment being extended for at least 1 month thereafter. Serology should be monitored again before the end of treatment and for 6 months after the end of treatment. This approach is provided as a guideline based on anecdotal experience and has not been the subject of a clinical trial.

Key points for systemic mycoses

- Systemic mycoses are not usually treated primarily by dermatologists.
- Most opportunistic mycoses are seen in immunocompromised patients.
- Skin lesions in most endemic mycoses such as paracoccidioidomycosis probably result from lung dissemination.
- They occasionally exhibit direct skin invasion following infiltration of organisms or indirect skin manifestations such as erythema nodosum or multiforme, probably from immune complex deposition.
- Although many patients with cutaneous cryptococcal infection probably develop skin involvement as a result from internal spread, some cases of primary cutaneous cryptococcus do exist.
- Anecdotal evidence suggests that itraconazole or fluconazole might be effective in such cases.
- A number of controlled clinical trials for the treatment of systemic mycoses are currently underway by the US Mycosis Study Group and the EORTC.

References

1. Mahgoub ES, Murray IG. *Mycetoma*. London: William Heinemann Medical, 1973.
2. Mariat F. Sur la distribution geographique et la repartition des agents des mycetomes. *Bull Soc Path Exot* 1963;**56**:35–45.
3. Hay RJ, Mackenzie DWR. Mycetoma (Madura foot) in the United Kingdom – a survey of 44 cases. *Clin Exp Dermatol* 1983;**8**:553–62.
4. Hay RJ, Mahgoub ES, Leon G *et al.* Mycetoma. *J Med Vet Mycol* 1992;**30**(Suppl. 1):41–9.
5. Boiron P, Locci R, Goodfellow M *et al.* Nocardia, nocardiosis and mycetoma. *Med Mycol* 1998;**36**(Suppl. 1):26–37.
6. Welsh O, Salinas MC, Rodriguez MA. Treatment of eumycetoma and actinomycetoma. *Curr Top Med Mycol* 1995;**6**:47–71.

7. Ramam M, Garg T, D'Souza P *et al.* A two-step schedule for the treatment of actinomycotic mycetomas. *Acta Derm Venereol* 2000;**80**:378–80.

8. Gugnani HC, Ezeanolue BC, Khalil M *et al.* Fluconazole in the therapy of tropical deep mycoses. *Mycoses* 1995;**38**:485–8.

9. Paugam A, Tourte-Schaefer C, Keita A *et al.* Clinical cure of fungal madura foot with oral itraconazole. *Cutis* 1997;**60**:191–3.

10. Lee MW, Kim JC, Choi JS, Kim KH, Greer DL. Mycetoma caused by *Acremonium falciforme*: successful treatment with itraconazole. *J Am Acad Dermatol* 1995;**32**:897–900.

11. Hay RJ. Therapeutic potential of terbinafine in subcutaneous and systemic mycoses. *Br J Dermatol* 1999;**141**(Suppl. 56):36–40.

12. Subrahmanyam M. Intra-arterial chemotherapy for mycetoma of the foot. *Br J Surg* 1995;**82**:643.

13. Ghosh A, Chakrabarti A, Sharma VK, Singh K, Singh A. Sporotrichosis in Himachal Pradesh (north India). *Trans R Soc Trop Med Hyg* 1999;**93**:41–5.

14. Conias S, Wilson P. Epidemic cutaneous sporotrichosis:report of 16 cases in Queensland due to mouldy hay. *Aust J Dermatol* 1998;**39**:34–7.

15. Pappas PG, Tellez I, Deep AE *et al.* Sporotrichosis in Peru: description of an area of hyperendemicity. *Clin Infect. Dis* 2000;**30**:65–70.

16. Tobin EH, Jih WW. Sporotrichoid lymphocutaneous infections: etiology, diagnosis and therapy. *Am Fam Phys* 2001;**63**:326–32.

17. Kauffman CA. Old and new therapies for sporotrichosis. *Clin Infect Dis* 1995;**21**:981–5.

18. Noguchi H, Hiruma M, Kawada A. Case report. Sporotrichosis successfully treated with itraconazole in Japan. *Mycoses* 1999;**42**:571–6.

19. Karakayali G, Lenk N, Alli N, Gungor E, Artuz F. Itraconazole therapy in lymphocutaneous sporotrichosis: a case report and review of the literature. *Cutis* 1998;**61**:106–7.

20. Kauffman CA, Pappas PG, McKinsey DS *et al.* Treatment of lymphocutaneous and visceral sporotrichosis with fluconazole. *Clin Infect Dis* 1996;**22**:46–50.

21. Cabezas C, Bustamante B, Holgado W, Begue RE. Treatment of cutaneous sporotrichosis with one daily dose of potassium iodide. *Pediatr Infect Dis J* 1996;**15**:352–4.

22. Kauffman CA, Hajjeh R, Chapman SW. Practice guidelines for the management of patients with sporotrichosis. For the Mycoses Study Group. Infectious Diseases Society of America. *Clin Infect Dis* 2000;**30**:684–7.

23. Bargman H. Successful treatment of cutaneous sporotrichosis with liquid nitrogen:report of three cases. *Int J Dermatol* 1995;**38**:285–7.

24. Minotto R, Bernardi CD, Mallmann LF *et al.* Chromoblastomycosis: a review of 100 cases in the state of Rio Grande do Sul, Brazil. *J Am Acad Dermatol* 2001;**44**:585–92.

25. Bonifaz A, Carrasco-Gerard E, Saul A. Chromoblastomycosis: clinical and mycologic experience of 51 cases. *Mycoses* 2001;**44**:1–7.

26. Esterre P, Inzan CK, Ramarcel ER *et al.* Treatment of chromomycosis with terbinafine: preliminary results of an open pilot study. *Br J Dermatol* 1996;**134**(Suppl. 46):33–6.

27. Tanuma H, Hiramatsu M, Mukai H *et al.* Case report. A case of chromoblastomycosis effectively treated with terbinafine. Characteristics of chromoblastomycosis in the Kitasato region, Japan. *Mycoses* 2000;**43**:79–83.

28. Guerriero C, De Simone C, Tulli A. A case of chromoblastomycosis due to *Phialophora verrucosa* responding to treatment with fluconazole. *Eur J Dermatol* 1998;**8**:167–8.

29. Kombila M, Gomez de Diaz M, Richard Lenoble D *et al.* Chromoblastomycosis in Gabon. Study of 64 cases. *Sante* 1995;**5**:235–44.

30. Kullavanijaya P, Rojanavanich V. Successful treatment of chromoblastomycosis due to *Fonsecaea pedrosoi* by the combination of itraconazole and cryotherapy. *Int J Dermatol* 1995;**34**:804–7.

31. Hiruma M, Kawada A, Yoshida M, Kouya M. Hyperthermic treatment of chromomycosis with disposable chemical pocket warmers. Report of a successfully treated case, with a review of the literature. *Mycopathologia* 1993;**122**:107–14.

32. Kumarasinghe SP, Kumarasinghe MP. Itraconazole pulse therapy in chromoblastomycosis. *Eur J Dermatol* 2000;**10**:220–2.

33. Poirriez J, Breuillard F, Francois N *et al.* A case of chromomycosis treated by a combination of cryotherapy, shaving, oral 5–fluorocytosine, and oral amphotericin B. *Am J Trop Med Hyg* 2000:**63**:61–3.

34. Bonifaz A, Martinez-Soto E, Carrasco-Gerrard E, Peniche J. Treatment of chromoblastomycosis with itraconazole, cryosurgery and a combination of both. *Int J Dermatol* 1997;**36**:542–7.

35. Patel P, Ramanathan J, Kayser M, Baran J Jr. Primary cutaneous cryptococcosis of the nose in an immunocompetent woman. *J Am Acad Dermatol* 2000;**43**:344–5.

36. Noble RC, Fajardo LF. Primary cutaneous cryptococcosis: review and morphologic study. *Am J Clin Pathol* 1972;**57**:13–22.

37. Antony SA, Antony SJ. Primary cutaneous cryptococcus in nonimmunocompromised patients. *Cutis* 1995;**56**:96–8.

38. Hamann ID, Gillespie RJ, Ferguson JK. Primary cryptococcal cellulitis caused by *Cryptococcus neoformans* var. gattii in an immunocompetent host. *Aust J Dermatol* 1997;**38**:29–32.

39. Sanchez P, Bosch RJ, de Galvez MV *et al.* Cutaneous cryptococcosis in two patients with acquired immuno-deficiency syndrome. *Int J STD AIDS* 2000;**11**:477–80.

40. Coker LR, Swain R, Morris R, McCall CO. Disseminated cryptococcosis presenting as pseudofolliculitis in an AIDS patient. *Cutis* 2000;**66**:207–10.

41. Naka W, Masuda M, Konohana A *et al.* Primary cutaneous cryptococcosis and *Cryptococcus neoformans* serotype D. *Clin Exp Dermatol* 1995;**20**:221–5.

42. Glassman SJ, Hale MJ. Cutaneous cryptococcosis and Kaposi's sarcoma occurring in the same lesions in a patient with the acquired immunodeficiency syndrome. *Clin Exp Dermatol* 1995;**20**:480–6.

Part 3: The evidence

Section D: Infestations

Editor: Berthold Rzany

37
Scabies

Ian F Burgess

Background
Definition

Scabies is an itchy immune hypersensitivity reaction to infestation of the skin by the mite *Sarcoptes scabiei*. Adult female mites burrow through the skin at the junction of the stratum corneum and the prickle cell layer, where they lay their eggs. Burrows then move out progressively towards the skin surface with the stratum corneum. Adult males and juvenile mites (larvae and nymphs) live mostly at the skin surface but may make temporary burrows for moulting from one development stage to another.

Infestation of immune-competent people is most common on the hands, digits and finger webs, and on the wrists. The flexor surfaces of the elbows, the axillae, ankles, buttocks, breasts and male genitalia may also be infested. In the elderly, infants and the immunocompromised the infestation may be more diffuse, including the head and neck, and palms and soles.

Incidence/prevalence

We found no recent published data on incidence or prevalence from any developed country. Scabies is a common public health problem in developing countries, where prevalence may exceed 50% in some communities, and prevalence has been estimated at 300 million cases worldwide.[1] Older studies have shown that prevalence is highest in teenagers and schoolchildren.[2–4] However, incidence has increased recently in the institutionalised elderly. Historical data from Denmark show that epidemic cycles arise at 15–20-year intervals.[2]

Aetiology/risk factors

Transmission of scabies mites occurs during relatively prolonged skin–skin contact. The infection is most frequent in communities with long-term conditions of overcrowding, and increases following social disruption. Reduction of immune competence increases the risk of contracting infestation, with a concomitant risk of high mite numbers. We found no evidence that hygiene influences risk, although good hygiene may ameliorate symptomatic presentation.[5]

Prognosis

Scabies is not life threatening, but the severe, persistent itch and secondary infections may be debilitating and disfiguring. Long-term infestations are inherently immunodepressive and in susceptible people may lead to development of a form of the disease in which large numbers of mites inhabit hyperkeratotic plaques. These shed skin plaques may be a source of reinfection and transmission.[6] In some circumstances scabies infected with haemolytic streptococci may result in acute glomerulonephritis.[5]

Diagnosis

A diagnosis of active infestation is confirmed only by finding mites, mite ova or faecal pellets (scybala). Mite burrows in the skin, the distribution of papular lesions and bilateral itch not affecting the head, chest or back are indicative but are not confirmation of an active infestation. Nodular lesions around the axillae, navel or on the penis or scrotum are pathognomonic, but may persist for months after cure.

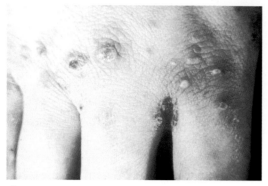

a)

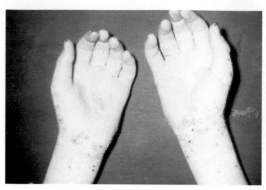

b)

Figure 37.1   a) Papules, pustules and impetaginisation in the vicinity of scabies burrows and b) excoriated rash and papules on the wrists in simple scabies

Aims of treatment

The aim of treatment is to eliminate infestation by killing or removing all mites and their eggs.

Outcomes

There are no established standard criteria for making a diagnosis or judging treatment success. Trials used different methods, and in many cases the method was not stated. Treatment success should be given as the percentage of people completely cleared of scabies mites, ova or faecal pellets in skin scrapings viewed under magnification. Clinical success includes elimination of papular and vesicular eruptions and pruritus. Ideally, outcomes should be assessed 28 days after the start of treatment. This allows lesions to heal. If treatment fails, eggs hatch within 3 days and emerging mites become mature 9–10 days later.

Methods of search

1. The initial search conducted for a systematic review compiled in 1999[7] used the following primary sources: Cochrane Central Register of Controlled Trials; Medline 1966 to 1997;

Embase 1974 to 1997; records of military trials from the UK, US and Russia, and the specialist register of the Cochrane Diseases Group.
2. Clinical evidence search, May 2000
3. Medline update search for evidence-based dermatology, January 2002
4. Hand searching of relevant journals

QUESTIONS

How successful are topical treatments for scabies? For example, would a topical treatment be suitable for treating newly diagnosed scabies in a 16-year-old girl? (Figure 37.1)

Insecticide-based pharmaceutical products
Benefits

We found one systematic review (search date 1997) that examined four trials. In each case a single application of treatment was given unless stated otherwise. One study (150 adults and children) compared 5% permethrin cream with 10% crotamiton cream (a non-insecticide) and 1% lindane lotion.[8] It used clinical features as the measure of success. The results showed that permethrin was slightly, but not significantly, more likely to cure (49/50 (98%)) people with permethrin versus 44/50 (88%) with crotamiton; relative risk (RR) 1·11, 95% confidence intervals (CI) 1·0–1·2). The same study also found permethrin to be significantly more effective than lindane: permethrin cured 49/50 (98%) whereas lindane cured only 12/50 (24%) people (RR 4·08, CI 2·5–6·7).[8] A single randomised controlled trial (RCT) comparing 5% permethrin cream with 10% crotamiton cream evaluated cure by elimination of parasites.[9] It found permethrin to be more effective after 14 and 28 days. After 14 days 33/47 (70%) of people in the permethrin group and 41/47 (87%) in the crotamiton group still had lesions. At this point 10 people in the crotamiton group were withdrawn from the study because their infestation was exacerbated. However, after 28 days 42/47 (89%) people in the permethrin group were free from parasites compared with 28/47 (60%) in the crotamiton group (RR 1·5, CI 1·2–1·9).[9] This study also recorded patients' subjective reports on the persistence of pruritus, which was found to be closely related to effectiveness of the treatments.

Two trials compared the effect of 5% permethrin cream with that of 1% lindane lotion. A small study (46 people) found fewer people improved 14 days after using permethrin (13/23 (57%) versus lindane 20/23 (87%); P<0·02), but a significantly better rate of cure, by parasitological examination, for permethrin at 28 days (21/23 versus 15/23; P<0·025, RR 1·4, CI 1·0–1·9).[10] A larger trial (467 people) did not identify parasites but recorded a significant decrease in the number of lesions persisting in both groups after 14 ± 3 days. At 28 ± 7 days success rates were 181/199 (91%) after using 5% permethrin cream, compared with 176/205 (86%) after using 1% lindane lotion (P = 0·18, RR 1·06, CI 0·9–1·1).[11] At final assessment, significantly fewer of the permethrin group (27/194 (14%)) had persistent itch compared with 49/197 (25%) of the lindane group (P = 0·007).[11]

The systematic review identified no RCTs comparing 0·5% malathion, in either aqueous or alcohol vehicles, with other treatments. Case series and one quasi-randomised trial suggest that it is effective, with a cure rate of over 80% at 4 weeks.[12–14]

Drawbacks

Only minor adverse effects have been reported for most insecticides. The exception is lindane, for which there are extensive reports of effects related to overdosing and absorption.[15,16] Despite recognised neurotoxicity, lindane is still widely used, partly because alternatives are not readily available in many countries. Lindane passes transdermally during treatment and other exposures, and may be stored in fatty tissues and excreted in breast milk.[17] Acute exposure to lindane during scabies treatment has potentiated seizures in people on medication that reduces seizure threshold.[18,19] Therefore, lindane appears to be contraindicated for those undergoing therapy for HIV infection,[18] or attention deficit hyperactivity disorder using amphetamine,[19] and in those who suffer from epileptiform seizures. Concern has been expressed that lindane may be a risk factor for triggering of seizures in epileptics because it may alter liver cell function. Lindane does cause oxidative stress but does not appear to modify liver microsomal function, and in experimental systems these effects were mitigated by prior treatment with phenobarbital.[20,21] Consequently, those being treated with barbiturates may be at lower risk of suffering side-effects from lindane. However, it is not clear whether people receiving anticonvulsant drugs in general are at greater risk of having seizures if exposed to lindane.

Various studies have shown that the solvent vehicle plays an important role in the rate of transdermal absorption of lindane.[22,23] Additionally, much of the drug can also be absorbed as the treatment is washed off because a depot of lindane builds up in the stratum corneum.[23–25] In many countries, scabicides are still applied after a hot bath but the resultant peripheral vasodilation is likely to enhance transdermal absorption. A related increase in passage of lindane through the dermis has been identified if soap and hot water are used to remove the acaricide at the end of the treatment process. Absorption can be minimised if cool water alone is used to remove residues of lindane products before bathing.[25] An investigation of the absorption of permethrin and lindane through human cadaver skin *in vitro* found that lindane achieved a rate of 2 microgram/hour/cm^2 in less than 5 hours, whereas the rate for permethrin was one-tenth of this after 10 hours. However, fresh guinea pig skin absorbed both at the same rate.[26]

Most RCTs have reported no serious adverse events using these topical insecticide-based products. One RCT reported five serious adverse events, two possibly associated with permethrin (rash and diarrhoea) and three possibly associated with lindane use (pruritic rash, papules and diarrhoea).[11] Post-marketing surveillance of permethrin use in the USA from 1990 to 1995 found six adverse events per 100 000 units of product (equivalent to one central nervous system adverse event for each 500 000 units of permethrin used).[27] Case series based on community intervention studies have reported a burning paraesthesia as one of the most frequent adverse events following permethrin use, particularly in the immunodeficient.[27,28] A burning sensation was the most frequent adverse event, although not significantly so, in the largest RCT, with 23 events in 233 people following application of 5% permethrin, compared with 12/232 after 1% lindane lotion ($P = 0.08$).[11]

Comment
Generally, it is believed that all mites and their eggs are killed soon after treatment. Confirmation of cure is therefore difficult because mites may not be detectable in post-treatment skin scrapings. It is therefore impossible to determine success until sufficient time has passed to permit the various lesions resulting from the infestation to heal. Many people show considerable improvement after 14 days but a definitive clinical cure cannot be concluded until about 28 days after treatment, when all lesions present at the time of treatment should either be healed or resolving, without new lesions developing.

Three of the RCTs were conducted in developing countries. The fourth study was divided between the USA and Mexico.[11] It is not known whether scabies mites may be more susceptible to treatment in communities where treatments are not generally available but it is likely that prior exposure to acaricidal chemicals may select for reduced sensitivity in mites in developed countries, and some cases of suspected resistance, particularly to lindane, have been recorded.[27,29]

Lindane products are still used against scabies in most western countries, despite its relative toxicity. In the UK the only lindane product was withdrawn on commercial grounds. The former market-leading product in the USA is now no longer produced for the same reason.

Implications for clinical practice
The evidence indicates that permethrin is more effective than crotamiton, lindane and malathion, and has been associated with fewer side-effects than lindane. However, the high cost of permethrin may limit its use in some communities. Permethrin is probably more likely to be effective with one application than are other insecticides but a second treatment may be necessary for all.[30]

Non-insecticide-based acaricides
Benefits
Randomised studies comparing the non-insecticide antiscabies agent crotamiton with

insecticide-based treatments were described above.

We found one trial (158 adults and children) comparing 25% benzyl benzoate with sulphur ointment (concentration of sulphur not given) in a community study in India.[31] In this study patients were first scrubbed in a bath; the treatments were then applied three times in 24 hours (morning, night, next morning). Assessments were made at approximately 5-day intervals. No significant difference was found between the treatments regarding improvement of lesions at 9–10 days (benzyl benzoate 68/89 (76%) versus 45/69 (65%) with sulphur; RR 1·17, CI 1·0–1·4). At this time, if lesions remained the patients were treated again so that by 14–15 days improvement of symptoms in the benzyl benzoate group was 81/89 (91%) compared with 67/69 (97%) for sulphur (RR 0·94, CI 0·9–1·0), which was also not significantly different.

Non-controlled studies and case studies have indicated a variable effectiveness for both benzyl benzoate (20% emulsion,[32] 25% emulsion,[14] 25% cream[33]) and sulphur ointment (5%,[35] 6%,[34] or 10%[32,35]). Activity of these acaricides is related to the concentration of active drug in the vehicle and the number of times they are applied. In general, benzyl benzoate appears to require a minimum of two applications and sulphur may require several applications over one week or longer.[36]

We found a single RCT evaluated by the systematic review comparing pork fat containing 1% salicylic acid and cold cream as ointment vehicles for delivery of sulphur.[37] The numbers in this study were small (51 confirmed cases) and differences of efficacy could have been due to chance effects. Every participant applied the sulphur ointment on three consecutive nights and then again three days later. Evaluations were made on the tenth day after the last treatment. This study is more relevant for the side-effects observed, described below.

We found that other non-insecticide active materials have only been described in non-randomised studies and case series. One non-randomised study comparing 5% sulphur ointment, 1% lindane cream, 25% benzyl benzoate cream, 10% crotamiton lotion, and 0·2% nitrofurazone in a water-soluble ointment, found nitrofurazone was least effective, with a 70% cure rate.[33] A case series of 20 patients using the same nitrofurazone ointment produced "complete clinical cure" in 80% of cases.[38]

Monosulfiram is now little used either as a liquid (25% before dilution for use) or a soap. Most studies are of poor quality and more than 50 years old, and more recent case studies show a high incidence of side-effects (see below). Thiabendazole has been used as a 5% and a 10% cream applied over several days. In one case series, 5/19 (26%) were still infested after 5% cream was used twice daily for 5 days. The remaining patients were cured after a further 5 days of treatment.[39] Another case series, in which 10% cream was used, achieved 80% success after 5 days.[40]

Drawbacks

Generally, only minor adverse reactions have been reported for non-insecticide treatments for scabies. Most of these have been related to skin irritation, often following repeated or multiple applications of the formulation. The RCT comparing vehicles for sulphur ointment[37] did not provide adequate data for a full analysis of effects. Side-effects were reported in patients and close contacts within 6 days of first being treated with either cold cream or pork fat with 1% salicylic acid: pruritus (31% versus 60%), xerosis (24% versus 34%), burning sensation (12% versus 17%), erythema (10% versus 2%), and keratosis (2% versus 15%).[37] Where sulphur is used in developed countries it is normally applied in petroleum jelly and similar skin reactions have been reported as side-effects from case studies and series.[36,41] Similar irritant reactions occur with repeat treatments using benzyl benzoate, particularly if naturally derived rather than synthetic material is used.[36,42] In one RCT approximately 25% of people reported an increase in pruritus and dermatitis after treatment with two applications of 10% benzyl benzoate.[43]

Monosulfiram has been associated with a systemic adverse event in a number of case reports in which the people developed dermal oedema, flushing, sweating and tachycardia, especially after ingesting alcohol within 24 hours of treatment.[44–46] This reaction occurs because monosulfiram is chemically related to disulfiram, used in the treatment of alcoholism (Antabuse).

Multiple applications of crotamiton can result in dermatitis and there is one report of a suspected link with methaemaglobinaemia.[16,36,47]

Comments

Most studies in this group are not comparable because of differences in the formulations used, the concentrations of the active substances and the duration or number of applications. Evidence for activity is limited in each case, and it is possible that some of the effectiveness is partially related to a physical effect, for example sulphur in a heavy greasy base may physically trap and subsequently remove developmental stages of the mite from the skin surface. The mode of action of crotamiton is not understood and there is some doubt about both its acaricidal and antipruritic activities. Similar questions may apply to all of the non-insecticide-based treatments. The fact that these treatments are cheap means that they are more likely to be used in developing countries where source materials may be less well characterised. Most of these compounds have been in use for around 50 years and there is some suspicion that resistance is developing in some areas.[16]

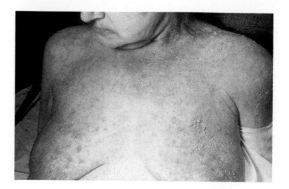

Figure 37.2 Hyperkeratotic crusts may develop in abnormal sites. With permission from Institute of Dermatology

Implications for clinical practice

All of these products are likely to require 2–4 applications and are not particularly cosmetic. They may therefore suffer from compliance problems. However, the low cost and relative safety, apart from skin irritancy, make non-insecticide-based acaricides attractive alternatives to insecticide-based products where mites may have developed resistance or if cost is an issue.

How successful are oral treatments for scabies? Would an oral treatment be suitable for treating an 82-year-old resident in a nursing home? (Figure 37.2)

Orally administered treatments
Benefits

We found one systematic review examining two small RCTs, one of which had inadequate follow up. A placebo-controlled RCT (55 adults and children) found that significantly more people treated with ivermectin, 200 microgram/kg, (23/29 (79%)) were free from symptoms at 7 days compared with those treated with placebo (2/26 (8%) RR 10·3, CI 2·7–39·6). The code was then broken and the controls and all patients who had not improved received ivermectin.[48] A comparative RCT (44 people) found no significant difference in improvement of lesions between ivermectin, 100 microgram/kg, (16/23 (70%)) and benzyl benzoate 10%, applied twice over 2 days (10/21 (48%)) at 30 days (RR 1·46, CI 0·9–2·5).[43]

We also found one RCT (85 people) comparing ivermectin, 200 microgram/kg, with 5% permethrin cream, evaluated at 1, 2, 4 and 8 weeks.[49] In this study a single dose of ivermectin relieved symptoms in significantly fewer people (28/40 (70%)) than permethrin (44/45 (98%) RR 0·72, CI 0·6–0·9), but when a second dose of treatment was given after 2 weeks there was no significant difference in the improvement rate between the ivermectin group (38/40 (95%)) and the permethrin group, in which everyone was cured . A second RCT (53 people, 43 completing the study) found ivermectin, 150–200 microgram/kg, to be statistically equivalent to 1% lindane lotion.[50] After 15 days 14/19 (74%) had improved with ivermectin, compared with 13/24 (46%) treated with lindane (RR 1·36, CI 0·9–2·1). At 29 days all but one person in each group were cured (18/19 (95%) with ivermectin versus 23/24 (96%) with lindane; RR 0·99, CI 0·9–1·1).

Drawbacks

All the RCTs were too small to provide adequate safety data for use of ivermectin against scabies, particularly in children. Ivermectin has been used extensively in community control programmes for onchocerciasis and filariasis and there have been few reports of serious adverse events.[51,52] There has been one report of a significant increase in mortality rate in a psychogeriatric unit (15/42 (36%); $P = 0.001$) within 6 months of ivermectin use compared with controls in the same care facility over a 3-year period.[53] However, each resident in the unit had previously received several applications of other scabies treatments, including lindane and permethrin. Use of ivermectin in the elderly in other countries has not resulted in any similar increase in mortality.[54]

Comment

Ivermectin has been licensed for use against scabies only in France. However, its use on a named-patient basis has become widespread as a component of treatment for hyperkeratotic scabies in which it is often difficult to kill all the mites because of the limited penetration of the plaques by topical acaricides. In this condition, ivermectin can reach trophic mites by incorporation in the living cell layer on which the mites feed. However, ivermectin is unlikely to have any effect on mite eggs, and failures of treatment have been reported unless either dosing is repeated or a topical scabicide is used concurrently.[55–57] So far no proper dosing studies using ivermectin have been performed, and the relative underdosing using both ivermectin and benzyl benzoate in one study indicates how important a contribution to knowledge this would be.[43]

Implications for practice

A reliable and safe oral treatment is the most attractive option for dosing and compliance with scabies treatment. Ivermectin has not yet been evaluated sufficiently to determine the most appropriate dosing regimen, but it can be a useful adjunct to conventional treatment approaches.

Additional comment

The evidence for effectiveness of scabies treatments is still largely rudimentary and the majority of studies have employed inadequate criteria for diagnosis and evaluation of efficacy. What evidence exists indicates that none of the topical products is reliable with a single application. The limited evidence available for ivermectin is far from the aspirations expressed by those dealing with problems of long-term infestation. Consequently, further investigation is required for this and other treatments to determine adequate drug regimens.

Key points

- Permethrin and lindane are probably effective in scabies treatment, although lindane has been withdrawn from some markets and has a higher potential for toxicity. Malathion may be effective but more evidence is required.
- Crotamiton, benzyl benzoate, and sulphur show insufficient evidence of efficacy, as do nitrofurazone, monosulfiram, and thiabendazole.
- There is currently insufficient evidence of the effectiveness of ivermectin from small trials. Case studies indicate that it may be effective if used with a topical agent. A proper dose regimen evaluation is required.

References

1. Stein DH. Scabies and pediculosis. *Curr Opin Pediatr* 1991;**3**:660–6.

2. Christopherson J. The epidemiology of scabies in Denmark, 1900 to 1975. *Arch Dermatol* 1978;**114**:747–50.

3. Church RE, Knowlesden J. Scabies in Sheffield: a family infestation. *BMJ* 1978;i:761.

4. Palicka P. The incidence and mode of scabies transmission in a district of Czechoslovakia (1961–1979). *Folia Parasitol* 1982;**29**:51–9.

5. Burgess I. *Sarcoptes scabiei* and scabies. *Adv Parasitol* 1994;**33**:235–92.

6. Carslaw RW, Dobson RM, Hood AJK *et al.* Mites in the environment of cases of Norwegian scabies. *Br J Dermatol* 1975;**92**:333–7.

7. Walker GJA, Johnstone PW. Treating scabies. In: Cochrane Collaboration. *Cochrane Library*, Issue 4. Oxford: Update Software, 1999.

8. Amer M, El-Gharib I. Permethrin versus crotamiton and lindane in the treatment of scabies. *Int J Dermatol* 1992;**31**:357–8.

9. Taplin D, Meinking TL, Chen JA *et al.* Comparison of crotamiton 10% cream (Eurax) and permethrin 5% cream (Elimite) for the treatment of scabies in children. *Pediatr Dermatol* 1990;**7**:67–73.

10. Taplin D, Meinking TL, Porcelain SL *et al.* Permethrin 5% dermal cream: a new treatment of scabies. *J Am Acad Dermatol* 1986;**15**:995–1001.

11. Schultz MW, Gomez M, Hansen RC *et al.* Comparative study of 5% permethrin cream and 1% lindane lotion for the treatment of scabies. *Arch Dermatol* 1990;**126**:167–70.

12. Hanna NF, Clay JC, Harris JRW. *Sarcoptes scabiei* infestation treated with malathion liquid. *Br J Vener Dis* 1978;**54**:354.

13. Thianprasit M, Schuetzenberger R. Prioderm lotion in the treatment of scabies. *Southeast Asian J Trop Med Public Health* 1984;**15**:119–21.

14. Burgess I, Robinson RJ, Robinson J *et al.* Aqueous malathion 0·5% as a scabicide:clinical trial. *BMJ* 1986;**292**:1172.

15. Schmutz JL, Barbaud A, Trechot P. Intoxication aigue au lindane chez 3 enfants. *Ann Dermatol Venereol* 2001;**128**:799.

16. Elgart ML. A risk-benefit assessment of agents used in the treatment of scabies. *Drug Saf* 1996;**14**:386–93.

17. Schinas V, Leontsinidis M, Alexopoulos A *et al.* Organochlorine pesticide residues in breast milk from southwest Greece: associations with weekly food consumption patterns of mothers. *Arch Environ Health* 2000;**55**:411–17.

18. Solomon BA, Haut SR, Carr EM *et al.* Neurotoxic reaction to lindane in an HIV-seropositive patient. An old medication's new problem. *J Fam Pract* 1995;**40**:291–6.

19. Cox R, Krupnick J, Bush N *et al.* Seizures caused by concomitant use of lindane and dextroamphetamine in a child with attention deficit hyperactivity disorder. *J Miss State Med Assoc* 2000;**41**:690–2.

20. Simon Giavarotti KA, Rodrigues L, Rodrigues T *et al.* Liver microsomal parameters related to oxidative stress and antioxidant systems in hyperthyroid rats subjected to acute lindane treatment. *Free Radic Res* 1998;**29**:35–42.

21. Videla LA, Arisi AC, Fuzaro AP *et al.* Prolonged phenobarbital pretreatment abolishes the early oxidative stress component induced in the liver by acute lindane intoxication. *Toxicol Lett* 2000;**115**:45–51.

22. Dick IP, Blain PG, Williams FM. The percutaneous absorption and skin distribution of lindane in man. I. In vivo studies. *Hum Exp Toxicol* 1997;**16**:645–51.

23. Dick IP, Blain PG, Williams FM. The percutaneous absorption and skin distribution of lindane in man. II. In vitro studies. *Hum Exp Toxicol* 1997;**16**:652–7.

24. Lange M, Nitzsche K, Zesch A. Percutaneous absorption of lindane in healthy volunteers and scabies patients.

Dependency of penetration kinetics in serum upon frequency of application, time and mode of washing. *Arch Dermatol Res* 1981;**271**:387–99.

25. Zesch A, Nitsche K, Lange M. Demonstration of the percutaneous resorption of a lipophilic pesticide and its possible storage in the human body. *Arch Dermatol Res* 1982;**273**:43–9.

26. Franz TJ, Lehman PA, Franz SF *et al.* Comparative percutaneous absorption of lindane and permethrin. *Arch Dermatol* 1996;**132**:901–5.

27. Meinking TL, Taplin D. Safety of permethrin *v* lindane for the treatment of scabies. *Arch Dermatol* 1996;**132**:959–62.

28. Carapetis JR, Connors C, Yarmirr D *et al.* Success of a scabies control program in an Australian Aboriginal community. *Pediatr Infect Dis J* 1996;**15**:1056–7.

29. Hernandez-Perez E. Resistance to antiscabietic drugs. *J Am Acad Dermatol* 1983;**8**:121–2.

30. Roberts DT, ed. Lice & scabies. A health professional's guide to epidemiology and treatment. London: Public Health Laboratory Service, 2000:25.

31. Gulati PV, Singh KP. A family based study on the treatment of scabies with benzyl benzoate and sulphur ointment. *Indian J Dermatol Venereol Lepr* 1978;**44**:269–73.

32. Srivastava BC, Chandra R, Srivastava VK *et al.* Epidemiological studies of scabies and community control. *J Commun Dis* 1980;**12**:134–8.

33. Amer M, El-Bayoumi, Rizik MK. Treatment of scabies: preliminary report. *Int J Dermatol* 1981;**20**:289–90.

34. Henderson C. Community control of scabies. *Lancet* 1991;**337**:1548.

35. Kenawi MZ, Morsy TA, Abdalla KF *et al.* Treatment of human scabies by sulfur and permethrin. *J Egypt Soc Parasitol* 1993;**23**:691–6.

36. Burns DA. The treatment of human ectoparasite infection. *Br J Dermatol* 1991;**125**:89–93.

37. Avila-Romay A, Alvarez-Franco M, Ruiz-Maldonado R. Therapeutic efficacy, secondary effects, and patient acceptability of 105% sulfur in either pork fat or cold cream for the treatment of scabies. *Pediatr Dermatol* 1991;**8**:64–6.

38. Chowdhury SPR. Nitrofurazone in scabies. *Lancet* 1977;**i**:152.

39. Biagi F, Delgado Y, Garnica R. First therapeutic trials with thiabendazole cream. *Int J Dermatol* 1974;**13**:102–3.

40. Hernandez-Perez E. topically applied thiabendazole in the treatment of scabies. *Arch Dermatol* 1976;**112**:1400–1.

41. Orkin M, Maibach HI. Treatment of today's scabies. In: Orkin M, Maibach HI, eds. *Cutaneous infestations and insect bites.* New York: Marcel Dekker, 1986:103–8.

42. Temesvart E, Soos GY, Podamy B *et al.* Contact urticaria provoked by Balsam of Peru. *Contact Dermatitis* 1978;**4**:65–8.

43. Glaziou P, Cartel JL, Alzieu P *et al.* Comparison of ivermectin and benzyl benzoate for treatment of scabies. *Trop Med Parasitol* 1993;**44**:331–2.

44. Plouvier B, Lemoine X, de Coninck P *et al.* Antabuse effect following topical application based on monosulfiram. *Nouvelle Presse Med* 1982;**11**:3209.

45. Blanc D, Deprez P. Unusual adverse reaction to an acaricide. *Lancet* 1990;**335**:1291–2.

46. Burgess I. Adverse reactions to monosulfiram. *Lancet* 1990;**336**:873.

47. Arditti J, Jouglard J. Cutaneous overdose with crotamiton and suspicion of methaemoglobinaemia. *Bull Med Legale Toxicol* 1978;**21**:661–2.

48. Macotela-Ruiz E, Pena-Gonzalez G. Treatment of scabies with oral ivermectin. *Gac Med Mex* 1993;**129**:210–15.

49. Usha V, Gopalakrishnan Nair TV. A comparative study of oral ivermectin and topical permethrin cream in the treatment of scabies. *J Am Acad Dermatol* 2000;**42**:236–40.

50. Chouela EN, Abeldano AM, Pellerano G *et al.* Equivalent therapeutic efficacy and safety of ivermectin and lindane in the treatment of human scabies. *Arch Dermatol* 1999;**135**:651–5.

51. Pacque M, Munoz B, Greene BM *et al.* Safety of and compliance with community-based ivermectin therapy. *Lancet* 1990;**335**:1377–80.

52. De Sole G, Remme J, Awadzi K *et al.* Adverse reactions after large-scale treatment of onchocerciasis with ivermectin: combined results from eight community trials. *Bull World Health Organ* 1989;**67**:707–19.

53. Barkwell R, Shields S. Deaths associated with ivermectin treatment of scabies. *Lancet* 1997;**349**:1144–5.

54. Diazgranados JA, Costa JL. Deaths associated with ivermectin treatment of scabies. *Lancet* 1997;**349**:1698.

55. Corbet EL, Crossley I, Holton J *et al*. Crusted ("Norwegian") scabies in a specialist HIV unit: successful use of ivermectin and failure to prevent nosocomial transmission. *Genitourin Med* 1996;**72**:115–17.

56. Meinking TL, Taplin D, Hermida JL *et al*. The treatment of scabies with ivermectin. *N Engl J Med* 1995;**333**:26–30.

57. Aubin F, Humbert P. Ivermectin for crusted (Norwegian) scabies. *N Engl J Med* 1995;**332**:612.

38
Head lice

Ian F Burgess and Ciara S Dodd

Background
Definition
Head lice (*Pediculus capitis*) are blood-feeding insects that are obligate ectoparasites of socially active humans. All stages of the life cycle infest the scalp where the adult insects attach their eggs to the hair shafts. The juvenile forms (nymphs) are essentially miniature versions of adults and there is no distinct larval stage.

Incidence/prevalence
We found no data on incidence and no recent published prevalence data from any developed country. Anecdote suggests that prevalence has increased in the past decade in most communities in the UK, US and other countries where pediculicides are in use.

Aetiology/risk factors
Observational studies indicate that infections occur most frequently in children of school age, although there is no evidence of a link with school attendance. We found no evidence that either hygiene or hairstyle influence risk or that lice prefer clean hair to dirty hair.

Prognosis
This infection is essentially harmless. However, the stigma associated with head lice and the psychological trauma experienced by some people in their efforts to eliminate the infection greatly outweigh the physical impact of the infestation. Sensitisation reactions to louse saliva and faeces may cause local irritation and erythema. Secondary infection of scratches may occur. Lice have been identified as primary mechanical vectors of scalp pyoderma caused by streptococci and staphylococci usually found on the skin.[1]

Diagnosis
Only finding living lice can confirm a diagnosis of active infestation. Eggs glued to hairs, whether hatched (nits) or unhatched, are not proof of active infection because dead eggs may appear viable for weeks. Itching, resulting from multiple bites, is not diagnostic but may increase the index of suspicion.

Aims of treatment
The aim of treatment is to eliminate infestation by killing or removing all head lice and their eggs.

Outcomes
Treatment success is given as the percentage of people completely cleared of head lice. There are no standard criteria for judging treatment success. Trials used different methods, and in many cases the method was not stated. Few studies are pragmatic.

Method of search
- The Cochrane Infectious Diseases Group at the Liverpool School of Tropical Medicine performed the initial search for a systematic review compiled in July 1998, updated February 2001 (Search date: February 2001; primary sources: Cochrane Central Register

of Controlled Trials, Medline, Embase, BIDS SC, Biosis (biological abstracts database), and Toxline).

- Dermatological Evidence update search July 2001.
- Hand searching of relevant journals.

QUESTIONS

How successful are treatments for head lice?

Case scenario 1

A 10-year-old girl with shoulder-length hair is diagnosed with head louse infestation. How easy would it be to treat her?

Insecticide-based pharmaceutical products
Efficacy

We found two systematic reviews.[2,3] The first (search date March 1995, seven randomised controlled trials (RCTs), 1808 people) of 11 insecticide products included lindane, carbaryl, malathion, permethrin and other pyrethroids in various vehicles.[3] Two RCTs were identified as showing that only permethrin produced clinically significant differences in the rate of treatment success; both compared lindane (1% shampoo) with permethrin (1% crème rinse).[4,5] Permethrin was found to be more effective (lindane versus permethrin; odds ratio (OR) for not clearing head lice 15·2, 95% confidence interval (CI) 8·0–28·8).

The more recent systematic review (search date May 1998, updated February 2001) set stricter criteria for RCTs and rejected all but four trials.[2] It excluded both studies on which the earlier review was based. One RCT (63 people) looked at the effect of permethrin (1% crème rinse) compared with the base formulation minus the permethrin (placebo). It found that, after 7 days, permethrin was more effective against head lice than a placebo (29/29 people had no lice with permethrin compared with 3/34 with placebo;

relative risk (RR) 11·3, CI 3·9–33·4; number needed to treat (NNT) 1, CI 0·03–0·3). Two weeks after treatment, fewer people who had received permethrin were infected with head lice compared with the placebo group (1/29 (4%) versus 22/24 (92%); RR 0·04, CI 0·006–0·3; NNT 1, CI 4–172).[6] One RCT (115 people) compared malathion (0·5% alcoholic lotion) with the vehicle base as placebo. At 1 week, fewer people treated with malathion were found to have head lice compared with the placebo group (3/65 (5%) versus 26/47 (55%); RR 0·08, CI 0·03–0·3; NNT 2, CI 4–39).[7] One quasi-randomised study (22 people) comparing synergised pyrethrin (0·16% mousse) with permethrin (1% crème rinse) found that, at 6 days, people treated with pyrethrin had no lice compared with permethrin (17/19 versus 3/3; RR 0·89, CI 0·8–1·0; NNT 10, CI 1–1·3).[8]

Drawbacks

Only minor adverse effects have been reported for most insecticides. The exception is lindane, for which there are extensive reports of effects related to overdosing (treatment of scabies), and absorption (treatment of head lice). Lindane passes transdermally during treatment of head lice,[9] but we found no reports of adverse effects in this setting.

We found no confirmed reports of adverse effects from therapeutic exposure to the organophosphorus compound, malathion. A recent randomised open volunteer study (32 people) examined transdermal absorption of malathion from four head louse treatment products available in the UK.[10] Urinalysis for malathion metabolites found 0·2–3·2% of the applied dose was eliminated in urine before decreasing to baseline values by 96 hours. Erythrocyte cholinesterase levels were clinically unaffected, irrespective of dose or whether the skin was excoriated.

Pyrethroid insecticides are listed as contraindicated for people with ragweed allergy but we found only one report of an anaphylactoid reaction to a head louse treatment product.[11]

Comments

Follow up for 6 days is inadequate because louse eggs normally take 7 days to hatch. In cases where a second application of insecticide is required it should be given 7 days after the first treatment. Most investigators agree that assessment for absence of infestation at 14 days after treatment is appropriate to determine the primary endpoint of a study.

The three trials comparing chemical treatments included in the most recent systematic review were conducted in developing countries, where insecticide treatments were not regularly available.[2] This may have resulted in greater efficacy, because the insects had not been subjected to any kind of selection pressure.

No RCT has yet considered that the formulation of a pediculicide might affect its activity. Studies *in vitro* suggest that other components of products (for example terpenoids and solvents) may contribute significantly to pediculicide activity, in some cases more than the insecticide itself.[12]

Resistance to one or more insecticides has now been identified in several countries.[13–19] There are no data available to indicate the prevalence of resistance, and most studies have collected insects from only a few problem cases in making their evaluation of resistance. These cases are unlikely to be representative of the population at large. However, one RCT (193 people) compared malathion (0·5% lotion with terpenoids) with phenothrin (0·3% lotion) in a community where lice were identified *in vitro* as being tolerant of phenothrin.[13] One day after treatment more people treated with phenothrin had lice (8/95 (8%) versus 59/98 (60%); RR 0·14, CI 0·07–0·3; NNT 2, CI 4–14) and this difference had increased by day 7 (6/95 (6%) versus 40/98

(41%); RR 0·15, CI 0·07–0·3; NNT 3, CI 3–15). However, some children not free from lice on day 1 had become louse free by day 7 in both groups, suggesting some parental intervention had influenced the results. Nevertheless, this study indicates that resistance to pyrethroid insecticide may have influenced around 60% of the treatments.

Implications for practice

Evidence for any insecticide-based pediculicide is limited, although permethrin has a greater body of evidence in its support, having come somewhat later to market than the others. However, all insecticides now in use are subject to the effects of insecticide resistance, which varies considerably both within and between countries. Available data are insufficient to judge this factor other than on a case-by-case basis.

Mechanical removal of lice or viable eggs by combing
Efficacy

We found one systematic review that evaluated louse removal by combing compared with insecticide treatment, but none evaluating nit combing to remove eggs. Three studies compared the effectiveness of insecticide treatments and wet combing with conditioner. The first, a community-based pragmatic RCT (72 people) included in the systematic review, compared "bug-busting" (wet combing with conditioner) with two applications of 0·5% malathion 7 days apart.[20] Seven days after treatment, fewer people using malathion had lice compared with those using "bug-busting" (9/40 (23%) versus 20/32 (63%); RR 1·27, CI 0·2–0·7; NNT 3, CI 2–5). A second small RCT, in which a trained hairdresser performed the first combing treatment or applied the insecticide product, compared a single application of permethrin (1% crème rinse) with "bug-busting".[21] After 14 days more people treated with permethrin still had lice

(8/11 (73%) versus 8/14 (57%); RR 1·27, CI 0·7–2·3; NNT 6, CI 0·4–1·4). An unpublished community-based pragmatic RCT (275 people), (SSL International, personal communication, 1998) compared single applications of phenothrin 0·2% lotion with both phenothrin 0·5% mousse and "bug-busting" in an area where resistance to pyrethroid insecticides was subsequently identified. Insecticide treatments were assessed at 4, 7, 10 and 14 days, with the primary endpoint determined at 14 days, and combing was assessed at 14, 21 and 28 days with the primary endpoint determined either after 28 days or if lice were discovered earlier. Fewer people treated with phenothrin lotion still had lice when compared with those treated with phenothrin mousse (77/107 (72%) versus 84/105 (80%); RR 0·9, CI 0·8–1·0; NNT 12, CI 1–1·3) and those using "bug-busting" (77/107 (72%) versus 49/63 (78%); RR 0·9, CI 0·8–1·1; NNT 17, CI 0·9–1·3). Analysis of ovicidal failure showed that if a second application of insecticide had been given after 7 days the effectiveness of the lotion would have increased compared with both mousse (45/107 (42%) versus 74/105 (71%); RR 0·6, CI 0·5–0·8; NNT 4, CI 1·3–2·2) and "bug-busting" (45/107 (42%) versus 49/63 (78%); RR 0·54, CI 0·4–0·7; NNT 3, CI 1·4–2·4). We found four RCTs comparing different pediculicides in combination with nit combing, but only one included a non-combing control group and none included a combing-only group.[22–24] All had significant methodological flaws.

Drawbacks

We found no evidence of drawbacks from combing alone, apart from discomfort for both the carer and the person being combed. Potential drawbacks exist for wet combing with conditioner, which requires conditioning crème rinses to be left on the scalp for prolonged periods, because adverse reactions to hair-conditioning agents have occurred after normal limited cosmetic use. Reactions include allergic contact dermatitis, urticaria, urticaria with systemic symptoms and angioedema.[25–29]

Comment

All three studies comparing insecticide treatments with combing were performed in areas where some level of resistance to the insecticide employed was either recognised before commencing the study or else identified as part of the study. As a result, the potential effectiveness of the insecticides was limited. Studies evaluating nit combing as an adjunct to insecticide treatment, used combs that differed considerably in material and construction so it was difficult to attribute efficacy, or lack of it, to either the pediculicide or the comb. An *in vitro* study (IF Burgess, unpublished) has found that many so-called "nit combs" cannot remove nits from hairs drawn between the teeth.

Implications for clinical practice

Although combing may seem an attractive, simple and safe treatment method, there is no real evidence that it is effective, especially when practised by carers who may have little skill in the method. What little evidence is available indicates that insecticide-based products are more likely to be effective if applied twice with an interval of 2 weeks, even in areas where insecticide resistance has developed. No doubt the success of currently used insecticides will diminish with time but combing requires better evidence of success before it will replace chemical treatments for the majority of patients.

Herbal treatments and essential oils

Some activity against lice and their eggs has been identified *in vitro*, and in uncontrolled studies, both for essential oils and their constituent terpenoids.[12, 30–33]

We found no systematic reviews, RCTs, or cohort studies evaluating herbal treatments or essential oils for head lice, and no evidence of drawbacks, although a potential for toxic effects has been recognised for several essential oils.[30]

Herbal and other alternative therapies have become more popular with the general public, despite a lack of evidence for efficacy in this application. Although terpenoids are a major constituent of the active component of some registered products, most alternative therapies use these chemicals at low concentrations to reduce the risk of side-effects. However, such low doses will inevitably select for resistant strains of lice and some resistance to terpenoids has already been observed in the UK (IF Burgess, unpublished).

What is the best method for diagnosing louse infection?

Case scenario 2

Head louse infections have been reported on some of the classmates of a 9-year-old girl. A few empty louse eggshells are visible on her hair and she scratches occasionally. How can this evidence of what may be a past infection be distinguished from an active infestation? Is detection combing or direct observation the most efficient way for finding lice? (Figures 38.1 and 38.2).

Efficacy

We found no systematic reviews and no RCTs evaluating detection methods. One observational study (224 people) compared traditional scalp inspection with wet combing with conditioner. Wet combing found more cases of louse infection in a school population than scalp inspection (49/224 (22%) versus 33/224 (15%); RR 1·5, CI −1·0–2·1; NNT 14, CI 0·5–1). However, inspection claimed to identify a further 13 cases that were not confirmed either by

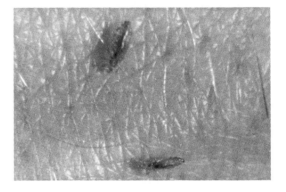

Figure 38.1 Head lice are difficult to see against human skin

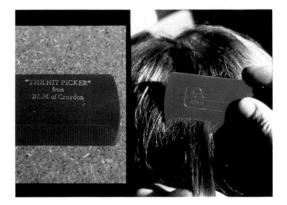

Figure 38.2 Detection combing for head lice using a plastic detection comb

combing or by follow up examination 2 weeks later.[34] An unpublished randomised trial has found that dry detection combing is more sensitive than either scalp inspection or shampooing followed by straining the rinse water to find lice washed from the hair (Dr Cynthia Guzzo, personal communication, 2001). One RCT of treatments found dry combing with a detection comb to be more effective than visual inspection in identifying positive cases before treatment (25/25 (100%) versus 12/25 (48%); RR 2·08, CI 1·3–3·1; NNT 2, CI 0·3–0·7).[21]

Comment

Accurate diagnosis of an active head louse infection is fundamental to deciding whether treatment is needed. In the past, the presence of apparently viable louse eggs close to the scalp was considered sufficient evidence of an active infection. Now only the presence of mobile stages is considered adequate evidence.[2] A recent cohort study (50 people) confirmed that the presence of eggs close to the scalp is a limited risk factor. Children screened by direct observation of the scalp, and found only to have louse eggs, were evaluated again 14 days later. Those with five eggs or more within 6 mm of the scalp were more likely to develop an active infection than those with fewer than five eggs (7/22 versus 2/28; RR 4·5, CI 1·0–19·4). It was concluded that many children are excluded from school or treated unnecessarily and that repeated examinations to determine whether an infection develops would be more beneficial.[35]

Unnecessary treatments and school exclusions also arise because caregivers and health professionals misdiagnose items found in the hair. An observational study evaluating 614 samples of presumed head lice found that only 364 (59%) were louse related, showing that better diagnostic tools are required.[36]

Implications for practice

Accurate diagnosis is essential for developing an appropriate treatment strategy. Treatment should only be given if living lice are found. Too often children are exposed to insecticides unnecessarily because a parent finds a few empty louse eggshells in the hair. However, if a child has never had head lice before, an infection may run for several weeks before it is discovered by chance, simply because there is no overt sign of the infestation.[12] Prescribers should, therefore, always ask for evidence of active infection, in the form of a louse stuck to a piece of paper, before deciding on treatment.

Key points

- Permethrin, malathion and synergised pyrethrins are probably effective against head lice, provided resistance is not present. There is limited evidence for older insecticides like lindane, which have now been withdrawn in most countries. All trials had methodological flaws.
- There is insufficient evidence of the effectiveness of combing alone or in comparison with insecticide treatment for either removing lice or nit combing.
- There is no evidence on the effects of herbal treatments and essential oils as alternative treatments for head lice.
- Combing with a plastic detection comb appears to be the most effective method for finding live lice, but methods for diagnosing louse infection have been little studied.

References

1. Taplin D, Meinking TL. Infestations. In: Schachner LA, Hansen RC, eds. *Pediatric Dermatology*, vol 2. New York: Churchill Livingstone, 1988:1465–93.

2. Dodd C. Interventions for treating head lice. In: Cochrane Collaboration. *Cochrane Library*. Issue 3. Oxford: Update Software, 2001.

3. Vander Stichele RH, Dezeure EM, Bogaert MG. Systematic review of clinical efficacy of topical treatments for head lice. *BMJ* 1995;**311**:604–8.

4. Brandenburg K, Deinard AS, Di Napoli J *et al*. 1 percent permethrin cream rinse *v*. 1 percent lindane shampoo in treating pediculosis capitis. *Am J Dis Child* 1986;**140**: 894–6.

5. Bowerman JG, Gomez MP, Austin RD *et al*. Comparative study of permethrin 1% crème rinse and lindane shampoo for the treatment of head lice. *Pediatr Inf Dis J* 1987;**6**:252–5.

6. Taplin D, Meinking TL, Castillero PM *et al*. Permethrin 1% crème rinse for the treatment of *Pediculus humanus* var. capitis infestation. *Pediatr Dermatol* 1986;**3**:344–8.

7. Taplin D, Castillero PM, Spiegel J *et al*. Malathion for treatment of *Pediculus humanus var.* capitis infestation. *JAMA* 1982;**247**:3103–5.

8. Burgess IF, Brown CM, Burgess NA. Synergized pyrethrin mousse, a new approach to head lice eradication: efficacy in field and laboratory studies. *Clin Ther* 1994;**16**:57–64.

9. Ginsburg CM, Lowry W. Absorption of gamma benzene hexachloride following application of Kwell shampoo. *Pediatr Dermatol* 1983;**1**:74–6.

10. Dennis GA, Lee PN. A phase I volunteer study to establish the degree of absorption and effect on cholinesterase activity of four head lice preparations containing malathion. *Clin Drug Invest* 1999;**18**:105–15.

11. Culver CA, Malina JJ, Talbert RL. Probable anaphylactoid reaction to a pyrethrin pediculocide shampoo. *Clin Pharmacol* 1988;**7**:846–9.

12. Burgess I. Malathion lotions for head lice:a less reliable treatment than commonly believed. *Pharm J* 1991;**247**:630–2.

13. Chosidow O, Chastang C, Brue C et al. Controlled study of malathion and d-phenothrin lotions for *Pediculus humanus* var. capitis-infested schoolchildren. *Lancet* 1994;**344**:1724–7.

14. Rupes V, Moravec J, Chmela J et al. A resistance of head lice (*Pediculus capitis*) to permethrin in Czech Republic. *Cent Eur J Public Health* 1995;**1**:30–2.

15. Mumcuoglu KY, Hemingway J, Miller J et al. Permethrin resistance in the head louse *Pediculus capitis* from Israel. *Med Vet Entomol* 1995;**9**:427–32.

16. Burgess IF, Brown CM, Peock S et al. Head lice resistant to pyrethroid insecticides in Britain [letter]. *BMJ* 1995;**311**:752.

17. Downs AMR, Stafford KA, Harvey I et al. Evidence for double resistance to permethrin and malathion in head lice. *Br J Dermatol* 1999;**141**:508–11.

18. Pollack RJ, Kiszewski A, Armstrong P et al. Differential permethrin susceptibility of head lice sampled in the United States and Borneo. *Arch Pediatr Adolesc Med* 1999;**153**:969–73.

19. Lee SH, Yoon KS, Williamson M et al. Molecular analyses of kdr-like resistance in permethrin-resistant strains of head lice, *Pediculus capitis*. *Pestic Biochem Physiol* 2000;**66**:130–43.

20. Roberts RJ, Casey D, Morgan DA et al. Comparison of wet combing with malathion for treatment of head lice in the UK: a pragmatic randomised controlled trial. *Lancet* 2000;**356**:540–4.

21. Bingham P, Kirk S, Hill N et al. The methodology and operation of a pilot randomized control trial of the effectiveness of the Bug Busting method against a single application insecticide product for head louse treatment. *Public Health* 2000;**114**:265–8.

22. Bainbridge CV, Klein GI, Neibart SI et al. Comparative study of the clinical effectiveness of a pyrethrin-based pediculicide with combing versus a permethrin-based pediculicide with combing. *Clin Pediatr Phila* 1998;**37**:17–22.

23. Clore ER, Longyear LA. A comparative study of seven pediculicides and their packaged nit combs. *J Pediatr Health Care* 1993;**7**:55–60.

24. Hipolito RB, Mallorca FG, Zuniga Macaraig ZO ot al. Head lice infestation: single drug versus combination therapy with one percent permethrin and trimethoprim/ sulfamethoxazole. *Pediatrics* 2001;**107**:E30.

25. Korting JC, Pursch EM, Enders F et al. Allergic contact dermatitis to cocamidopropyl betaine in shampoo. *J Am Acad Dermatol* 1992;**27**:1013–15.

26. Niinimaki A, Niinimaki M, Makinen-Kiljunen S et al. Contact urticaria from protein hydrolysates in hair conditioners. *Allergy* 1998;**53**:1070–82.

27. Schalock PC, Storrs FJ, Morrison L. Contact urticaria from panthenol in hair conditioner. *Contact Dermatitis* 2000;**43**:223.

28. Pasche-Koo F, Claeys M, Hauser C. Contact urticaria with systemic symptoms caused by bovine collagen in hair conditioner. *Am J Contact Dermatol* 1996;**7**:56–7.

29. Stadtmauer G, Chandler M. Hair conditioner causes angioedema. *Ann Allergy Asthma Immunol* 1997;**78**:602.

30. Veal L. The potential effectiveness of essential oils as a treatment for headlice, *Pediculus humanus capitis*. *Complementary Therapies in Nursing and Midwifery* 1996;**2**:97–101.

31. Priestley CM, Burgess IF, Williamson EM. Comparison of activity of insecticidal monoterpenoids on human lice and their eggs. In: *Natural Products Research in the New Millenium*. International Congress, Sept 2000, ETH Zurich, Abstract P2A/77.

32. Gauthier R, Agoumi A, Gourai M. Activité d'extraits de *Myrtus communis* contre *Pediculus humanus capitis*. *Plantes Med Phytother* 1989;**23**:95–108.

33. Schuld M, Jungen C. Control of lice and nits with NeemAzal-FT. In: Kleeberg H, Micheletti V, eds. *Practice

oriented results on use and production of neem ingredients and pheromones, IV. Wetzlar: Trifolio-M GmbH, 1996.

34. De Maeseneer J, Blikland I, Willems S *et al.* Wet combing versus traditional scalp inspection to detect head lice in schoolchildren: observational study. *BMJ* 2000;**321**:1187–8.

35. Williams LK, Reichart A, MacKenzie WR *et al.* Lice, nits and school policy. *Pediatrics* 2001;**107**:1011–15.

36. Pollack RJ, Kiszewski AE, Spielman A. Overdiagnosis and consequent mismanagement of head louse infestations in North America. *Pediatr Infect Dis J* 2000;**19**:689–93.

39
Insect bites

Michael Kulig and Jacqueline Müller-Nordhorn

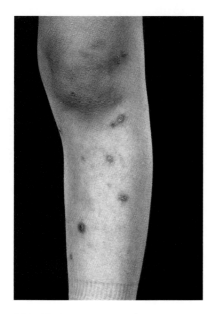

Figure 39.1 Patient with insect bites

Background
Definition

Insect bites or stings such as mosquito bites or Hymenoptera stings in general induce immediate and delayed cutaneous reactions. These vary from the common immediate wheal-and-flare reaction and delayed papules to the rare bullous eruptions and Arthus-type reactions. Insect stings of the order Hymenoptera (bees or vespids such as wasps (yellow jackets) and hornets) can also cause allergic reactions. Allergic reactions range from large local reactions through severe systemic reactions to an anaphylactic shock syndrome.

Incidence/prevalence

The prevalence of allergic sensitisation to Hymenoptera venoms as indicated by the presence of specific IgE in unselected populations ranges from 12 to 18%.[1] Systemic reactions to Hymenoptera stings as assessed in surveys are reported to be 0·3–5% in general and selected populations.[1–11] The number of deaths from allergic reactions to Hymenoptera stings occurring per year is 0·09–0·45 per million inhabitants.[1,10]

Aetiology/risk factors

Immediate cutaneous reactions to insect bites are mediated by antisaliva IgE induced by the injection of the insect saliva.[12] Reactions to Hymenoptera stings are caused by the venom of the stinging insect and can be either toxic (local reaction) or allergic (large local reaction, mild or severe systemic reaction). Patients who have been diagnosed with hypersensitivity to Hymenoptera venoms (positive skin-prick test and/or presence of specific IgE) as well as patients with a previous history of systemic reactions to Hymenoptera stings are at higher risk for systemic allergic reactions than non-sensitised subjects.[1,13–25]

Prognosis

The risk of severe systemic reaction to Hymenoptera stings cannot be sufficiently and accurately predicted by "diagnostic" tests such as the skin-prick test or the determination of specific IgE to the venom of the stinging insect.

Several controlled trials and observational studies investigated the risk of recurrent systemic reactions after Hymenoptera re-stings in subjects with a history of systemic reactions. The reported recurrence rate ranged from 14% to 76%.[1,13,14,18–20,22–27] The risk of systemic reactions after a re-sting varied according to the severity of the initial reaction. If the initial reaction was severe, a risk of recurrent systemic reactions of 49–76% was observed,[1,18,28] compared with 14–41% after mild initial reactions.[1,13,18,21] For children, the risk of recurrent allergic symptoms is lower.[29]

Aims of treatment

- To reduce the severity and duration of symptoms
- To prevent recurrence of systemic reaction to Hymenoptera insect stings

Outcomes

- Severity and duration of symptoms (itching, pain, swelling, local and systemic reactions such as urticaria, angioedema, hypotension, bronchospasm, anaphylactic shock)
- Recurrence rate of systemic reaction to Hymenoptera insect stings
- Adverse effects of treatment

Search methods

Search and appraisal (May 2001) of:

- Medline (1966 to May 2001)
- Embase (1974 to May 2001)
- Cochrane Library to issue 2, 2001
- skin databases of the Cochrane Skin Group

In addition we screened the reference lists of the retrieved articles.

QUESTIONS

How effective is symptomatic treatment after mosquito bites?

Case scenario 1

A 23-year-old woman reported itching and pain in her left leg several hours after a mosquito bite. What treatment would best relieve the patient's symptoms?

Efficacy

We found no systematic review.

Oral antihistamines versus placebo

We found two randomised controlled trials (RCTs) of oral cetirizine versus placebo given prophylactically to 23 healthy adult volunteers and to 18 patients with previous dramatic cutaneous reactions.[30,31] A significant decrease in wheal size and pruritus was found in the healthy subjects at 15 minutes after the controlled bites, and in the previously reacting patients at 15 minutes and 24 hours after the controlled bites. In a non-randomised controlled trial, oral ebastine was administered before controlled mosquito exposure to 25 adults with previous cutaneous reactions.[32] A significant decrease in bite size and pruritus was found at 15 minutes after the controlled bites.

Topical treatments versus placebo

We found two RCTs in adults with previous immediate cutaneous reactions of ammonium solution (n = 25) and of a topical homeopathic treatment ("Prrrikweg gel" n = 100).[33,34] The ammonium solution significantly relieved symptoms after bites (itching, burning and/or pain) whereas no significant effect was observed with the homoeopathic gel.

Drawbacks

In RCTs, sedation was reported for 18% (two patients) who received cetirizine, and for 8% (one patient) who received placebo,[30,31] and for 21% (six patients) treated with ebastine, and 7%

(two subject) who received placebo.[32] No skin irritation or other side-effects occurred in patients after the application of topical treatments.[33,34]

Comment

The reduction of symptoms caused by insect bites has been evaluated for just two of the many oral antihistamines available. The effect of intravenous antihistamines (dimetindene maleate versus clemastine) in patients allergic to "insects" was investigated in an RCT of only eight patients.[35]

How effective is symptomatic treatment after Hymenoptera stings?

Efficacy

We found no systematic reviews, RCTs or other studies that evaluated symptomatic treatment of local and systemic toxic and/or allergic reactions after stings by bees, wasps or hornets (Hymenoptera). However, in many studies investigating the effect of venom immunotherapy, case series are reported about the treatment of potentially life-threatening adverse systemic reactions to the insect venom (similar treatment to that of anaphylaxis from any other cause).

Pinching versus scraping off the bee sting left in the skin

We found one RCT of two volunteers who either pinched or scraped off honeybee stings (20 stings in each group). The wheal response was greater for stings removed by pinching than those removed by scraping (80 mm^2 versus 74 mm^2) but the difference was not statistically significant.[36]

Drawbacks

We found no systematic reviews, RCTs or other interventional studies that reported any adverse effects.

Comment

The evaluation of the symptomatic treatment of allergic reactions to insect stings was addressed in a number of non-systematic reviews, although the recommendations in these reviews were not based on scientific evidence.[37–40] Despite the absence of systematic and reliable evidence in the specific context of insect stings, we want to emphasise the importance of treating anaphylactic reactions to insect venoms in the same way as anaphylaxis from any other cause.[37–40] An emergency kit for self-medication has been recommended for patients with a known history of systemic reactions.[41–43]

Is subcutaneous venom immunotherapy (VIT) effective in preventing systemic reactions to Hymenoptera stings?

Efficacy

We found one systematic review.[44] In this review, studies of different designs were combined (randomised/non-randomised; placebo-controlled/ other control groups; before/after VIT trials). We have therefore included the results of the individual studies in the following sections. The reported pooled effect of all eight studies in the meta-analysis was a significant protective effect of VIT against systemic reaction after re-stings (odds ratio: 2·2, 95% confidence intervals 1·72–2·81).[44]

VIT versus placebo/no treatment/other treatment

We found two RCTs. In the first RCT, 59 adults with a history of systemic reactions after stings and a positive skin-prick test received VIT for 6–10 weeks.[14] A significantly reduced incidence of systemic reactions after controlled sting challenges was observed in the VIT group compared with the placebo group (5% versus 58%) and with a group that received whole-body extract (64%). In the second trial, 74 children with a history of systemic reactions and a positive skin-prick test were randomised to VIT or no treatment. Occurrence of field insect stings were observed for the subsequent 2 years. The difference in recurrence rates was not significant between the VIT group (6%) and the no-treatment group (17%).[19]

We found two non-randomised controlled trials. In the first,[24] the incidence of recurrent systemic reactions was compared in 271 patients who underwent VIT, no VIT or incomplete VIT (stopped against physicians' advice). The incidence of systemic reactions after re-stings was 4% in the VIT group, 27% in the incomplete-VIT group and 50% in the no-VIT group. No statistical analyses were performed. In the second trial, VIT was compared with therapy with bee whole-body extract in 56 patients with bee-sting hypersensitivity. A significant reduction in the incidence of recurrent systemic reactions after field stings in patients treated with VIT was observed (25% versus 75%).[45]

Effect of VIT during ongoing VIT

We found 27 non-randomised non-controlled trials (before–after comparisons) that examined the recurrence rates of systemic allergic reactions to inhospital sting challenges or field stings in patients with a history of systemic reactions after Hymenoptera stings and venom sensitisation confirmed by positive skin-prick test and/or presence of specific IgE. The recurrence rate in re-stung patients ranged from 0% to 38% (one trial of 19 patients reported a rate of 58%).[18,24,45–69]

Recurrence of systemic reaction to stings after stopping VIT

We found 19 non-randomised non-controlled trials that examined the recurrence rates of systemic allergic reactions to inhospital sting challenges or field stings in patients with a history of systemic reactions after Hymenoptera stings and venom sensitisation confirmed by positive skin-prick test and/or presence of specific IgE. The recurrence rate in re-stung patients ranged from 0% to 27%.[24,48,53,60,70–82]

In children

One randomised trial showed no significant effect of VIT in children.[19] One observational prospective study in 29 honeybee-hypersensitive children and adolescents (4–20 years of age) reported recurrence rates of systemic reactions of 3% at 1 year and of 14% at 2 years after stopping VIT.[82] Another study reported little benefit of VIT in children who had had only local reactions.[26]

Drawbacks

We found 39 reports on the safety of VIT. The treatment protocols are very different in the single studies. The duration and number of injections differed, as well as the doses during the initial phase. We included only studies with the usual maintenance dose of 100 micrograms. The rate of systemic allergic reactions per treated patient during VIT ranged from 0% to 39% (two trials with ≤12 patients reported rates of 50% and 64%, respectively). We pooled the data by simply adding up the numbers, without any study weighting; we calculated the rate of systemic reactions to be 16% (961/5971 patients). If reported separately, the rate of systemic reactions in honeybee-sensitive patients treated with honeybee venom ranged from 0% to 45% (one trial with 11 patients reported a rate of 64%). After pooling, we calculated a rate of 27% (453/1697 patients). The rate of systemic reactions in wasp-sensitive patients treated with wasp venom ranged from 0% to 34%. After pooling we calculated a rate of 14% (329/2383 patients).[14,28,50,51,56,60,64–69,83–108]

Comments

Because Hymenoptera venom hypersensitivity is potentially life threatening, it seems unethical to perform double-blind, placebo-controlled trials. This may explain why we found only two RCTs and few non-randomised controlled studies but many non-randomised non-controlled prospective or retrospective studies evaluating the effect of VIT. In nearly all studies the effect of VIT was evaluated by measuring the recurrence rates of systemic reactions to re-stings in patients with previous systemic events. Patients with a known history of systemic reactions are at risk of potentially life-threatening reactions to re-stings. In those non-randomised non-controlled trials, it is implicitly assumed that the effect of VIT can be evaluated by comparing the recurrence rates during or after VIT with the recurrence rates in observational studies investigating the natural course of Hymenoptera hypersensitivity (see Prognosis). Another implicit assumption is that the risk for recurrence remains unchanged over time. Many of the trials have addressed the question of when to discontinue VIT, but we found no good and reliable evidence.

One of the two randomised placebo-controlled trials included children who were not randomised properly to the treatment and the analysis was not reported separately for the two allocation groups.[19] Since baseline data were similar, the pooled results do not seem to be biased.

Does pretreatment with antihistamines reduce the risk of adverse effects of VIT?

Efficacy

We found no systematic review.

Four RCTs have compared pretreatment with oral antihistamines with placebo in VIT.

- In 140 patients cetirizine significantly reduced local adverse reactions but not systemic adverse reactions.[109]
- In 54 patients fexofenadine significantly reduced local adverse reactions but not systemic adverse reactions.[110]
- In one RCT (n = 52) terfenadine significantly reduced local adverse reactions but not systemic reactions.[111]
- In the second RCT (n = 121) terfenadine significantly reduced both systemic adverse reactions and local adverse reactions during the first week.[112]

Drawbacks

Side-effects of the antihistamine pretreatment were reported in only one of the above RCTs: headache in 2% (2/82) and nausea in 1% (1/82) of the patients who received terfenadine, and fatigue in 3% (1/39) of those who received placebo.

Comment

The few data that exist suggest that the efficacy of VIT is not affected by anti-histamine premedication.[113]

Key points

- We found good evidence evaluating oral antihistamines given prophylactically (but only cetirizine and ebastine) versus placebo and little evidence evaluating topical treatment for insect-bite reactions.
- We found no reliable evidence on symptomatic treatment of Hymenoptera stings and only one trial evaluating removing the honeybee sting with pinching versus scraping. Treatment of adverse systemic reactions to insect stings with antihistamines and steroids was reported in case series. Anaphylactic reactions were treated similarly to anaphylactic reactions from other causes.

Because reactions to the venom of stinging insects are potentially life threatening, we emphasise that, despite the absence of systematic and reliable evidence, systemic reactions should be treated as one would treat anaphylaxis from any other cause. An emergency kit for self-medication is recommended for patients with a known history of systemic reactions.

- We found good evidence evaluating the effect of VIT. However, because of the potentially life-threatening nature of Hymenoptera venom hypersensitivity, it seems unethical to perform double-blind, placebo-controlled trials. Therefore our evaluation had to be based mainly on lower-level evidence – non-randomised, non-controlled interventional studies.
- We found good evidence that pretreatment with oral antihistamines in VIT reduces local reactions, but inconclusive evidence that it reduces systemic reactions.

References

1. Müller UR: Epidemiology of insect sting allergy. *Epidemiol Clin Allergy Monogr Allergy* 1993;**31**:131–46.

2. Fernandez J, Blanca M, Soriano V *et al*. Epidemiological study of the prevalence of allergic reactions to Hymenoptera in a rural population in the Mediterranean area. *Clin Exp Allergy* 1999;**29**:1069–74.

3. Grigoreas C, Galatas ID, Kiamouris C, Papaioannou D. Insect-venom allergy in Greek adults. *Allergy* 1997;**52**:51–7.

4. Novembre E, Cianferoni A, Bernardini R *et al*. Epidemiology of insect venom sensitivity in children and its correlation to clinical and atopic features. *Clin Exp Allergy* 1998;**28**:834–8.

5. Bjornsson E, Janson C, Plaschke P *et al*. Venom allergy in adult Swedes: a population study. *Allergy* 1995;**50**:800–5.

6. Chafee FH. The prevalence of bee sting allergy in an allergic population. *Acta Allergologica* 1970;**25**:292–3.

7. Settipane GA, Newstead GJ, Boyd GK. Frequency of Hymenoptera allergy in an atopic and normal population. *J Allergy Clin Immunol* 1972;**50**:146–50.

8. Settipane GA, Boyd GK. Prevalence of bee sting allergy in 4,992 boy scouts. *Acta Allergologica* 1970;**25**:286–91.

9. Golden DBK, Addison BI, Gadde J *et al*. Prospective observations on stopping prolonged venom immunotherapy. *J Allergy Clin Immunol* 1989;**84**:162–7.

10. Charpin D, Birnbaum J, Vervloet D. Epidemiology of hymenoptera allergy. *Clin Exp Allergy* 1994;**24**:1010–15.

11. Valentine MD. Anaphylaxis and stinging insect hypersensitivity. *JAMA* 1992;**268**:2830–3.

12. Reunala T, Brummer-Korvenkontio H, Palosuo T. Are we really allergic to mosquito bites. *Ann Med* 1994;**26**:301–6.

13. Blaawu PJ, Smithuis LOMJ. The evaluation of the common diagnostic methods of hypersensitivity for bee and yellow jacked venom by means of an in-hospital insect sting. *J Allergy Clin Immunol* 1985;**75**:556–62.

14. Hunt KJ, Valentine Md, Sobotka AK *et al*. A controlled trial of immunotherapy in insect hypersensitivity. *N Engl J Med* 1978;**299**:157–61.

15. Mauriello PM, Barde SH, Georgitis JW, Reisman RE. Natural history of large local reactions from stinging insects. *J Allergy Clin Immunol* 1984;**74**:494–8.

16. Müller UR. *Insect Sting Allergy: Clinical Picture, Diagnosis and Treatment*. Stuttgart: Fischer, 1990.

17. Graf DF, Schuberth KC, Kagey-Sobotka A *et al*. The development of negative skin tests in children treated with venom immunotherapy. *J Allergy Clin Immunol* 1984;**73**:61–8.

18. Reisman RE. Natural history of insect sting allergy: relationship of severity of symptoms of initial sting anaphylaxis to re-sting reaction. *J Allergy Clin Immunol* 1992;**90**:335–9.

19. Schuberth KC, Lichtenstein LM, Sobotka AK *et al*. Epidemiologic study of insect allergy in children. II. Effect of accidental stings in allergic children. *J Pediatr* 1983;**102**:361–5.

20. Van der Linden PW, Hack CE, Struyvenberg A, Kees J, van der Zwan JK. Intentional diagnostic sting challenges: an important medical issue. *J Allergy Clin Immunol* 1994;**94**:563–4.

21. Van der Zwan J, van der Linden P. Anaphylactic reactions to bee or wasp stings: results of 308 sting provocations. *Schweiz Med Wochenschr* 1991;**121** (Suppl. 40/I):62.

22. Mosbech H, Christensen J, Dirksen A, Söborg M. Insect allergy. Predictive value of diagnostic tests: a three-year follow-up study. *Clin Allergy* 1986;**16**:433–40.

23. Parker JL, Santrach PJ, Dahlberg MJE, Yunginger JW. Evaluation of Hymenoptera-sting sensitivity with deliberate sting challenges: inadequacy of present diagnostic methods. *J Allergy Clin Immunol* 1982;**69**:200–7.

24. Reisman RE, Dvorin DJ, Randolph CC, Georgitis JW. Stinging insect allergy: natural history and modification with venom immunotherapy. *J Allergy Clin Immunol* 1985;**75**:735–40.

25. Settipane GA, Chafee FH. Natural history of allergy to Hymenoptera. *Clin Allergy* 1979;**9**:385.

26. Valentine MD, Schuberth KC, Sobotka AK et al. The value of immunotherapy with venom in children with allergy to insect stings. *New Engl J Med* 1990;**323**:1601–3.

27. Van der Linden P-WG, Struyvenberg A, Kraaijenhagen RJ et al. Anaphylactic shock after insect-sting challenge in 138 persons with a previous insect-sting reaction. *Ann Intern Med* 1993;**118**:161–8.

28. Van der Zwan JC, Flinterman J, Jankowski IG, Kerckhaert JAM. Hyposensitisation to wasp venom in six hours. *BMJ* 1983;**287**:1329.

29. Schuberth KC, Lichtenstein LM, Kagey-Sobotka A, Szklo M, Kwiterovich KA, Valentine MD. Epidemiologic study of insect allergy in children. II Effect of accidental stings in allergic children. *J Pediatr* 1983;**102**:361–5.

30. Reunala T, Lappalainen P, Brummer-Korvenkontico H et al. Cutaneous reactivity to mosquito bites: effect of cetirizine and development or anti-mosquito antibodies. *Clin Exp Allergy* 1991;**2**:617–22.

31. Reunala T, Brummer-Korvenkontico H, Karppinen A et al. Treatment of mosquito bites with cetirizine. *Clin Exp Allergy* 1993;**23**:72–5.

32. Reunala T, Brummer-Korvenkontico H, Petman L et al. Effect of ebastine on mosquito bites. *Acta Derm Venereol* 1997;**77**:315–16.

33. Zhai H, Packman EW, Maibach HI. Effectiveness of ammonium solution in relieving type I mosquito bite symptoms: a double-blind, placebo-controlled study. *Acta Derm Venereol* 1998;**78**:297–8.

34. Hill N, Stam C, van Haselen RA. The efficacy of prrrikweg gel in the treatment of insect bites: a double-blind, placebo-controlled clinical trial. *Pharm World Sci* 1996;**18**:35–41.

35. Zimmermann B, Fischer H. Antipruriginöse bzw. antiallergische Therapie. *Fortschr Med* 1981;**99** (35):1–3.

36. Visscher PK, Vetter RS, Camazine S. Removing bee stings. *Lancet* 1996;**348**:301–2.

37. Jerrard DA. ED management of insect stings. *Am J Emerg Med* 1996;**14**:429–33.

38. Reisman RE. Current concepts: insect stings. *N Engl J Med* 1994;**331**:523–7.

39. Valentine MD. Insect venom allergy: diagnosis and treatment. *J Allergy Clin Immunol* 1984;**73**:299–304.

40. Am College of Allergy, Asthma & Immunology: Insect stings. *Ann Allergy Asthma Immunol* 1998;**80**:453–5.

41. Müller U, Mosbech H, Blaauw P et al. Emergency treatment of allergic reactions to Hymenoptera stings. *Clin Exp Allergy* 1991;**21**:281–8.

42. Müller U, Mosbech H, Aberer W et al. Adrenaline for emergency kits. *Allergy* 1995;**50**:783–7.

43. Tryba M, Ahnefeld FW, Barth J et al. Acute therapy of anaphylactoid reactions: Results of an interdisciplinary consensus conference. *Allergo J* 1994;**3/4**:211–24.

44. Ross RN, Nelson HS, Finegold I. Effectiveness of specific immunotherapy in the treatment of Hymenoptera venom hypersensitivity: a meta-analysis. *Clin Ther* 2000;**22**:351–8.

45. Müller U, Thurnherr U, Ratrizzi R, Spiess J, Hoigner. Immunotherapy in bee sting hypersensitivity. *Allergy* 1979;**34**:369–78.

46. Blaawu PJ, Smithuis OLMJ, Elbers ARW. The value of an in-hospital insect sting challenge as a criterion for application or omission of venom immunotherapy. *J Allergy Clin Immunol* 1996;**98**:39–47.

47. Golden DBK, Kagey-Sobotka A, Valentine MD, Lichtenstein LM. Dose dependence of Hymenoptera venom immunotherapy. *J Allergy Clin Immunology* 1981;**67**:370–4.

48. Keating MU, Sobotka AK, Hamilton RG, Yunginger JW. Clinical and immunologic follow-up of patients who stop venom immunotherapy. *J Allergy Clin Immunol* 1991;**88**:339–48.

49. Mosbech H, Malling H-J, Biering I et al. Immunotherapy with yellow jacket venom. *Allergy* 1986;**41**:95–103.

50. Müller U, Helbling A, Berchtold E. Immunotherapy with honeybee venom and yellow jacket venom is different regarding efficacy and safety. *J Allergy Clin Immunol* 1992;**89**:529–35.

51. Przybilla B, Ring J, Grießhammer B, Braun-Falco O. Schnellhyposensibilisierung mit Hymenopterengiften. *DMW* 1987;**112**:416–24.

52. Yunginger JW, Paull BR, Jones RT, Santrach PJ. Rush venom immunotherapy program for honeybee sting sensitivity. *J Allergy Clin Immunol* 1979;**63**:340–7.

53. Bousquet J, Knani J, Velasquez G *et al.* Evolution of sensitivity to Hymenoptera venom in 200 allergic patients followed for up to 3 years. *J Allergy Clin Immunol* 1989;**84**:944–50.

54. Kochuyt AM, Stevens EA. Safety and efficacy of a 12-week maintenance interval in patients treated with Hymenoptera venom immunotherapy. *Clin Exp Allergy* 1994;**24**:35–41.

55. Nataf P, Guinnepain MT, Herman D. Rush venom immunotherapy: a 3-day programme for Hymenoptera sting allergy. *Clin Allergy* 1984;**14**:269–75.

56. Bäurle G, Schwarz W. Hymenopteren-Allergie: Stellenwert des allergenspezifischen IgG bei der Therapie. *DMW* 1983;**108**:1351–5.

57. Golden DBK, Kagey-Sobotka A, Valentine MD, Lawrence M, Lichtenstein ML. Prolonged maintenance interval in Hymenoptera venom immunotherapy. *J Allergy Clin Immunol* 1981;**67**:482–4.

58. Kampelmacher MJ, van der Zahn JC. Provocation test with a living insect as a diagnostic tool in systemic reactions to bee and wasp venom: a prospective study with emphasis on the clinical aspects. *Clin Allergy* 1987;**17**:317–27.

59. Malling HJ, Djurup R, Sondergarard I, Weeke B. Clustered immunotherapy with yellow jacket venom. evaluation of the influence of time interval on *in vivo* and *in vitro* parameters. *Allergy* 1985;**40**:373–83.

60. Urbanek R, Karitzky D, Forster J. Die Hyposensibilisierungsbehandlung mit reinem Bienengift. *DMW* 1978;**103**:1656–60.

61. Adolph J, Dehnert I, Fischer JF, Wenz W. Results of hyposensitization with bee and wasp venom. *Z Erkrank Atm Org* 1986;**166**:119–24.

62. Bernstein DI, Mittman RJ, Kagen SL, Korbee L, Enrione M, Bernstein L. Clinical and immunologic studies of rapid venom immunotherapy in Hymenoptera-sensitive patients. *J Allergy Clin Immunol* 1989;**84**:951–9.

63. Bousquet J, Müller UR, Dreborg S *et al.* Immunotherapy with Hymenoptera venoms. Position Paper of the Working Group on Immunotherapy of the European Academy of Allergy and Clinical Immunology. *Allergy* 1987;**42**:401–13.

64. Golden DBK, Valentine MD, Kagey-Sobotka A, Lichtenstein LM. Regimens of Hymenoptera venom immunotherapy. *Ann Intern Med* 1980;**92**:620–4.

65. Tarhini H, Knani J, Michel FB, Bousquet J. Safety of immunotherapy administered by a cluster schedule. *J Allergy Clin Immunol* 1992;**89**:1198–9.

66. Wyss M, Scheitlin T, Stadler BM, Wäthrich B. Immunotherapy with aluminum hydroxide absorbed insect venom extracts (Alutard SQ): immunologic and clinical results of a prospective study over 3 years. *Allergy* 1993;**48**:81–6.

67. Birnbaum J, Charpin D, Vervloet D. Rapid Hymenoptera venom immunotherapy: comparative safety of three protocols. *Clin Exp Allergy* 1993;**23**:226–30.

68. Golden BK, Kwiterovich KA, Sobotka AK *et al.* Discontinuing venom immunotherapy: outcome after five years. *J Allergy Clin Immunol* 1996;**97**:579–87.

69. Gillman SA, Cummins LH, Kozak PP, Hoffman DR. Venom immunotherapy: comparison of "rush" *v* "conventional" schedules. *Ann Allergy* 1980;**45**:351–4.

70. Thurnheer U, Müller U, Stoller A, Lanner A, Hoigné R. Venom immunotherapy in Hymenoptera sting allergy. Comparison of rush and conventional hyposensitization and observations during long-term treatment. *Allergy* 1983;**38**:465–75.

71. Haugaard L, Norregaard OFH, Dahl R. In-hospital sting challenge in insect venom-allergic patients after stopping venom immunotherapy. *J Allergy Clin Immunol* 1991;**87**:699–702.

72. Müller U, Berchtold E, Helbing A. Honeybee venom allergy: results of a sting challenge 1 year after stopping successful venom immunotherapy in 86 patients. *J Allergy Clin Immunol* 1991;**87**:702–9.

73. Van Halteren HK, van der Linden P-WG, Burgers JA, Bartelink AKM. Discontinuation of yellow jacket venom immunotherapy: follow-up or 75 patients by means of deliberate sting challenge. *J Allergy Clin Immunol* 1997;**100**:767–70.

74. Golden DBK, Sobotka AK, Lichtenstein LM. Survey of patients after discontinuing venom immunotherapy. *J Allergy Clin Immunol* 2000;**105**:385–90.

75. Golden DBK, Kwiterovich KA, Sobotka AK. Discontinuing venom immunotherapy: extended observations. *J Allergy Clin Immunol* 1998;**101**:298–305.

76. Golden DBK, Kwiterovich KA, Valentine MD, Kagey-Sobotka A, Lichtenstein LM. Risk and benefit of discontinuing venom immunotherapy (VIT) after 5 years. *J Allergy Clin Immunol* 1991;**87**:237.

77. Graft DF, Schoenwetter WF. Insect sting allergy: analysis of a cohort of patients who initiated venom immunotherapy from 1978 to 1986. *Ann Allergy* 1994;**73**:481–5.

78. Harries MG, Kemeny DM, Youlten LJF, Mills MM, Lessof MH. Skin and radioallergosorbent tests in patients with sensitivity to bee and wasp venom. *Clin Allergy* 1984;**14**:407–12.

79. Lerch E, Müller U. Long-term protection after stopping venom immunotherapy: results of re-stings in 200 patients. *J Allergy Clin Immunol* 1998;**101**:606–12.

80. Reisman RE. Duration of venom immunotherapy: relationship to the severity or symptoms of initial insect sting anaphylaxis. *J Allergy Clin Immunol* 1993,**92**:831–6.

81. Golden BKG, Johnson K, Addison BI, Valentine MD, Kagey-Obotka A, Lichtenstein LM. Clinical and immunologic observations in patients who stop venom immunotherapy. *J Allergy Clin Immunol* 1986;**77**:435–42.

82. Urbanek R, Forster J, Kuhn W, Ziupa J. Discontinuation of bee venom Immunotherapy in children and adolescents. *J Pediatr* 1985;**107**:367–71.

83. Brehler R, Wolf H, Kätting B *et al.* Safety of a two-day ultrarush insect venom immunotherapy protocol in comparison with protocols of longer duration and involving a larger number of injections. *J Allergy Clin Immunol* 2000;**105**:1231–5.

84. Chipps BE, Valentine MD, Sobotka AK *et al.* Diagnosis and treatment of anaphylactic reactions to Hymenoptera stings in children. *J Pediatr* 1980;**97**:177–84.

85. Diez Gómez ML, Gancedo SQ, de Pàramo BJ. Venom immunotherapy: tolerance to a 3–day protocol of rush-immunotherapy. *Allergol Immunopathol* 1995;**23**:277–84.

86. Fender G, Veltman G. Beobachtungen zum Ablauf der Schnellhyposensibilisierung mit Insektengift unter besonderer Berücksichtigung der Lokalreaktion, als Beitrag zur Risikominimierung. *Z Hautkr* 1983;**58**:357.

87. Mellerup MT, Hahn GW, Poulsen LK, Malling H-J. Safety of allergen-specific immunotherapy. Relation between dosage regimen, allergen extract, disease and systemic side-effects during induction treatment. *Clin Exp Allergy* 2000;**30**:1423–39.

88. Mosbech H, Müller U. Side-effects of insect venom immunotherapy: results from an EAACI multicenter study. *Allergy* 2000;**55**:1005–10.

89. Lockey RF, Turkeltaub PC, Olive ES *et al.* The Hymenoptera venom study. III: Safety of venom immunotherapy. *J Allergy Clin Immunol* 1990;**86**:775–80.

90. Nataf P, Guinnepain MT, Herman D. Rush venom immunotherapy: a 3-day programme for Hymenoptera sting allergy. *Clin Allergy* 1984;**14**:269–75.

91. Rueff F, Reißig J, Przybilla B. Nebenwirkungen der Schnellhyposensibilisierung mit Hymenopteragift. *Allergo J* 1997;**6**(Suppl 1):59–64.

92. Treudler R, Tebbe B, Orfanos CE. Standardized rapid hyposensitization with purified Hymenoptera venom in wasp venom allergy. Prospective study of development of tolerance and side-effect profile. *Hautarzt* 1997;**48**:734–9.

93. Youlten LJ, Atkinson BA, Lee TH. The incidence and nature of adverse reactions to injection immunotherapy in bee and wasp venom allergy. *Clin Exp Allergy* 1995;**25**:159–65.

94. Westall GP, Thien FC, Czarny D *et al.* Adverse events associated with rush Hymenoptera venom immunotherapy. *Med J Aust* 2001;**174/5**:227–30.

95. Laurent J, Smiejan JM, Bloch-Morot E *et al.* Safety of Hymenoptera venom rush immunotherapy. *Allergy* 1997;**52**:94–6.

96. Adolph J, Dehnert I, Fischer JF, Wenz W. Ergebnisse der Hyposensibilisierung mit Bienen- und Wespengift. *Z Erkrank Atm Org* 1986;**166**:119–24.

97. Glowenia HJ, Schulz KH. Die Bienen-und Wespengiftallergie. *Therapiewoche* 1981;**31**:6371.

98. Grimm I. Die kausale Behandlung der Insektengiftallergie. *Z Hautkr* 1982;**57**:78.

99. Jarisch R. Die Bienengiftallergie (Modell einer IgE-mediierten Soforttypallergie). *Wien klin Wschr* 1980;**92** (Suppl. 122):3.

100. Maucher OM, Grau M, Hartmann M, Schöpf E. Klinische Erfahrung bei der Testung und Hyposensibilisierung mit gereinigtem Bienen-und Wespengift. *Allergol* 1981;**4**:67.

101. Müller U, Lanner A, Schmid P, Bischof M, Dreborg S, Hoigné R. A double blind study on immunotherapy with chemically modified honey bee venom: monomethoxy polyethylene glycol-coupled versus crude honey bee venom. *Int Arch Allergy Appl Immunol* 1985;**77**:201.

102. Müller U, Thurnheer U, Stoller R, Gäleryäz D, Hoigné R. Neue Gesichtspunkte bei der Diagnose und Behandlung allergischer Allgemeinreaktionen nach Insektenstichen. *Schweiz med Wschr* 1981;**111**:106.

103. Miyachi SM, Lessof MH, Kemeny DM. Evaluation of bee sting allergy by skin tests and serum antibody assays. *Int Arch Allergy Appl Immunol* 1979;**60**:148.

104. Näßlein H, Köstler C, Gläck H, Baenkler HW, Kalden JR. Diagnostik und Therapie der Bienen-und Wespengiftallergie. *Therapiewoche* 1984;**34**:421.

105. Reisman RE, Arbesman CE, Lazell M. Clinical and immunological studies of venom immunotherapy. *Clin Allergy* 1979;**9**:167.

106. Rocklin RE, Alfano N, Sabotka AK, Rosenwasser LJ, Findlay SR. Low incidence of systemic reactions during venom immunotherapy. *J Allergy Clin Immunol* 1982;**69**: 125.

107. Schwartz HJ, Golden DB, Lockey RF. Venom immunotherapy in the Hymenoptera-allergic pregnant patient. *J Allergy Clin Immunol* 1990;**85**:709–12.

108. Small P, Barrett D, Biskin N. Venom immunotherapy – a critical evaluation of *in vitro* techniques. *Ann Allergy* 1983;**50**:256.

109. Herman D, Melac M. Effect of pretreatment with cetirizine on side effects from rush-immunotherapy with honey bee venom. *Allergy* 1996;**51**:68.

110. Reimers A, Hari Y, Müller U. Reduction of side-effect from ultrarush immunotherapy with honeybee venom by pretreatment with fexofenadine: a double-blind, placebo-controlled trial. *Allergy* 2000; **55**:483–7.

111. Berchtold E, Maibach R, Müller U. Reduction of side effects from rush-immunotherapy with honey bee venom by pretreatment with terfenadine. *Clin Exp Allergy* 1992;**22**:59–65.

112. Brockow K, Kiehn M, Riethmüller C, Vieluf D, Berger J, Ring J. Efficacy of antihistamine pretreatment in the prevention of adverse reactions to Hymenoptera immunotherapy: A prospective, randomized, placebo-controlled trial. *J Allergy Clin Immunol* 1997;**100**: 458–63.

113. Müller U, Hari Y, Berchtold E. Premedication with antihistamines may enhance efficacy of specific-allergen immunotherapy. *J Allergy Clin Immunol* 2001;**107**:81–6.

Part 3: The evidence

Section E: Disorders of pigmentation

Editor: Berthold Rzany

40
Vitiligo

Cinzia Masini and Damiano Abeni

Background
Definition

Vitiligo is an acquired disorder of pigmentation affecting mainly the skin, where the loss of functioning melanocytes results in white patches. The hair and, rarely, the eyes or other organs and systems may be also affected. The most common form of vitiligo is symmetrical, usually affecting the skin around the orifices, the genitals, sun-exposed areas such as the face and hands, and friction areas such as extensor surfaces of the limbs. The rare segmental type affects only one area of the body.

Incidence/prevalence

Vitiligo is a common skin disorder, affecting about 0·5% of the general population, irrespective of ethnic origin.[1-3] Anyone of any age can develop vitiligo, but generally the disease begins between the ages of 2 and 40 years. In a Dutch study, 50% of participants reported the onset of the disease before the age of 20 years.[4]

Aetiology

There appears to be a genetic predisposition to vitiligo, consistent with a polygenic disorder, and up to one-third of patients report a family history of hypopigmentation.[5,6] No definitive precipitating factor responsible for initiating vitiligo has been established, and the basic pathogenesis in general still remains unknown. Current hypotheses range from intrinsic melanocyte dysfunction and/or death to destruction mediated by autoantibodies. Many vitiligo patients also exhibit other autoimmune disorders and the presence of serum melanocyte-specific autoantibodies appears to correlate with the extent and activity of the disease.[7,8]

The development of vitiligo patches over friction areas may be due to Koebner phenomenon in response to local trauma.

Prognosis

Although neither lethal nor symptomatic, the effects of vitiligo can be cosmetically and psychologically devastating. We found only one retrospective study dealing with prognostic issues. The course of the disease is fairly unpredictable, but often progressive (in more than 80% of patients).[9] Periods of slow or rapid enlargement of the lesions, arrest in depigmentation, and spontaneous or partial repigmentation can occur. Spontaneous repigmentation, probably sunlight induced, is usually also a sign that the patient will respond to medical therapy. On the other hand, as the main reservoir of vital melanocytes is the hair follicle, glabrous skin and hair-bearing skin in which terminal hairs are clearly depigmented does not respond to medical therapies.

Aims of treatment

- To achieve partial or total repigmentation, at least for body areas that the patients estimate as "most significant", with minimal adverse effects
- To improve the patient's quality of life

Relevant outcomes

- Patient-rated clinical response: improvement in quality of life, repigmentation

- Doctor-rated clinical response: success rate in terms of repigmentation (>75%) or depigmentation (100%), long-term repigmentation rate
- Side-effects of treatment

Methods of search

We searched for randomised controlled trials (RCTs) or at least controlled trials of currently available medical and surgical treatments in the *Cochrane Library* and Cochrane Central Register of Controlled Trials, Medline and Embase, with the keywords "vitiligo" and "treatment". We also searched for "controlled trial", "meta-analysis", "systematic review", "practice guideline", "quality of life" and "prognosis". The search was completed in February 2002, and all the relevant papers found were critically appraised and included. Reference search of the key papers was performed.

A protocol by Barrett and Whitton on "Interventions for vitiligo" is in the Cochrane Database of Systematic Reviews. Two systematic reviews and a meta-analysis from which practice guidelines for the treatment of vitiligo were developed, by Njoo and coworkers, were published in the Evidence-based Dermatology section of *Archives of Dermatology*.

We found 10 additional controlled clinical studies published after the completion of the systematic reviews (December 1997). Only two studies addressed quality of life as an outcome.

QUESTIONS

What are the effects of medical treatment in vitiligo?

Case scenario

A 26-year-old woman reports a 10-year history of depigmented areas. Clinical examination reveals symmetrically distributed depigmented areas affecting the sun-exposed areas, mainly upper arms, face and neck (Figure 40.1).

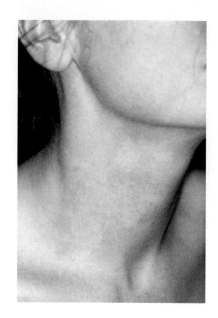

Figure 40.1   Neck with irregular-shaped depigmented areas in a 26-year-old woman with vitiligo

Phototherapy and photochemotherapy
Efficacy

Photochemotherapy is well established in the treatment of vitiligo, with different modalities essentially related to geographical area (solar exposure) and available equipment.

A meta-analysis[10] has found that the odds ratio (OR) versus placebo (the odds of a patient receiving the active therapy achieving >75% repigmentation compared with a patient receiving the placebo) was significant for oral methoxsalen plus sunlight (OR 23·4; 95% confidence interval (CI) 1·3–409.9), oral psoralen plus sunlight (OR 19.9; CI 2·4–166·3) and oral trioxsalen plus sunlight (OR 3·7; CI 1·2–11·2).

Two randomised double-blind right–left comparative studies on a total of 80 patients have shown that concurrent topical calcipotriol potentiates the efficacy of PUVAsol (oral psoralen plus sunlight)[11] or PUVA,[12] achieving earlier pigmentation with a lower total UVA dosage. A further RCT on 135 patients compared (left–right) the efficacy of a combination of fluticasone propionate and UVA with that of either used alone, and showed that combination treatment is more effective,[13] although efficacy remains low (only 13% patients achieving >75% repigmentation) because of the low basic efficacy of the two treatments (UVA alone or corticosteroid alone) in patients with extensive symmetrical vitiligo.

The meta-analysis and one further trial[14] found that topical or oral khellin and phenylalanine were not effective as photosensitisers in vitiligo therapy (there was no difference between active drug and placebo).

The case series included in the meta-analysis showed that the percentage of patients achieving >75% repigmentation was 63% for narrowband UVB, 57% for broadband UVB, 51% for oral methoxsalen plus UVA and 43% for oral bergapten (a furanocoumarin contained in bergamot orange) plus UVA.[10] The differences between the mean success rates reported were not significant. A controlled trial on a device producing a focused beam of UVB (microphototherapy)[15] found >75% repigmentation in five of eight subjects with segmental vitiligo treated for 6 months. A right–left comparison trial on 24 patients showed that PUVB is as effective as PUVA in the treatment of extensive symmetrical vitiligo.[16]

Drawbacks

Photochemotherapy necessitates close monitoring for acute toxicity and cutaneous carcinogenic effects. Oral methoxsalen plus UVA was associated with the highest incidence of side-effects. Severe phototoxic reactions (mainly associated with topical psoralen or oral methoxsalen plus UVA) can be avoided by carefully monitoring UV exposure. Nausea (reported in 29% of the patients treated with methoxsalen) can be reduced by taking food.[10] It seems that wearing UVA-opaque glasses for 24 hours after psoralen ingestion makes the risk of cataract development negligible. Liver and renal function tests and ophthalmologic examination should be repeated annually.[17]

In patients with psoriasis, long-term PUVA therapy was associated with an increased risk of skin cancer.[18,19] Although the risk seems to be lower in patients with vitiligo (possibly because of the lower cumulative dosages and/or darker skin types), guidelines for maximum cumulative PUVA doses should follow those recommended for psoriasis.[20] Both PUVA and UVB therapies should not be continuous, to minimise carcinogenic potential.

No systemic or local side-effects are reported for UVB therapy, except for erythema, pruritus and xerosis. Long-term side-effects and risk for skin carcinogenesis are unknown.[10] Side-effects of topical calcipotriol were negligible in the two trials reported.[11,12] Abnormal liver function tests were observed in 17% of patients using oral khellin.[10]

Comment/implications for clinical practice

The mean treatment duration of phototherapies and photochemotherapies varied from 6 months to 2 years. Since phototherapy is time-consuming and patients must remain motivated for long periods, monitoring of compliance is relevant but seldom reported in trials. Moreover, we found no trials considering quality of life as an outcome, except for a case series of 51 children treated with narrowband UVB.[21] These issues need to be better assessed in further studies. Also, follow up studies are needed to assess the persistence of therapy-induced repigmentation.

Corticosteroids
Efficacy

Topical class 3 corticosteroids have been shown to be effective in localised vitiligo, with a pooled OR of 14·3 (CI 2·4–83·7); pooled ORs showed non-significant differences between topical class 4 or intralesional corticosteroids and their respective placebos.[10] Treatment duration in the trials varied from 5 to 8 months, and strongly depended on the response: when no response occurred after 2–3 months, therapy was stopped.

The efficacy of oral corticosteroids in generalised vitiligo was low, with fewer than 20% of patients achieving >75% repigmentation in 4–24 months.[10]

Drawbacks

Atrophy was the most common side-effect with local corticosteroids, mainly induced by intralesional and class 4 corticosteroids. Side-effects, mainly moon face, weight gain and acne, were frequent with oral corticosteroids.[10]

Comment/implications for practice

Topical and systemic corticosteroids have been used to treat localised and generalised vitiligo, respectively. These drugs are relatively effective and have well-known side-effects. Only case series have been found on the use of oral corticosteroids.

Cognitive behavioural therapy
Efficacy

We found one controlled trial on 16 patients, showing effectiveness of cognitive behavioural therapy in improving the patient's quality of life[22]; this was one of only two trials addressing the disease and treatment implications from the patient's point of view.

Drawbacks

No drawbacks were reported.

Comment/implications for clinical practice

Studies that consider the effects of treatments on the quality of life and global health of the patients from the patient's point of view are much needed.

Melagenine, pseudocatalase, systemic antioxidant therapy

One small trial on 20 patients found no clinical differences between melagenine- and placebo-treated groups.[23] The effects of the other therapies, proposed on a theoretical basis, are unknown.[24]

What are the effects of surgical treatment?

In general, autologous transplantation methods are indicated for stable and/or focal lesions that are refractory to medical therapy.[24] Koebner phenomenon should be absent, and tendency for scar or keloid formation should be ascertained. "Stable" disease is not uniformly defined across the studies.

Even after successful grafting, depigmentation of the grafts may still occur during "reactivation" of the disease.[25]

Autologous non-cultured transplantation methods
Efficacy

One systematic review was found,[26] based on case series only (a total of 39 series, reporting on five different techniques). The highest success rates occurred with split-thickness grafting and suction blister epidermal grafting, with 87% of patients achieving >75% repigmentation (sample-size weighted averages, CI 82–91 and 83–90, respectively). With minigrafting, 68%

(CI 62–64) of the patients were successfully grafted. A trial comparing minigrafting and suction blister epidermal grafting[27] confirmed the results of the review, although the outcome measure was the proportion of patches instead of the proportion of patients. In a placebo-controlled trial on 18 patients, the addition of a melanotropin analogue applied topically on minigrafted patches did not improve the success of the minigrafting.[28]

Drawbacks

The most frequently reported side-effects were scar formation at the donor site (40% of patients) and cobblestone appearance over the recipient area (27%) for minigrafting; scar formation (12% of patients), milia (13%) and partial loss of grafts (11%) for split-thickness grafts, and hyperpigmentation at the donor site (28% of patients) for suction blister epidermal grafts.[26]

Comment/implications for practice

Minigrafting was reported to be the easiest and least expensive method, with the shortest duration procedure (45 minutes for 50 cm^2) and requiring minimal equipment. Suction blister epidermal grafting was the longest procedure, requiring up to 3 hours for blister formation and about half an hour for the grafting procedure itself.[26]

The data on surgical procedures should be interpreted with caution, as they are derived mainly from small case series. We found only one comparative trial,[27] with a questionable outcome measure.

Autologous cultured transplantation methods

Very little experience has been gained with culturing techniques, implying *in vitro* culturing of epidermis containing both melanocytes and keratinocytes (co-culture) or melanocytes alone. One systematic review updated to 1997 includes 10 case series reporting on five different techniques,[26] and two further series have reported on melanocyte grafting.[29,30]

Efficacy

The highest reported percentages of patients with >75% repigmentation (sample-size weighted averages) were 53% (CI 27–78) for co-cultured melanocyte and keratinocyte grafting (15 patients) and 48% (CI 39–56) for cultured melanocyte grafting (130 patients).[26] However, the results are fairly variable in the different series, a reflection of the different techniques, patient selection criteria and reported outcome measures, in addition to sample variability.

Drawbacks

No adverse effects are reported. Concern has been raised about the tumorigenic risk of culturing techniques when the culture media are supplemented with tumour promoters.

Comment/implications for practice

Specialised personnel and high-technology laboratory facilities are required.

What are the effects of depigmentation therapy?

Efficacy

Only case series were found, showing efficacy of monobenzylether of hydroquinone (monobenzone), a potent melanocytotoxic agent,[31] methoxyphenol (11/16 patients achieving total depigmentation) and Q-switched ruby laser (9/13 patients).[32]

Drawbacks

When applying monobenzone, patients should be warned about possible depigmentation at distant sites and of the skin of others (partners), and should be informed that bleaching is a permanent and irreversible process. Contact dermatitis and corneal and conjunctival melanosis have also been reported.[24]

Repigmentation occurred after total depigmentation was achieved, in 36% (CI 11–69) of patients treated with methoxyphenol cream and 44% (CI 14–79) of patients treated with Q-switched ruby laser.[32]

Comment/implications for clinical practice

Depigmentation therapy may be indicated in patients with extensive vitiligo (>80% of the body) or disfiguring lesions resistant to repigmentation therapies.[24]

Treatment with monobenzone normally requires 1–3 months to initiate a response and 6 months to 2 years may be required to complete therapy.[31]

Key points

- A meta-analysis of RCTs has found that psoralen plus sunlight and topical class 3 corticosteroids are effective when compared with placebo for treating generalised and localised vitiligo respectively. Photochemotherapy requires careful dosage and close monitoring for acute toxicity and long-term carcinogenic effects. Two RCTs have found that concurrent topical calcipotriol potentiates the efficacy of PUVA.
- Mainly case series have shown that PUVA and UVB are effective. Long-term side-effects of UVB are unknown.
- We found limited evidence (case series only) on the effectiveness of surgical treatments for selected patients and on the effectiveness of depigmentation therapy for vitiligo universalis.
- We found no evidence of efficacy for phenylalanine, topical or oral khellin and melagenine.

- We found treatments to have been evaluated mainly in the short term, with very few comparative trials. The maintenance value of therapies, and the assessment of patients' preferences, satisfaction and quality of life have not yet been adequately addressed. Patient compliance was seldom reported in the studies.
- Only a few studies reporting negative results with a therapy were found.

References

1. Jacobson DL, Gange SJ, Rose NR, Graham NM. Epidemiology and estimated population burden of selected autoimmune diseases in the United States. *Clin Immunol Immunopathol* 1997;**84**:223–43.

2. Das SK, Majumder PP, Chakraborty R, Majumdar TK, Haldar B. Studies on vitiligo. I. Epidemiological profile in Calcutta, India. *Genet Epidemiol* 1985;**2**:71–8.

3. Howitz J, Brodthagen H, Schwartz M, Thomsen K. Prevalence of vitiligo. Epidemiological survey on the Isle of Bornholm, Denmark. *Arch Dermatol* 1977;**113**:47–52.

4. Barrett C, Whitton M. Interventions for vitiligo. Protocol for Cochrane review. Cochrane Collaboration. *Cochrane Library*. Issue 1. Oxford: Update Software, 2002.

5. Bhatia PS, Mohan L, Pandey ON, Singh KK, Arora SK, Mukhija RD. Genetic nature of vitiligo. *J Dermatol Sci* 1992;**4**:180–4.

6. Kim SM, Chung HS, Hann SK. The genetics of vitiligo in Korean patients. *Int J Dermatol* 1998;**37**:908–10.

7. Naughton GK, Reggiardo D, Bystryn JC. Correlation between vitiligo antibodies and extent of depigmentation in vitiligo. *J Am Acad Dermatol*, 1986;**15**:978–81.

8. Harning R, Cui J, Bystryn JC. Relation between the incidence and level of pigment cell antibodies and disease activity in vitiligo. *J Invest Dermatol* 1991;**97**: 1078–80.

9. Hann SK, Chun WH, Park YK. Clinical characteristics of progressive vitiligo. *Int J Dermatol* 1997;**36**:353–5.

10. Njoo MD, Spuls PI, Bos JD, Westerhof W, Bossuyt PM. Nonsurgical repigmentation therapies in vitiligo. Meta-analysis of the literature. *Arch Dermatol* 1998;**134**:1532–40.

11. Parsad D, Saini R, Verma N. Combination of PUVAsol and topical calcipotriol in vitiligo. *Dermatology* 1998;**197**:167–70.

12. Ermis O, Alpsoy E, Cetin L, Yilmaz E. Is the efficacy of psoralen plus ultraviolet A therapy for vitiligo enhanced by concurrent topical calcipotriol? A placebo-controlled double-blind study. *Br J Dermatol* 2001;**145**:472–5.

13. Westerhof W, Nieuweboer-Krobotova L, Mulder PG, Glazenburg EJ. Left-right comparison study of the combination of fluticasone propionate and UV-A *v.* either fluticasone propionate or UV-A alone for the long-term treatment of vitiligo. *Arch Dermatol* 1999;**135**:1061–6.

14. Orecchia G, Sangalli ME, Gazzaniga A, Giordano F. Topical photochemotherapy of vitiligo with a new khellin formulation: preliminary clinical results. *J Dermatol Treat* 1998;**9**:65–9.

15. Lotti TM, Menchini G, Andreassi L. UV-B radiation microphototherapy. An elective treatment for segmental vitiligo. *J Eur Acad Dermatol Venereol* 1999;**13**:102–8.

16. Mofty ME, Zaher H, Esmat S *et al.* PUVA and PUVB in vitiligo – are they equally effective? *Photodermatol Photoimmunol Photomed* 2001;**17**:159–63.

17. Drake LA, Ceilley RI, Dorner W. Guidelines of care for phototherapy and photochemotherapy. American Academy of Dermatology Committee on Guidelines of Care. *J Am Acad Dermatol* 1994;**31**:643–8.

18. Stern RS, Laird N. The carcinogenic risk of treatments for severe psoriasis. Photochemotherapy follow-up study. *Cancer* 1994;**73**:2759–64.

19. Stern RS, Nichols KT, Vakeva LH. Malignant melanoma in patients treated for psoriasis with methoxsalen (psoralen) and ultraviolet A radiation (PUVA). The PUVA Follow-Up Study. *N Engl J Med* 1997;**336**:1041–5.

20. British Photodermatology Group guidelines for PUVA. *Br J Dermatol* 1994;**130**:246–255.

21. Njoo MD, Bos JD, Westerhof W. Treatment of generalized vitiligo in children with narrow-band (TL-01) UVB radiation therapy. *J Am Acad Dermatol* 2000;**42**:245–53.

22. Papadopoulos L, Bor R, Legg C. Coping with the disfiguring effects of vitiligo: a preliminary investigation into the effects of cognitive-behavioural therapy. *Br J Med Psychol* 1999;**72**:385–96.

23. Souto MG, Manhaes AMH, Milhomens CH, Succi ICB. Comparative study of melagenine and placebo for the treatment of vitiligo. *An Bras Dermatol* 1997;**72**: 237–9.

24. Njoo MD, Westerhof W. Vitiligo. Pathogenesis and treatment. *Am J Clin Dermatol* 2001;**2**:167–81.

25. Kim HY, Kang KY. Epidermal grafts for treatment of stable and progressive vitiligo. *J Am Acad Dermatol* 1999;**40**:412–17.

26. Njoo MD, Westerhof W, Bos JD, Bossuyt PM. A systematic review of autologous transplantation methods in vitiligo. *Arch Dermatol* 1998;**134**:1543–9.

27. Gupta S, Jain VK, Saraswat PK. Suction blister epidermal grafting versus punch skin grafting in recalcitrant and stable vitiligo. *Dermatol Surg* 1999;**25**:955–8.

28. Schwartzmann-Solon AM, Visconti MA, Castrucci AM. Topical application of a melanotropin analogue to vulgar vitiligo dermo-epidermal minigrafts. *Braz J Med Biol Res* 1998;**31**:1557–64.

29. Chen YF, Chang JS, Yang PY, Hung CM, Huang MH, Hu DN. Transplant of cultured autologous pure melanocytes after laser-abrasion for the treatment of segmental vitiligo. *J Dermatol* 2000;**27**:434–9.

30. Guerra L, Capurro S, Melchi F *et al.* Treatment of "stable" vitiligo by timed surgery and transplantation of cultured epidermal autografts. *Arch Dermatol* 2000;**136**: 1380–9.

31. Mosher DB, Parrish JA, Fitzpatrick TB. Monobenzylether of hydroquinone. A retrospective study of treatment of 18 vitiligo patients and a review of the literature. *Br J Dermatol* 1977;**97**:669–79.

32. Njoo MD, Vodegel RM, Westerhof W. Depigmentation therapy in vitiligo universalis with topical 4–methoxyphenol and the Q-switched ruby laser. *J Am Acad Dermatol* 2000;**42**:760–9.

41
Melasma

Asad Salim, Mónica Rengifo-Pardo, Sam Vincent and Luis Gabriel Cuervo-Amore

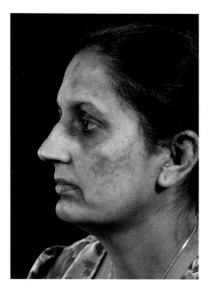

Figure 41.1   Patient with melasma

Background
Definition

Melasma is an acquired increased pigmentation of the skin, characterised by grey–brown symmetrical patches, mostly on the areas of the face exposed to the sun, but occasionally on the neck and forearms.[1] Its clinical and histological presentation does not differ between men and women, apart from differences in incidence (see below).

Incidence/prevalence

There are few studies showing the prevalence of melasma. A study done in Mexico[2] and another done in Peru[3] found that melasma accounted for 4–10% of new dermatology hospital referrals. Melasma was found to be the third most common pigmentary disorder of the skin in a survey of 2000 black people at a private clinic in Washington DC.[4] Melasma is thought to be more common in people of Hispanic origin who live in areas of high ultraviolet-light exposure and in Asian people.[5]

Aetiology

Melasma occurs most commonly during pregnancy, and has also been associated with the use of oral contraceptives containing oestrogens and/or progestogens, and with certain drugs such as hydantoin.[6–8] Sun exposure appears to be important for the development of melasma[9] and there also appears to be a familial predisposition.[9] Melasma may also affect men, especially those of Hispanic or Asian origin. A descriptive study in 27 men in Puerto Rico suggested that sunlight exposure and family history are the most important determinants for development of melasma in men.[10] The cause of melasma is unknown; hormonal mechanisms may be involved. Mild ovarian dysfunction has been considered as a cause after a study found increased levels of leutinising hormone and low levels of serum oestradiol in nine women with melasma.[11] A case-control study of 108 non-pregnant women with melasma found a significant association with increased thyroid antibodies in the blood.[12] Studies measuring levels of immunoreactive β-melanocyte stimulating hormone found normal levels in patients taking oral contraceptives, some of whom had melasma,[13] suggesting that the development of melasma is not related to melanocytic hormone.

Prognosis

Melasma usually persists for several years. It may present as odd streaking on the face, causing cosmetic disfigurement. Pregnancy-related melasma may persist for several months after delivery, and melasma related to hormonal treatments may persist for long periods after stopping oral contraceptives. Recurrences are common, particularly after re-exposure to the sun.[9] Response to the treatment can be variable, although dermal type melasma is less responsive than epidermal type (see below). The benefits of treatment may not be apparent for many months. Treatment is often unsatisfactory and has been associated with side-effects such as local irritation, scarring, contact dermatitis and residual patches of lighter colour on the skin – so-called "confetti pigmentation". Hydroquinone, one of the common depigmentation agents, has been particularly associated with exogenous ochronosis (deposit of brown, blue or black pigmentation in the skin and cartilage seen in sufferers of alkaptonuria, which is a rare inherited metabolic disorder) from prolonged use of strong concentrations.[14]

Diagnostic tests

Melasma is usually a clinical diagnosis. Microscopy studies suggest that there may be two main types of melasma[9]: the epidermal type, characterised by increased melanin pigmentation in the suprabasal layers of the epidermis, and the dermal type, characterised by increased melanin in the dermal macrophages, with associated milder epidermal hyperpigmentation. With mixed type, some areas show enhanced pigmentation, and some do not when examined with a Wood's light, revealing a mixture of dermal and epidermal melasma in the same person (see below).

This distinction may provide a clue to the expected treatment response. Dermal type has been found to be less responsive to conventional therapy.[5] An alternative way of establishing the type of melasma clinically is by using a source of ultraviolet A light such as a Wood's lamp.[15] Ultraviolet light lamps enhance the lesions in light-coloured skins (i.e. skin phototypes I–IV; see Box 41.1),[12] but may be of little use in dark-skinned people, in whom the enhancement is less prominent.

Box 41.1 Skin phototype

Skin phototype is a classification used to determine the risk of cutaneous sunburning and tanning tendency following exposure to ultraviolet radiation. It is useful in determining the dose regimens for phototherapy and photochemotherapy, an individual's susceptibility to photoageing and skin cancer, and the degree of photoprotection required. Phototypes are categorised in a range of I–VI.[16]

- Phototype I describes white people, those who always burn and never tan.
- Phototypes IV–VI describe darker people, from light brown to dark brown or black. These people have low sensibility to ultraviolet radiation and have a low risk of burning and react to exposure by tanning.

Aims of treatment

Treatments should aim to prevent the development of melasma, prevent or reduce the severity of recurrence, reduce affected areas, improving the cosmetic defect, and reduce time to clearance, with fewest possible side-effects.

Time for clearance is important as current treatments take several months to have any effect.

Relevant outcomes

- Improvement in patient satisfaction measures, and quality-of-life assessment measures during the time course of the intervention
- Clearance of lesions evaluated by objective methods (for example melasma area and severity index (MASI) or melasma area and melanin index (MAMI); see Box 41.2) or any other objective semiquantitative measures of disease
- Lightening of pigmentation (evaluated objectively by a colorimeter, for example)
- Adverse effects such as irregular pigmentation or irritation related to the interventions

Box 41.2 Melasma scoring indexes

MAMI

This is the melasma area and melanin index.[17] It is calculated as MASI (see below) but darkness and homogeneity are replaced by the single variable of melanin index. This variable is a measurement of colour at involved sites determined using a reflectance spectrophotometer.

MASI score

This is the melasma area and severity index.[18] The index evaluates four areas of the face: the forehead (f), the right (rm) and left malar (lm) regions and the chin (c). Each of the first three is weighted with 30% of the score, while the chin is weighted with 10% of the score. The extent of melasma in each area (A) is calculated and given a numerical value as follows:

0   no involvement
1   <10%
2   10–29%
3   30–49%
4   50–69%
5   70–89%
6   <90–100%.

Severity of melasma is described by a combination of two factors, darkness (D) and homogeneity (H), each evaluated on a scale of 0 to 4, and is calculated as follows:
$$MASI = 0{\cdot}3(D_f + H_f)A_f + 0{\cdot}3(D_{mr} + H_{mr})A_{mr} + 0{\cdot}3(D_{ml} + H_{ml})A_{ml} + 0{\cdot}1(D_c + H_c)A_c.$$

Methods of search

Medline 1966 to 3rd August 2001, EmBase 1980 to 3rd August 2001, *Cochrane Library* 2001 issue 3, Psycinfo 1970 to 3rd August 2001 and LILACs were searched for the terms "melasma", "chloasma" or "mask of pregnancy" as text words and/or keywords if present in the database. Randomised controlled trials (RCTs) were searched for first, using a filter; the remaining abstracts from the search were then scanned to see if any RCTs had been missed using the search filter. References from identified papers were searched. The results of the search were appraised by at least two of the authors.

QUESTIONS

How effective are preventive interventions in high-risk populations?

Case scenario 1

A Latin-American woman is planning to have children and is concerned about developing melasma. Her three sisters all developed melasma during pregnancy, which lasted for many years.

Efficacy

We found no studies assessing the effects of preventive measures (such as educational interventions to avoid sun exposure or use of prophylactic sunscreens) in high-risk populations.

Comment

Overall, expert opinion supports interventions aimed at reducing exposure to ultraviolet light, which may reduce the risk of developing melasma.

Key messages

We found no incontrovertible or solid evidence to support preventive interventions in high-risk populations. Current opinion, based on known risk factors, suggests that preventing exposure to ultraviolet light such as sunlight may reduce the risk of developing melasma.

Implications for clinical practice/categorisation

Unknown effectiveness.

How effective are therapeutic interventions in childbearing, pregnant and breastfeeding women?

Case scenario 2

A 30-year-old woman developed melasma in the 20th week of her first pregnancy. She is not on any medication and has not used an oral contraceptive in the past.

Efficacy

We found no studies in populations clearly identified as pregnant or breastfeeding women. Several studies did not clearly specify if included women were pregnant or became pregnant during follow up. When components used in the

study included those that are not recommended in childbearing women (i.e. retinoids) the study was considered to be done in non-pregnant or nursing populations and are discussed under the corresponding question.

Comment

Common expert opinion is that women under high risk of developing melasma should avoid exposure to sun or other sources of ultraviolet light. It would seem reasonable to consider the use of broad-spectrum sunscreen with solar protection factors (SPF) >15 in women at high risk of developing melasma.

Key messages

We found no good evidence to support any therapeutic intervention in childbearing, pregnant or breastfeeding women. Current opinion suggests that such women with melasma may benefit from using broad-spectrum sunscreens and avoiding exposure to ultraviolet light such as sunlight.

Implications for clinical practice/categorisation

Unknown effectiveness.

How effective are therapeutic interventions in non-childbearing women?

Case scenario 3

A 35-year-old woman presented with a 3-month history of melasma. She was taking an oral contraceptive, which she had recently stopped taking after a tubal ligation. She is an outdoor worker.

Sunscreens
Efficacy

We found no systematic reviews. We found one RCT[19] comparing sunscreens with placebo in women receiving hydroquinone. The study involved 59 non-pregnant Hispanic women in Puerto Rico. None of the participating women was taking contraceptive hormones and all had had melasma for 2–25 years. All women were prescribed a clearing solution of hydroquinone 3% in hydroalcoholic solvent twice daily. Women were randomised to a morning application of broad-spectrum sunscreen or vehicle (placebo) and were then followed for 3 months. Improvement, assessed subjectively by a physician, was similar with sunscreen (improvement in 26/27 (96%) women receiving sunscreen and hydroquinone compared with 21/26 (81%) women receiving placebo and hydroquinone; relative risk (RR) 1·19, 95% confidence intervals (CI) 0·98–1·46). Improvement rates assessed by participants were high in both groups (27/27 (100%) with sunscreen and hydroquinone compared with 25/26 (96%) with placebo and hydroquinone; absolute risk reduction (ARR) 4%, CI −1 to 18·9%). Six of the 59 women (10%) withdrew and 9/53 (17%) women suffered side-effects; the report did not mention which group these women were allocated to.

Comment

Sunscreens are commonly prescribed for melasma.

Key messages

We found limited evidence from a single RCT evaluating the effect of therapeutic sunscreens. It showed that during the 3-month follow up period, the majority of women receiving hydroquinone improved regardless of the addition of sunscreen to their treatment. The study did not describe if women used other strategies to avoid sunlight.

Implications for clinical practice/categorisation

Unknown effectiveness.

Topical corticosteroids
Efficacy

We found no systematic reviews. We found one trial of 17 participants (16 consecutive women and one man) followed for 3 months.[20] The trial compared the topical application of a 0·2% betamethasone 17-valerate cream with cream excipient (placebo). Randomisation was used to allocate the side of the face to which creams were applied. There was good improvement (subjectively defined by physician and participants) in eight people, eight of whom considered betamethasone to be better than placebo. Three considered they achieved moderate improvement with either betamethasone or placebo, and four people said they had no improvement at all. One person withdrew from the trial.

Drawbacks

The study reported no significant side-effects.[20]

Comment

Although the study reports that betamethasone was effective as a depigmenting agent ($P<0·05$), numbers were very small and 7/16 patients found no therapeutic difference between treatment and placebo.[20] There is controversy over the balance between benefits and harms of using topical steroids in the treatment of melasma.

Key messages

We found insufficient evidence to support the use of topical steroids in melasma. There is controversy over the use of topical steroids in melasma.

Implications for clinical practice/categorisation

Unknown effectiveness.

Topical retinoids
Efficacy

We found no systematic review. We found three RCTs.

In Caucasian people: The first RCT was done in 50 Caucasian women with facial melasma.[21] Pregnant or nursing women were excluded. Women attending tanning salons, having heavy sun exposure, or who had used systemic retinoids during the previous 6 months or topical retinoids during the previous month were excluded. The trial compared the daily use of topical 0.1% tretinoin with placebo (vehicle cream for tretinoin). The withdrawal rate was 24%. Insufficient baseline data was presented to determine if groups were comparable at baseline.

In Asian people: The second RCT[17] included 30 Thai people (26 women and 4 men) with facial melasma. It excluded pregnant and nursing women, and people who had used systemic retinoids in the previous 6 months or topical retinoids in the previous month. The RCT compared a titrated daily application of 0.05% isotretinoin gel with colour-matched vehicle used as placebo, for 40 weeks. There were no significant differences in the MASI or MAMI scores in the evaluations done at 2 weeks, 4 weeks and monthly for up to 40 weeks. The only two participants with dermal melasma were allocated to the isotretinoin group. Participants in both groups improved during the 40-week follow up.

In black people: One RCT in the US compared the daily application to the entire face of a cream with 0.1% tretinoin or placebo (vehicle) in 30 (29 women) Afro-American black people, followed for 40 weeks.[22] The MASI score was used to assess the severity of melasma. Darkness and homogeneity were also assessed. Colorimetry, photographic and histology studies were done before and after treatment. After 40 weeks people receiving tretinoin had higher rates of improvement in their mean ± SD MASI score (MASI score changed in the tretinoin group from 15.0 ± 1.8 at baseline to 10.2 ± 2 and in the vehicle group from 15.5 ± 2.6 to 13.9 ± 2.7 after 40 weeks of treatment ($P=0.03$).) Changes were assessed by an independent clinician, who found no significant differences between tretinoin and placebo after 24 weeks (improved or much improved: 11/15 (73%) with tretinoin compared with 6/13 (46%) with placebo; RR 1.6, CI 0.8–3.1).

Drawbacks

In Caucasian people: The first RCT described some causes for withdrawal such as cutaneous side-effects (3/25 (12%) with tretinoin compared with 0/25 with placebo). Worsening of melasma occurred in a woman from the tretinoin group. Moderate cutaneous reactions were more frequent with tretinoin (22/25 (88%)) than with placebo (7/24 (29%)) with placebo (RR 3.0, CI 1.6–5.7; number need to harm (NNH (see Table 10.1) 1.7, CI 1.3–3.1). Severe cutaneous reactions occurred only with tretinoin (4/25 (16%); NNH 6.3).[21]

In Asian people: The second RCT found similar withdrawals rates in both groups (4/15 (27%) with isotretinoin compared with 3/15 (20%) with placebo).[17] Mild transient erythema and/or peeling occurred only in the isotretinoin group (4/15 (27%) NNH 3.8).

In black people: The most frequently found side-effects in the third RCT were erythema and/or peeling (10/15 (67%) with tretinoin compared with 1/15 (7%) with placebo; RR 10, CI 1.5–68.7; NNH 1.7, CI 1.1–2.4) in the area of application.[22]

Comment

The withdrawal rate was high in the first RCT,[21] which compromised the validity of the results. Both RCTs have small samples, which make it difficult to draw conclusions with confidence. The RCT done in black people[22] may have had insufficient power to rule out an effect, as CIs for physician-assessed changes were broad. It is impossible to draw reliable conclusions on the effects of retinoids in Caucasian women. The trials done in Asian people[17] and black people[22] were small, so the finding of no differences does not rule out the possibility of a clinically important effect. Side-effects, however, were quite common in people receiving retinoids. It is unknown whether the use of sunscreens may have introduced any confounding.

Key messages

We found inconclusive evidence of an effect of retinoids in people with melasma, but side-effects were common.

Implications for clinical practice/categorisation

Unlikely to be beneficial.

Azelaic acid
Efficacy

We found no systematic reviews. One RCT done in the US (52 people: 45 non-pregnant or non-nursing women, 7 men; skin phototype IV, V or VI; clinical diagnosis of facial hyperpigmentation which could in some cases be caused by melasma) compared azelaic acid with placebo.[23] After 24 weeks the authors found a statistically significant decrease in the treatment group in pigmentary intensity as measured by chromometer analysis ($P = 0.039$) and investigators' subjective scale ($P = 0.021$). The study failed to differentiate at any stage those participants with melasma from those with other hyperpigmentation disorders, making it difficult to draw conclusions applicable to people with melasma.

We found one RCT and one non-randomised controlled trial comparing azelaic acid with hydroquinone. The RCT[24] was in 340 people with non-dermal melasma (17 men evenly distributed), and compared twice-daily 20% azelaic acid cream with twice-daily 2% hydroquinone cream for 24 weeks. It found that improvement (defined as a reduction of >50% in a score including area and pigmentation) was higher with azelaic acid (106/154 (69%) than with hydroquinone (88/161 (55%)); RR 1·26; CI 1·06–1·50; NNT 7, CI 4–30). The majority of patients were of skin phototypes III–VI. No subgroup analysis was done to determine if men had a different response to women. The non-randomised controlled trial[25] (60 women with skin phototypes I–IV, centromalar or facial distribution, followed for 24 weeks) included women with epidermal (72%) or mixed melasma (28%), in the age range 18–40 years. Thirty per cent of women were taking oral contraceptives. The trial compared 20% azelaic acid cream with 4% hydroquinone cream. All women were given sunscreen (details not provided) and were asked to apply azelaic acid on one side of their face and hydroquinone in the other side, twice daily for 24 weeks. No detail is provided to explain how interventions were concealed. Improvement was assessed subjectively by participants and evaluators. The study was completed by 85% of participants. Improvement was similar in women receiving azelaic acid (23/26 (88%) and hydroquinone (22/25 (88%); RR 1·0, CI 0·8–1·3).

Drawbacks

The study done in people with undifferentiated hyperpigmentation disorders[23] found that people using azelaic acid cream had a higher incidence of burning, particularly at weeks 4 and

12 ($P = 0.046$ and 0.021, respectively; detailed data not provided) and significantly higher stinging symptoms at week 4 ($P = 0.002$, detailed data not provided) than those using placebo.

In the comparison with hydroquinone, complaints of mild symptoms such as itching and burning were more frequent with azelaic acid (61/167 (37%)) than with hydroquinone (22/173 (12%); RR 3·0, CI 1·7–4·7; NNH 4, CI 3–6). Withdrawals related to intolerance (local irritation) occurred in both groups (4/167 (2%) with azelaic acid compared with 2/173 (1%) with hydroquinone). Marked irritation was more frequent with azelaic acid (15/167 (9%)) than with hydroquinione (2/173 (1%)); RR 7·8, CI 1·8–33·5; 12, CI 7–30).[24]

Comment
Results of the non-randomised clinical trial should be interpreted with caution as the authors did not describe strategies used to avoid bias, outcomes were assessed subjectively and no standardised or validated scales were used.

Key messages
Azelaic acid was found to be superior to 2% hydroquinone in achieving improvement in people with melasma. We found no solid evidence compared with placebo. Azelaic acid was associated with a higher incidence of side-effects.

Implications for clinical practice/categorisation
Unknown effectiveness (compared with placebo).

Likely to be beneficial (compared with hydroquinone).

Hydroquinone
Efficacy
We found no systematic review. We found one RCT, done between autumn and spring in Brazil (48 people, four men; age range 19–55 years).[26] Participating women were asked to use effective contraception during the trial. All participants had a clinical diagnosis of melasma with Wood's lamp evaluation. People using benzoyl peroxide, hydrogen peroxide or alcoholic cleansing agents were excluded. People suffering from alcohol or drug abuse, severe emotional problems, or irritation or wounds in the treatment area were also excluded. All participants received an SPF15 sunscreen. The intervention group received 4% hydroquinone cream applied twice daily, while the control group received placebo. Outcomes were assessed by subjective clinical evaluation and photography. After 12 weeks hydroquinone showed higher improvement rates (20/21 (95%) with hydroquinone versus 16/24 (67%) with placebo; RR 1·4, CI 1·06–1·9; NNT 3·5, CI 1·9–12·1). Total clearance of lesions was more frequent in people receiving hydroquinone (8/21 (38%) compared with placebo (2/24 (8%)) (RR 4·6, CI 1·1–19·2; NNT 3·4, CI 1·8–12·7). We found one RCT comparing hydroquinone with azelaic acid (see above).[24]

Drawbacks
The RCT[26] found adverse effects in six people using hydroquinone and five using placebo. Erythema was more frequent with hydroquinone (five people using hydroquinone, two using placebo). Contact dermatitis occurred in one person receiving hydroquinone. In the placebo group, two people reported acne, one skin dryness, one solar erythema and one cutaneous irritation. The RCT comparing azelaic acid with hydroquinone is described above.[24]

Comment
The trial was small and had exclusion criteria that should be considered when deciding on the applicability of the results. Hydroquinone (4%) plus sunscreen was found to be superior to placebo plus sunscreen in the RCT, while 2%

hydroquinone in comparison against azelaic acid was less effective.

Key messages

We found limited evidence from one RCT showing that the use of hydroquinone plus sunscreen was superior to the use of sunscreen and placebo.

Implications for clinical practice/categorisation

Likely to be beneficial (when used with sunscreen).

Glycolic acid
Efficacy

We found no systematic review. We found one randomised and one non-randomised trial. The RCT (10 non-pregnant and non-nursing Asian women with skin phototypes IV or V, suffering moderate-to-severe facial melasma) compared the use of peelings with glycolic acid on one side of the face versus no peelings on the other side.[27] All women received concomitant twice-daily applications of a cream containing 10% glycolic acid and 2% hydroquinone, as well as SPF15 sunscreen. An independent evaluator assessed the results using a Munsell colour chart and photographs. Participants also assessed the results. Treatments were randomly allocated to a side of the face, and no placebo was used to conceal the intervention. The physician evaluation found improvement in the side using peeling in all cases, and improvement in control sides in 8/10 cases.

The open non-randomised trial (16 women with skin phototypes II–VI, followed for 6 months) comparing glycolic acid peels against Jessner's solution found no differences in the two groups.[28] All women received nightly 0·05% tretinoin (preparation not specified) for 1–2 weeks and

daily applications of sunscreen. All women also received three peeling sessions, a month apart. Peelings were done using titrated doses of 70% glycolic acid applied to the right side of the face and Jessner's solution applied to the left side. Follow up was completed by 11 (68%) participants and no differences were found between groups.

Drawbacks

All participants in the RCT[27] experienced stinging and redness during and after each peeling session. One person developed an area of burn after the 20% glycolic acid peeling, resulting in a zone of hyperpigmentation which disappeared after 2 months. No significant differences between treatments were found.

Glycolic acid peelings were more frequently reported as more painful than Jessner's solution. One participant developed postinflammatory hyperpigmentation in the side receiving glycolic acid.[28]

Comment

The RCT may have been too small to rule out differences, and concealment may have been difficult to achieve because of the side-effects of the peelings.[27] The open non-randomised trial has major limitations that compromise the validity of the results. The design of the study is not the most appropriate to answer a clinical question referring to treatment effectiveness. Befor–after comparisons do not allow firm conclusions to be drawn, and comparisons with results of previous reports from different populations may be misleading.[28]

Key messages

We found insufficient evidence to assess the effects of glycolic acid.

Implications for clinical practice/categorisation

Unknown effectiveness.

Combined therapies
Efficacy

We found no systematic reviews. We found five RCTs. The first trial was an open RCT (50 Oriental people, 49 women, with non-dermal melasma and not taking oral contraceptives).[18] It compared the daily use of a cream containing 20% azelaic acid, 0·05% tretinoin and sunscreen, with a cream containing 20% azelaic acid and sunscreen, for a period of 6 months with monthly evaluations. The number of withdrawals was high and therefore it is difficult to draw conclusions. Furthermore, some outcome categories overlapped.

A second RCT[29] (65 dark-skinned people, skin phototypes >III, with hyperpigmentation, 44 (68%) of whom had melasma) compared a cream containing 20% azelaic acid cream plus 15–20% glycolic acid (first month only) plus sunscreen with 4% hydroquinone plus sunscreen; participants were followed for 24 weeks. There was no difference between the two groups in overall improvement, and reduction in lesion area, pigmentary intensity and disease severity were comparable in the two treatment groups.

A third RCT[30] in 40 Chinese women with pure epidermal melasma confirmed by Wood's lamp (age range not specified) compared the twice-daily application of a gel containing 2% kojic acid, 2% hydroquinone and 10% glycolic acid followed by a sunblock with titanium dioxide SPF15 with the twice-daily application of a control gel containing 2% hydroquinone and 10% glycolic acid, followed by sunblock with titanium dioxide SPF15. Randomisation was used to determine which side of the face would receive each intervention. Data from three women who withdrew were not included in the analysis. The frequency of >50% clearance of the melasma area was higher where kojic acid was used, although this difference was not significant (24/40 (60%) for the combined gel containing kojic acid versus 19/40 (48%) for the combined gel without kojic acid; RR 1·3, CI 0·8–1·9). When participating women assessed improvement, this was found to be better with the gel containing kojic acid.

The fourth RCT[31] included 38 non-childbearing women with skin phototype I–IV and melasma (type not specified). The study randomised affected areas of skin instead of people and was achieved using a list. The study compared a cream containing 12% alpha hydroxyacid (particular preparation not specified), 1% polypeptide ascorbate complex and titanium oxide photoprotector with a preparation containing titanium oxide photoprotector and the vehicle for the cream prepared to the same pH. It found that patient global assessment, which was measured using a visual analogue scale for area and pigmentation, improved in more women receiving active treatment than in those using the placebo preparation. However this difference did not quite reach significance (34/36 (94%) with the combination treatment versus 17/36 (47%) with placebo. RR 1·51, CI 0·96–2·40). Differences were significant for the melanic index measured using a Mexameter (mean melanic index 15·2 with active treatment versus 22·1 with placebo; $P<0·01$ at day 56).

The fifth RCT[32] (39 people with facial melasma, 5% of them with dermal melasma under Wood's light; 38 women, followed for 3 months) compared 2% hydroquinone and 5% glycolic acid gel with 2% kojic acid and 5% glycolic acid gel. This study compared interventions applied to the left or right side of the face. Outcomes were comparison of facial photographs taken using an ultraviolet filter, clinical evaluation, participants' impressions and decrease in affected area (no formal scales were used). There were no significant differences between groups (28% reduction with kojic acid and 21% reduction with hydroquinone).

Drawbacks

The reasons for withdrawals in the first RCT[18] are not clear. Numbers were similar in both groups (6/25 (24%) for the azelaic acid, tretinoin and sunscreen group versus 7/25 (28%) for the azelaic acid and sunscreen group; RR 0·9, CI 0·3–2·2).

In the second RCT[29] the azelaic acid group experienced significantly more burning and peeling. There were two withdrawals in azelaic acid group and four in the hydroquinone group. However, these were described as not being due to side-effects of the preparations.

All participants in the third RCT comparing a combination of hydroquinone and glycolic acid followed by sunblock with or without 2% kojic acid,[30] complained of redness, stinging and mild exfoliation in both sides of their face (randomisation was done for the side receiving each treatment). Three women withdrew from the study because of adverse effects on both sides of their face and were replaced by three other women.

In the fourth RCT comparing alpha hydroxyacid, polypeptide ascorbate complex and titanium oxide photoprotector with a preparation containing titanium oxide photoprotector,[31] one woman withdrew after 28 days because of depigmentation. However, no detail is provided on whether this happened on the intervention or control cheek. A second participant was excluded when it became apparent that she did not have melasma. In the active treatment group a higher frequency of erythema and burning feeling was reported and this persisted throughout follow up. However, no further details are provided.

In the fifth RCT[32] both treatments were described as being well tolerated, although all participants had some degree of skin irritation. Kojic acid gel was found to be a stronger irritant. No further detail was provided.

Comment

Methodological limitations compromise the validity of results found in the first RCT comparing azelaic acid, tretinoin and sunscreen with azelaic acid and sunscreen.[18]

With the second RCT comparing azelaic acid cream, glycolic acid and sunscreen with hydroquinone and sunscreen, it was not possible to determine if the response varied between people with melasma and people with other hyperpigmentation conditions.[29] It is therefore difficult to draw valid conclusions.

The third RCT comparing a gel containing kojic acid, hydroquinone, 10% glycolic acid followed by titanium dioxide sunblock, with a gel containing hydroquinone and glycolic acid followed by titanium dioxide sunblock had methodological limitations, which may compromise its validity, and the sample size may be insufficient to rule out an effect.[30]

The fourth RCT[31] did not provide detail on the melasma type. Melasma type has been associated with treatment response. The study does not give details of the kind of alpha hydroxyacid used and lacks detail of demographic data.

The fifth RCT does not allow one to look at variables but gives percentage improvements and P values. It concludes that the addition of 2% kojic acid gel to glycolic acid is as efficacious as 2% hydroquinone.[32] Addition of 2% kojic acid to a gel containing 10% glycolic acid and 2% hydroquinone further improves melasma. No additional side-effects were reported on the kojic acid side.[32]

We found one abstract[33] which did not provide sufficient detail to make a critical appraisal of the study methodology.

Key messages

Overall we found no good evidence of the effects of combined therapies compared with placebo or other preparations. The studies had methodological flaws that compromised the validity of the results, including small sample sizes.

Implications for clinical practice/categorisation

Unknown effectiveness (all combined preparations).

Laser therapies
Efficacy

We found no systematic review. We found one RCT[34] in eight dark-skinned people (skin phototype IV–VI) with dermal melasma diagnosed by Wood's lamp. The article does not provide any detail of the demographics of participants. All participants received a 14-day course of 0·05% tretinoin cream, 4% hydroquinone cream and 1% hydrocortisone cream, applied twice daily. All participants were asked to use a sunblock of SPF15 or higher. Participants had a 1 cm² area of the face exposed to one pass of the 950-microsecond pulsed carbon dioxide laser with a computerised pattern generation set at 300 mJ/cm². The intervention group received, in addition to the above, another pass with Q-switched alexandrite pigmented dye laser at a dose of 6 J/cm². The treated area was evaluated after 6 months. Normal skin was found in three participants of the intervention group and one of the control group. However, the sample size is too small to draw valid conclusions, and confounding factors such as the use of different sunblock preparations was not accounted for.

Drawbacks

Two participants in the control group suffered peripheral hyperpigmentation. As mentioned above, the small sample size does not allow firm conclusions to be drawn.

Comment

This RCT[34] is of particular interest because it evaluates one of the few interventions currently used for dermal melasma. Properly designed RCTs are needed to determine the effect of laser therapies in dermal melasma.

Key messages

We found insufficient evidence to evaluate the effect of laser therapies in the treatment of melasma.

Implications for clinical practice/categorisation

Unknown effectiveness.

Other treatments
Efficacy

We found no systematic review. We found one RCT[35] (Japan, 3-month follow up; 176 women and 2 men with diagnosis of melasma). Melasma was present in 136 people (76%) and pigmented contact dermatitis in 42 (24%). Specific results for melasma were available from the study report. The RCT compared oral vitamin E (50 people), vitamin C (45 people) and a combination of vitamins E and C (41 people). The study excluded pregnant women and people suffering from systemic diseases. After 12 weeks, physician-rated colour difference and photographic findings were used to assess changes. Using colour photographs, an improvement was noticed in 69% of those receiving a combination therapy of vitamins E and C, 60% of those receiving vitamin E and 50% of people receiving vitamin C. These differences did not reach statistical significance. In the objective clinical improvement evaluation,

72% of the participants in the combined-therapy group showed improvement compared with 63% in the vitamin E group and 44% in the vitamin C group. The difference between the combined-therapy and vitamin C groups reached statistical significance ($P < 0.05$).

Drawbacks

The Japanese RCT had 10 withdrawals.[35] One participant withdrew because of side-effects while 51 failed to complete the 12-week follow up. Five people in the group receiving vitamins E and C suffered side-effects: two had acne, one xerosis, one mild stomach upset and one metrorrhagia. Eight people in the vitamin E group complained of side-effects: four had acne, one stomach upset, one excessive perspiration and two menstrual abnormalities. Side-effects were reported by participants receiving vitamin C: four suffered acne, two hot flushes, one stomach upset and one seborrhoeic dermatitis.

Comments

The Japanese study did not have a placebo group, and all groups improved. Improvement was better in people receiving preparations containing vitamin E. A placebo-controlled study is needed to determine the effect of these compounds. Thirty-one people suffered side-effects, although it is not clear if this refers to people with chloasma or if it included people with other pigmentary disorders.

Key messages

We found limited evidence that the combination of vitamins C and E is better than vitamin C alone. We found no evidence of the effects of these therapies against placebo.

Implications for clinical practice/categorisation

Unknown effectiveness.

Case scenario 4

A 40-year-old Latin-American man living in California has had melasma for 3 months. It appeared after a beach holiday. He is not on any regular medication but has a family history of melasma.

Efficacy

We identified no studies assessing the effects of therapeutic interventions exclusively in men. Although several RCTs included a few men, none of them did a subgroup analysis, and none would have had sufficient power to find clinically relevant differences.

Comment

Based on expert opinion, the same treatments used in non-pregnant women may be considered appropriate in men with melasma.

Key messages

We found no evidence specifically evaluating the effects of treatment in men.

Implications for clinical practice/categorisation

Unknown effectiveness.

Implications of the available evidence

For consumers (the public)

Current opinion, based on known risk factors, suggests that measures preventing exposure to sunlight may reduce the risk of development and recurrence of melasma. From the available trial evidence therapies likely to be beneficial are azelaic acid and hydroquinone.

For clinical practice (healthcare providers)

From the available evidence, treatments likely to benefit patients with melasma are azelaic acid with sunscreens and 2–4% hydroquinone with sunscreens. The use of hydroquinone for melasma has been limited recently because of several case reports of it causing exogenous ochronosis. However, there were no reports of this side-effect in any studies with a follow up for up to 24 months.

We did not find convincing evidence for the effectiveness of topical retinoids, topical corticosteroids, glycolic acid, oral vitamins E or C, lasers or any combined therapies.

For research (research agencies and researchers)

We have found inconclusive evidence for the effectiveness of topical steroids, topical retinoids, glycolic acid and laser therapy. These are commonly used therapies for melasma in clinical practice and would require further RCTs to validate their use. Lasers offer a potential advantage over conventional therapies because time to clearance can be much reduced. We found only a few studies that looked at patient-based outcomes.

Key points

- No incontrovertible or solid evidence supports preventive interventions in high-risk populations. Current opinion, based on known risk factors, suggests that preventing exposure to sources of ultraviolet light such as sunlight may reduce the risk of developing melasma.
- No incontrovertible evidence supports any therapeutic intervention in pregnant or breastfeeding women. Current opinion suggests that such women with melasma may benefit from using broad-spectrum sunscreens and avoiding exposure to ultraviolet light such as sunlight.

- Limited evidence from a single RCT evaluating the effect of therapeutic sunscreens shows that during the 3-month study period, the majority of women using hydroquinone improved regardless of the addition of sunscreen to their treatment. The study did not describe whether women used other strategies to avoid sunlight.
- Evidence is insufficient to support the use of topical steroids in melasma. There is controversy over the use of topical steroids in melasma.
- An effect of retinoids on melasma has not been shown, but the available studies found that side-effects were common.
- Azelaic acid was found to be superior to 2% hydroquinone in achieving improvement in people with melasma. We found no solid evidence compared azelaic acid with placebo. Azelaic acid was associated with a higher incidence of side-effects.
- Limited evidence from one RCT suggests that hydroquinone plus sunscreen was better than sunscreen and placebo.
- Evidence is insufficient to assess the effects of glycolic acid.
- Overall we found no good evidence of the effects of combined therapies compared with placebo or other preparations. The studies had methodological flaws, including small sample sizes, that compromised the validity of results
- We found insufficient evidence to evaluate the effect of laser therapies in the treatment of melasma.
- We found limited evidence that a combination of vitamins C and E is better than vitamin C alone. We found no evidence of the effects of these therapies compared with placebo.
- No studies have assessed the effect of treatments specifically in men.

References

1. Newcomer VD. A melanosis of the face ('chloasma'). *Arch Dermatol* 1961;**83**:284–99.

2. Estrada-Castanon R, Torres-Bibiano B, Alarcon-Hernandez H *et al.* Epidemiología cutánea en dos sectores de atención mèdica en Guerrero, Mexico. *Dermato Rev Mex* 1992;**36**:29–34.

3. Failmezger C. Incidence of skin disease in Cuzco, Peru. *Int J Dermatol.*1992;**31**:560–1.

4. Halder RN, Grimes PE, McLaurin CI, Kress MA, Kennery JA Jr. Incidence of common dermatoses in a predominantly black dermatologic practice. *Cutis* 1983;**32**:388–90.

5. Pathak MA, Fitzpatrick TB, Kraus EW. Usefulness of retinoic acid in the treatment of melasma. *J Am Acad Dermatol.*1986;**15**:894–9.

6. Bleehem SS. Disorders of skin colour. In: Champion RH, Burton JL, Burns DA, Breathnach SM, eds. *Textbook of Dermatology, 6th ed.* Oxford: Blackwell Science, 1998:1753–1815.

7. Resnick S. Melasma induced by oral contraceptive drugs. *JAMA* 1967;**199**:601–5.

8. Escoda ECJ. Chloasma from progestational oral contraceptives. *Arch Dermatol* 1967;**87**:486.

9. Sanchez NP, Pathak MA, Sato S, Fitzpatrick TB, Sanchez JL, Minhm MC Jr. Melasma a clinical, light microscopic, ultrastructural and immunofluorescence study. *J Am Acad Dermatol* 1981;**4**:698–710.

10. Vazquez M, Maldonado H, Benaman C, Sanchez JL. Melasma in men: a clinical and histologic study. *Int J Dermatol* 1988;**27**:25–7.

11. Perez M, Samchez JL, Aguilo F. Endocrinologic profile of patients with idiopathic melasma. *J Invest Dermatol* 1983;**81**:543–5.

12. Lufti RJ, Fridmanis M, Misrunas AL. Association of melasma with thyroid autoimmunity and other thyroidal abnormalities and their relationship to the origin of melasma. *J Clin Endocrinol Metab* 1985;**61**:28–31.

13. Smith AG, Shuster S, Thody AJ *et al.* Chloasma, oral contraceptives, and plasma immunoreactive beta-melanocyte-stimulating hormone. *J Invest Dermatol* 1977:169–170.

14. Findley GH, Morrison JGL, Simon IW. Exogenous ochronosis and pigmented colloid milium from hydroquinone bleaching creams. *Br J Dermatol.* 1975;**93**:613–22.

15. Gilchrest BA, Fitzpatrick TB, Anderson RR, Parish JA. Localization of melanin pigmentation in the skin with Wood's lamp. *Br J Dermatol* 1977;**96**:245–8.

16. Fitzpatrick TB. Validity and practicality of sun-reaction types I–VI. *Arch Dermatol* 1988;**124**:869–71.

17. Leenutaphong V, Nettakul A, Rattanasuwon P. Topical isotretinoin for melasma in Thai patients: a vehicle-controlled clinical trial. *J Med Assoc Thai* 1999;**82**: 868–75.

18. Graupe K, Verallo RVM, Verallo V, Zaumseil RP. Combined use of 20% azelaic acid cream and 0·05% tretinoin cream in the topical treatment of melasma. *J Dermatol Treat* 1996;**7**:235–7.

19. Vazquez M, Sanchez JL. The efficacy of a broad-spectrum sunscreen in the treatment of melasma. *Cutis* 1983;**32**:92–6.

20. Neering H. Treatment of melasma (cholasma) by local application of a steroid cream. *Dermatologica* 1975;**151**:349–53.

21. Griffiths CE, Finkel LJ, Ditre CM, Hamilton TA, Ellis CN, Voorhees JJ. Topical tretinoin (retinoic acid) improves melasma. A vehicle-controlled, clinical trial. *Br J Dermatol* 1993;**129**:415–21.

22. Krimbrough-Green CK, Griffiths CEM, Finkel LJ *et al.* Topical retinoic acid (tretinoin) for melasma in black patients. *Arch Dermatol* 1994;**130**:727–33.

23. Lowe NJ, Rizk D, Grimes P, Billips M, Pincus S. Azealic acid 20% cream in the treatment of facial hyperpigmentation in darker-skinned patients. *Clin Ther* 1998;**20**:945–59.

24. Sivayathorn A, Verallo RV, Graupe K. 20% azelaic acid cream in the topical treatment of melasma: A double-blind comparison with 2% hydroquinone. *Eur J Dermatol* 1995;**5**:680–4.

25. Piquero-Martin J, Rothe de Arocha J, Beniamini Loker D. Estudio clínico doble ciego en el tratamiento del melasma entre ácido azelaico versus hidroquinona. *Med Cut I LA* 1988;**16**:511–14.

26. Ennes SBP, Paschoalick RC, Mota M. A double blind, comparative, placebo-controlled study of the efficacy and tolerability of 4% hydroquinone as a depigmenting agent in melasma. *J Dermatol Treat* 2000;**11**:173–9.

27. Lim JT, Tham SN. Glycolic acid peels in the treatment of melasma among Asian women. *Dermatol Surg* 1997;**23**:177–9.

28. Lawrence N, Cox SE, Brody HJ. Treatment of melasma with Jessner's solution versus glycolic acid: a comparison of clinical efficacy and evaluation of the predictive ability

of Wood's light examination. *J Am Acad Dermatol* 1997;**36**:589–93.

29. Kakita LS, Lowe NJ. Azelaic acid and glycolic acid combination therapy for facial hyperpigmentation in darker-skinned patients: A clinical comparison with hydroquinone. *Clin Ther* 1998;**20**:960–70.

30. Lim JT. Treatment of melasma using kojic acid in a gel containing hydroquinone and glycolic acid. *Dermatol Surg* 1999;**25**:282–4.

31. Poli F, Lakhdar H, Souissi R, Fiquet E, Chanez JF. Clinical evaluation of a depigmenting cream: Trio-D (R) in melasma of the face. *Nouv Dermatol* 1997;**16**:193–7.

32. Garcia A, Fulton JE Jr. The combination of glycolic acid and hydroquinone or kojic acid for the treatment of melasma and related conditions. *Dermatol Surg* 1996;**22**:443–7.

33. Pathak MA. Treatment of melasma with hydroquinone. *J Invest Dermatol* 1981;**76**:324.

34. Nouri K, Bowes L, Chartier T, Romagosa R, Spencer J. Combination treatment of melasma with pulsed CO_2 laser followed by Q-switched alexandrite laser:a pilot study. *Dermatol Surg* 1999;**25**:494–7.

35. Hayakawa R, Ueda H, Nozaki T *et al*. Effects of combination treatment with vitamins E and C on cholasma and pigmented contact dermatitis. A double blind controlled clinical trial. *Acta Vitaminol Enzymol* 1981;**3**:31–8.

Part 3: The evidence

Section F: Hair problems

Editor: Berthold Rzany

42
Male and female androgenetic alopecia

Hans Wolff

Background
Definition

The term androgenetic alopecia (AGA) describes a genetically determined condition leading to permanent loss of hair in men and women with normal levels of androgens. Synonyms are male and female pattern hair loss. Most men with AGA show a typical pattern of hair loss, often beginning at the temples and in the vertex area.[1-3] In contrast, most women with AGA have a diffuse thinning in the midline of the scalp.[4,5] In many, but not all, men and women the hair loss is accompanied by increased shedding of telogen hair, which is a reflection of shortened anagen growth phases.

Prevalence

AGA affects approximately 30% of men under 30 years of age, 50% under 50 years of age, and 70% under 70 years of age.[6] In women, the incidence before menopause is 5–10%, rising to 20–30% after the menopause.[7]

Aetiology

Microscopically, AGA is characterised by progressive shrinking of scalp hair follicles.[8] In many patients, AGA is accompanied by an acceleration of the hair growth cycle, as reflected by decrease of anagen and increase of telogen hair in the trichogram. However, some patients have a normal anagen/telogen ratio despite slowly progressive AGA. Whether and when a scalp hair follicle miniaturises is dependent on two factors: genetics and androgens. The genes responsible for shrinkage of a scalp hair follicle are not known. Each scalp hair follicle carries individual genetic information that determines whether and when it will develop a sensitivity towards androgens. Once a scalp hair follicle has become sensitive to androgens, it will progressively shrink over the next years. In men, the most important androgen driving AGA is dihydrotestosterone (DHT). Within the cells of the hair follicle, DHT is derived from its precursor testosterone by two enzymes: the 5-α-reductase types I and II.[9] DHT seems to be less important in women than in men.[10] In general, androgens can be considered potentially harmful and oestrogens potentially beneficial for scalp hair growth in women.

Prognosis

Without treatment, AGA progresses until all hair follicles that have developed a genetically determined sensitivity towards androgens are miniaturised. The extent of AGA depends on the number of hair follicles with genetic sensitivity to androgens. In its maximal expression, all hairs can be lost from the top of the scalp. In both men and women, occipital hair follicles never develop sensitivity to androgens; they are never lost in AGA.

Aims of treatment

Treatment of AGA has two major goals. First, it is important to reliably stop further hair loss. The term hair loss does not describe telogen effluvium but stands for permanent visible thinning of scalp hair density by miniaturisation of hair follicles. Second, some men and women benefit so strongly from treatment that they can regrow hair to a certain extent – their hair density can be increased by re-enlargement of individual hair follicles.

Relevant outcomes

- Stopping further hair loss: in a clinical study setting, this has to be documented after intervals of at least 1 year by microscopic methods such as hair counts or increase of hair weight in a representative area of hair loss.
- Increase of visible hair density: this has to be documented by standardised scalp hair photography.[11]

The change of anagen/telogen ratio does not reliably assess the efficacy of a treatment against further progression of AGA because not all men and women with AGA have abnormal anagen/telogen ratios. In addition, some patients with long-standing telogen effluvium never develop AGA.[12] Therefore, the trichogram cannot reliably measure the efficacy of a treatment against AGA.

Methods of literature search

In the PubMed database different search terms were used for male and female androgenetic alopecia. For male androgenetic alopecia the search terms were: "((androgenetic and alopecia) or (*male and pattern and baldness)) and (finasteride or minoxidil)." For female androgenetic alopecia the search terms were "((female and androgenetic and alopecia) or (female and pattern and baldness)) and (minoxidil or antiandrogen* or cyproteroneacetate or (cyproterone and acetate) or cyproteronacetate or estrogen* or oestrogen* or estradiol)."

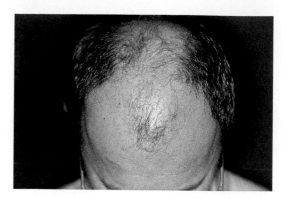

Figure 42.1 Typical male pattern hair loss in a 28-year-old patient

QUESTIONS

Which topical or systemic treatment can stop further hair loss and increase hair density in men?

Case scenario 1

The patient is a 28-year-old German computer specialist with a 3-year history of gradual hair loss starting at the temples and now also involving the top of the scalp (Figure 42.1).

Topical minoxidil for men with AGA
Efficacy

We found no systematic review. Several randomised controlled trials (RCTs) show that minoxidil 2% or 5% solution applied twice daily can increase test area hair counts and hair weights in men with AGA.[13–17]

Drawbacks

In approximately 5% of men, minoxidil causes redness and itching of the scalp skin. In most men this effect seems to be non-specific irritation by polyethylene glycol or other solvents; in some, however, specific type IV allergy against minoxidil is possible. Patients sometimes attribute specific systemic effects such as hypotension or increase of heart rate to minoxidil, but this is implausible because serum concentrations of minoxidil are very low after twice-daily topical administration.

Comment

Minoxidil 5% solution applied twice daily is a safe and effective topical treatment for AGA in men. There are no conclusive data on how often minoxidil solution can reliably stop hair loss and increase visible regrowth of hair in men. One of the possible mechanisms is improvement of the microcirculation in the dermal papilla.[18,19]

Implications for clinical practice

Minoxidil 5% solution can stop hair loss in many men, but hair loss resumes when the applications are stopped. There are no systemic side-effects.

Systemic finasteride for men with AGA
Efficacy

We found no systematic review. The 2-year results of the largest RCT were published by Kaufman et al.[20] The international multicentre clinical trial of more than 1500 patients demonstrated a significant increase of hair counts in the finasteride treatment group after 1 year (+ 86 hairs per 5.1 cm^2 test area versus –21 hairs in the placebo group). In the second year, there was stabilisation of the increased hair count in the finasteride group. Men on placebo had a progressive loss of hair count in the vertex test area. Men who were switched from finasteride to placebo after 1 year lost the hair gained under finasteride. Therefore, as with other medical treatments for AGA, finasteride needs to be taken permanently to show therapeutic benefit. Visible hair density was also documented by a standardised camera device.[11] After 1 and 2 years the before and after pictures were judged by an expert panel of dermatologists who were blinded to the treatment modality. After 1 year, 48% of men in the finasteride treatment group had visibly increased hair density in the vertex area, compared with 7% in the placebo group. After 2 years of treatment, 66% of the men in the finasteride group had visibly increased hair density, compared with only 7% in the placebo group.[20]

Other RCTs have demonstrated that finasteride significantly improves the anagen/telogen ratio[21] and has also positive effects on the frontal hair line.[22] On the basis of recently published 5-year data,[23] hair loss can be stopped in 90% of men taking finasteride, compared with 25% in the placebo group. In addition to stoppage of hair loss, an increase in hair density was seen in 48% of the men in the finasteride group, compared with 6% of men in the placebo group after 5 years of the study.

Drawbacks

There were no side-effects on liver, kidney or any other internal organ.[20] Serum hormones were unaffected, with the exception of a desired 70% decline in DHT and a compensatory 10% increase in testosterone. Sexual side-effects were reported in both the finasteride and the placebo group: decrease of libido 1.9% versus 1.3%; decrease of potency 1.4% versus 0.9%; decrease of ejaculate volume 1.0% versus 0.4%. Although the differences between the finasteride and placebo groups were small and statistically not significant,[20] finasteride must be considered capable of causing such effects in some men. A separate study found sperm function parameters to be unaltered by finasteride 1 mg.[24]

Comment

Finasteride 1 mg is a safe and effective drug for the treatment of AGA in men. Finasteride inhibits the enzyme 5-α-reductase type II, thereby preventing the intracellular conversion of testosterone to its more active metabolite DHT.[25] In men, DHT is essential for the development of AGA, and finasteride decreases DHT by 70%, both in the scalp skin and in serum.[26]

Implications for practice

Finasteride 1 mg can stop hair loss (for at least 5 years) in 90% of men treated while it is being taken. Systemic side-effects such as reduction of libido and potency are infrequent (1–2%) and often transient.

> Which topical or systemic treatment can stop further hair loss and increase hair density in women?

Case scenario 2

The patient is a 35-year-old teacher with a 5-year history of gradual hair loss starting at the midline of her scalp (Figure 42.2). Her mother also had thin hair; her father was bald.

Topical minoxidil for women with AGA
Efficacy

We found no systematic review. Several RCTs demonstrate that minoxidil 2% solution applied twice daily can increase test area hair counts and hair weights in women with AGA.[16,27,28] Most trials were done for at least 1 year. When effective, minoxidil solution increased visible hair density within 6 months. After 6 months, no further increase should be expected. A large American multicentre study involved 308 women with AGA; 256 women completed the trial. In the minoxidil group, there was an increase of 23 non-vellus hairs in a 1 cm^2 test area, compared with 11 hairs in the placebo group. By investigator assessment, no woman in the study had "dense" regrowth of hair; 13% of the minoxidil treated women had "moderate" regrowth of hair and 50% had "minimal" regrowth of hair, compared with 6% and 33% respectively, in the placebo group.[27]

Drawbacks

Minoxidil causes redness and itching of the scalp skin in approximately 5% of women. In most women this effect seems to be non-specific irritation by polyethylene glycol or other solvents; in some, however, specific type IV allergy against minoxidil is possible. Patients sometimes attribute specific systemic effects such as hypotension or increase of heart rate to minoxidil, but the very low serum concentrations of minoxidil after twice-daily topical administration make this implausible.

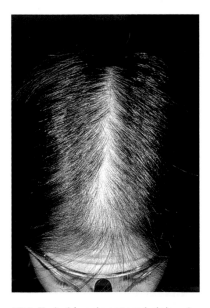

Figure 42.2 Typical female pattern hair loss in a 35-year-old patient.

Comment

Minoxidil 2% solution applied twice daily is a safe and effective topical treatment for AGA in some women while it is used. Minoxidil solution can reliably stop hair loss and increase obviously visible regrowth of hair in 10–20% of women.

Implications for clinical practice

Currently, minoxidil 2% solution is the only effective way to treat AGA in women. There are no systemic side-effects.

Systemic oestrogens and/or antiandrogens for women with AGA
Efficacy

Because oestrogens have many antiandrogenic actions, it is thought that they might have a positive influence on hair growth. Antiandrogens such as cyproterone acetate and chlormadinone acetate directly block the androgen receptor. However, most women with AGA have normal oestrogen and androgen levels.[29] Therefore, positive effects of oestrogens and/or antiandrogens on hair growth are questionable. There are no systematic reviews. Recently, one RCT compared the efficacies of the antiandrogen cyproterone acetate, 52 mg daily on days 1–20 of the cycle with twice-daily 2% minoxidil application in 66 women with AGA Ludwig I (67%), II (31%) and III (2%). The study duration was 1 year and each treatment group consisted of 33 women. The main outcome was number of strong hair (>40 micrometer in diameter) in a test area as detected by the phototrichogram. After 1 year, hair counts in the 0.32 cm^2 test area were -2.4 ± 6.2 in the cyproterone acetate group and $+6.5 \pm 9.0$ hairs in the minoxidil group.[30] Thus, 2% minoxidil was significantly more effective than cyproterone acetate.

Drawbacks

Systemic 17-beta-oestrogens are thought to slightly increase the risk of breast cancer and, particularly in women with coagulation disorders, deep venous thrombosis.

Comment

In theory, women using oestrogens and/or antiandrogens might benefit from treatment. However, as yet there is no convincing evidence that oestrogens and/or antiandrogens can stop or delay AGA.

Implications for practice

There are no convincing data showing efficacy of systemic oestrogens or antiandrogens in women with AGA. Therefore, we are reluctant to treat women with AGA with systemic hormones that increase the risk of deep venous thrombosis and fatal embolism.

Key points

Men with AGA

- Topical minoxidil 2% or 5% solution applied twice daily to the scalp is effective for many men with AGA, but hair loss resumes when the applications cease. The RCTs reported are too small to establish percentages for successful stoppage of hair loss and frequency of visible regrowth of hair.
- Large RCTs show that systemic therapy with finasteride 1 mg per day can stop further hair loss in 90% and increase visible hair density in 48% of treated men. However, hair loss resumes when treatment is stopped.

Women with AGA

- Topical minoxidil 2% solution applied twice daily to the scalp is moderately effective for some women with AGA.
- One RCT using modern methods of hair growth evaluation showed that the systemic antiandrogen cyproterone acetate is less effective than 2% minoxidil solution.

References

1. Norwood OT. Male pattern baldness classification and incidence. *South Med J* 1975;**68**:1359–65.
2. Sinclair R. Male pattern androgenetic alopecia. *BMJ* 1998;**317**:865–9.

3. Whiting DA. Male pattern hair loss: current understanding. *Int J Dermatol* 1998;**37**:561–6.

4. Ludwig E. Classification of the types of androgenetic alopecia (common baldness) occurring in the female sex. *Br J Dermatol* 1977;**97**:247–54.

5. Olsen EA. Female pattern hair loss. *J Am Acad Dermatol* 2001;**45**:S70–80.

6. Hamilton JB. Patterned loss of hair in man: types and incidence. *Ann NY Acad Sci* 1951;**53**:708–28.

7. Birch MP, Messenger JF, Messenger AG. Hair density, hair diameter and the prevalence of female pattern hair loss. *Br J Dermatol* 2001;**144**:297–304.

8. Paus R, Cotsarelis G. The biology of hair follicles. *N Engl J Med* 1999;**341**:491–7.

9. Bayne EK, Flanagan J, Einstein M *et al.* Immunohistochemical localization of type 1 and 2 5alpha-reductase in human scalp. *Br J Dermatol* 1999;**141**:481–91.

10. Sawaya ME, Price VH. Different levels of 5alpha-reductase type I and II, aromatase, and androgen receptor in hair follicles of women and men with androgenetic alopecia. *J Invest Dermatol* 1997;**109**:296–300.

11. Canfield D. Photographic documentation of hair growth in androgenetic alopecia. *Dermatol Clin* 1996;**14**:713–21.

12. Whiting DA. Chronic telogen effluvium: increased scalp hair shedding in middle-aged women. *J Am Acad Dermatol* 1996;**35**:899–906.

13. Katz HI, Hien NT, Prawer SE, Goldman SJ. Long-term efficacy of topical minoxidil in male pattern baldness. *J Am Acad Dermatol* 1987;**16**:711–18.

14. De Groot A, Nater JP, Herxheimer A. Minoxidil: hope for the bald? *Lancet* 1987;**329**:1019–22.

15. Rushton DH, Unger WP, Cotteril PC *et al.* Quantitative assessment of 2% topical minoxidil in the treatment of male pattern baldness. *Clin Exp Dermatol* 1989;**14**:40–6.

16. Savin RC, Atton AV. Minoxidil. Update on its clinical role. *Dermatol Clin* 1993;**11**:55–64.

17. Price VH, Menefee E, Strauss PC. Changes in hair weight and hair count in men with androgenetic alopecia, after application of 5% and 2% topical minoxidil, placebo, or no treatment. *J Am Acad Dermatol* 1999;**41**:717–21.

18. Lachgar S, Charveron M, Gall Y, Bonafe JL. Minoxidil upregulates the expression of vascular endothelial growth factor in human hair dermal papilla cells. *Br J Dermatol* 1998;**138**:407–11.

19. Yano K, Brown LF, Detmar M. Control of hair growth and follicle size by VEGF-mediated angiogenesis. *J Clin Invest* 2001;**107**:409–17.

20. Kaufman KD, Olsen EA, Whiting D *et al.* Finasteride in the treatment of men with androgenetic alopecia (male pattern hair loss). *J Am Acad Dermatol* 1998;**36**:578–89.

21. Van Neste D, Fuh V, Sanchez-Pedreno P *et al.* Finasteride increases anagen hair in men with androgenetic alopecia. *Br J Dermatol* 2000;**143**:804–10.

22. Leyden J, Dunlap F, Miller B *et al.* Finasteride in the treatment of men with frontal male pattern hair loss. *J Am Acad Dermatol* 1999;**40**:930–7.

23. The Finasteride Male Pattern Hair Loss Study Group. Long-term (5–year) multinational experience with finasteride 1 mg in the treatment of men with androgenetic alopecia. *Eur J Dermatol* 2002;**12**:38–49.

24. Overstreet JW, Fuh VL, Gould J *et al.* Chronic treatment with finasteride daily does not affect spermatogenesis or semen production in young men. *J Urol* 1999;**162**:1295–300.

25. Rittmaster RS. Finasteride. *N Engl J Med* 1994;**330**:120–5.

26. Drake L, Hordinsky M, Fiedler V *et al.* The effects of finasteride on scalp skin and serum androgen levels in men with androgenetic alopecia. *J Am Acad Dermatol* 1999;**41**:550–4.

27. DeVillez RL, Jacobs JP, Szpunar CA, Warner ML. Androgenetic alopecia in the female. Treatment with 2% topical minoxidil solution. *Arch Dermatol* 1994;**130**:303–7.

28. Olsen EA. Topical minoxidil in the treatment of androgenetic alopecia in women. *Cutis* 1991;**48**:243–8.

29. Orme S, Cullen DR, Messenger AG. Diffuse female hair loss: are androgens necessary? *Br J Dermatol* 1999;**141**:521–3.

30. Vexiau P, Chaspoux C, Boudou P *et al.* Effects of minoxidil 2% *v.* cyproterone acetate treatment on female androgenetic alopecia: a controlled, 12-month randomized trial. *Br J Dermatol* 2002;**146**:992–9.

43

Alopecia areata

Rod Sinclair and Catherine E Scarff

Background
Definition
Alopecia areata is an autoimmune, non-scarring disorder of hair growth affecting genetically predisposed individuals. It is characterised by circular bald areas that contain pathognomonic exclamation-mark hairs and which occur on any hair-bearing area of the body.[1] Severe disease may produce total loss of scalp hair (alopecia totalis) or universal loss of body hair (alopecia universalis).

Incidence/prevalence
The true incidence and prevalence of alopecia areata is unknown. It is estimated that 1·7% of the population will experience an episode of alopecia areata during their lifetime.[2] Alopecia areata accounts for 2% of new dermatological outpatient department attendances in the UK and US.[3] While alopecia areata can develop at any age, 30–40% of cases appear before 21 years of age and 20–30% after 40 years of age.[4] The condition occurs in equal incidence in both sexes. The percentage of patients with alopecia areata that go on to develop alopecia totalis/universalis is not known, but estimates range from 7% to 30%.[5]

Aetiology
Alopecia areata is an organ-specific autoimmune disease with genetic predisposition and environmental trigger.[6] The rate of concordance among monozygotic twins is about 55% and overall approximately 20% of patients have a positive family history.[5] A large number of potential environmental triggers have been evaluated, including emotional stress, pregnancy and intercurrent infections. However, no definite associations have been identified.[7]

Prognosis
Regrowth from an initial patch occurs within 6 months in 33% of cases, and within 1 year in 50%; however, 33% never recover from the initial episode.[8] Almost every patient will develop further patches if followed for long enough.[4]

Adverse prognostic factors include age less than 10 years at time of first episode, ophiasis pattern or total alopecia, poor response to previous treatment and the presence of associated atopy, nail dystrophy or Down's syndrome.[9] The duration of alopecia areata prior to treatment is also thought to be an independent prognostic factor.[10]

Diagnostic tests
The diagnosis of alopecia areata is a clinical one. Rarely a biopsy is required to exclude other forms of hair loss. The hallmarks of an active lesion are a dense lymphocytic infiltrate around the anagen hair bulbs and uniform miniaturisation of terminal hairs into vellus-like hairs.[11] Telogen hairs are not inflamed and there are decreased numbers of terminal anagen hairs.

Aims of treatment
The aim of treatment is to improve the patient's quality of life either by achieving cosmetically acceptable hair regrowth, or by encouraging the

patient to live with their hair loss. Unfortunately, the environmental events that trigger episodes of alopecia areata are unknown, and so relapse can be neither predicted nor prevented. Treatment is often unsatisfactory and is centred around the provision of emotional support to distressed patients and their families.

Methods of search

- Clinical evidence search and appraisal (May 2001)
- Supplementary search of Medline from 1966 to 2002
- Other references obtained from reference lists in all identified review articles and relevant sections of textbooks of dermatology

QUESTIONS

What are the effects of treatment for patchy alopecia areata?

Case scenario 1

Sarah is 22 years old and has two patches of alopecia areata over the frontal and parietal scalp that have been present for 8 months (Figure 43.1). At the age of 10 she developed alopecia totalis that regrew spontaneously after 9 months. At the age of 14 she developed a solitary patch of alopecia areata that regrew after two intralesional injections of triamcinolone acetonide 6 weeks apart.

She has a past history of atopy, her mother has idiopathic hypothyroidism, and a great aunt had become totally bald after receiving a telegram notifying her of her husband's death in the second world war. Sarah's only recent stress was breaking up with her boyfriend of 4 years, however, that occurred after the hair loss had begun.

On this occasion, three intralesional injections of triamcinolone acetonide 6 weeks apart had led

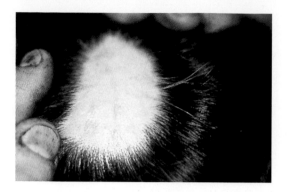

Figure 43.1   Patchy alopecia areata

to dermal atrophy, but no regrowth. A trial of 1% dithranol for 12 weeks had produced skin pigmentation, but no regrowth.

She was sensitised to 2% diphencyprone, applied in a Finn chamber to the scalp. Two weeks later 0·0001% diphencyprone in acetone was applied to one patch. Diphencyprone was reapplied each week, with the concentration adjusted to produce itch, erythema and scale (without vesiculation) that lasted 24–48 hours. After 8 weeks she was using 0·1% diphencyprone. She had occipital lymphadenopathy. Hair was regrowing in the treated patch, but not the control patch. Treatment was extended to include the control patch. After 24 weeks both patches had completely regrown and she remained in remission at the post-treatment follow up visit 6 months later.

Intralesional corticosteroids
Benefits

We found no systematic reviews. One randomised controlled trial (RCT) and one observational comparison study confirm that intradermal injections of triamcinolone acetonide, 5 mg/ml by a needle-less injector, produced rapid regrowth of hair in a high proportion of subjects with limited disease, within 4–6 weeks.

Versus placebo

In a report of 84 patients using normal-saline controls, 86% of patients treated with triamcinolone responded, compared with only 7% of control patients.[12] Injections of triamcinolone acetonide, 0·1 ml of 5 mg/ml, were given at weekly or two-weekly intervals on three occasions. The number of injections was determined by the size of the area of alopecia, with each injection producing a tuft of hair approximately 0·5 cm². Ninety-two per cent of patients with localised disease showed regrowth at 6 weeks, compared with 61% of those with alopecia totalis. This decreased to 71% at 12 weeks for alopecia areata and 28% for patients with alopecia totalis.

Versus each other

In an observational study comparing triamcinolone acetonide and triamcinolone hexacetonide involving 34 areas of alopecia in 11 patients, 64% of the sites injected with triamcinolone acetonide and 97% of the sites injected with triamcinolone hexacetonide regrew.[13]

Harms

Haemorrhage can occur at the puncture site but can easily be controlled with pressure.[12] No case of persistent atrophy of skin was seen. Plasma cortisol level was measured in one patient and showed significant suppression, raising the possibility of a systemic effect.[12]

Comment/implications for clinical practice

Despite the lack of RCTs, intradermal injection of triamcinolone acetonide in concentrations ranging from 2·5 to 10 mg/ml by either needle or a needle-less injector is the most widely used first-line treatment for patch alopecia areata. Rapid hair regrowth is achieved in a high proportion of subjects within 4–6 weeks. Dermal atrophy is common, but usually self-limiting.

Topical immunotherapy

Three agents have been used for topical immunotherapy: dinitrochlorobenzene, diphencyprone and squaric acid dibutyl ester (SADBE). All are applied topically at weekly intervals following initial sensitisation.

Benefits

We found one systematic review of published case series on the use of topical immunotherapy with diphencyprone, which concluded that 50–60% of patients achieve a worthwhile response. Patients with limited disease have higher response rates than patients with alopecia totalis/universalis.[14]

Versus placebo

We found no RCTs. In the largest series reported to date of diphencyprone in the treatment of alopecia areata, 148 consecutive patients were evaluated for unilateral regrowth following unilateral treatment.[15] At 32 months, cosmetically significant regrowth was obtained in 17·4% of those with alopecia totalis/universalis, in 60·3% of those with 75–99% hair loss, in 88·1% of those with 50–74% hair loss and in 100% of those with 25–49% hair loss. The only other independent predictor of treatment response was age of onset of alopecia areata, with older age of onset portending a better prognosis.[16] Relapse after achievement of cosmetically significant regrowth occurred in 62.6% after 37 months' follow up and was not prevented by maintenance therapy.[16]

Versus each other

A controlled trial compared SADBE, diphencyprone, minoxidil and placebo in patients with patchy alopecia areata involving less than 40% of the scalp.[17] The study involved 119 patients and was continued for at least 6 months. No significant differences were found between the different therapies used and placebo.

Harms

Dinitrochlorobenzene is mutagenic on the Ames test.[18] A moderately severe allergic contact dermatitis is necessary for success of the therapy,[19] which if severe may necessitate temporary suspension of treatment. Tender regional lymphadenopathy is common, but usually mild and self-limiting. Generalised dermatitis is uncommon but may necessitate permanent cessation. Contact urticaria, vitiligo and erythema multiforme have been reported.[20] Dinitrophenol, a metabolite of dinitrochlorobenzene, has been reported to cause hepatic and renal changes, convulsive seizures and hyperthermia.[21]

Comment/implications for clinical practice

Diphencyprone is not licensed in the USA. Immunotherapy for alopecia areata is only available in specialist treatment centres. We found no RCTs on the use of topical immunotherapy; however, a number of studies have demonstrated unilateral hair regrowth after unilateral treatment. This protocol conforms to the published investigational guidelines for alopecia areata.[14] In almost all case series, patients with limited disease have higher response rates than patients with alopecia totalis/universalis. In contrast to other studies, Shapiro et al.[22] found that a long duration of disease did not necessarily preclude a positive response to treatment with diphencyprone. Tosti et al. concluded from their work that transferring non-responder patients with alopecia totalis or universalis to other therapies is generally useless.[23]

Topical corticosteroids
Benefits

Topical steroids have been used widely, but there is only one well conducted RCT with adequate patient numbers to support their use. In the RCT, which involved 70 patients using 0·2% desoximetasone for 12 weeks, there was a trend to more regrowth in the treatment group, but the complete regrowth rates were higher in the placebo group.[24] In an observational study 0·2% fluocinolone acetonide was used under night-time occlusion. Of the 47 patients, of whom only 28 were evaluable, 17 (61%) achieved a satisfactory clinical response after 6 months.[25]

Harms

Side-effects of topical therapy include folliculitis, hypertrichosis, acneiform eruption and the potential for long-lasting local atrophy and telangiectasia.[25]

Comment

Topical corticosteroids are unlikely to be beneficial, except possibly in young children who have relatively thin skin. When used, the treatment should be used continuously for a minimum of 3 months.

PUVA

Photochemotherapy involves oral ingestion of psoralen capsules before exposure to UVA radiation. Treatment is performed three times a week, the dose of UVA being increased gradually.

Benefits

We found no systematic reviews or RCTs. A retrospective audit of 10 years of experience with PUVA showed an effective success rate of 6·3% for disease less severe than the totalis state.[26]

Harms

Potential risks include sunburn, irritation, accelerated photodamage and future development of lentigo, non-melanoma skin cancer and melanoma.[26]

Implications for clinical practice

PUVA is likely to be beneficial for only a small number of people. The time commitment involved in attending three times a week for up to 6 months, and the potential to induce skin cancer, make this therapy unattractive to most patients. PUVA is contraindicated in children because of the possible increase in risk of future development of melanoma.

Anthralin (dithranol)

Anthralin (dithranol) therapy is thought to act as a contact irritant and possibly also as an immunomodulator. Case series suggest that it needs to be applied on a daily basis in a sufficiently high concentration to produce skin irritation.

Benefits

We found no systematic reviews or RCTs. An uncontrolled, unblinded case series involving 68 patients with extensive alopecia areata suggested that up to 25% of patients with patchy alopecia areata may achieve regrowth, compared with 14% with hair loss >75%. New hair growth was generally seen within 3 months if the treatment was effective, although it may take more than double this time to achieve a cosmetically acceptable response.[27]

Harms

Side-effects include irritation, scaling, folliculitis and regional lymphadenopathy. Patients need to protect treated areas from sun exposure. Reversible staining of the skin occurs, and contact with the eyes must be avoided.[20]

Comment/implications for clinical practice

Anthralin is less effective than contact immunotherapy, but readily available and simple to prescribe.

Topical minoxidil
Benefits

We have found no systematic reviews.

Versus placebo

We have found 10 RCTs comparing various concentrations of topical minoxidil with placebo. Early reports suggested a significantly increased frequency of regrowth in patchy but not total alopecia areata,[28–34] although subsequent RCTs failed to confirm these results.[35,36]

Versus betamethasone

This incompletely reported study suggested that there was a higher response rate to 5% minoxidil than to 0·005% betamethasone dipropionate. Both were said to be superior to placebo but strict numbers and statistical analysis were not reported.[37]

Harms

Systemic side-effects are rare with topical minoxidil, and are generally only seen when it is combined with penetration enhancers. Irritant contact dermatitis is seen in fewer than 10%. Allergic contact dermatitis reaction is rare.[28]

Comment

Minoxidil is unlikely to be beneficial. It is a non-specific hair-growth stimulant with an unknown mechanism of action. Any effect it may have in alopecia areata is not immunologically based.

Cryosurgery
Benefits

We found no systematic reviews and no RCTs. We found a single partially controlled case series of 112 patients with patchy alopecia areata covering <25% of the scalp. Seventy-two patients with a total of 237 lesions received a 2–3-second application of a cotton swab dipped in liquid nitrogen.[38] Two freeze–thaw cycles were applied once weekly for 4 weeks. New hair growth was seen in over 60% of the involved area in over 97% of patients treated with liquid nitrogen, which was statistically significant compared with the results of the non-treatment group.

Harms

Side-effects include skin irritation, vesiculation and blistering. Temporary hyperpigmentation and permanent hypopigmentation can also occur.

Comment/implications for clinical practice

Cryosurgery is unlikely to be useful. It is not suitable for people with darkly pigmented skin.

Aromatherapy
Benefits

We found one RCT. The use of aromatherapy was compared with carrier oils alone in a randomised double-blind controlled trial over 7 months.[39] Treatment with the essential oils cedarwood, lavender, thyme and rosemary oils massaged into the scalp every night was seen to be significantly more effective than treatment with carrier oil alone, with an improvement rate of 44%. While the patients were randomised, treatment groups were small and disease severity was not specified. This result awaits confirmation.

Harms

None were found.

Comment/implications for clinical practice

Aromatherapy is unlikely to be successful.

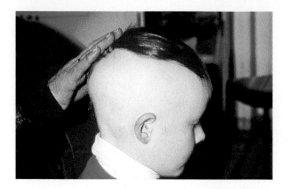

Figure 43.2   Alopecia areata in an oophiasis pattern

> What are the management options for severe chronic alopecia areata (including alopecia totalis and universalis)?

Case scenario 2

Michael is 15 years old. At the age of 13 he developed a solitary patch of alopecia areata. Two weeks after intradermal injection of triamcinolone, 5 mg/ml, he developed diffuse generalised hair shedding and within 10 days was totally bald (Figure 43.2). Three months later he began to lose his eyebrows, eyelashes and ultimately every hair on his body was lost. Unable to cope with the teasing at school, he had not attended for the previous 8 weeks. A general assumption by his teachers was that he was away from school receiving chemotherapy.

A reducing course of oral prednisolone (starting dose 0·75 mg/kg) led to complete regrowth within 6 weeks. The prednisolone was ceased after 8 weeks. He remained in remission for 4 months, changed schools and performed well at his work, before a new patch appeared. He refused intralesional corticosteroids, as he related the progression to totalis on the previous occasion to the injection. Topical immunotherapy was commenced with diphencyprone. Within 12 weeks the patch regrew and the therapy was ceased. Eight months later, following a mild upper respiratory tract infection, he relapsed and within 3 weeks had progressed to alopecia totalis/universalis once again. A second course of prednisolone failed to stimulate any regrowth. Topical immunotherapy over 6 months failed to initiate regrowth. Michael bought a wig, but found it uncomfortable to wear due to the heat in summer. In sympathy a friend at school shaved his head. Michael wore glasses with ordinary glass to disguise the loss of eyebrows and protect his eyes from dust etc. He elected to have intralesional corticosteroids into the eyebrows, which produced patch regrowth, around which he pencilled in his eyebrows. No other treatment was sought.

Topical immunotherapy
Benefits
We found one systematic review, no RCTs, but numerous case series.[21,22,40,41] Response rates for patients with severe disease vary from 2% to 50%.

Harms
These are identical to those listed for topical immunotherapy for patchy alopecia areata.

Comment/implications for clinical practice
In all the case series reported, patients with severe alopecia areata and in particular alopecia totalis/universalis responded less frequently to topical immunotherapy. While the response rates are lower when patients have severe alopecia areata, these patients are often highly motivated and prepared to trial the therapy regardless. A minimum trial of 6 months is required. Initial therapy to half the head and only treating the opposite half after demonstrable regrowth is advocated.

Systemic corticosteroids
Oral prednisolone or dexamethasone or intravenous methylprednisolone will stimulate hair regrowth in most but not all patients if used in high enough dosage. It has been suggested that the initial dose threshold for oral prednisolone is 0.8 mg/kg, which is then decreased slowly over 6–8 weeks.

Benefits
We found no systematic reviews or RCTs. Numerous case series have been reported but these are not directly comparable because of different patient selection, dose scheduling and duration of therapy. Winter et al.[42] treated 18 patients with prednisolone on alternate days at doses adjusted according to the clinical response (usually 2–4 times the daily adrenal replacement dose, and up to 80–120 mg on alternate days in unresponsive patients). A progressively increasing dose of prednisolone was required to maintain cosmetically acceptable hair growth and most patients experienced a rapid hair loss after discontinuation of prednisolone therapy.[42] Oral steroids used in combination with topical and intralesional steroids have shown benefit in non-randomised trials.[43] The use of topical and intralesional steroids allowed for more rapid lowering of oral doses and thus minimisation of side-effects. Seven of 15 patients treated with oral steroids showed regrowth of most or all of their hair, with an average remission of 32 months.[43] Pulse therapy was used in 32 patients with widespread alopecia areata.[44] Doses of 300 mg prednisolone at 4-week intervals for a minimum of four doses were given to 27 patients. Least success was noted in women and patients with alopecia areata for more than 2 years. Complete or cosmetically acceptable hair regrowth was seen in 14 patients, with response evident on average after 2.4 months and cosmetically acceptable at 4 months. Of eight patients who received pulses of 1000 mg, three had cosmetically acceptable hair growth at 6–9 months.[44]

Harms

Weight gain with cushingoid facies are the main side-effects.[43] Prolonged therapy with oral corticosteroids may retard growth, demineralise bones, and lead to premature fusion of the bony epiphyses. Nausea and polymenorrhoea can occur with pulsed steroid therapy.[44]

Comment/implications for clinical practice

Most patients offered systemic corticosteroids decline to take them because of the potential systemic side-effects and the high relapse rate. Some patients do regrow hair and have sustained remissions following a brief course of systemic corticosteroids, however they are in the minority. Well over 50% of those who regrow hair with systemic corticosteroids relapse on dose reduction or within a few months of ceasing therapy. Long-term high-dose systemic corticosteroids are not recommended for alopecia areata.

Ciclosporin
Benefits

We found no systematic reviews or RCTs for oral ciclosporin. In a small case series, six patients received oral ciclosporin, 6 mg/kg/day for 12 weeks.[45] All patients had some regrowth, however cosmetically acceptable regrowth occurred in only two of five patients with alopecia totalis/universalis and in the single patient with patchy alopecia areata. All patients had relapsed within 3 months of stopping therapy. A randomised study of 26 patients with alopecia totalis or universalis compared topical 10% ciclosporin daily with photochemotherapy three times a week and intravenous thymopentin, 50 mg three times a week every 3 months over 9 months.[23] All patients had previously been unresponsive to sensitising therapy for at least 12 months. None of the patients in the study had any cosmetic clinical improvement by the end of the study.

Harms

In the case series of six patients receiving oral ciclosporin the side-effects were mild and transient.[45] Davies et al. reported on two patients who had first developed alopecia areata while taking ciclosporin.[46] While the precise mechanism is unknown, alopecia areata can occur in patients who are least partially immunosuppressed.

Comment/implications for clinical practice

The effectivness of oral ciclosporin for alopecia areata is unknown. A dose of 6 mg/kg/day is a high dose of ciclosporin and would require very careful monitoring for renal and other toxicity. The relapse rates on discontinuation of therapy are high, and there is a reluctance to use long-term therapy because of cost and cumulative side-effects. Topical ciclosporin is ineffective.

Other therapies
Benefits

Inosine pranobex at a dose of 50 mg/kg/day for 6 months was ineffective in one series[47] and slightly helpful in another.[48]

The combination of SADBE immunotherapy at weekly intervals and interferon alfa $3\cdot0 \times 10^{-6}$ IU intramuscularly, daily for 15 days, three times a week for 2 weeks, then once a week for 2 months) seemed to be better than SADBE alone.[49]

Harms

Flu-like symptoms were observed in patients receiving interferon alfa.[49] No clinically significant side-effects attributable to inosine pranobex were reported.[48]

Comment/implications for clinical practice

The low response rate in alopecia totalis should be explained to patients before commencing experimental treatments.

What are the treatment options for alopecia areata in children?

Case scenario 3

Anthony developed 20-nail dystrophy at the age of 30 months. Six months later he developed a single patch of alopecia areata. Nightly topical application of 0·05% clobetasol dipropionate cream to the patch led to regrowth within 6 weeks, with no obvious cutaneous atrophy. There was some mild associated hypertrichosis of the forehead, which resolved within 6 months of stopping the cream.

Anthony had no family history of alopecia areata, and no history of atopy. Three years later, he re-presented with four patches of alopecia areata, each about 3 cm in diameter. In the intervening time his father had developed alopecia areata of the beard area. Six months of topical corticosteroids therapy failed to stimulate regrowth, but cutaneous atrophy occurred and the treatment was stopped. Topical anthralin therapy was tried for a further 6 months with no result. Topical minoxidil was then tried for 6 months, during which time the alopecia progressed to approximately 50% scalp involvement. The suggestion of intralesional corticosteroids was met with panic and tears, and it was obvious he would need to be physically restrained if this was going to be used. Topical immunotherapy with diphencyprone was tried for 6 months. During this time he progressed to alopecia totalis.

All therapy was ceased. Anthony got a wig. Two years later all the hair spontaneously regrew and he then remained in remission for the following 3 years before being lost to follow up.

Topical corticosteroids

Topical corticosteroids are discussed under the section on patchy alopecia areata.

Benefits

In an observational study of 48 patients, children aged 3–10 years had a higher response rate to topical corticosteroids than did adults.[25]

Topical immunotherapy
Benefits

We found no systematic reviews. We found one RCT that involved small numbers of children. Tosti et al.[17] compared SADBE, diphencyprone, minoxidil and placebo, finding a significant relationship between the age of the patients and the results. Complete hair regrowth was seen in 71·3% of adults, but only 38·9% of children.

We found two case series. Schuttelaar et al.[50] treated 26 children with diphencyprone weekly for a period of 3–12 months. Sixteen subjects had alopecia areata totalis, the others having patchy disease only. Eighty-four per cent of children showed hair regrowth, 32% of the total being cosmetically acceptable. Where treatment failed (0–5% hair growth), it was recommended not to continue treatment for longer than 1 year as hair growth is not promoted by continued treatment. Orecchia et al.[51] treated 28 unresponsive children under the age of 13 years with SADBE for 12 months. Thirty-two per cent of patients achieved complete or cosmetically acceptable regrowth and a further 21% achieved significant regrowth.

Harms

Schuttelaar et al. noted the problem of psychological dependence on the diphencyprone in certain children and parents, who asked to continue treatment after regrowth had been achieved, fearing a relapse.[50] As with previous studies, itching, erythema and scaling were noted side-effects. Swelling of regional lymph nodes was common and disappeared after discontinuation of treatment.[51]

Comment/implications for clinical practice

Topical immunotherapy has been used in children as young as 4 years by a number of investigators. Taking into consideration that the development of alopecia areata before the age of 10 years is an independent adverse prognostic indicator, side-effects and efficacy seem to be similar to those seen in adults. Efficacy is also influenced by extent of disease, associated nail changes and atopy.

Topical minoxidil

Topical minoxidil has not been trialed in children. Systemic absorption and systemic side-effects may be more likely to occur in children.

Key points

Patchy alopecia areata

- The spontaneous remission rate in alopecia areata is high, which makes evaluation of treatment in the absence of RCTs very difficult.
- No treatment alters the natural history of alopecia areata.
- We found no good evidence in support of non-drug treatment.
- Small RCTs have shown that intralesional injection of triamcinolone acetonide can effectively stimulate regrowth of patchy alopecia areata. Transient atrophy is common. Treatment can be repeated at 4–6 weekly intervals if necessary. We were not able to find data on long-term efficacy.
- One RCT demonstrated that potent topical corticosteroids are marginally more effective than placebo in patchy alopecia areata when used continuously for a minimum of 3 months. In observational case series, children between the ages of 3 and 10 years appear most likely to respond.
- We found one systematic review but no RCTs on the use of topical immunotherapy. A number of studies have demonstrated unilateral hair regrowth after unilateral treatment. This protocol has been favoured for evaluation of topical immunotherapy because of the inability to blind patients. The systematic review of published case series on the use of topical immunotherapy with diphencyprone concluded that 50–60% of patients achieve a worthwhile response. Patients with limited disease have higher response rates than those with alopecia totalis/universalis.
- We found insufficient evidence on the use of topical minoxidil, topical anthralin therapy, PUVA, aromatherapy, cryosurgery and ciclosporin A.

Alopecia totalis/universalis

- The prognosis for spontaneous or assisted regrowth is poor.
- In all RCTs, extent of disease is an adverse prognostic factor for regrowth.

Childhood alopecia areata

- In most RCTs an early age of onset is an adverse prognostic factor for regrowth.
- Topical corticosteroids therapy may be more effective in children than in adults.
- Intralesional injection of corticosteroids is unsuitable for use in children. Most children will not tolerate repeated injections, limiting the usefulness of intralesional corticosteroids.
- Prolonged therapy with oral corticosteroids may retard growth, demineralise bones, and lead to premature fusion of the bony epiphyses.
- PUVA is contraindicated in children because of the possible increase in risk of future development of melanoma.

References

1. Safavi K, Muller SA, Suman VJ, Moshell AN, Melton LJ. Incidence of alopecia areata in Olmsted County, Minnesota, 1975 through 1989. *Mayo Clin Proc* 1995;**70**:628–33.

2. Olsen EA. Hair disorders. In: Freedberg IM, Eisen AZ, Wolff K *et al.*, eds. *Fitzpatrick's Dermatology in General Medicine*, 5th ed. Vol 1. New York: McGraw-Hill. 1999:737–9.

3. Dawber RPR, de Berker D, Wojnarowska F. Disorders of hair. In: Champion RH, Burton JL, Burns DA, Breathnach SM, eds. *Textbook of Dermatology*, 6th ed. Vol 4. Oxford: Blackwell Science 1998:2919–27.

4. Messenger AG, Simpson NB. Alopecia areata. In: Dawber RPR, ed. *Diseases of the Hair and Scalp*. Oxford: Blackwell Science 1997:338–69.

5. Muller SA, Winkelmann RK. Alopecia areata. *Arch Dermatol* 1963;**88**:290–7.

6. Green J, Sinclair R. Genetics of alopecia areata. *Aus J Dermatol* 2000;**41**:213–18.

7. McDonagh AJG, Messenger AG. Alopecia areata. *Clin Dermatol* 2001;**19**:141–7.

8. Walker SA, Rothman S. Alopecia areata. a statistical study and consideration of endocrine influences. *J Invest Dermatol* 1950;**14**:403–13.

9. Sinclair RD, Banfield CC, Dawber RPR. *Handbook of Diseases of the Hair and Scalp*. Oxford: Blackwell Science 1999:75–84.

10. van der Steen PHM, van Baar HMJ, Happle R, Boezeman JBM, Perret CM. Prognostic factors in the treatment of alopecia areata with diphenylcyclopropenone. *J Am Acad Dermatol* 1991;**24**:227–30.

11. Weedon D. Diseases of cutaneous appendages. In: *Skin Pathology*. Edinburgh: Churchill Livingstone 1997:381–424.

12. Abell E, Munro DD. Intralesional treatment of alopecia areata with triamcinolone acetonide by jet injector. *Br J Dermatol* 1973;**88**:55–9.

13. Porter D, Burton J. A comparison of intralesional triamcinolone hexacetomide and triamcinolone acetonide in alopecia areata. *Br J Dermatol* 1971;**85**:272–3.

14. Olsen E, Hordinsky M, McDonald-Hull S *et al.* Alopecia areata investigational assessment guidelines. National Alopecia Areata Foundation. *J Am Acad Dermatol* 1999;**40**:242–6.

15. Rokshar CK, Shupack JL, Vafai JJ, Washenik K. Efficacy of topical sensitizers in the treatment of alopecia areata. *J Am Acad Dermatol* 1998;**39**:751–61.

16. Wiseman MC, Shapiro J, MacDonald N, Lui H. Predictive model for immunotherapy of alopecia areata with diphencyprone. *Arch Dermatol* 2001;**37**:1063–8.

17. Tosti A, De Padova MP, Minghetti G, Veronesi S. Therapies versus placebo in the treatment of patchy alopecia areata. *J Am Acad Dermatol* 1986;**15**:209–10.

18. Swanson NA, Mitchell AJ, Leahy MS, Headington JT, Diaz LA. Topical treatment of alopecia areata. *Arch Dermatol* 1981;**117**:384–7.

19. Daman LA, Rosenberg EW, Drake L. Treatment of alopecia areata with dinitrochlorobenzene. *Arch Dermatol* 1978;**114**:1036–8.

20. Madani S, Shapiro J. Alopecia areata update. *J Am Acad Dermatol* 2000;**42**:549–66.

21. de Prost Y, Paquez F, Touraine R. Dinitrochlorobenzene treatment of alopecia areata. *Arch Dermatol* 1982;**118**:542–5.

22. Shapiro J, Tan J, Ho V, Abbott F, Tron V. Treatment of chronic severe alopecia areata with topical diphenylcyclopropenone and 5% minoxidil: a clinical and immunopathological evaluation. *J Am Acad Dermatol* 1993;**29**.729–35.

23. Tosti A, Bardazzi F, Guerra L. Alopecia totalis: Is treating non-responder patients useful? *J Am Acad Dermatol* 1991;**24**:455–6.

24. Charuwichitratana S, Wattanakrai P, Tanrattanakorn S. Randomized double-blind placebo-controlled trial in the treatment of alopecia areata with 0·25% desoximetasone cream. *Arch Dermatol* 2000;**136**:1276–7.

25. Pascher F, Kurtin S, Andrade R. Assay of 0·2% fluocinolone acetonide cream for alopecia areata and totalis. *Dermatologica* 1970;**141**:193–202.

26. Taylor CR, Hawk JLM. PUVA treatment of alopecia areata partialis, totalis and universalis: audit of 10 years' experience at St John's Institute of Dermatology. *Br J Dermatol* 1995;**133**:914–18.

27. Feidler-Weiss VC, Buys CM. Evaluation of anthralin therapy in the treatment of alopecia areata. *Arch Dermatol* 1987;**123**:1491–3.

28. Feidler-Weiss VC, West DP, Fu TS *et al.* Alopecia areata treated with topical minoxidil. *Arch Dermatol* 1984;**120**: 457–63.

29. Vanderveen EE, Ellis CN, Kang S *et al.* Topical minoxidil for hair regrowth. *J Am Acad Dermatol* 1984;**11**:416–21.

30. Frentz G. Topical minoxidil for extended areata alopecia. *Acta Derm Venereol* 1985;**65**:172–5.

31. Shi Y-P. Topical minoxidil in the treatment of alopecia areata and male-pattern alopecia. *Arch Dermatol* 1986;**122**:506.

32. Fiedler-Weiss VC. Topical minoxidil solution (1% and 5%) in the treatment of alopecia areata. *J Am Acad Dermatol* 1987;**16**:745–8.

33. Fiedler-Weiss VC, West DP, Buys CM, Rumsfield JA. Topical minoxidil dose-response effect in alopecia areata. *Arch Dermatol* 1986;**122**:180–2.

34. Price V. Double-blind, placebo-controlled evaluation of topical minoxidil in extensive alopecia areata. *J Am Acad Dermatol* 1987;**16**:730–6.

35. White SI, Friedmann PS. Topical minoxidil lacks efficacy in alopecia areata. *Arch Dermatol* 1985;**121**:591.

36. Vestey JP, Savin JA. A trial of 1% minoxidil used topically for severe alopecia areata. *Acta Derm Venereol* 1986;**66**:179–80.

37. Feidler VC. Alopecia areata: Current therapy. *J Invest Dermatol* 1991;**96**(Suppl.):69.

38. Lei Y, Nie Y-F, Zhang J-M, Liao D-Y, Li H-Y. Effect of superficial hypothermic cryotherapy with liquid nitrogen on alopecia areata. *Arch Dermatol* 1991;**127**:1851–2.

39. Hay I, Jamieson M, Ormerod A. Randomized trial of aromatherapy. *Arch Dermatol* 1998;**134**:1349–52.

40. Happle R, Hausen BM, Wiesner-Menzel L. Diphencyprone in the treatment of alopecia areata. *Acta Derm Venereol* 1983;**63**:49–52.

41. van der Steen PHM, van Baar HMJ, Perret CM, Happle R. Treatment of alopecia areata with diphenylcyclopropenone. *J Am Acad Dermatol* 1991;**24**:253–7.

42. Winter RJ, Kern F, Blizzard RM. Prednisolone therapy for alopecia areata. *Arch Dermatol* 1976;**112**:1549–52.

43. Unger WP, Schemmer RJ. Corticosteroids in the treatment of alopecia totalis. *Arch Dermatol* 1978;**114**:1486–90.

44. Sharma VK. Pulsed administration of corticosteroids in the treatment of alopecia areata. *Int J Dermatol* 1996;**35**:133–6.

45. Gupta AK, Ellis CN, Cooper KD *et al.* Oral cyclosporin for the treatment of alopecia areata. *J Am Acad Dermatol* 1990;**22**:242–50.

46. Davies MG, Bowers PW. Alopecia areata arising in patients receiving cyclosporine immunosuppression. *Br J Dermatol* 1995;**132**:827–9.

47. Berth-Jones J, Hutchinson PE. Treatment of alopecia totalis with a combination of inosine pranobex and diphencyprone compared to each treatment alone. *Clin Exp Dermatol* 1991;**16**:172–5.

48. Galbraith GMP, Thiers BH, Jensen J, Hoehler F. A randomised double-blind study of inosiplex (Isoprinosine) therapy in patients with alopecia totalis. *J Am Acad Dermatol* 1987;**16**:977–83.

49. Pipoli M, D'Argento V, Coviello C, Dell'Osso A, Mastrolonardo M, Vena GA. Evaluation of topical immunotherapy with squaric acid dibutylester, systemic interferon alpha and the combination of both in the treatment of chronic severe alopecia areata. *J Dermatol Treat* 1995;**6**:95–8.

50. Schuttelaar M-LA, Hamstra JJ, Plinck EPB *et al.* Alopecia areata in children: treatment with diphencyprone. *Br J Dermatol* 1996;**135**:581–5.

51. Orecchia G, Malagoli P. Topical immunotherapy in children with alopecia areata. *J Invest Dermatol* 1995;**104**(Suppl.):35S–36S.

Part 3: The evidence

Section G: Leg ulceration

Editor: Berthold Rzany

44
Venous ulcers

Jonathan Kantor and David J Margolis

Background
Definition

Venous ulcers are wounds that usually occur in a gaiter distribution of the lower leg (Figure 44.1). They are associated with increased pressure in the superficial venous system of the lower legs during ambulation, and are possibly related to failure of the calf muscle pump to return venous flow effectively.[1]

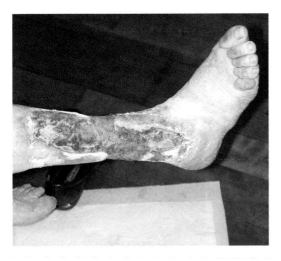

Figure 44.1   Venous ulcer of the lower extremity (case scenario 1)

Incidence/prevalence

A recent study utilising the General Practice Research Database found the incidence of venous ulcers in people over 65 years of age in the UK to be 0·76 (95% confidence interval (CI) 0·71–0·83) per 100 person-years for men and 1·42 (1·35–1·48) for women.[1] Venous ulcers therefore represent a major public health problem.

Aetiology

Venous ulcers result from poor venous return. It is hypothesised that the calf muscle pump fails to return blood flow effectively. These wounds may also be associated with varicose veins and other venous disease. In addition, arterial disease and diabetes may also complicate the clinical picture of venous leg ulceration.[2]

Prognosis

Many venous ulcers heal within 24 weeks of care, but the proportion healed after 24 weeks varies widely between studies. There are multiple risk factors for venous ulcers failing to heal, including the age of the wound, the size of the wound, a history of vein surgery, and arterial insufficiency.[2] There is also a significant risk of recurrence in patients who have had a single venous ulcer in the past.[3]

Aims of treatment

The aims of treatment are to improve the rate of healing and to increase the likelihood that a patient will heal over a given period of time.

Relevant outcomes

Relevant outcomes include the proportion of wounds healed by the end of the study and the rate of healing.

Methods of search

Medline and the Cochrane Database of Systematic Reviews were searched for the terms "venous ulcer" and "heal" or "treat". Current issues of *Clinical Evidence* were reviewed for relevant additions,[3] and bibliographies of relevant articles and systematic reviews were also reviewed.

QUESTIONS

What therapies are effective for curing venous leg ulcers?

Case scenario 1

A 56-year-old woman has a 25 × 6 cm ulcer on the medial side of the left ankle (Figure 44.1). The ulcer's red base is covered with yellowish fibrinous debris. On the edges are some signs of re-epithelialisation. The left lower leg was oedematous before use of a limb compression stocking. The limb shows signs of chronic venous insufficiency – pigmentation, enlargement of the cutaneous veins and fibrosis. What therapies would be effective for curing a venous leg ulcer?

Compression
Benefits

Compression of the lower extremities is one of the oldest and most widely used treatments for venous ulcers. Methods of compression vary and include stockings, multilayer bandages, high-pressure compression boots, and an Unna boot.

A Cochrane collaborative review has evaluated the role of compression in the treatment of venous ulcers.[4] This review included 22 trials using a number of different compression methods. Six trials compared compression with no compression, and demonstrated a clear benefit of compression over no compression. Of these, three trials evaluated compression using an Unna boot versus no compression. Two of the three studies demonstrated a benefit of compression.[5,6] Three additional studies compared compression bandages with

non-compressive bandages and demonstrated a benefit of compression bandages. Of note, the results of only four of these six trials were statistically significant, although the preponderance of evidence suggests that compression results in a greater chance of healing than no compression.

Three trials compared elastic high-compression bandages with inelastic low-compression bandages.[7] Pooled results from these studies evaluated in the Cochrane review suggest that the relative risk of healing with elastic high-compression bandages over inelastic low-compression bandages was 1·54 (CI 1·19–2·00).

Four trials compared multilayer high-compression bandages with single-layer (low) compression.[8] A pooled analysis of these studies demonstrated a relative risk of healing of 1·41 (CI 1·11–1·80) when using multilayer compression bandages rather than single-layer bandages.

Four trials compared multilayer high-compression bandages with inelastic high-compression bandages (Unna boot and short-stretch bandages). No statistically significant differences were shown between these types of high-compression therapy. Similarly, studies comparing other types of high-compression therapy, including the four-layer Charing Cross bandage system, did not show statistically significant differences between the different types of high-compression therapies.

Complications

Complication rates are not usually noted in trials, partly because compression therapy is generally benign. Inexpertly applied high compression could lead to soft tissue damage, the development of additional wounds, and potentially amputation, although the chance of this occurring is remote.

Comment

Compression has been the mainstay of therapy for venous ulcers, and with good reason. Compression has been shown to have a clear benefit over no compression. Moreover, the evidence suggests that a high level of compression (>25 mmHg) lends a clear benefit over low-level compression. Therefore, treatment with minimally compressive bandages, while better than nothing, is less than ideal. Depending on location and the skill of the provider, different types of high-compression bandage (Unna boot, multilayer elastomeric compression) can be used effectively. The method used to apply these bandages is important, and there is some suggestion that the ability to apply compression bandages effectively varies widely among nurses. Compression therapy should not be used in patients with an impeded blood supply to the lower extremities, whether from diabetes or arterial disease. Infection, however, has not been shown to be a contraindication to compression.

Implications for clinical practice

Compression should represent the cornerstone of the clinical management of patients with venous ulcers. Most studies evaluating novel therapies for venous ulcers use compression as the standard care regimen. Those caring for patients with venous ulcers should be sure that they use sufficient compression, namely more than 25 mmHg of compression to the lower leg. This can be accomplished either with multilayer bandages or an Unna boot, depending on the preference and training of the provider.

Pentoxifylline
Benefits

Pentoxifylline is a trisubstituted xanthine derivative that has been used to treat a variety of systemic disorders, most notably intermittent claudication.[9] Theoretically, its beneficial effects in vaso-occlusive disease could extend to therapy for venous ulcers, and so several studies have explored the potential benefits of pentoxifylline in treating patients with venous leg ulcers.

A Cochrane collaborative review has addressed the efficacy of pentoxifylline for the treatment of venous ulcers.[10] Nine trials including 572 patients were included in the Cochrane review. Of note, only five of the trials included compression therapy in both the pentoxifylline and placebo groups. One of the included trials compared pentoxifylline with defibrotide rather than placebo, and was therefore excluded from the meta-analysis used to evaluate the potential benefit of pentoxifylline.

Combining the data from the eight trials that compared pentoxifylline (in varying doses) with placebo, pentoxifylline demonstrated a beneficial effect. The relative risk of healing with pentoxifylline versus placebo was 1·41 (CI 1·19–1·66). A separate examination of just the trials that compared pentoxifylline plus compression with placebo plus compression also showed a benefit of pentoxifylline therapy with a relative risk of 1·30 (CI 1·10–1·54). Most of the studies used the probability of healing by 24 weeks as the endpoint.

Complications

Pentoxifylline therapy is associated with an increased risk of side-effects, mostly gastrointestinal in nature. This increase in adverse events was not, however, statistically significant (relative risk 1·25; CI 0·87–1·80).

Comment

Given the pooled results of these clinical trials, it appears that pentoxifylline is beneficial as an adjuvant treatment for venous ulcers. Of note, some of the studies included in the meta-analysis conducted by the Cochrane group did not individually show statistical significance. Moreover, the dose of pentoxifylline used in the studies varied, and there is a legitimate question regarding the optimal dosing for the treatment of patients with venous ulcers. For example, in the study by Falanga et al., the dose of pentoxifylline used was greater than that used to treat intermittent claudication (800 mg versus 400 mg three times daily).[9]

In some of the studies included in the Cochrane meta-analysis patients did not necessarily receive compression as standard care. Even including these studies, however, pentoxifylline therapy was shown to be more beneficial than placebo, resulting in a higher proportion of patients healed by the study endpoint. However, it is important to note that this was a relative benefit, and that the relative benefit of pentoxifylline over placebo persisted even for patients treated with compression. Since compression therapy has been shown to increase the baseline chance of healing, patients treated with pentoxifylline should always be treated with compression therapy as well.

Implications for clinical practice

Pentoxifylline has been shown to increase the relative risk of healing by 30% over compression therapy alone, although this benefit may be as low as 10% or as high as 54%. Clinicians must ultimately decide whether this potential benefit is worth both the practical and the financial cost of pentoxifylline.

Skin grafting
Benefits

Most venous ulcers respond well to compression therapy. However, a minority of wounds fail to heal with compression therapy alone. One of the options available to the healthcare provider is to treat the wound with a skin graft. Grafts can include full-thickness, partial-thickness, allogeneic (cultured), and artificial skin grafts.

The use of skin grafts for the treatment of venous ulcers is the subject of a Cochrane collaborative review.[11] Two trials evaluated split-thickness autografts, three trials evaluated cultured keratinocyte allografts, one compared artificial skin with a dressing, and one compared artificial skin with a split-thickness skin graft.

The two small studies evaluating split-thickness autografts were pooled by the Cochrane group, but the results did not show a significant benefit of skin grafting.[11] Both studies were small, and used different placebo treatments.

Graftskin (Apligraf) is a bilayered skin equivalent that includes both dermal and epidermal components.[12] It is manufactured by harvesting neonatal foreskins and extracting both keratinocytes and fibroblasts, which are then separately cultured to create the epidermal and dermal components, respectively. Graftskin has been studied for the treatment of venous leg ulcers.[13,14] In a study that enrolled 240 patients, the percentage of ulcers healed after 24 weeks was significantly higher in those treated with Graftskin plus standard care (compression) than in those treated with compression alone (57% versus 40%).[15] Notably, secondary analyses evaluating the relative efficacy of Graftskin in wounds of more than one year's duration demonstrated that the benefit of Graftskin was most significant for patients with older wounds (47% versus 19%). Among patients with wounds of less than one year's duration, there was no statistically significant difference in the percentage healed after 24 weeks between those treated with Graftskin and those treated with placebo (66% versus 73%). The Cochrane group analysed this trial data and concluded that the relative risk of healing with artificial skin versus standard dressings is 1·29 (CI 1·04–1·60).

Three studies compared cultured keratinocyte allografts with standard dressings. A pooled analysis of these trials conducted by the Cochrane group did not demonstrate a significant benefit of allografts over control dressings, and the relative risk of healing with the keratinocyte allografts was 1·42 (CI 0·71–2·84). These were all small trials and may have been underpowered to demonstrate an effect.

A single study compared tissue-engineered skin with a split-thickness allograft, but failed to show any significant benefit of either treatment.[16] Note, however, that this study was small and was conducted before the newest tissue-engineered skin became available.

Complications

Risk of infection, bleeding and other tissue damage is inherent in any autologous skin grafting procedure. Moreover, there is always an inherent risk that the donor site will prove difficult to heal as well.

Using cultured autologous keratinocytes is likely to delay of treatment because it takes several weeks for the cells to be cultured. Moreover, patients need to undergo a skin biopsy in order to provide the laboratory with the necessary cells.[11]

Artificial skin theoretically could be cultured from samples that are infected with viruses, including HIV. Given the aggressive screening associated with this harvesting, however, the chance of infection is remote, although it does remain a possibility that the allogeneic human cells were taken from an HIV-positive but seronegative donor.[17]

Comment

While autologous skin grafts are occasionally used in some centres to aid the closure of recalcitrant wounds, the difficulties associated with harvesting the donor graft, as well as the complexities associated with inducing closure of

the grafted site (in addition to the donor site), mean that this procedure cannot be undertaken lightly. Similarly, use of autologous cultured keratinocytes is a time-consuming, expensive and complex process that demands multiple patient visits and a laboratory capable of culturing the autologous keratinocytes.

Artificial skin for the treatment of venous ulcers is not in widespread use. This may because of the substantial cost involved. This concern has been addressed in an economics study.[18]

Implications for clinical practice

While most clinicians would not treat all venous ulcers with skin grafts, patients who have wounds recalcitrant to compression therapy could be considered for skin grafts as an adjunct to improve their likelihood of healing. Of the available skin grafting methods, the use of artificial skin appears to be the most promising, conferring a 29% increase in the likelihood of healing by 24 weeks and an increased rate of healing. These results are based on a randomised controlled trial in patients with recalcitrant venous ulcers.[17] However, the significant costs associated with this therapy, as well as the theoretical risk of viral infection and the existence of only a single trial supporting its use, means that clinicians need to think carefully before treating patients with artificial skin.

Vitamins and minerals
Benefits

Few practitioners dispute the importance of adequate nutrition for promoting wound healing. However, despite the assumption that vitamin and mineral supplements may aid in healing these wounds, few studies have addressed the potential benefits of supplementation in a rigorous fashion. Vitamin C supplements are often prescribed for patients with chronic wounds. Presumably, the well-known effects of excessive ascorbic acid deprivation, as seen in scurvy, include a susceptibility to non-healing wounds. Some reports have evaluated the use of vitamin C as an adjunctive wound-healing agent, with mixed results, and failed to demonstrate a clear benefit of vitamin C supplements in patients with chronic wounds of all types.[19,20]

Zinc has been used for more than a century as a topical adjunct for the care of chronic wounds.[21] Unna believed that the zinc paste in his boots had a beneficial effect on healing; however, it now appears more likely that the continued popularity of the Unna boot for patients with venous leg ulcers stems from its compressive effects on the lower leg in patients with venous ulcers.[22] Oral zinc for the treatment of venous ulcers has been addressed in a Cochrane collaborative review evaluating six trials of oral zinc therapy, most of which failed to show a beneficial effect of therapy.[23] Five of these studies included patients with venous ulcers. The doses of zinc varied across studies. A study by Greaves et al. failed to demonstrate a significant benefit of oral zinc therapy, with a relative risk of healing of 1·5 (CI 0·28–7·93).[24] The remaining studies also failed to show a benefit of zinc therapy.[23,25,26]

Topical zinc has also been evaluated as a treatment for venous ulcers. One study suggested that topical zinc oxide improves healing in both arterial and venous ulcers.[21] However, a study in porcine skin suggested that the only beneficial action of zinc on the wound bed was that it inhibited bacterial growth.[27]

Several studies have addressed the efficacy of rutinoids in decreasing the oedema associated with venous insufficiency.[28–33] Results appear to be promising, and these drugs may be useful in patients with venous ulcers, since these wounds generally cannot heal in the setting of persistent oedema. Moreover, reducing the oedema of venous insufficiency may reduce the likelihood of future wounds.

Complications
There are few side-effects associated with vitamin or mineral therapy for venous ulcers.

Comment
Despite a marked lack of supporting evidence, one of the tenets of good wound care, at least in the US, is supplementary vitamin C and zinc. This is largely a result of the relatively benign nature of these treatments, as well as their modest cost.

No studies have effectively evaluated the role of daily multivitamins in patients with chronic wounds. Another unexplored therapy is iron supplementation. An adequate tissue iron level is needed for appropriate metabolic functioning, and indeed mildly decreased iron levels may be associated with hair loss.[34] Since granulation tissue represents an environment of rapid cell proliferation, it is possible that wound healing may be sensitive to mildly decreased levels of iron, although this has yet to be demonstrated.

Implications for clinical practice
Given the prevalence of malnourishment among adults with chronic wounds, the low cost of vitamin C and zinc, and the low incidence of side-effects associated with supplementary water-soluble vitamins and minerals, it would certainly be reasonable to provide vitamin C and zinc supplements to patients. However, little evidence exists to support this practice, and clinicians should not feel compelled to provide patients with vitamins and minerals, particularly those who appear to be nutritionally replete.

Laser therapy
Benefits
Laser therapy, using a variety of different lasers, has been proposed as an adjunct therapy for venous leg ulcers. Low-level lasers have been shown to stimulate cellular function, leading to

increased protein synthesis and fibroblast and macrophage proliferation.

Laser therapy for venous ulcers is the subject of a Cochrane collaborative review which included four trials.[35] Two trials compared laser therapy with sham laser, and failed to detect a significant difference in healing between the groups.[36,37] The results of these studies were pooled in the Cochrane review and failed to demonstrate a significant benefit of laser therapy, with a relative risk of 1·21 (CI 0·73–2·03). One study compared three types of laser therapy and found that a combination of laser and infrared light resulted in significantly more wounds being healed than using non-coherent unpolarised red light alone, with a relative risk of healing of 2·4 (CI 1·12–5·13). The study endpoint was healing after 9 months. Another very small study comparing low-level laser therapy with ultraviolet light in six patients failed to show a significant difference between the groups.

Harms
Laser therapy, including low-level laser therapy, may be associated with adverse effects, including burns and retinal damage, although these complications occur very rarely when therapy is administered by well-trained and experienced staff.

Comment
The studies evaluating the potential effect of low-level laser therapy for the treatment of venous ulcers included a total of only 139 patients. Moreover, the types of laser, power and duration of follow up varied across the studies. Some of these studies used very short endpoints, and it is possible that potential benefits were missed because the studies failed to follow patients for long enough. Moreover, there is some suggestion that laser therapy may have an effect on endpoints other than chance of healing, for example pain at the wound site and the amount of granulation tissue,[38] although this remains an area in need of further investigation.

Implications for clinical practice
There is currently insufficient evidence to support the use of low-level laser therapy in treating venous ulcers. Only one study showed a benefit of laser therapy.

Intermittent pneumatic compression
Benefits
Intermittent pneumatic compression has been used for a number of indications, and is currently employed in the US as an adjunctive for the prophylaxis of nosocomial deep vein thrombosis. Since the underlying cause of venous ulceration is postulated to involve deficient blood return in the calf muscle pump, it has been suggested that intermittent pneumatic compression could improve the healing rates of venous ulcers by improving venous return.

Intermittent pneumatic compression for the treatment of venous ulcers has been the subject of a Cochrane collaborative review.[39] This review evaluated four randomised controlled trials of intermittent pneumatic compression for the treatment of venous ulcers. One trial of 45 patients compared intermittent pneumatic compression plus standard limb compression with standard limb compression alone, and found a significant benefit in the intermittent pneumatic compression plus standard compression group, with a relative risk of healing of 11·4 (CI 1·6–82). Two other small trials (including 75 people altogether) failed to find a significant benefit of intermittent pneumatic compression plus standard compression over standard compression alone. Notably, the duration of therapy with intermittent pneumatic compression in these trials varied considerably. Moreover, the study endpoints differed substantially, ranging from 3 to 6 months. Results of these trials were therefore not pooled by the Cochrane group. One small study compared intermittent pneumatic compression alone (i.e. without standard compression) with standard compression, and failed to show a significant difference between the groups. The *Clinical Evidence* group pooled the results of a study published after the systematic review with the results of the above studies but failed to demonstrate a significant benefit of intermittent pneumatic compression.[3,40]

Complications

There are few real complications with intermittent pneumatic compression – as long as the equipment is properly set up, patients would not be expected to suffer any injuries.

Comment

As with many of the so-called adjunctive therapies for venous ulcers, there is little literature on the effectiveness of intermittent pneumatic compression. It certainly seems that intermittent pneumatic compression may be beneficial as an adjunct to standard limb compression, but this has yet to be demonstrated conclusively. The largest study, of 45 patients, did demonstrate a benefit, but the standard compression used was graduated compression stockings, in contrast to the Unna boot used in another study that failed to show a significant difference in the proportion of ulcers healed after 6 months.[41] Of note, both studies demonstrated an increase in the actual rate of healing, suggesting that the different study endpoints (3 versus 6 months) may have played a role in the differing results.

It is therefore possible that intermittent pneumatic compression could be an effective adjunct to standard compression, but further study – ideally a large randomised controlled trial – is needed before this can be known conclusively. Moreover, it is important to explore whether intermittent pneumatic compression would result in a slightly more rapid healing of wounds already destined to heal within a several-month period, or whether it could potentially increase the likelihood of wounds healing that would otherwise fail to heal after months of therapy.

The size of the equipment means that the patient must remain in a single place for the duration of therapy. The equipment is also costly.

Implications for clinical practice

Intermittent pneumatic compression may increase the rate of wound healing for patients already treated with standard compression, but further study is needed for this to be demonstrated conclusively. Moreover, there is no suggestion that wounds that would fail to heal with standard compression alone are more likely to heal with intermittent pneumatic compression. Therefore, unless the equipment for intermittent pneumatic compression is already available, it is unlikely to be beneficial to begin this therapy in most patients with venous ulcers.

Therapeutic ultrasound
Benefits

Therapeutic ultrasound has been proposed as a potential adjunct for therapy of venous ulcers. A Cochrane collaborative review has evaluated the role of ultrasound in venous ulcers.[42] Seven studies were included in the review, none of which demonstrated a significant difference in healing rates, although some studies did show a trend towards a benefit of ultrasound. Because of study heterogeneity – including population, duration of follow up, and ultrasound therapy – the results were not pooled by the Cochrane group.

Complications

Studies did not usually assess adverse effects of ultrasound. Some mild local reactions may occur in patients treated with therapeutic ultrasound. Moreover, ultrasound does require repeated office (or home), which may affect the patient's quality of life.

Comment

There is little evidence to support the routine use of therapeutic ultrasound in patients with venous ulcers. As with other therapies, an important question – whether ultrasound would increase the chance of healing ulcers that would otherwise fail to heal – was not addressed by the studies. The trend towards a benefit of ultrasound in several of the studies is certainly promising, although further research is needed, particularly in patients who have wounds recalcitrant to standard compression therapy.

Implications for clinical practice

There is insufficient evidence to recommend that therapeutic ultrasound be adopted into clinical practice for the treatment of venous ulcers. Further well-designed trials are needed before this modality should be widely adopted.

What therapies are effective in reducing the risk of recurrence of venous leg ulcers?

Compression
Benefits

Compression therapy has been demonstrated to be an effective therapy for increasing the likelihood that a patient with venous ulcers will heal after 12 to 24 weeks. Since many venous ulcer patients have recurrent ulcers even after they have successfully healed, a pressing question remains as to whether continued compression after wound healing could reduce the likelihood of recurrent venous ulcer formation.

A Cochrane collaborative review has evaluated compression as a treatment for preventing the recurrence of venous ulcers.[43] This systematic review did not find any studies directly comparing the incidence of recurrent ulcers in patients who did and did not use compression. Two studies were included in the systematic review: one study compared medium- and high-compression stockings, and did not find a significant difference between recurrence rates in these two groups. The other study compared two different types of medium-compression stockings and did not find any significant differences between the two groups. The studies did in fact examine the differences in recurrence rates between patients who were and were not compliant with compression stockings, but this did demonstrate that patients who were non-compliant with compression were more likely to have recurrent ulcerations.[43]

Another study conducted after this systematic review also addressed this issue, and found that compression stockings reduced the risk of recurrence of venous ulceration.[3,44] This study of 153 people found that wearing compression stockings significantly reduced the risk of recurrence of venous ulcers at 6 months, with a relative risk reduction of 54% (CI 24–72%).

Complications

Complication rates are not usually noted in trials, partly because compression therapy is generally benign. Inexpertly applied high compression could lead to soft tissue damage, the development of additional wounds, and potentially amputation, although the chance of this occurring is remote.

Comment

One study has shown that compression reduces the risk of recurrent venous ulceration. Two studies that compared different types of compression found that non-compliant patients had a higher rate of recurrence than those who were compliant with any type of compression regimen. While these data may seem to suggest that ulcers may recur in patients who do not use compression, there are other confounding factors that need to be addressed before this conclusion can be drawn. For example, non-compliant patients may be more or less likely to have serious wounds or to comply with other elements of wound care, including nutrition and avoiding trauma.

The findings of the recent trial, coupled with the implications of the non-compliant patients' increased rate of recurrence from earlier trials and the biological plausibility of this therapy mean that compression is likely to reduce the risk of recurrence of venous leg ulcers. Finally, compression therapy to prevent recurrence is considered by most wound care experts to be "standard therapy". It might not be ethically justified to conduct a trial comparing limb compression with no limb compression for prevention of recurrent ulceration.

Implications for clinical practice

Compression appears to reduce the risk of recurrent venous ulceration, and should be recommended for all patients with a history of venous leg ulcers as long as they do not have any other conditions that would make this therapy potentially harmful (for example arterial disease).

Key points

- Limb compression is the mainstay of therapy for venous leg ulcers and several studies have shown that compression offers a clear benefit over no compression.
- Pentoxifylline as an adjuvant therapy to limb compression has been shown to increase the likelihood of healing.
- Skin equivalents as an adjuvant therapy to limb compression are associated with an increased likelihood of healing.

- The use of long-term limb compression therapy for those with a healed venous leg ulcer is associated with a decreased rate of recurrence, although poor compliance does compromise the effectiveness of this treatment.

References

1. Margolis DJ, Bilker W, Santanna J, Baumgarten M. Venous leg ulcer: Incidence and prevalence in the elderly. *J Am Acad Dermatol* 2002;**46**:381–6.

2. Margolis DJ, Berlin JA, Strom BL. Risk factors associated with the failure of a venous leg ulcer to heal. *Arch Dermatol* 1999;**135**:920–6.

3. Nelson EA, Cullum N, Jones J. Venous leg ulcers. *Clin Evid* 2001;**6**:1502–13.

4. Cullum N, Nelson EA, Fletcher AW, Sheldon TA. Compression for venous leg ulcers. In: Cochrane Collaboration. *Cochrane Library*. Issue 3. Oxford: Update Software, 2002.

5. Kikta MJ, Schuler JJ, Meyer JP et al. A prospective, randomized trial of Unna's boots versus hydroactive dressing in the treatment of venous stasis ulcers. *J Vasc Surg* 1988;**7**:478–83.

6. Rubin JR, Alexander J, Plecha EJ, Marman C. Unna's boot v polyurethane foam dressings for the treatment of venous ulceration. A randomized prospective study. *Arch Surg* 1990;**125**:489–90.

7. Gould DJ, Campbell S, Newton H, Duffelen P, Griffin M, Harding EF. Setopress v Elastocrepe in chronic venous ulceration. *Br J Nurs* 1998;**7**:66–73.

8. Nelson EA. Compression bandaging in the treatment of venous leg ulcers. *J Wound Care* 1996;**5**:415–18.

9. Margolis DJ. Pentoxifylline in the treatment of venous leg ulcers. *Arch Dermatol* 2000;**136**:1142–3.

10. Jull AB, Waters J, Arroll B. Oral pentoxifylline for treatment of venous leg ulcers. In: Cochrane Collaboration. *Cochrane Library*. Issue 3. Oxford: Update Software, 2002.

11. Jones JE, Nelson EA. Skin grafting for venous leg ulcers. In: Cochrane Collaboration. *Cochrane Library*. Issue 3. Oxford: Update Software, 2002.

12. Veves A, Falanga V, Armstrong DG, Sabolinski ML. Graftskin, a human skin equivalent, is effective in the

management of noninfected neuropathic diabetic foot ulcers: a prospective randomized multicenter clinical trial. *Diabetes Care* 2001;**24**:290–5.

13. Falanga V, Sabolinski M. A bilayered living skin construct (APLIGRAF) accelerates complete closure of hard-to-heal venous ulcers. *Wound Repair Regen* 1999;**7**:201–7.

14. Falanga V, Pearce W, Milstone L, Atillasoy ES. Graftskin in the treatment of venous leg ulcers: a prospective study. *Wound Repair Regen* 2001;**9**:147–51.

15. Dolynchuk K, Hull P, Guenther L et al. The role of Apligraf in the treatment of venous leg ulcers. *Ostomy Wound Manage* 1999;**45**:34–43.

16. Mol MA, Nanninga PB, van Eendenburg JP, Westerhof W, Mekkes JR, van Ginkel CJ. Grafting of venous leg ulcers. An intraindividual comparison between cultured skin equivalents and full-thickness skin punch grafts. *J Am Acad Dermatol* 1991;**24**:77–82.

17. Falanga V, Margolis D, Alvarez O, et al. Rapid healing of venous ulcers and lack of clinical rejection with an allogeneic cultured human skin equivalent. Human Skin Equivalent Investigators Group. *Arch Dermatol* 1998;**134**: 293–300.

18. Schonfeld WH, Villa KF, Fastenau JM, Mazonson PD, Falanga V. An economic assessment of Apligraf (Graftskin) for the treatment of hard-to-heal venous leg ulcers. *Wound Repair Regen* 2000;**8**:251–7.

19. Margolis DJ, Cohen JH. Management of chronic venous leg ulcers: a literature-guided approach. *Clin Dermatol* 1994;**12**:19–26.

20. Margolis DJ, Lewis VL. A literature assessment of the use of miscellaneous topical agents, growth factors, and skin equivalents for the treatment of pressure ulcers. *Dermatol Surg* 1995;**21**:145–8.

21. Brandrup F, Menne T, Agren MS, Stromberg HE, Holst R, Frisen M. A randomized trial of two occlusive dressings in the treatment of leg ulcers. *Acta Derm Venereol* 1990;**70**:231–5.

22. Margolis DJ, Berlin JA, Strom BL. Which venous leg ulcers will heal with limb compression bandages? *Am J Med* 2000;**109**:15–19.

23. Wilkinson EA, Hawke CI. Oral zinc for arterial and venous leg ulcers. In: Cochrane Collaboration. *Cochrane Library*. Issue 3. Oxford: Update Software, 2002.

24. Greaves MW, Ive FA. Serum-zinc and healing of venous leg ulcers. *Lancet* 1972;**2**:1261.

25. Phillips A, Davidson M, Greaves MW. Venous leg ulceration: evaluation of zinc treatment, serum zinc and rate of healing. *Clin Exp Dermatol* 1977;**2**:395–9.

26. Hallbook T, Lanner E. Serum-zinc and healing of venous leg ulcers. *Lancet* 1972;**2**:780–2.

27. Agren MS, Franzen L, Chvapil M. Effects on wound healing of zinc oxide in a hydrocolloid dressing. *J Am Acad Dermatol* 1993;**29**:221–7.

28. Clement DL. Management of venous edema: insights from an international task force. *Angiology* 2000;**51**: 13–17.

29. Pedersen FM, Hamberg O, Sorensen MD, Neland K. Effect of O-(beta-hydroxyethyl)-rutoside (Venoruton) on symptomatic venous insufficiency in the lower limbs. *Ugeskr Laeger* 1992;**154**:2561–3.

30. Nocker W, Diebschlag W, Lehmacher W. A 3-month, randomized double-blind dose-response study with O-(beta-hydroxyethyl)-rutoside oral solutions. *Vasa* 1989;**18**:235–8.

31. Nocker W, Diebschlag W. Dose-response study with O-(beta-hydroxyethyl)-rutoside oral solution. *Vasa* 1987; **16**:365–9.

32. Bergqvist D, Hallbook T, Lindblad B, Lindhagen A. A double-blind trial of O-(beta-hydroxyethyl)-rutoside in patients with chronic venous insufficiency. *Vasa* 1981;**10**:253–60.

33. van Cauwenberge H. Double-blind study of the efficacy of a soluble rutoside derivative in the treatment of venous disease. *Arch Int Pharmacodyn Ther* 1972;**196** (Suppl.): 8–13.

34. Van Neste DJ, Rushton DH. Hair problems in women. *Clin Dermatol* 1997;**15**:113–25.

35. Flemming K, Cullum N. Laser therapy for venous leg ulcers. In: Cochrane Collaboration. *Cochrane Library*. Issue 3. Oxford: Update Software, 2002.

36. Lundeberg T, Malm M. Low-power HeNe laser treatment of venous leg ulcers. *Ann Plast Surg* 1991;**27**: 537–9.

37. Malm M, Lundeberg T. Effect of low power gallium arsenide laser on healing of venous ulcers. *Scand J Plast Reconstr Surg Hand Surg* 1991;**25**:249–51.

38. Sugrue ME, Carolan J, Leen EJ, Feeley TM, Moore DJ, Shanik GD. The use of infrared laser therapy in the treatment of venous ulceration. *Ann Vasc Surg* 1990;**4**: 179–81.

39. Mani R, Vowden K, Nelson EA. Intermittent pneumatic compression for treating venous leg ulcers (Cochrane Review). In: Cochrane Collaboration. *Cochrane Library*. Issue 3. Oxford: Update Software, 2002.

40. Schuler JJ, Maibenco T, Megerman J. Treatment of chronic venous leg ulcers using sequential gradient intermittent pneumatic compression. *Phlebology* 1996;**11**:111–16.

41. McCulloch JM, Marler KC, Neal MB, Phifer TJ. Intermittent pneumatic compression improves venous ulcer healing. *Adv Wound Care* 1994;**7**:22–4, 26.

42. Flemming K, Cullum N. Therapeutic ultrasound for venous leg ulcers. In: Cochrane Collaboration. *Cochrane Library*. Issue 3. Oxford: Update Software, 2002.

43. Nelson EA, Bell-Syer SE, Cullum NA. Compression for preventing recurrence of venous ulcers. In: Cochrane Collaboration. *Cochrane Library*. Issue 3. Oxford: Update Software, 2002.

44. Vandongen YK, Stacey MC. Graduated compression elastic stockings reduce lipodermatosclerosis and ulcer recurrence. *Phlebology* 2000;**15**:33–7.

Part 3: The evidence

Section H: Less common skin disorders

Editor: Michael Bigby

45

Cutaneous lupus erythematosus

Susan Jessop and David Whitelaw

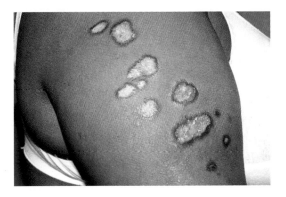

Figure 45.1 Lesions of discoid lupus erythematosus, showing scarring and changes in pigmentation

Background
Definition

Systemic lupus erythematosus (SLE) is a multisystem inflammatory disease characterised by the presence of a wide variety of autoantibodies. Skin involvement is common, being present in 55–90% of cases.[1] The characteristic skin lesions can be divided into acute, subacute and chronic subsets.[2] The acute forms include the malar (butterfly) rash, papular lesions, urticaria, vasculitic lesions, hair loss and painless mouth ulcers. Subacute cutaneous lupus erythematosus (SCLE) is an uncommon form of cutaneous lupus, described as a clinical subset by Sontheimer in 1979.[3] Chronic discoid lupus erythematosus (DLE) tends to be the most persistent of the skin lesions and may lead to unsightly scarring. It is most frequently seen as an isolated entity, but may also occur in people with the systemic form of lupus.

Lupus panniculitis (also known as lupus profundus), neonatal lupus, lupus tumidus and bullous lupus are less commonly encountered forms of the disease.

Incidence/prevalence

Accurate figures are difficult to obtain because different methods have been used in the reported studies. Reported prevalence rates vary from 12·5 per 100 000 in England to 50·8 per 100 000 in certain groups in the US.[4] Many series are hospital based and probably do not reflect the true incidence. African–American, Chinese and Malaysian women appear to be the populations with the highest prevalence. Published figures suggest an increasing incidence, but this may be because of greater awareness of the condition.

Aetiology

Lupus seems to result from an interaction between genetic, hormonal and environmental factors.[5] SLE is known to be associated with the production of a large range of autoantibodies. In certain specific subsets, such as neonatal lupus, their role in pathogenesis is now clearly established. The greatest risk factor is female sex (the female:male ratio is 9:1), and the highest prevalence is in the child-bearing age group. There is now evidence to suggest that oestrogens stimulate the immune system, which may be the reason for this observation. The genetic hypothesis is supported by the familial clustering of lupus[6] and the association of certain HLA types with particular subsets of lupus.[7]

Evidence for a viral aetiology has not been conclusive.[8]

Prognosis

Mortality is associated with severe systemic disease, and is highest with renal and central nervous system involvement.

Skin involvement, while not associated with mortality *per se*, frequently produces scarring, with considerable morbidity, both physical and psychological.

Diagnostic tests

Diagnosis of cutaneous lupus can generally be made by clinical examination, skin biopsy being used to confirm the diagnosis when the clinician is in doubt. Autoantibody tests (such as antinuclear antibody titre) may be positive in cutaneous lupus but do not necessarily imply systemic disease. Specific antibodies, notably antiRo antibody, are strongly associated with certain subsets, such as SCLE and neonatal lupus.

Aims of treatment

The aim of treatment is to stop the inflammatory process so that the lesion does not enlarge or cause further damage. The erythema (redness) and thickening should disappear but thinning of the skin, hair loss and increased or decreased pigmentation may persist.

Relevant outcomes

- Improvement in redness, thickness or scaling of lesions
- Change in extent of lesions
- Total clearing
- No change or worsening of skin lesions (redness, thickness or size)
- Development of new lesions
- Scarring may persist although no new lesions appear

Methods of search

We searched the *Cochrane Library* (2001), Medline (1966 to June 2001), Embase (1988 to 2001) and the Cochrane Central Register of Controlled Trials. We included all randomised controlled trials (RCTs) and controlled trials. Where no controlled trials were found, we report briefly on observational studies.

QUESTIONS

> What are the effects of antimalarial treatment in cutaneous lupus?

Chloroquine or hydroxychloroquine

Benefits

We found one systematic review.[9]

We found one RCT involving 39 people with DLE and 19 with SCLE, in which hydroxychloroquine, 400–1200 mg/day, was compared with acitretin, 50 mg/day, over 8 weeks.[10] The groups in the two treatment arms were equal for age, sex and extent of disease, but SCLE was more strongly represented in the chloroquine group. Complete clearing or marked improvement occurred approximately equally in the two groups (50% versus 46%). Four patients dropped out because of treatment side-effects (all in the acitretin arm) and three because of total clearing of lesions (all in the hydroxychloroquine arm).

We found three RCTs of chloroquine in non-life-threatening SLE. In the Canadian study, people taking hydroxychloroquine for SLE were randomised to continue the drug (n = 25) or to take placebo (n = 22).[11] At 6 months 16 of the 22 on placebo and 9 of 25 in the active arm had experienced disease flares, a 2·5-fold increase in flares in the untreated participants. Skin lesions were not specifically described. Williams compared hydroxychloroquine, 400 mg/day, with placebo in 71 people with mild SLE over 48 weeks.[12] Although the study was designed to determine the effect of the trial drug on joint disease, cutaneous, neurological and cardiopulmonary systems were also evaluated. Placebo and active groups both improved but overall there was no significant difference in the outcome of skin lesions between the two groups at any stage in the study. The third RCT involved 23 participants, 11 randomised to receive chloroquine, and 12 to receive placebo.[13] The chloroquine group showed less skin activity than the placebo group (9% compared with 42%; 95% confidence interval 9–74%). Overall, patients taking chloroquine experienced fewer flares and required lower doses of steroids. The nature of the skin lesions was not documented.

We found one double-blind but non-randomised trial comparing hydroxychloroquine with placebo in DLE.[14] Forty-nine people were treated for 1 year, 24 with hydroxychloroquine and 25 with placebo. Results at both 3 and 12 months indicated that hydroxychloroquine was superior to placebo.

We found many observational trials of chloroquine or hydroxychloroquine in cutaneous lupus.[15–21] Christiansen reviewed 13 case series up to 1956 and added his own, giving data on a total of 414 people treated in these studies. He noted that 265 (64%) experienced complete clearing or marked improvement. His series was notable for the duration of treatment (18–53 weeks) and the careful description of outcome, but was flawed by the absence of a parallel control group and the high dose of chloroquine (500–750 mg daily).

Harms

In the study of Ruzicka *et al.* adverse events were described in 17 of 30 patients taking hydroxychloroquine.[10] Symptoms included dry skin (n = 8), itching (n = 5) and gastrointestinal disturbance (n = 5). The most frequent side-effects described by Kraak *et al.* were gastrointestinal (eight in hydroxychloroquine arm versus three in placebo arm), and cutaneous (four in hydroxychloroquine arm versus three in placebo arm).[14] However, in addition they identified one person who developed a severe retinopathy while taking hydroxychloroquine. This person had taken chloroquine previously for several years and had taken a high dose of hydroxychloroquine (1200 mg) during the trial. A valuable discussion on retinal toxicity is presented by Houpt.[22] A review of the systemic toxicity of chloroquine found little to support regular blood monitoring.[23] A meta-analysis of toxicities places the toxicity of antimalarials in perspective.[24]

Comments

We found only two controlled trials, one of them randomised, on the use of antimalarials for DLE. The RCT was flawed by the short duration and by the inclusion of people with SCLE in unequal numbers in the two study groups. We found three RCTs of chloroquine in mild SLE, but little information about skin lesions was reported. The older observational studies lacked a parallel control group but patients were carefully followed up for longer and included large numbers of people. Dosage tended to be unacceptably high by current standards. We have not found evidence of a difference between hydroxychloroquine and chloroquine in the treatment of cutaneous lupus or any information on this disorder regarding dosage in relation to either efficacy or toxicity.

Amodiaquine and quinacrine
Benefits

We found no RCTs or controlled trials. Wallace has reviewed the literature on quinacrine, finding 20 observational trials.[25] In these studies, 209 of 771 people (27%) with lupus erythematosus showed an excellent response. However, the cutaneous subsets and outcome measures were not clearly defined. Smaller observational studies of amodiaquine have been published.[26,27]

Harms

Reported side-effects were headache, dizziness, gastrointestinal symptoms, raised liver enzymes, pustular eruption of the face, severe insomnia, retinal damage (in people previously taking chloroquine) and leucopenia.

Combinations of antimalarials
Benefits

We found no controlled trials, but three observational trials of the combination of chloroquine and quinacrine in people with chronic cutaneous lupus. A total of 77 people were treated, with 51 (66%) showing marked improvement or clearing.[28-30] Success with this combination has also been the subject of a case report.[31]

Harms

Yellow skin discoloration, photophobia, insomnia and nausea were noted by some people but did not usually require withdrawal of treatment.

Intralesional antimalarials
Benefits

We found no controlled trials. We found two observational studies of intralesional chloroquine in a total of 23 people with DLE, with benefit noted in 11.[32,33]

Harms

Local inflammation occurred in one lesion.

> What are the effects of steroids in cutaneous lupus?

Topical steroids
Benefits

We found two RCTs of potent topical steroids. The first study compared two potent topical steroids: 0·025% fluocinolone acetonide and 0·1% betamethasone valerate used for 3 weeks. Symmetrical skin lesions were used, and the participants were randomised to use the creams on the right or left side of the body. Betamethasone valerate appeared to be superior in 15 of 25 (60%) participants.[34]

In a 12-week crossover study, 0·05% fluocinonide (a potent steroid cream) was compared with 1% hydrocortisone (a low-potency steroid cream).[35] After 6 weeks, an excellent response was seen in 10 of 37 people (27%) using fluocinonide and in 4 of 41 people (10%) using hydrocortisone cream. This suggests that high-potency steroid cream is more effective than low-potency steroid cream.

We found one controlled trial. Bjornberg and Hellgren used the symmetrical skin lesion design to compare fluocinolone acetonide with ointment base; 17 of 20 people (85%), showed greater improvement with the steroid than with base alone.[36]

We found six observational studies of topical steroids.[37-42] A total of 263 people were treated in these trials, 220 (84%) of whom experienced complete clearing or marked improvement in the treated areas.

Harms

Skin irritation was noted by three people using hydrocortisone, and a burning sensation by one person using fluocinolone.[35] No side-effects were reported in the other controlled trials. In the uncontrolled trial of methylprednisolone aceponate in 322 people with various dermatoses, local side-effects such as burning, itching, pain and inflammation were observed in 22 people (7%).[38] Toxicity of topical steroids has been reviewed by Cornell.[43]

Comments

All the controlled trials of topical steroid were of short duration but the evidence does appear to support the use of potent topical steroids in DLE.

Although topical steroid use may be associated with skin atrophy, it is probably relatively unimportant in DLE, which produces severe scarring and atrophy in itself.

Oral steroids
Benefits
We found no RCT of oral steroids in cutaneous lupus. We found one observational study.[44] A "very good result" was reported in two of 25 people (8%), suggesting that oral steroids were not beneficial. There is a case series of 15 people with DLE treated successfully with a combination of antimalarial and oral steroid drugs.[45]

Harms
"Mild cushingoid features" were noted in two people taking oral steroids during the above study.[44] A wide range of toxicities have been ascribed to oral steroids, reviewed by Werth.[46]

Comments
There is not sufficient evidence to judge the efficacy of oral steroids in cutaneous lupus.

Clinical experience suggests that oral steroids are rarely beneficial in treating chronic cutaneous lupus.

Intralesional steroids
Benefits
We found no RCT. We found five case series, involving 114 people. There was marked improvement or clearing in 91 participants (80%).[47–50]

Harms
Skin thinning (atrophy) was noted in a few people in the above studies.[44,48]

What are the effects of other oral agents in cutaneous lupus?

Azathioprine
Benefits
We found no RCTs or controlled trials. Callen[51] has published the largest observational study. All six patients had been treated unsuccessfully with less toxic agents prior to azathioprine. Three people experienced complete clearing or marked improvement at a dose of 250 mg per day.

A number of case reports describe successful treatment of DLE with azathioprine.[52–54]

Harms
Callen reported fever, pancreatitis, disturbed liver function and skin infections in his study.[51] Side-effects associated with the long-term use of azathioprine in rheumatic diseases are reviewed by Speerstra et al.[55]

Comments
There is insufficient evidence to determine the efficacy of azathioprine in cutaneous lupus.

Clofazimine
Benefits
We found no RCTs or controlled trials. We found four observational studies. A total of 31 of 50 people (62%) with chronic cutaneous lupus showed marked improvement on clofazimine at a dose ranging from 100 mg three times weekly to 100 mg/day.[56–59]

Harms
A pink or red discoloration and darkening of the skin resulting from the deposition of clofazimine has been recorded by several authors. Dry skin and keratosis pilaris were reported by Mackey and Barnes.[58] Jakes[59] reported a transient rise in transaminases. Arbiser and Moschella have reviewed the toxicity of clofazimine.[60]

Comments

Evidence for efficacy of clofazimine is lacking and it is not possible to reach any conclusion on the value of this preparation.

Dapsone
Benefits

We found no RCTs or controlled trials of dapsone in lupus erythematosus. Belief in the efficacy of dapsone is based on a number of observational studies. These studies report on a total of 55 people with various forms of cutaneous lupus.[61–63] Marked improvement was noted in 22 people (50%). The use of dapsone has also been reported in several case reports and particularly in people with unusual forms of lupus, such as bullous lupus and urticarial vasculitis.[64–69] Dosage varied from 25 to150 mg/day.

Harms

Side-effects described ranged from nausea, vomiting, headache and fatigue to haemolysis, methaemoglobinaemia, and leucopenia. Mok *et al.* have reviewed the toxicity of dapsone.[70]

Comments

There is inadequate evidence to guide clinical practice.

Long-term remission without maintenance therapy is rare.[71] Dapsone may have a specific role in bullous lupus but this has not been established in clinical trials.

Gold
Benefits

We found no RCTs or other controlled trials. We found several large observational studies with a total of 550 participants.[72–75]

Wright described an observational study of 76 people treated with gold and followed for 10 years.[72] Participants were not identified as having DLE but appear to have had some form of chronic cutaneous lupus. Of the 76 participants, 28 were described as cured, 26 as showing marked improvement and 9 as having failed to improve. Pascher reported on 46 patients with DLE, 54% showing clearing or a marked improvement.[75]

An observational study reported the effect of a newer gold preparation, auranofin, in 23 people with DLE over 1 year.[76] A marked improvement was seen in eight participants.

Harms

Twenty-one adverse events were described in the 76 participants of Wright's study.[72] These included 10 skin eruptions (two purpuric), and four episodes of fever. Dalziel reported frequent gastrointestinal side-effects, with diarrhoea in 10 of 23 people taking auranofin.[76]

Gold has been extensively used in rheumatoid arthritis and a meta-analysis examining its toxicity has been published.[24]

Comment

There is insufficient evidence to evaluate the effects of gold in cutaneous lupus. Apart from not being controlled, the older studies are impaired by the lack of clear clinical definition and outcome measures.

Methotrexate
Benefits

We found no RCTs but one controlled trial of methotrexate in systemic lupus. Carneiro and Sato in their double-blind study reported that 12 of 20 patients in the active arm and 16 of 21 in the placebo arm had cutaneous lesions, declining to three in the active arm but remaining unchanged in the placebo group.[77] The skin lesions and outcome measures are not described. We found small observational studies and case reports describing improvement in skin lesions of lupus.[78–86]

Harms

Problems encountered with methotrexate in these studies included dyspepsia, a rise in transaminases (55% reported by Carneiro and Sato[77]) and an increased rate of infection. Three of 12 patients withdrew from Wilson and Abeles'[79] study because of side-effects – thrombocytopenia and elevated liver enzymes in one, persistent nausea and elevated liver enzymes in a second and recurring mouth ulcers in a third.[79] Transient malaise was also reported. A thorough discussion of methotrexate toxicity has been published by McKendry.[87]

Comments

The evidence for an improvement of skin lesions is too limited to allow any conclusions to be drawn.

Phenytoin

An open trial of phenytoin in 93 patients with DLE reported an excellent or very good response in 98% of cases.[88]

Retinoids
Benefits

We found one RCT involving 39 people with DLE and 19 with SCLE, in which hydroxychloroquine, 400–1200 mg/day, was compared with acitretin, 50 mg/day, over 8 weeks,[10] described above in the section on hydroxychloroquine. We found three uncontrolled trials of oral retinoids (etretinate or acitretin) in chronic cutaneous lupus. A total of 64 people were treated, and 46 (72%) cleared or experienced marked improvement.[89–91]

Several case reports report the successful use of retinoids in DLE and SCLE.[92–97] We found one case report describing the successful use of topical retinoid in DLE.[98]

Harms

Retinoids are teratogenic. Side-effects were recorded more commonly with acitretin (27 of 28 people) than with chloroquine.[10] Symptoms were predominantly cutaneous, with dry lips, dry skin, scaling of the skin, itching and hair loss being most common. Raised serum triglycerides was noted in five of 18 people. All improved with dose reduction and resolved when therapy was discontinued. Retinoid toxicity has been reviewed by Lowe and David.[99]

Comments

There is insufficient evidence to assess the value of retinoids in cutaneous lupus. The available evidence suggests that efficacy is similar to that of hydroxychloroquine, but that side-effects appear to be more frequent.

Thalidomide
Benefits

We found no RCTs or controlled trials. The evidence for efficacy relies on a number of observational studies and a large number of case reports. The open trials, in general (but not universally), have included patients resistant to the conventional therapies of antimalarials and topical steroids.

Knop et al. reported an observational study of 60 patients with DLE resistant to conventional therapy.[100] Sixty-five per cent showed complete clearing, with a further 25% having some response with 3–5 months' treatment. When treatment was stopped, 50% relapsed. Stevens et al. reported similar results in 16 patients with a variety of lesions including DLE, SCLE, and malar rash; half the patients had SLE.[101] Thirteen (71%) experienced complete clearing. Similar results have been reported by Samsoen *et al.*,[102] Atra and Sato,[103] Ordi-ros *et al.*,[104] Duong *et al.*,[105] Hasper[106] and Naas and Faber.[107] The number of patients in these trials ranged from seven to 23 and the period of completed treatment varied from weeks to years. Duong *et al.* reported on patients who had been on treatment for 8–9 years. Low-dose maintenance therapy (50–100 mg/day) successfully controlled disease in the majority of cases.

Harms

Thalidomide is teratogenic.

Knop *et al.* reported some degree of drowsiness in all patients, and other series reported rates of 20–50%.[100] Paraesthesias were frequent in the study of Knop *et al.* but only one patient (<1%) developed the electromyographical changes of peripheral neuropathy. A recent review found the incidence of peripheral neuropathy to range from 1 to 70%.[108] Other neurological side-effects reported have been dizziness, vertigo, dreams and mood changes. Rarely was it necessary to stop the drug. Calabrese and Fleischer have reviewed the side-effects of thalidomide.[109]

Comments

There is inadequate evidence to guide clinicians in the use of thalidomide in lupus, although published studies do suggest that thalidomide may have a role in the person with disease resistant to other agents.

Implications for clinical practice

Current recommendations for people taking thalidomide include patient education, a 3-monthly clinical examination, and electrophysiological studies, if indicated. Women must be counselled on the risks of fetal abnormality if they should become pregnant. Women of child-bearing age must use effective contraception while taking this agent.

Vitamin E (tocopherol)
Benefits

We found no RCTs but six observational trials and case reports involving a total of 154 patients with various skin lesions.[110–115] Forty-one patients improved, 102 remained unchanged and 11 deteriorated. Apart from a small series in 1992, there are no recent reports on the use of vitamin E.[115]

Comments

There is insufficient evidence to recommend the use of vitamin E in the treatment of skin lesions in lupus.

Other oral agents
Benefits

We found no RCTs or controlled trials of other oral agents in cutaneous lupus. There are many case reports describing success in individuals or small numbers of patients. Favourable case reports describe cefuroxime,[116] cyclophosphamide,[117] ciclosporin A,[118,119] cytarabine,[120] interferon alfa (parenteral and intralesional),[121,122] intravenous immunoglobulin,[123,124] chimeric monoclonal antibodies,[125] mycophenolate mofetil,[126] and pulses of methylprednisolone.[127] An open trial of sulfasalazine in 13 patients with cutaneous lupus demonstrated an excellent or good response in eight,[128] and there is a favourable case report on the treatment of DLE with sulfasalazine.[129]

De Pitá *et al.* could not reproduce the favourable response to immunoglobulins – of their seven patients with SCLE none responded to this therapy.[130]

Comments

So few patients were involved in the reports mentioned above that it is not possible to make any comments.

What are the effects of non-drug treatments in cutaneous lupus?

Sunscreens
Benefits
We found one double-blind intra-individual trial on the efficacy of sunscreens in the treatment of the skin lesions in SLE. People using three different commercially available sunscreens were tested with ultraviolet light. Protective efficacy varied from 100% to <30%.[131] We found one further open-label study.[132] In this trial broad-spectrum sunscreen decreased skin disease activity significantly over an 8-week period.

Comments
There is insufficient evidence to guide the clinician in the use of sunscreens.

Surgery
Benefits
We found no RCTs or controlled trials. We found six reports describing 17 patients treated with either dermabrasion or excision and grafting.[133–138] Results were favourable in all cases, but with four patients suffering recurrences.

Comments
Insufficient data are available to comment.

Ultraviolet light
Benefits
We found one controlled trial of UVA1 (350–440 nm) in 11 people with systemic lupus.[139] Disease activity was measured by the SLEDAI score, a 24-item score that measures SLE activity,[140] but skin lesions were not specifically described. A non-significant improvement in Raynaud's phenomenon and rash (type not specified) was noted.

We found several observational studies and case reports. McGrath found that people with systemic lupus treated with low-dose UVA irradiation showed benefit in constitutional and musculoskeletal complaints. Skin lesions did not worsen but were not formally assessed.[141] There was a further favourable case report of UV treatment in SLE.[142] Sonnischen successfully treated a person with DLE.[143] We also found case reports describing the successful use of extracorporeal photopheresis in cutaneous lupus.[144–146]

Harms
No adverse events were reported in the above studies.

Comments
Although the trial reported by Polderman et al.[139] was double blind, the findings cannot be interpreted with confidence because the numbers were small and the two arms (nine active treatment, two placebo) were disproportionate.

There is currently insufficient evidence to comment on the use of this modality. There is no evidence to indicate the relative risk of inducing a flare in this light-sensitive disorder.

Laser treatment
Benefits
We found no RCTs or controlled trials. We found one case series and five case reports.[147–152] Clearing or marked improvement was noted in 12 of a total of 20 people with cutaneous lupus, using either pulsed dye or argon laser.

Harms
Transient pigmentation was seen in some people.

Key points

- We found very few RCTs on the treatment of cutaneous lupus and only a few controlled trials.
- We found many observational studies, some involving large numbers of people, followed for several years, particularly relating to older treatments.
- We found limited evidence that potent topical steroids, chloroquine and acitretin are beneficial in cutaneous lupus.

References

1. Yell JA, Mbuagbaw J, Burge SM. Cutaneous manifestations of systemic lupus erythematosus. *Br J Dermatol* 1996;**135**:355–62.

2. Gilliam JN, Sontheimer RD. Distinctive cutaneous subsets in the spectrum of lupus erythematosus. *J Am Acad Dermatol* 1981;**4**:471–5.

3. Sontheimer RD, Thomas JR, Gilliam JN. Subacute cutaneous lupus erythematosus: a cutaneous marker for a distinct lupus erythematosus subset. *Arch Dermatol* 1979;**115**:1409–15.

4. Hochberg MC. The epidemiology of systemic lupus erythematosus. In: Wallace DJ, Hahn BH, eds. *Dubois' Lupus Erythematosus*. Philadelphia: Lea and Febiger, 1993:49–57.

5. Isenberg DA. Systemic lupus erythematosus: Immunopathogenesis and the card game analogy. *J Rheumatol* 1997;**24**:62–6.

6. Arnett FC. The genetic basis of lupus erythematosus. In: Wallace DJ, Hahn BH, eds. *Dubois' Lupus Erythematosus*. Philadelphia: Lea and Febiger, 1993:13–36.

7. Millard TP, McGregor JM. Molecular genetics of cutaneous lupus erythematosus. *Clin Exp Dermatol* 2001;**26**:184–91.

8. Vaughan JH. Viruses and autoimmune disease. *J Rheumatol* 1996;**23**:1831–3.

9. Jessop S, Whitelaw D, Jordaan F. Drugs for discoid lupus erythematosus (Cochrane Review). In: *Cochrane Collaboration*. Cochrane Library. Issue 1. Oxford: Update Software, 2001.

10. Ruzicka T, Sommerburg C, Goerz G, Kind P, Mensing H. Treatment of cutaneous lupus erythematosus with acitretin and hydroxychloroquine. *Br J Dermatol* 1992;**127**:513–18.

11. Canadian Hydroxychloroquine Study Group. A randomised study of the effect of withdrawing hydroxychloroquine sulphate in systemic lupus erythematosus. *N Engl J Med* 1991;**324**:150–4.

12. Williams HJ, Egger MJ, Singer JZ *et al.* Comparison of hydroxychloroquine and placebo in the treatment of mild systemic lupus erythematosus. *J Rheumatol* 1994;**21**: 1457–62.

13. Meinao IM, Sato EI, Andrade LE, *et al.* Controlled trial with chloroquine diphosphate in systemic lupus erythematosus. *Lupus* 1996;**5**:237–41.

14. Kraak JH, van Ketel WG, Prakken JR. The value of hydroxychloroquine (Plaquenil) for the treatment of chronic discoid lupus erythematosus: a double blind trial. *Dermatologica* 1965;**130**:293–305.

15. Christiansen JV. Treatment of lupus erythematosus with chloroquine. *Br J Dermatol* 1957;**69**:158–68.

16. Brodthagen H. Hydroxychloroquine (Plaquenil) in the treatment of lupus erythematosus. *Acta Derm Venereol* 1959;**39**:233–7.

17. Crissey JT, Murray PF. A comparison of chloroquine and gold in the treatment of lupus erythematosus. *Arch Dermatol* 1956;**74**:69–72.

18. Galla F. L'idrossiclorochina nel trattamento dell'eritematodes cronico. *Minerva Dermatologica* 1961;**36**:99–101.

19. Goode P. Plaquenil in the treatment of cutaneous lupus erythematosus. *Br J Dermatol* 1958;**70**:176–8.

20. Tye MJ, Schiff BL, Collins SF, Baler GR, Appel B. Chronic discoid lupus erythematosus. Treatment with Daraprim and chloroquine diphosphate (Aralen). *New Engl J Med* 1954;**251**:52–5.

21. Kuhn A, Richter-Hinz D, Oslislo C *et al.* Lupus erythematosus tumidus. *Arch Dermatol* 2000;**136**: 1033–41.

22. Houpt JB. A rheumatologist's verdict on the safety of chloroquine versus hydroxychloroquine. *J Rheumatol* 1999;**26**:1864–7.

23. Sontheimer R. Questions answered and a $1 million question raised concerning lupus erythematosus tumidus. *Arch Dermatol* 2000;**136**:1044–9.

24. Felson DT, Anderson JJ, Meenan RF. The comparative efficacy and toxicity of second-line drugs in rheumatoid arthritis. Results of two metaanalyses. *Arthritis Rheum* 1990;**33**:1449–59.

25. Wallace DJ. The use of quinacrine (Atabrine) in rheumatic diseases: A reexamination. *Semin Arthritis Rheum* 1989;**18**:282–96.

26. Maguire A. Amodiaquine hydrochloride in the treatment of chronic discoid lupus erythematosus. *Lancet* 1962;**31**:665–7.

27. Leeper RW, Allende MF. Antimalarials in the treatment of discoid lupus erythematosus. *Arch Dermatol* 1956;**73**:50–7.

28. Feldmann R, Salomon D, Saurat JH. The association of the two antimalarials chloroquine and quinacrine for treatment-resistant chronic and subacute cutaneous lupus erythematosus. *Dermatology* 1994;**189**:425–7.

29. Lipsker D, Piette JC, Cacoub P, Godeau P, Frances C. Chloroquine-quinacrine association in resistant cutaneous lupus. *Dermatology* 1995;**190**:257–8.

30. Tye MJ, White H, Appel B, Ansell HB. Lupus erythematosus treated with a combination of quinacrine, hydroxychloroquine and chloroquine. *N Engl J Med* 1959;**260**:63–5.

31. Von Schmiedeberg S, Ronnau AC, Schuppe HC *et al.* Combination of antimalarial drugs mepacrine and chloroquine in therapy refractory cutaneous lupus erythematosus. *Hautarzt* 2000;**51**:82–5.

32. Everett MA, Coffey CM. Intradermal administration of chloroquine for discoid lupus erythematosus and lichen sclerosis et atrophicus. *Arch Dermatol* 1961;**83**:977–9.

33. Pelzig A, Witten VH, Sulzberger MB. Chloroquine for chronic discoid lupus erythematosus. *Arch Dermatol* 1961;**83**:146–8.

34. Bjornberg A, Hellgren L. Topical treatment of chronic discoid lupus erythematosus with betamethason-17-valerate and fluocinolone acetonie – a double blind study. *Indian J Dermatol* 1966;**12**:17–18.

35. Roenigk HH, Martin JS, Eichorn P, Gilliam JN. Discoid lupus erythematosus. Diagnostic features and evaluation of topical corticosteroid therapy. *Cutis* 1980;**25**:281–5.

36. Bjornberg A, Hellgren L. Treatment of chronic discoid lupus erythematosus with fluocinolone acetonide ointment. *Br J Dermatol* 1963;**75**:156–60.

37. Bjornberg A, Hellgren L. Treatment of chronic discoid lupus erythematosus with betamethasone-17, 21 dipropionate. *Curr Ther Res* 1976;**19**:442–3.

38. Haneke E. Long-term treatment with 6 α-methylprednisolone aceponate. *J Eur Acad Dermatol Venereol* 1994;**3**:S19–S22.

39. Jansen GT, Dillaha CJ, Honeycutt WM. Discoid lupus erythematosus. *Arch Dermatol* 1965;**92**:283–5.

40. Marsden CW. Fluocinolone acetonide 0·2% cream – a co-operative clinical trial. *Br J Dermatol* 1968;**80**:614–17.

41. Mitchell AD, Mitchell DM. Fluocinolone acetonide in the treatment of chronic discoid lupus erythematosus. *Lancet* 1962;**2**:359.

42. Reymann F. Treatment of discoid lupus erythematosus with betamethasone-valerate cream 1%. *Dermatologica* 1974;**149**:65–8.

43. Cornell RC. Topical glucocorticoids in dermatology. *Curr Opin Dermatol* 1995;193–7.

44. Callen JP. Chronic cutaneous lupus erythematosus. *Arch Dermatol* 1982;**118**:412–16.

45. Alexander S, Cowan MA. The treatment of chronic discoid lupus erythematosus with a combination of antimalarial and corticosteroid drugs. *Br J Dermatol* 1961;**73**:359–61.

46. Werth VP. Glucocorticoids in dermatology. *Curr Opin Dermatol* 1993;195–9.

47. Ferguson Smith JF. Intralesional triamcinolone as an adjunct to antimalarial drugs in the treatment of chronic discoid lupus erythematosus. *Br J Dermatol* 1962;**74**:350–3.

48. James APR. Intradermal triamcinolone acetonide in localized lesions. *J Invest Dermatol* 1980;**34**:175–6.

49. Kraak JH. Lokale behandeling van chronische (lupus) erythematodes. *Ned T Geneesk* 1964;**108**:1305–6.

50. Rowell NR. Treatment of chronic discoid lupus erythematosus with intralesional triamcinolone. *Br J Dermatol* 1962;**74**:354–7.

51. Callen J, Spencer LV, Burruss JB, Holtman J. Azathioprine. *Arch Dermatol* 1991;**127**:515–22.

52. Ashinoff R, Werth VP, Franks AG. Resistant discoid lupus erythematosus of palms and soles: successful treatment with azathioprine. *J Am Acad Dermatol* 1988;**19**:961–5.

53. Shehade S. Successful treatment of generalised discoid skin lesions with azathioprine. *Arch Dermatol* 1986;**122**:376–7.

54. Tsokos GC, Caughman SW, Klippel JH. Successful treatment of generalised discoid skin lesions with azathioprine. *Arch Dermatol* 1985;**121**:1323–5.

55. Speerstra F, Th Boerbooms AM, Van de Putte LBA *et al.* Side-effects of azathioprine treatment in rheumatoid arthritis: analysis of 10 years of experience. *Ann Rheum Dis* 1982;**41**(Suppl.):37–9.

56. Dupré A, Bonafé JL, Lassére J, Albarel N, Christol B. Traitement du lupus érythémateux chronique par le lampréne. *Ann Dermatol Venereol* (Paris) 1978;**105**:423–5.

57. Krivanek J, Paver WKA, Kossard S. (Lamprone) in the treatment of discoid lupus erythematosus. *Dermatol* 1976;**17**:108–10.

58. Mackey JP, Barnes J. Clofazimine in the treatment of discoid lupus erythematosus. *Br J Dermatol* 1974;**91**:93–6.

59. Jakes JT, Dubois EL, Quismorio FP. Antileprosy drugs and lupus erythematosus. *Ann Intern Med* 1982;**97**:788.

60. Arbiser JL, Moschella SL. Clofazimine:A review of its medical uses and mechanisms of action. *J Am Acad Dermatol* 1995;**32**:241–7.

61. Coburn PR, Shuster S. Dapsone and discoid lupus erythematosus. *Br J Dermatol* 1982;**106**:105–6.

62. Lindskov R, Reymann F. Dapsone in the treatment of cutaneous lupus erythematosus. *Dermatologica* 1986;**172**:214–17.

63. Ruzicka T, Goerz G. Dapsone in the treatment of lupus erythematosus. *Br J Dermatol* 1981;**104**:53–56.

64. Bohm I, Bruns A, Schupp G, Bauer R. ANCA-positive lupus erythematodes profundus. Successful therapy with low dosage dapsone. *Hautarzt* 1998;**49**:403–7.

65. Hall RP, Lawley TJ, Smith HR, Katz SI. Bullous eruption of systemic lupus erythematosus. Dramatic response to dapsone therapy. *Ann Intern Med* 1982;**97**:165–70.

66. Holtman JH, Neustadt DH, Klein J, Callen JP. Dapsone is an effective therapy for the skin lesions of subacute cutaneous lupus erythematosus and urticarial vasculitis in a patient with C2 deficiency. *J Rheumatol* 1990;**17**: 1222–5.

67. McCormack LS, Elgart ML, Turner MLC. Annular subacute cutaneous lupus erythematosus responsive to dapsone. *J Am Acad Dermatol* 1984;**11**:397–401.

68. Neri R, Mosca M, Bernacchi E, Bombardieri S. A case of SLE with acute, subacute and chronic cutaneous lesions successfully treated with dapsone. *Lupus* 1999; **8**:240–3.

69. Tsutsui K, Imai T, Hatta N *et al*. Widespread pruritic plaques in a patient with subacute cutaneous lupus erythematosus and hypocomplementemia: response to dapsone therapy. *J Am Acad Dermatol* 1996;**35**: 313–15.

70. Mok CC, Lau, CS, Wong RW. Toxicities of dapsone in the treatment of cutaneous manifestations of rheumatic diseases. *J Rheumatol* 1998;**25**:1246–7.

71. Duna GF, Cash JM. Treatment of refractory cutaneous lupus erythematosus. *Rheum Clin North Am* 1995;**21**:99–115.

72. Wright CS. Ten years experience in the treatment of lupus erythematosus with gold compounds. *Arch Dermatol Syph* 1936;**33**:413–29.

73. Rutledge WU. Lupus erythematosus. Treatment with gold preparations. *Arch Dermatol Syph* 1931;**23**:874–83.

74. Strandberg J. Six years' experience of the treatment of lupus erythematosus with gold compounds. *Acta Med Scand* 1931;**75**:296–317.

75. Pascher F. Treatment of lupus erythematosus with calciferol, antibiotics and gold preparations. *Arch Dermatol Syph* 1950;**61**:906–12.

76. Dalziel K, Going G, Cartwright PH *et al*. Treatment of chronic discoid lupus erythematosus with an oral gold compound (auranofin). *Br J Dermatol* 1986;**115**:211–16.

77. Carneiro JR, Sato EI. Double blind, randomized, placebo-controlled clinical trial of methotrexate in systemic lupus erythematosus. *J Rheumatol* 1999;**26**:1275–9.

78. Gansauge S, Breitbart A, Rinaldi N, Schwarz- Eywill M. Methotrexate in patients with moderate systemic lupus erythematosus (exclusion of renal and central nervous system disease). *Ann Rheum Dis* 1997;**56**:382–5.

79. Wilson J, Abeles M. A 2 year, open ended trial of methotrexate in systemic lupus erythematosus. *J Rheumatol* 1994;**21**:1674–7.

80. Arfi S, Numeric P, Grollier L, Panelatti G, Jean Baptiste G. Treatment of corticodependent systemic lupus erythematosus with low dose methotrexate. *Rev Med Intern* 1995;**16**:885–90.

81. Davidson JR, Graziano FM, Rothenberg RJ. Methotrexate therapy for severe systemic lupus erythematosus. *Arthritis Rheum* 1987;**30**:1195–6.

82. Garcia G, Portales G, Nebro F *et al*. Effectiveness of the treatment of systemic lupus erythematosus with methotrexate. *Med Clin* (Barc) 1993;**101**:361–4.

83. Bohm L, Uerlich M, Bauer R. Rapid improvement of subacute cutaneous lupus erythematosus with low-dose methotrexate. *Dermatology* 1997;**194**:307–8.

84. Rothenberg RJ, Graziano FM, Grandone JT *et al*. The use of methotrexate in steroid-resistant systemic lupus erythematosus. *Arthritis Rheum* 1988;**31**:612–15.

85. Walz LeBlanc BAE, Dagenais P, Urowitz MB, Gladman DD. Methotrexate in systemic lupus erythematosus. *J Rheum* 1994;**21**:836–8.

86. Bottomley WW, Goodfield M. Methotrexate for the treatment of severe mucocutaneous lupus erythematosus. *Br J Dermatol* 1995;**133**:311–14.

87. McKendry RJR. The remarkable spectrum of methotrexate toxicities. *Rheum Dis Clin North Am* 1997; **23**:939–45.

88. Rodriguez-Castellanos MA, Rubio JB, Gomez JFB, Mendonza AG. Phenytoin in the treatment of discoid lupus erythematosus. *Arch Dermatol* 1995;**131**:620–1.

89. Grupper C, Berretti B. Lupus erythematosus and etretinate. In: Cunliffe W, Miller A, eds. *Retinoid Therapy: a Review of Clinical and Laboratory Research.* Lancaster: MTP Press, 1984:73–81.

90. Ruzicka T, Meurer M, Braun-Falco O. Treatment of cutaneous lupus erythematosus with etretinate. *Acta Derm Venereol* 1985;**65**:324–9.

91. Ruzicka T, Meurer M, Bieber T. Efficiency of acitretin in the treatment of cutaneous lupus erythematosus. *Arch Dermatol* 1988;**124**:897–902.

92. Furner BB. Subacute cutaneous lupus erythematosus. Response to isotretinoin. *Int J Dermatol* 1990;**29**:587–90.

93. Green SG, Piette WW. Successful treatment of hypertrophic lupus erythematosus with isotretinoin. *J Am Acad Dermatol* 1987;**17**:364–8.

94. Marks R. Lichen planus and cutaneous lupus erythematosus. In: Lowe N, Marks R, eds. *Retinoids.* London: Martin Dunitz, 1995:143–7.

95. Newton RC, Jorizzo JL, Solomon AR *et al* Mechanism-oriented assessment of isotretinoin in chronic or subacute cutaneous lupus erythematosus. *Arch Dermatol* 1986;**122**:170–6.

96. Rubenstein DJ, Huntley AC. Keratotic lupus erythematosus: treatment with isotretinoin. *J Am Acad Dermatol* 1986;**14**:910–14.

97. Shornick JK, Formica N, Parke AL. Isotretinoin for refractory lupus erythematosus. *J Am Acad Dermatol* 1991;**24**:49–52.

98. Seiger E, Roland S, Goldman S. Cutaneous lupus treated with topical tretinoin: A case report. *Cutis* 1991:**47**:351–5.

99. Lowe NJ, David M. Toxicity. In: Lowe N, Marks R, eds. *Retinoids. A Clinician's Guide.* London: Martin Dunitz, 1998;149–65.

100. Knop J, Bonsmann G, Happle R *et al.* Thalidomide in the treatment of sixty cases of chronic discoid lupus erythematosus. *Br J Derm* 1983;**108**:461–6.

101. Stevens RJ, Andujar C, Edwards CJ *et al.* Thalidomide in the treatment of the cutaneous manifestations of lupus erythematosus: experience in sixteen consecutive patients. *Br J Rheumatol* 1997;**36**:353–9.

102. Samsoen M, Grosshans E, Basset A. La thalidomide dans le traitement du lupus àrythémateux chronique. *Ann Dermatol Venereol* 1980;**107**:515–23.

103. Atra E, Sato EI. Treatment of the cutaneous lesions of systemic lupus erythematosus with thalidomide. *Clin Exp Rheumatol* 1993;**11**:487–93.

104. Ordi-Ros J, Cortes F, Cucurull E *et al.*Thalidomide in the treatment of cutaneous lupus refractory to conventional therapy. *J Rheumatol* 2000;**27**:1429–33.

105. Duong DJ, Spigel T, Moxley RT *et al.* American experience with low dose thalidomide therapy for severe cutaneous lupus erythematosus. *Arch Dermatol* 1999;**135**:1079–87.

106. Hasper MF. Chronic cutaneous lupus erythematosus. Thalidomide treatment of 11 patients. *Arch Dermatol* 1983;**119**:812–15.

107. Naafs B, Faber WR. Thalidomide therapy. An open trial. *Int J Dermatol* 1985;**24**:131–4.

108. Tseng S, Pak G, Washenik K *et al.* Rediscovering thalidomide:a review of its mechanism of action, side effects and potential uses. *J Am Acad Dermatol* 1996;**35**:969–79.

109. Calabrese L, Fleischer AB. Thalidomide: Current and potential clinical applications. *Am J Med* 2000;**108**:487–95.

110. Morgan J. A note on the treatment of lupus erythematosus with vitamin E. *Br J Dermatol* 1951;**63**:224–5.

111. Burgess JF, Pritchard JE. Tocopherols (Vitamin E). Treatment of lupus erythematosus: preliminary report. *Arch Dermatol Syph* 1948;**57**:953–64.

112. Pascher F, Sawicky HH, Silverberg MF *et al.* Tocopherol (vitamin E) for discoid lupus erythematosus and other dermatoses. *J Invest Dermatol* 1951;**17**:261–2.

113. Sawicky HH. Therapy of lupus erythematosus. *Arch Dermatol Syph* 1950;**61**:906–9.

114. Sweet RD. Vitamin E in collagenoses. *Lancet* 1948;**ii**:310–11.

115. Yell JA, Burge S, Wojnarowska F. Vitamin E and discoid lupus erythematosus. *Lupus* 1992;**1**:303–5.

116. Rudnicka L, Szymanska E, Walecka I, Slowinska M. Long-term cefuroxime axetil in subacute cutaneous lupus erythematosus. A report of three cases. *Dermatology* 2000;**200**:129–31.

117. Schulz EJ, Menter MA. Treatment of discoid and subacute lupus erythematosus with cyclophosphamide. *Br J Dermatol* 1971;**85**:S7, 60–6.

118. Yell JA, Burge SM. Cyclosporin and discoid lupus erythematosus. *B J Dermatol* 1994;**131**:132–3.

119. Saeki Y, Ohshima S, Kurimoto I, Miura H, Suemura M. Maintaining remission of lupus erythematosus profundus (LEP) with cyclosporin A. *Lupus* 2000;**9**:390–2.

120. Yung RL, Richardson BC. Cytarabine in systemic lupus erythematosus. *Arth Rheum* 1995;**38**:1341–3.

121. Thivolet J, Nicolas JF, Kanitakis J *et al.* Recombinant interferon alpha 2a is effective in the treatment of discoid and subacute cutaneous lupus erythematosus. *Br J Dermatol* 1990;**122**:405–9.

122. Martinez J, de Misa RF, Torrelo A, Ledo A. A low-dose intralesional interferon alpha for discoid lupus erythematosus. *J Am Acad Dermatol* 1992;**26**:494–96.

123. Généreau T, Chosidow O, Danel C, Chérin P, Herson S. High-dose intravenous immunoglobulin in cutaneous lupus erythematosus. *Arch Dermatol* 1999;**135**:1124–5.

124. Piette JC, Frances C, Roy S, Papo T, Godeau P. High-dose immunoglobulins in the treatment of refractory cutaneous lupus erythematosus:open trial in 5 patients (abstract). *Arth Rheum* 1995;**38**(Suppl. 9):S304.

125. Prinz JC, Meurer M, Reiter C *et al.* Treatment of severe cutaneous lupus erythematosus with a chimeric CD4 monoclonal antibody, cM-T412. *J Am Acad Dermatol* 1996;**34**:244–52.

126. Goyal S, Nousari HC. Treatment of resistant discoid lupus erythematosus of the palms and soles with mycophenolate mofetil. *J Am Acad Dermatol* 2001;**45**:142–4.

127. Goldberg JW, Lidsky MD. Pulse methylprednisolone therapy for persistent subacute cutaneous lupus. *Arth Rheum* 1984;**27**:837–8.

128. Artuz F. Efficacy of sulphasalazine in discoid lupus erythematosus. *Int J Dermatol* 1996;**35**:746–8.

129. Carmichael AJ, Paul CJ. Discoid lupus erythematosus responsive to sulphasalazine. *Br J Dermatol* 1991;**125**:291.

130. De Pitá O, Bellucci AM, Ruffelli M, Girardelli CR, Puddu P. Intravenous immunoglobulin therapy is not able to efficiently control cutaneous manifestations in patients with lupus erythematosus. *Lupus* 1997;**6**:415–17.

131. Stege H, Budde MA, Grether-Beck S, Krutmann J. Evaluation of the capacity of sunscreens to photoprotect lupus erythematosus patients by employing the photoprovocation test. *Photoderm Photoimmunol Photomed* 2000;**16**:256–9.

132. Callen JP, Roth DE, McGrath C, Dromgoole SH. Safety and efficacy of a broad-spectrum sunscreen in patients with discoid or subacute cutaneous lupus erythematosus. *Cutis* 1991;**47**:130–2.

133. Cornbleet T, Barsky S, Hoit L. Discoid lupus erythematosus scars treated by plastic surgery. *Arch Dermatol* 1957;**74**:219.

134. Neuman Z, Shulman J, Ben-hur N. Successful skin grafting in discoid lupus erythematosus. *Ann Surg* 1961;**154**:142–4.

135. Friederich HC. Hautverschiebung und hautverpflanzung beim lupus erythematodes integumentalis chronicus. *Hautarzt* 1969;**20**:119–22.

136. Kurwa AR, Evans AJ. Discoid lupus erythematosus treated by dermabrasion. *Br J Dermatol* 1970;**101**:S53.

137. Schiödt M. Local excision in the treatment of oral discoid lupus erythematosus. *Acta Derm Venereol Suppl* 1978;**59**:274–6.

138. Ratner D, Skouge JW. Discoid lupus erythematosus scarring and dermabrasion: a case report and discussion. *J Am Acad Dermatol* 1990;**22**:314–16.

139. Polderman MC, Huizinga, TW, Le-CessieS, Pavel S. UVA-1 cold light treatment of SLE: a double blind, placebo controlled crossover trial. *Ann Rheum Dis* 2001;**60**:112–15.

140. Bombardier C, Gladman DD, Urowitz MB, Caron D, Chang CH. Derivation of the SLEDAI. A disease activity index for lupus patients. The Committee on Prognosis Studies in SLE. *Arthritis Rheum* 1992;**35**:630–40·

141. McGrath H. Ultraviolet A1 irradiation decreases clinical disease activity and autoantibodies in patients with systemic lupus erythematosus. *Clin Exp Rheumatol* 1994;**12**:129–35.

142. Molina JF, McGrath H. Longterm ultraviolet-A1 irradiation therapy in systemic lupus erythematosus. *J Rheum* 1997;**24**:1072–4.

143. Sonnichsen NH, Meffert V, Kunzelmann V, Audring H. UVA1 therapy of subacute cutaneous lupus erythematosus. *Hautarzt* 1993;**44**:723–5.

144. Richter HI, Krutmann J, Goerz G. Extracorporeal photopheresis in therapy-refractory disseminated discoid lupus erythematosus. *Hautarzt* 1998;**49**: 487–91.

145. Wollina U, Looks A. Extracorporeal photochemotherapy in cutaneous lupus erythematosus. *J Eur Acad Dermatol Venereol* 1999;**13**:127–30.

146. Knobler RM, Graninger W, Graninger W, Lindmaier A, Trautinger F, Smolen JS. Extracorporeal photochemotherapy for the treatment of systemic lupus erythematosus. A pilot study. *Arthritis Rheum* 1992;**35**:319–24.

147. Raulin C, Schmidt C, Hellwig S. Cutaneous lupus erythematosus-treatment with pulsed dye laser. *Br J Dermatol* 1999;**141**:1046–50.

148. Gupta G, Roberts DT. Pulsed dye laser treatment of subacute cutaneous lupus erythematosus. *Clin Exp Dermatol* 1999;**24**:498–9.

149. Núñez M, Boixeda P, Miralles ES, de Misa RF, Ledo A. Pulsed dye laser treatment of telangiectatic chronic erythema of cutaneous lupus erythematosus. *Arch Dermatol* 1996;**132**:354–5.

150. Zachariae H, Bjerring P, Cramers M. Argon laser treatment of cutaneous vascular lesions in connective tissue diseases. *Acta Derm Venereol* 1952;**68**:179–82.

151. Nurnberg W, Algermissen B, Hermes B, Henz BM, Kolde G. Erfolgreiche behandlung des chronisch diskoiden lupus erythematodes mittels argon-laser. *Hautarzt* 1996;**47**:767–70.

152. Kuhn A, Becker-Wegerich PM, Ruzicka T, Lehmann P. Successful treatment of discoid lupus erythematosus with argon laser. *Dermatology* 2000;**201**:175–7.

46
Dermatomyositis

Jeffrey P Callen

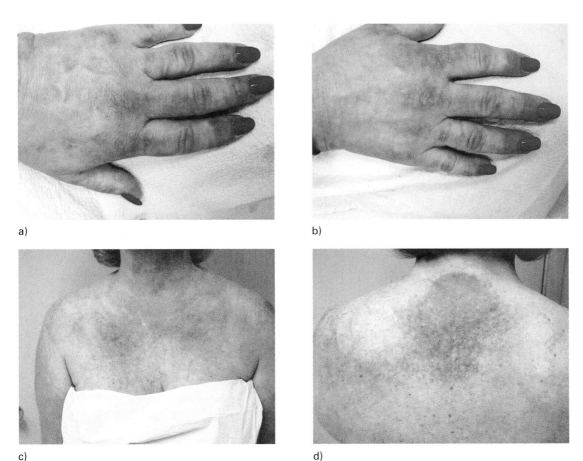

a)

b)

c)

d)

Figure 45.1 This patient presented for the evaluation and treatment of her skin condition, which had been present for the past 6 months. A previous biopsy had revealed an interface dermatitis and her antinuclear antibody was positive. A working diagnosis of lupus erythematosus was made. Treatment with sunscreens and topical corticosteroids were ineffective. Hydroxychloroquine administration resulted in a severe cutaneous drug reaction that required hospitalisation

Background
Definition

Dermatomyositis is one of the idiopathic inflammatory myopathies.[1-3] In a set of criteria to aid in the diagnosis and classification of dermatomyositis and polymyositis, first proposed in 1975 by Bohan and Peter,[4] four of the five criteria are related to the muscle disease:

1. Progressive proximal symmetrical weakness
2. Elevated muscle enzymes
3. Abnormal electromyogram (EMG)
4. Abnormal muscle biopsy
5. Presence of compatible cutaneous disease

It has subsequently been recognised that there are many patients with compatible cutaneous disease who do not have initial manifestations of their muscles as defined by clinical weakness and elevated enzymes. Some of these patients have subtle changes on biopsy, EMG or magnetic resonance imaging studies at diagnosis; some develop these changes and possibly clinical manifestations later, while a small group of patients never seem to develop clinical muscle disease. Sontheimer[5] has used the term "amyopathic dermatomyositis" for those patients without muscle weakness and with normal muscle enzymes for at least 2 years in the absence of disease modifying therapies such as corticosteroids and/or immunosuppressive agents.

Incidence/prevalence

Dermatomyositis is a rare disorder. It may be slightly more frequent in women, but all races are affected. It has been estimated that dermatomyositis or its related condition polymyositis occur in 5·5 patients per million. However, this figure includes patients with polymyositis and dermatomyositis and most likely does not include patients with amyopathic dermatomyositis.

Aetiology

The aetiology of dermatomyositis is unknown. Probably the mechanism behind the skin disease differs from that of the muscle disease.

Prognosis

In the patient with amyopathic dermatomyositis the prognosis is good in the absence of malignancy. For patients with muscle disease, the prognosis depends on the severity of the muscle disease, the presence of lung disease, oesophageal dysfunction and/or malignancy. Children and adolescents with dermatomyositis often develop calcinosis, which can result in disability or discomfort.

Diagnostic tests

The diagnosis of amyopathic dermatomyositis is confirmed by clinical–pathological correlation. The pattern of the skin disease is relatively characteristic and when an interface dermatitis is demonstrated on skin biopsy the diagnosis may be relatively firm. Classically, the diagnosis of dermatomyositis is confirmed by the presence of typical muscle symptoms and findings, together with elevated muscle enzymes, or an abnormal EMG and/or an abnormal muscle biopsy. Magnetic resonance imaging is becoming widely available and abnormalities of this test might be useful in diagnosis.

Aims of treatment

Treatment provides control of the muscle inflammation and allows the patient to return to normal function; the patient might otherwise become disabled from the weakness. The skin disease is often symptomatic and is cosmetically displeasing, therefore the goal of therapy is to relieve the symptoms and improve the patient's self-image and ability to interact with other people. Some patients with dermatomyositis have an associated malignancy, and treatment of the malignancy might in some patients result in a control of the disease process. In children with dermatomyositis, treatment also aims to prevent calcinosis, or to eradicate calcinosis if it does occur.

Relevant outcomes

Return of the patient to normal muscle function and improvement in the quality of life for those with skin disease only are important measures of outcome. In addition, identification and treatment of a potential malignancy is important.

Methods of search

The databases of the Cochrane Skin Group, the *Cochrane Library* to issue 2, 2001, Medline and Embase between 1968 and July 2001 were searched for articles that were trials of therapy of skin disease, or dermatomyositis, or the relationship of dermatomyositis to malignancy. Both Embase and Medline were searched using the Ovid search engine at Nottingham University. The searches involved the following terms:

- the relationship of dermatomyositis to cancer (malignancy, neoplasia)
- treatment of skin disease in patients with dermatomyositis (idiopathic inflammatory myopathy, polymyositis, juvenile dermatomyositis) .
- treatment of dermatomyositis with any of the following agents: antimalarials (hydroxychloroquine, chloroquine), corticosteroids (prednisone, methylprednisolone), dapsone, thalidomide, methotrexate, mycophenolate mofetil, azathioprine, intravenous immune globulin (IVIG), probenecid, alendronate, diltiazem, coumadin and sunscreens.

QUESTIONS

What is the risk of malignancy in the patient with dermatomyositis or amyopathic dermatomyositis (ADM) and how should the patient with dermatomyositis/ADM be assessed for possible cancer?

The data are clearer today than they were in 1975 when I first became interested in this issue. However, there are conflicting reports that probably related to the lack of precision in the definition and classification of the patient with dermatomyositis or polymyositis. Population-based studies from Scandinavia clearly demonstrate an increase in the risk of cancer in dermatomyositis, while the modest increase in polymyositis is explained primarily by diagnostic suspicion bias and is not reflected in an increase in mortality (see Table 46.1). It is also clear that these patients are at increased risk for ovarian cancer.[6-12] What is not clear is whether these data are applicable to other populations such as Southeast Asians, African–Americans or other ethnic groups.

A recent study from Australia[13] calls into question much of the data that has been based on clinical diagnosis. It does appear that dermatomyositis and polymyositis are not the same disease and that their histopathological abnormalities differ significantly and are recognisable by muscle pathologists. Therefore, there may exist a group of patients who were thought to have polymyositis but who might be classified as having dermatomyositis *sine* dermatitis. This concept is intriguing and might explain why some studies have shown little difference in the prevalence/incidence of malignancy in the two groups. In addition, the existence of this subset might well explain some of the differences that are observed in the studies of therapy (see below).

It is not known whether the increased cancer association is also valid for patients with amyopathic dermatomyositis because the only published data are individual case reports and small case series. One of the difficulties regarding this issue relates to the manner in which ADM is diagnosed. If one applies the criteria of Sontheimer,[5] then in my view there are few if any patients with this condition, because either the patient has not been studied in enough detail (magnetic resonance imaging, muscle biopsy, etc.) or the patient has been treated with a corticosteroid and/or systemic corticosteroids.

Several studies have suggested that there might be certain clinical features that are associated

Table 46.1 What is the risk of malignancy in patients with dermatomyositis or a myopathic dermatomyositis?

Study	Population-based?	Patients with CA in the DM/ADM group	Patients with CA in the PM group	Statistically different?	Comment(s)
Sigurgeirsson et al.[6]	Yes	59/392	37/396	Both groups had elevated rate v controls. Cancer mortality raised only in DM	Ovarian cancer increased 17-fold Authors suggest increase in PM due to more extensive evaluation
Airio et al.[7]	Yes	19/71	12/175	SIR DM: 6·5 PM: 1·0	Risk rises with age, slight risk for overlap patients Non-melanoma skin cancers, myelofibrosis, polycythemia vera, in situ cervical cancer and 12 preceding cancers eliminated Overrepresentation of ovarian cancer
Chow et al.[8]	Yes	31/203	26/336	SIR DM: 3·8 PM: 1·7 reduced to 1·0 by 3rd year following diagnosis	Excess lymphoma/leukaemia Surveillance for prolonged periods may not be needed
Hill et al.[9]	Yes	115/618	95/914	SIR DM: 3·0 PM: 1·3	Plan for evaluation based on the results of their study suggested data derived from Swedish, Finnish and Danish studies, but included additional follow up from Denmark and Finland
Buchbinder et al.[13]	Yes, population-based, retrospective cohort study based on pathological findings	36/85	57/321	OR all cases: 2·6 DM 6·2 PM: 2·0 IBM: 2·4 JDM: 29·0 Myositis with CTD: 4·6	Authors feel diagnosis of DM possible without the presence of a rash, based on the changes observed in the muscle biopsy Increased malignancy rate found in all groups, including children

(Continued)

Table 46.1 (*Continued*)

Study	Population-based?	Patients with CA in the DM/ADM group	Patients with CA in the PM group	Statistically different?	Comment(s)
Stockton et al.[20]	Yes	50/286 Women: 30/189 Men: 20/97	40/419 Women: 28/244 Men 12/175	SIR DM: 7·7 PM: 2·1	27 patients with DM and 31 with PM had cancer before DM/PM diagnosed; not known whether any of these patients had metastatic disease at the time of diagnosis Increase in ovarian, cervical and lung cancer in DM and in Hodgkin's disease in PM found
Manchul et al.[21]	No; CC study	11/31 (5 antecedent, 4 concurrent, 2 subsequent)	8/40 (3 antecedent, 4 concurrent, 1 subsequent)	P<0·01 (rheumatic controls) P<0·001 (other controls) OR and confidence intervals reported	Controls included cases of skin cancer Issues about classification for the presence or absence of skin disease
Lakhanpal et al.[22]	No; CC study	11/50	18/65	Not statistically different between groups or v controls	Mayo Clinic studies continue to lack a demonstrable relationship of myositis and cancer Authors suggest that extensive evaluation is not needed
Lyon et al.[23]	CC study	1/40	4/64	No difference v controls (siblings)	Two cases in the control group had skin cancer and should not have been included in the analysis. These patients had a small number of cancers
Zantos et al.[24]	Meta-analysis of 4 CC cohort studies	97/513	56/565	OR DM: 4·4 PM: 2·1	Increased malignancy in the preceding and subsequent 4 years
Marie et al.[25]	No; CC study elderly v younger patients (> 65)	10/11 elderly	1/12 – elderly ?/28	11/23 v 5/56 P<0·0001	The patient with "PM" and malignancy had muscle biopsy changes similar to that expected for DM but lacked a dermatitis

(Continued)

Table 46.1 *(Continued)*

Study	Population-based?	Patients with CA in the DM/ADM group	Patients with CA in the PM group	Statistically different?	Comment(s)
Pautas et al.[26]	No; CC study elderly v younger patients (>65)	–	–	5/21 v 2/21 Not significant	
Chen et al.[27]	CC	16/91 (0/20 ADM)	2/14	$P = 0.08$	Malignancy was more common in patients over 45; NPC was the most common cancer (SIR 22·2 v 2·8 for general population) Malignancy inversely correlated with interstitial lung disease
Callen et al.[28]	No	7/27 (3 occurred concurrently and 1 within 1 year of DM diagnosis; 3 had prior cancer)	1/31 (Hodgkin's disease preceded polymyositis by 5 years)	$P<0.05$	Early study suggesting presence of skin disease associated with cancer
Tymms and Webb[29]	No	7/36	9/69	Not done	Patients with cancer-associated DM/PM were 10–12 years older Strong association in only 8 patients (4 DM, 4 PM)
Cox et al.[30]	No	23/53	–	Not tested	20 patients had an association of cancer and myositis; most discovered by a directed search High prevalence of ovarian cancer in women and lung cancer in men
Cherin et al.[11]	No	12/56 (6 ovarian cancers in 45 women)	12/84	Not tested	First group to suggest that ovarian cancer is overrepresented

(Continued)

Table 46.1 (*Continued*)

Study	Population-based?	Patients with CA in the DM/ADM group	Patients with CA in the PM group	Statistically different?	Comment(s)
Davis and Ahmed[31]	Cross-sectional retrospective review	–	–	–	14 patients with ovarian cancer, 12 with DM and 2 with PM in an analysis of all Mayo cases from 1950 to 1995
Koh et al.[32]	No	15/40	2/35	P<0·01	Cancer association in older patients, also affected the mortality rate. NPC third most common cancer
Maoz et al.[33]	No	9/20	4/15	SIR 12·6 for concurrent and subsequent cancers, but only 4·2 for subsequent cancers alone	–
Benbassat et al.[34]	No	10/39	3/21	Not done	Prevalence of cancer increased with age
Winkelmann et al.[35]	No	Unknown	Unknown	Not done	16/289 patients had cancer. Authors conclude that extensive evaluation is not necessary
Moss and Hanelin[36]	No	2/28	0/15	Not done	Focus on negative value of screening by radiological tests
Scaling et al.[10]	No	4/22 (3 ovarian)	1/3 (patient also had myasthenia gravis) cervical *in situ* cancer	Not done	One of the first reports to note a high prevalence of ovarian cancer. Many of these patients had no pelvic examination during initial hospitalisation
Duncan et al.[37]	No	10/39 had a total of 12 cancers	–	–	4 patients with antecedent cancer presented with metastatic disease at the time of DM diagnosis. Non-directed malignancy search was not of value. Paraneoplastic course was rare
Bonnetblanc et al.[38]	No	34/118 (7 antecedent, 22 concurrent, 5 subsequent)	–	Not tested	2 patients with oesophageal cancer, 3 with ovarian occurred concurrently

(Continued)

Table 46.1 (Continued)

Study	Population-based?	Patients with CA in the DM/ADM group	Patients with CA in the PM group	Statistically different?	Comment(s)
Peng et al.[39]	No	27/104	–	–	NPC occurred in 12 patients in this Taiwanese study
Whitmore et al.[14]	No	6/19 overall (4/12 with ADM;2/7 with DM)	–	–	First linkage of cancer with ADM
Ang et al.[40]	No	12/28	–	ADM v DM Defined as weakness v no weakness, not significant Defined by clinical or laboratory evidence of myositis, $P = 0.0083$	6/12 had NPC, malignancy occurs in ADM

ADM, amyopathic dermatomyositis; CC, case control; DM, dermatomyositis; CTD, connective tissue disease; IBM, inclusion body myositis, JDM = juvenile dermatomyositis; NPC, nasopharyngeal carcinoma; OR, odds ratio; PM, polymyositis; SIR, standardised incidence ratio with a greater risk of malignancy. Fudman and Schnitzer[15] reported that patients with dermatomyositis who had a normal creatine kinase had a poor prognosis. Three of their seven patients had malignancy. However, Montagna et al.[16] found that 5/17 patients with elevated creatine kinase had malignancy compared with 3/9 with normal creatine kinase. The presence of cutaneous vasculitis may also be associated with an increased risk of malignancy. Feldman et al.[17] found clinical evidence of vasculitis manifest as dermal or subcutaneous nodules, periungual infarcts or digital ulceration in seven of 76 patients. Two of these patients had cancer, compared with four of those without vasculitis. In addition, the vasculitic lesions occurred primarily in patients with dermatomyositis (six of seven patients). However, the number of patients in these reports is small and therefore the conclusions reached need affirmation in larger studies. Recently, Hunger et al.[18] reported that the prevalence of neoplasia was greater when there was histopathological evidence of vasculitis in the skin biopsy: four of their five patients with vasculitis had cancer, compared with three of their 18 patients without vasculitis ($P<0.05$). The number of patients in these studies is too small to firmly conclude that vasculitis or normal creatine kinase are markers of malignancy in patients with dermatomyositis.

Another issue that is discussed almost universally in the case-control studies is whether the use of immunosuppressive drugs is associated with an elevated risk of subsequent malignancy. In all of the Scandinavian studies[6–9] it appears that there is no increase in the prevalence of malignancy in the patients that have been treated with an immunosuppressive agent; however, there are many individual case reports of subsequent malignancy in dermatomyositis patients. Several reports[19] have linked the use of methotrexate with Epstein–Barr virus associated lymphoma. Some but not all of these patients can have a spontaneous

resolution of their lymphoma when the drug therapy is stopped.

The search for malignancy in patients with dermatomyositis should include a careful history, physical examination and standard laboratory evaluation (complete blood count, comprehensive metabolic panel, chest radiograph and stool haematest). Any abnormalities found should be thoroughly investigated. In addition, testing should include tests that would be ordered in a "healthy" person of the same age, sex and race as of the patient with newly diagnosed dermatomyositis (for example it is recommended that persons over 50 years of age have a colonoscopy). Data from the recent studies by Hill et al.[9] and Stockton et al.[20] suggest that for a Caucasian patient with dermatomyositis CT scan of the chest and abdomen, and stool haematest should be performed. In women, pelvic CT and mammography are justified. Tests that are recommended for any person of the patient's age should also be performed (for example colonoscopy in patients over 50 years of age). For patients with polymyositis a chest radiograph and urinalysis should be performed at the time of diagnosis. It appears that continued surveillance is necessary for patients with dermatomyositis, but perhaps not for those with polymyositis. However, what testing should be done beyond age-specific cancer screening is not clear, and the clinician must form a plan in the absence with supporting data. Lastly, nasopharyngeal cancer is much more common in the Asian patient within southeast Asia, and therefore a careful ENT evaluation is needed. It is not known if Asian patients who live elsewhere also harbour this increased risk of nasopharyngeal cancer.

Are there effective treatments for dermatomyositis?

The following are some quotes from "major" dermatologic texts that deal with treatment of patients with dermatomyositis:

- "Most forms of polymyositis and dermatomyositis are approached in a similar manner. Corticosteroids are the main pillar of drug therapy. ... However, early use of corticosteroid-sparing drugs should be considered, including combined therapy, from onset. The main drugs for combined therapy are methotrexate, azathioprine and antimalarials."[41]
- "Systemic glucocorticoids remain the traditional first line therapy for classic dermatomyositis."[42]
- "Treatment with corticosteroids is required in almost all cases, the dose depending upon the degree of activity."[43]
- "Prednisone is the therapeutic mainstay."[44]

All of the above authorities recommend corticosteroids as first-line therapy, and relatively high doses are generally suggested. In addition, the early use of a corticosteroid-sparing agent is often proposed, with methotrexate or azathioprine being the most frequently suggested agents. Do we know that these medications are effective, what the proper dosing should be, when a second-line agent should be introduced, which agent should be utilised and what the likelihood of success is? Unfortunately, as is illustrated in Table 46.2, the evidence available to answer these questions is poor. It is unclear whether the rate of remission is affected by corticosteroids, whether they are used in high or low doses. In addition, there is little evidence regarding these therapeutic manoeuvres for the treatment of cutaneous disease that might accompany dermatomyositis. Well-controlled randomised trials for this disease are lacking, and even the ones that have been conducted often lack power, or have design flaws or potential biases. Many of the studies have included patients with malignancy-associated myositis, a condition that is believed to respond less well than dermatomyositis. In addition, most studies mix dermatomyositis and polymyositis patients in their analysis, and it has become evident that these disorders are probably different in their pathogenesis and most likely have a differential response to therapy.

Current recommendations

It seems that there are no strong data that support the use of corticosteroids in dermatomyositis, whether considering the muscle component, systemic disease such as pulmonary involvement or the skin disease. Despite this, most authorities state that corticosteroids are a mainstay of therapy. Therefore, it seems prudent to use corticosteroids for as short a period of time as is possible, substituting a steroid-sparing agent early in the course of treatment. Which of the agents to use is, in my view, dependent on the clinician's comfort level with the specific agent. Observations from individual case reports and small case series suggest that for skin disease, hydroxychloroquine, methotrexate and mycophenolate mofetil are effective corticosteroid-sparing agents.

IVIG has been the subject of a randomised controlled trial (RCT) and was found to be effective for both the muscle disease and the skin disease in patients with dermatomyositis refractory to corticosteroids and immunosuppressive agents. However, at least one open-label analysis reported that only seven of 19 patients treated with IVIG improved. Also, there has been the suggestion that patients with dermatomyositis have an increased risk of hydroxychloroquine reactions, which may be severe at times. This issue has not been adequately tested.

What about the therapy for juvenile dermatomyositis? This condition is complicated in two major ways. First, patients with juvenile dermatomyositis are more prone to calcinosis and second they may be permanently disabled by contractures. The results of retrospective

Table 46.2 Treatments for patients with dermatomyositis

Agent/study	Treatments compared/studied	Type of study	Outcome	Comment(s)
Corticosteroids				
Winkelmann et al.[35]	CS therapy	Retrospective review of DM and PM Primary endpoint: outcome of myositis	High-dose regimen (>50 mg/d) favoured	No statistical analysis Mixture of patients Identified some with an acute, fulminant course
Carpenter et al.[45]	Low- v high-dose prednisone (<10 mg/d v >20 mg/d) Daily 50 mg v alternate day	Retrospective CCS age-, sex-matched PM patients	No difference in survival	Doses selected to represent "high" dose may be too low to be clinically meaningful
Uchino et al.[46]	100 mg prednisone IVCS v OCS	Retrospective review of patients with PM	Alternate-day regimen more effective: 21/30 v 9/17	Groups not comparable groups Some patients with cancer probably included
Klein-Gitleman et al.[47]		Retrospective comparison of 10 patients	IVCS more costly, but more effective	Small group of patients No statistical analysis
Immunosuppressives				
Mosca et al.[48]	CS alone v CS with immunosuppressive	Retrospective analysis	CS first-line therapy	–
Metzger et al.[49]	MTX for CS-resistant DM/PM Initial dose 10–15 mg/wk, raised to 30–50 mg/wk (IV or IM)	Retrospective analysis of 22 patients (13 DM, 9 PM)	17/22 had improvement in strength or cutaneous lesions Steroid-sparing	Minor, reversible toxicity
Al-Mayouf et al.[50]	IV MP with MTX MTX given early v late	6 JDM in each group	0/6 v 2/6 developed calcinosis	Small trial
Fisher et al.[51]	CS and MTX for JDM	Retrospective analysis of open-label experience in 35 patients	Mild calcinosis in 5 patients	Calcinosis associated with longer time to diagnosis, longer duration of elevated muscle enzymes and longer disease duration

(Continued)

Table 46.2 *(Continued)*

Agent/study	Treatments compared/studied	Type of study	Outcome	Comment(s)
Bunch *et al.*[52]	Prednisone 60 mg/d plus AZA 2 mg/kg/d *v* prednisone plus placebo	3 month DB-PC trial 16 patients with PM	No significant differences	–
Bunch[53]	Long-term follow up of previous study	Unblinded continuance for 3 years	Significant benefit in AZA group	Often 8 weeks before affect of immunosuppressive agent noted
Villalba *et al.*[54]	Oral weekly MTX and daily AZA *v* IV MTX with leucovorin rescue	Randomised, open-label crossover study 18 PM and 11 DM	ITT analysis showed trend in favour of oral combination	Toxicity slightly more common in IV group
Joffe *et al.*[55]	Prednisone, MTX or AZA analysed	Retrospective analysis: 113 patients with a variety of types of IIM	All agents effective in some patients Advantage of AZA *v* MTX could not be determined	Certain subsets of patients respond less well: IBM, those with MSAs PM responds less well than DM, some patients crossed over from AZA to MTX and vice versa; equal numbers responded to each agent
Ramirez *et al.*[56]	Prednisone initially in 23. AZA (23), MTX (4), CYT (7), TBI (1)	Retrospective analysis of 25 patients with DM (17) or PM (1) or overlap (6) or PM with Ca (1)	15/22 treated with AZA and prednisone had excellent response 1 with prednisone alone and one with no treatment responded	Stepwise approach to treatment with prednisone and early AZA then other immunosuppressive if there is failure suggested
Tausche and Meurer[57]	MMF alone or with IVIG	Open-label 4 patients	Three-quarters improved	One patient had cancer-associated DM
Sinoway and Callen[58]	Chlorambucil for DM	Open-label 5 patients	Steroid sparing	Assessment of myositis primarily
Adams *et al.*[59]	Fludarabine 20 mg/m²/for 3 days per month for 6 months recalcitrant PM or DM	Open-label 7 PM, 9 DM patients	Improved: 4 Unchanged: 7 Failures: 5	A subset of patients respond to this agent

(Continued)

Table 46.2 (*Continued*)

Agent/study	Treatments compared/studied	Type of study	Outcome	Comment(s)
Heckmatt et al.[60]	CYA for JDM (2·5–7·5 mg/kg/d)	Open-label, retrospective analysis of 14 patients	All had a lower steroid dose, and increased strength	AZA failed in 10 patients
Qushmaq et al.[61]	CYA mean dose 3·5 mg/kg/d	Retrospective analysis of 6 patients (4 PM, 2 DM)	Steroid sparing	No controls
Vencovsky et al.[62]	CYA 3–3·5 mg/kg/d v MTX 7·5–15 mg/wk with folic acid	Randomised, but not masked Mixture of PM and DM patients	Improvement equal Steroid sparing	Analysis of reports in the literature Small group Mixture of patients
Plasmapheresis				
Dau[63]	Plasmapheresis with prednisone and CYT or chlorambucil: 15 PM, 11 DM, 7 SDM, 1 each with RA or SS and myositis	Open-label retrospective analysis of 35 patients with disease recalcitrant to prednisone and various immunosuppressive agents	Increased strength in 32 patients No comment on effect on skin disease	All patients received the procedure and drugs that might be expected to be effective without pheresis
Miller et al.[64]	Plasma exchange or leukapheresis v placebo	RCT of 39 patients with PM/DM	Equal effect to sham pheresis	Prior open-label trails had been positive
Cherin et al.[65]	Plasma exchange	Retrospective, multicentre analysis of 24 PM and 33 DM patients in France	Significant improvement in acute myopathy only	PE given with albumin replacement in this study Must be combined with an immunosuppressive agent
IVIG				
Cherin et al.[66]	IVIG for PM/DM 1 g/kg/d for 2 days each month (n = 3) or 0·4 g/kg/d for 5 days each month (n = 7)	Open-label of 14 PM and 6 DM patients	Statistically significant improvement in strength and decrease in dose of steroids in 15 patients	Toxicity in 4 patients consisted of fever, sweating, headaches, delirium or vomiting
Dalakas et al.[67]	IVIG v placebo for 3–6 months	DB-PC trial with crossover of 15 patients with DM	Statistically significant benefit for IVIG	Skin disease, strength, muscle biopsy improved

(*Continued*)

Table 46.2 (*Continued*)

Agent/study	Treatments compared/studied	Type of study	Outcome	Comment(s)
Al-Mayouf et al.[68]	IVIG for JDM	Open label 18 JDM patients	Steroid sparing	Small trial Multiple regimens used
Gottfried et al.[69]	IVIG for DM	Open-label trial of 19 patients (4 with cancer)	7 responders Non-responders had severe skin and muscle disease, presence of MSA or cancer	IVIG monotherapy in some patients, used after immunosuppressive agents in some and with immunosuppressive in some sIL-2R levels decreased with response
Miscellaneous				
Hollingsworth et al.[70]	"Intensive immunosuppression" Initial phase ALG: 15 daily infusions of 750 mg, plus prednisone 150 mg/d tapering to 20 mg/d over 10 days and AZA 2·5 mg/kg/d (max. 150 mg) Maintenance phase: AZA and prednisone adjusted to disease activity	Open-label study of 12 patients	9/12 improved	Mixed group of patients included, including perhaps 3 with malignancy Toxicity was common
Treatments of cutaneous disease of DM				
Woo et al.[71]	Hydroxychloroquine for cutaneous lesions of DM	Retrospective, multicentre analysis of 7 patients	Steroid sparing in 2 patients. CR in 3 patients	No toxicity noted in these patients
Zieglschmid-Adams et al.[72]	MTX for DM (7) or ADM (3), initial dose 7·5 or 9·2 mg/wk raised to 14·2 or 20 mg/wk for DM or ADM	Retrospective analysis	9/10 had improvement of skin disease	Mild, reversible toxicity in 7 patients Liver biopsy in 4 patients, 2 had hepatic fibrosis (grade IIIA)

(*Continued*)

Table 46.2 *(Continued)*

Agent/study	Treatments compared/studied	Type of study	Outcome	Comment(s)
Kasteler and Callen[73]	MTX for DM Eventual dose 2.5–30 mg/wk	Retrospective analysis 13 patients	CR – 4 PR – 9 Steroid-sparing	Minimal toxicity
Gelber et al.[74]	MMF for recalcitrant DM	Open label 4 patients	Steroid sparing	–

ALG, antilymphocyte globulin; ADM, amyopathic dermatomyositis; AZA, azathioprine; CA, Calcium; CCS, clinical case series; CR, complete response; CS, corticosteroids; CYA, ciclosporin; CYT, cyclophosphamide; DB-PC, double-blind, placebo-controlled; DM, dermatomyositis; IBM, inclusion body myositis; IIM, idiopathic inflammatory myopathy; ITT, intention-to-treat; JDM, juvenile dermatomyositis; MSA, myositis-specific antibodies; OCS, oral CS; IM, intramuscular; IV, intravenous; IVCS, intravenous corticosteroids; IVIG, intravenous immunoglobulin; MMF, mycophenolate mofetil; MP, methylprednisolone; MTX, methotrexate; PM, polymyositis; RCT, randomised controlled trial; RA, rheumatoid arthritis; SDM, sclerodermatomyositis; SIL-2R, soluble interluekin-2 receptor; SS, Sjogren's syndrome; PR, partial response; TBI, total body irradiation case series suggest that the use of early "aggressive" therapy will limit the possibility of calcinosis. However, there are no studies that clearly demonstrate the veracity of this statement. Klein-Gitleman et al.[47] believe that high-dose, intravenous pulsed methylprednisolone limits the risk and severity of calcinosis. However, adequate RCTs have not yet corroborated this belief. It does appear that whatever the treatment, combination with physical therapy will prevent contractures from developing and that even if contractures occur, the use of physical therapy might improve the long-term disability. Once established, calcinosis may resolve spontaneously after a period of months to years; however, there are multiple individual case reports and some small series suggesting that various therapies, including warfarin, diltiazem and probenecid, are effective in reversing the calcinosis.

References

1. Callen JP. Dermatomyositis. Lancet 2000;355:53–7.

2. Plotz PH, Rider LG, Targoff IN, Raben N, O'Hanlon TP, Miller FW. NIH conference. Myositis: immunologic contributions to understanding cause, pathogenesis, and therapy. Ann Intern Med 1995;122:715–24.

3. Targoff IN. Dermatomyositis and polymyositis. Curr Prob Dermatol 1991;3:131–80.

4. Bohan AB, Peter JB. Polymyositis and dermatomyositis. N Engl J Med 1975;292:344–7;403–7.

5. Sontheimer RD. Cutaneous features of classic dermatomyositis and amyopathic dermatomyositis. Curr Opin Rheumatol 1999;11:475–82.

6. Sigurgeirsson B, Lindelof B, Edhag O, Allender O. Risk of malignancy in patients with dermatomyositis or polymyositis. N Engl J Med 1992;326:363–7.

7. Airio A, Pukkala E, Isomaki H. Elevated cancer incidence in patients with dermatomyositis: A population based study. J Rheumatol 1995;22:1300–3.

8. Chow WH, Gridley G, Mellemkjaer L, McLaughlin JK, Olsen JH, Fraumeni JF Jr. Cancer risk following polymyositis and dermatomyositis: a nationwide cohort study in Denmark. Cancer Causes Control 1995;6:9–13.

9. Hill CL, Zhang Y, Sigurgeirsson B et al. Frequency of specific cancer types in dermatomyositis and polymyositis: a population-based study. Lancet 2001;357: 96–100.

10. Scaling ST, Kaufman RH, Patten BM. Dermatomyositis and female malignancy. Obstet Gynecol 1979;54:474–7.

11. Cherin P, Piette J-C, Herson S et al. Dermatomyositis and ovarian cancer: A report of 7 cases and literature review. J Rheumatol 1993;20:1897–9.

12. Whitmore SE, Rosenshein NB, Provost TT. Ovarian cancer in patients with dermatomyositis. Medicine 1994;73: 153–60.

13. Buchbinder R, Forbes A, Hall S, Dennett X, Giles G. Incidence of malignant disease in biopsy-proven inflammatory myopathy: a population-based cohort study. Ann Intern Med 2001;134:1087–95.

14. Whitmore SE, Watson R, Rosenshein NB, Provost TT. Dermatomyositis sine myositis: Association with malignancy. J Rheumatol 1996;23:101–5.

15. Fudman EJ, Schnitzer TJ. Dermatomyositis without creatine kinase elevation: A poor prognostic sign. Am J Med 1986;80:329–32.

16. Montagna GL, Manzo C, Califanc E, Tirri R. Absence of elevated creatine kinase in dermatomyositis does not exclude malignancy. Scand J Rheumatol 1988;17:73–4.

17. Feldman D, Hochberg MC, Zizic TM, Stevens MB. Cutaneous vasculitis in adult polymyositis/ dermatomyositis. J Rheumatol 1983;10:85–9.

18. Hunger RE, Durr D, Brand CU. Cutaneous leukocytoclastic vasculitis in dermatomyositis suggests malignancy. Dermatology 2001;202:123–6.

19. Kamel OW, van de Rijn M, Weiss LM et al. Reversible lymphomas associated with Epstein-Barr virus occurring during methotrexate therapy for rheumatoid arthritis and dermatomyositis. N Engl J Med 1993;328:1317–21.

20. Stockton D, Doherty VR, Brewster DH. Risk of cancer in patients with dermatomyositis or polymyositis, and follow-up implications: a Scottish population-based cohort study. Br J Cancer 2001;85:41–5.

21. Manchul LA, Jin A, Pritchard KI et al. The frequency of malignant neoplasms in patients with polymyositis-dermatomyositis: A controlled study. Arch Intern Med 1985;145:1835–9.

22. Lakhanpal S, Bunch TW, Ilstrup DM, Melton LJ III. Polymyositis-dermatomyositis and malignant lesions:

Does an association exist. *Mayo Clin Proc* 1986;**61**:645–54.

23. Lyon MG, Bloch DA, Hollak B, Fries JF. Predisposing factors in polymyositis-dermatomyositis: results of a nationwide survey. *J Rheumatol* 1989;**16**:1218–24.

24. Zantos D, Zhang Y, Felson D. The overall and temporal association of cancer with polymyositis and dermatomyositis. *J Rheumatol* 1994;**21**:1855–9.

25. Marie I, Hatron P-Y, Levesque H *et al.* Influence of age on characteristics of polymyositis and dermatomyositis in adults. *Medicine* 1999;**78**:139–47.

26. Pautas E, Cherin P, Piette J-C *et al.* Features of polymyositis and dermatomyositis in the elderly: A case-control study. *Clin Exp Rheumatol* 2000;**18**:241–4.

27. Chen Y-J, Wu C-Y, Shen J-L. Predicting factors of malignancy in dermatomyositis and polymyositis: a case-control study. *Br J Dermatol* 2001;**144**:825–31.

28. Callen JP, Hyla JF, Boles GG, Kay DR. The relationship of dermatomyositis and polymyositis to internal malignancy. *Arch Dermatol* 1980;**116**:295–8.

29. Tymms KE, Webb J. Dermatopolymyositis and other connective tissue diseases: A review of 105 cases. *J Rheumatol* 1985;**12**:1140–8.

30. Cox NH, Lawrence CM, Langtry JA, Ive FA. Dermatomyositis. Disease associations and an evaluation of screening investigations for malignancy. *Arch Dermatol* 1990;**126**:61–5.

31. Davis MDP, Ahmed I. Ovarian malignancy in patients with dermatomyositis and polymyositis: A retrospective analysis of fourteen cases. *J Rheumatol* 1997;**37**:730–3.

32. Koh ET, Seow A, Ong B, Rattnagopal P, Tjia H, Shng HH. Adult onset polymyositis/dermatomyositis: clinical and laboratory features and treatment response in 75 patients. *Ann Rheum Dis* 1993;**52**:857–61.

33. Maoz CM, Langevitz P, Livneh A *et al.* High incidence of malignancies in patients with dermatomyositis and polymyositis: An 11-year analysis. *Sem Arthritis Rheum* 1998;**27**:319–24.

34. Benbassat J, Gefel D, Larholt K, Sukenik S, Morgenstern V, Zlotnick A. Prognostic factors in polymyositis/dermatomyositis: A computer assisted analysis of ninety-two cases. *Arthritis Rheum* 1985;**28**:249–55.

35. Winkelmann RK, Mulder DW, Lambert EH, Howard FM, Diessner GR. Course of dermatomyositis-polymyositis: Comparison of untreated and cortisone-treated patients. *Mayo Clin Proc* 1968;**43**:545–56.

36. Moss AA, Hanelin LG. Occult malignant tumors in dermatologic disease. *Radiology* 1977;**123**:69–71.

37. Duncan AG, Richardson JB, Klein JB, Targoff IN, Woodcock TM, Callen JP. Clinical, serologic, and immunogenetic studies in patients with dermatomyositis. *Acta Derm Venereol* 1990;**71**:312–16.

38. Bonnetblanc JM, Bernard P, Fayol J. Dermatomyositis and malignancy: a multicenter cooperative study. *Dermatologica* 1990;**180**:212–16.

39. Peng J-C, Sheen T-S, Hsu M-M. Nasopharyngeal carcinoma with dermatomyositis: Analysis of 12 cases. *Arch Otolaryngol Head Neck Surg* 1995;**121**:1298–301.

40. Ang P, Sugeng MW, Chua SH. Classical and amyopathic dermatomyositis seen at the National Skin Centre of Singapore: a 3-year retrospective review of their clinical characteristics and association with malignancy. *Ann Acad Med Singapore* 2000;**29**:219–23.

41. Catoggio LJ. Inflammatory Muscle Disease. Management. In: Klippel JH, Dieppe PA, eds. *Rheumatology, 2nd ed.* London: Mosby, 1998:7.

42. Sontheimer RD. Dermatomyositis. In: Freedberg IM, Eisen AZ, Wolff K, Austen KF, Goldsmith LA, Katz SI, Fitzpatrick TB, ed. *Fitzpatrick's Dermatology in General Medicine, 5th ed.* New York: McGraw-Hill, 1999:2018–20.

43. Rowell NR, Goodfield MJD. The connective tissue diseases. In: Champion RH, Burton JL, Burns DA, Breathnach SM, ed. *Textbook of Dermatology, 6th ed.* Oxford: Blackwell Science, 1998:2564–5.

44. Provost TT, Flynn JA. Dermatomyositis. In: Provost TT, Flynn JA, eds. *Cutaneous Medicine.* Toronto: BC Decker Inc., 2001:82–103.

45. Carpenter JR, Bunch TW, Engel AG, O'Brien PC. Survival in polymyositis. Corticosteroids and risk factors. *J Rheumatol* 1977;**4**:207–14.

46. Uchino M, Araki S, Yoshida O, Uekawa K, Nagata J. High single-dose alternate day corticosteroid regimens in treatment of polymyositis. *J Neurol* 1985;**232**:175–8.

47. Klein-Gitleman MS, Waters T, Pachman LM. The economic impact of intermittent high-dose intravenous

versus oral corticosteroid treatment of juvenile dermatomyositis. *Arthritis Care Res* 2000;**13**:360–8.

48. Mosca M, Neri R, Pasero G, Bombardieri S. Treatment of the idiopathic inflammatory myopathies: A retrospective analysis of 63 Caucasian patients longitudinally followed at a single center. *Clin Exp Rheumatol* 2000;**18**:451–6.

49. Metzger AL, Bohan A, Goldberg LS, Bluestone R, Pearson SM. Polymyositis and dermatomyositis: Combined methotrexate and corticosteroid therapy. *Ann Intern Med* 1974;**81**:182–9.

50. Al-Mayouf SM, Laxer RM, Schneider R, Silverman ED, Feldman BM. Intravenous immunoglobulin therapy for juvenile dermatomyositis: efficacy and safety. *J Rheumatol* 2000;**27**:2498–503.

51. Fisher RE, Liang MG, Fuhlbrigge RC, Yalçındag A, Sundel RP. Aggressive management of juvenile dermatomyositis results in improved outcome and decreased incidence of calcinosis. *J Am Acad Dermatol* 2002;**47**:505–11.

52. Bunch TW, Worthington JW, Combs JJ, Ilstrup DM, Engel AG. Azathioprine and prednisone for polymyositis: A controlled, clinical trial. *Arthritis Rheum* 1980;**92**:365–9.

53. Bunch TW. Prednisone and azathioprine for polymyositis: Long-term follow-up. *Arthritis Rheum* 1981;**24**:45–8.

54. Villalba L, Hicks JE, Adams EM *et al.* Treatment of refractory myositis: a randomized crossover study of two new cytotoxic regimens. *Arthritis Rheum* 1998;**41**:392–9.

55. Joffe MM, Love LA, Leff RL *et al.* Drug therapy of the idiopathic inflammatory myopathies: predictors of response to prednisone, azathioprine, and methotrexate and a comparison of their efficacy. *Am J Med* 1993;**94**:379–87.

56. Ramirez G, Asherson RA, Khamashta MA, Cervera R, D'Cruz D, Hughes GRV. Adult-onset polymyositis-dermatomyositis: Description of 25 patients with emphasis on treatment. *Sem Arthritis Rheum* 1990;**20**:114–20.

57. Tausche AK, Meurer M. Mycophenolate mofetil for dermatomyositis. *Dermatology* 2001;**202**:341–3.

58. Sinoway PA, Callen JP. Chlorambucil: An effective corticosteroid-sparing agent for patients with recalcitrant dermatomyositis. *Arthritis Rheum* 1993;**36**:319–28.

59. Adams EM, Pucino F, Yarboro C *et al.* A pilot study: Use of fludarabine for refractory dermatomyositis and

polymyositis, and examination of endpoint measures. *J Rheumatol* 1999;**26**:352–60.

60. Heckmatt J, Saunders C, Peters AM *et al.* Cyclosporine in juvenile dermatomyositis. *Lancet* 1989;i(8646):1063–6.

61. Qushmaq KA, Chalmers A, Esdaile JM. Cyclosporin A in the treatment of refractory adult polymyositis/dermatomyositis: Population based experience in 6 patients with literature review. *J Rheumatol* 2000;**27**:2855–9.

62. Vencovsky J, Jarosova K, Machacek S *et al.* Cyclosporine A versus methotrexate in the treatment of polymyositis and dermatomyositis. *Scand J Rheumatol* 2000;**29**:95–102.

63. Dau PC. Plasmapheresis in idiopathic inflammatory myopathy: experience with 35 patients. *Arch Neurol* 1981;**38**:544–52.

64. Miller FW, Leitman SF, Cronin ME *et al.* Controlled trial of plasma exchange and leukapheresis in polymyositis and dermatomyositis. *N Engl J Med* 1992;**326**:1380–4.

65. Cherin P, Auperin I, Bussel A, Pourrat J, Herson S. Plasma exchange in polymyositis and dermatomyositis: A multicenter study of 57 cases. *Clin Exp Rheumatol* 1995;**13**:270–1.

66. Cherin P, Herson D, Wechsler B *et al.* Efficacy of intravenous gammaglobulin therapy in chronic refractory polymyositis and dermatomyositis: An open study with 20 adult patients. *Am J Med* 1991;**91**:162–8.

67. Dalakas MC, Illa I, Dambrosia JM *et al.* A controlled trial of high-dose intravenous immune globulin infusions as treatment for dermatomyositis. *N Engl J Med* 1993;**329**:1993–2000.

68. Al-Mayouf S, Al-Mazyed A, Bahabri S. Efficacy of early treatment of severe juvenile dermatomyositis with intravenous methylprednisolone and methotrexate. *Clin Rheumatol* 2000;**19**:138–41.

69. Gottfreid I, Seeber A, Anegg B, Rieger A, Stingl G, Volc-Platzer B. High dose intravenous immunoglobulin (IVIG) in dermatomyositis: clinical responses and effect on sIL-2R levels. *Eur J Dermatol* 2000;**10**:29–35.

70. Hollingsworth P, Tyndall ADV, Ansell BM *et al.* Intensive immunosuppression versus prednisolone in the treatment

of connective tissue diseases. *Ann Rheum Dis* 1982;**41**:557–62.

71. Woo TY, Callen JP, Voorhees JJ, Bickers DB, Hanno R, Hawkins C. Cutaneous lesions of dermatomyositis are improved by hydroxychloroquine. *J Am Acad Dermatol* 1984;**10**:592–600.

72. Zieglschmid-Adams ME, Pandya AG, Cohen SB, Sontheimer RD. Treatment of dermatomyositis with methotrexate. *J Am Acad Dermatol* 1995;**32**:754–7.

73. Kasteler JS, Callen JP. Low-dose methotrexate administered weekly is an effective corticosteroid-sparing agent for the treatment of cutaneous lesions of dermatomyositis. *J Am Acad Dermatol* 1997;**36**: 67–71.

74. Gelber AC, Nousari HC, Wigley FM. Mycophenolate mofetil in the treatment of severe skin manifestations of dermatomyositis: a series of 4 cases. *J Rheumatol* 2000;**27**:1542–5.

47

Bullous pemphigoid

Maria Roest, Vanessa Venning, Nonhlanhla Khumalo, Gudula Kirtschig and Fenella Wojnarowska

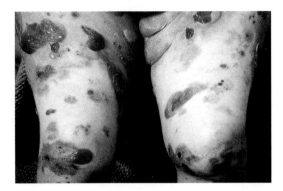

Figure 47.1 Crusted erosions and large haemorrhagic bullae

Background
Definition

Bullous pemphigoid (BP) is an acquired non-scarring autoimmune subepidermal bullous disease characterised by tense blisters. Circulating IgG autoantibodies (rarely IgA and IgE) bind to BP230 and BP180 antigens, which are components of the hemidesmosome adhesion complex found in the basement membrane zone of the skin. Direct antibody and antigen interaction, local activation of complement and release of cytokines lead to loss of dermoepidermal adherence and formation of subepidermal blisters.[1] Blistering typically occurs on the flexures although BP may be generalised or localised to one site such as the lower legs. Erosions and blisters occur on the mucous membranes, particularly the mouth, in about 50% of cases. Blister formation may be preceded by pruritus or an urticarial or eczematous rash, which may precede the blistering rash for many months.

Incidence/prevalence

BP is the most common autoimmune blistering disease in the West, with an estimated incidence of 6–7 cases per million population per year in France and Germany.[2,3] It tends to affect the elderly and there is no sex preponderance.

Aetiology

No clear aetiological factors have been identified. There are anecdotal reports of BP being preceded by local cutaneous trauma such as surgery and exposure to ionising or ultraviolet radiation. BP has been reported in association with malignancies, although most large studies have concluded that there is no increased risk of malignancy in patients with BP in western countries compared with controls.[4]

Prognosis

The majority of patients with BP will have disease remission within 5 years.[5] Both treated and untreated BP shows a chronic relapsing course.

Aims of treatment

The aims of treatment are to achieve short-term healing of skin and mucous membrane lesions, longer term disease remission, and to improve quality of life with minimal adverse effects of treatment.

Outcomes

- rate of healing of blisters and suppression of new blister formation
- effect on quality of life
- duration of remission after stopping treatment
- complications of disease
- adverse effects of treatment, including mortality

Methods of search

Randomised controlled trials (RCTs) were identified from searches of Medline and Embase up to I January 2001. All RCTs on interventions for BP confirmed by immunofluorescence studies were included.

QUESTIONS

What are the effects of corticosteroids?

A systematic review of treatments for BP[6] identified only six RCTs, with a total of 293 patients.

Topical corticosteroids
Benefits

We found one RCT published in abstract form[7] with few clinical details. Three small open-label uncontrolled studies ≤20 subjects each[8-10] demonstrated that potent topical steroids produced suppression and healing of blisters with low relapse rates in patients with localised and mild disease, although follow up periods were variable.

Harms

Skin infection, skin atrophy and evidence of systemic absorption was noted by Zimmermann et al.[8]

Comment

Although evidence is limited, the relatively few side-effects associated with topical corticosteroids would support their use as first-line agents in localised and mild BP.

Systemic corticosteroids
Benefits

Two small RCTs looked at the effects of systemic corticosteroids alone. We found no RCTs comparing systemic corticosteroids with placebo. One trial compared biologically equivalent doses of different corticosteroids: methylprednisolone, 1·17 mg/kg/day, and prednisolone methylsulphobenzoate, 1·16 mg/kg/day.[11] Another trial compared different doses of prednisolone: 0·75 mg/kg/day with 1·25 mg/kg/day.[12] Both trials found no statistical difference in effectiveness of treatment.

Harms

Higher doses of prednisolone were associated with more side-effects, including infection, hepatic and renal impairment, cerebrovascular accident, hypertension, heart failure and death.

Comment

Systemic corticosteroids are considered standard treatment for BP, although only a few small non-controlled trials have been carried out. Higher doses of corticosteroids are associated with increased morbidity and mortality.

Does combination treatment offer any advantage over corticosteroid monotherapy?

Benefits

We found three non-blinded RCTs. Burton et al.[13] compared prednisolone, 30–80 mg/day, alone and in combination with azathioprine, 2·5 mg/kg/day. The addition of azathioprine resulted in a 45% reduction in prednisolone dose over a 3-year period.[13] Roujeau et al. compared prednisolone, 0·3 mg/kg/day, alone and in combination with plasma exchange. They found that less than half the total prednisolone dose was required in the plasma exchange group.[14] Disease control was achieved within weeks in both groups – in the plasma exchange group with a mean ± SD dose of 0·52 ± 0·28 mg/kg/day and in the prednisolone-only group with 0·97 ± 0·33 mg/kg/day. Guillaume *et al.* compared prednisolone 1 mg/kg/day alone or in combination with either azathioprine (100 mg for body weight <60 kg and 150 mg for body weight <60 kg) or plasma exchange.[15] This trial failed to confirm any benefit of combination therapy over prednisolone alone.

Harms

The addition of azathioprine and/or plasma exchange did not increase the incidence of side-effects; in fact, similar side-effect profiles were seen in the studies of Burton *et al.*[13] and Roujeau *et al.*[14] Guillaime *et al.* commented that most side-effects could be attributed to corticosteroids, but details were not supplied.

Comment

In the study by Burton *et al.*[13] there was no definition of "disease control" and little clinical data were available, although patients were followed up for 3 years. We noted that the decision to include patients in this trial was made by the consultant after prednisolone had been started to suppress new blisters. The plasma exchange trial[15] excluded patients over 80 years of age. Low doses of prednisolone (0·3 mg/kg/day) were used in both treatment groups although, on average, higher doses were required to achieve disease control. With the current available evidence the value of combination treatment remains doubtful.

Are antimicrobials useful?

Benefits

One (non-placebo) RCT compared prednisolone, 40–80 mg/day, alone with tetracycline, 2 g/day in four divided doses, plus nicotinamide, 1500 mg/day in three divided doses.[16] This trial suggested no statistically significant difference in treatment response between the two groups.

Harms

More serious side-effects (including death due to sepsis) were noted in the prednisolone group. One patient with established renal impairment in the tetracycline/nicotinamide group developed acute tubular necrosis, although concomitant medications included aspirin and ibuprofen.

Comments

This was a small trial of 18 patients, with an unclear method of randomisation and a high dropout rate. At 10 months three patients remained in the steroid group and five in the tetracycline group.

Key points

- Few RCTs on systematic review of treatments for BP were identified.
- The available evidence is inadequate to allow confident recommendation of optimal treatment.
- A less aggressive approach to therapy with low doses of corticosteroids may be sufficient for disease control and appears to be associated with less morbidity and mortality.
- Tetracyclines and nicotinamide may be effective but larger trials are needed to compare this therapy with low-dose prednisolone.
- The benefits of azathioprine and plasma exchange are difficult to assess.

Additional chapters on Cicatrical pemphigoid and Epidermolysis bullosa acquisita by Maria Roest are published on the book website http://www.evidbasedderm.com.

References

1. Sams WM Jr, Gammon WR. Mechanism of lesion production in pemphigus and pemphigoid. *J Am Acad Dermatol* 1982;**6**:431–52.

2. Bernard P, Vaillant L, Labeille B *et al*. Incidence and distribution of subepidermal autoimmune bullous diseases in three French regions. *Arch Dermatol* 1995;**131**:48–52.

3. Zillikens D, Wever S, Roth A *et al*. Incidence of autoimmune subepidermal blistering dermatoses in a region of Central Germany. *Arch Dermatol* 1995;**131**:957–8.

4. Venning VA, Wojnarowska F. The association of bullous pemphigoid and malignant disease: a case control study. *Br J Dermatol* 1990;**123**:439–45.

5. Venning V, Wojnarowska F. Lack of predictive factors for the course of bullous pemphigoid. *J Am Acad Dermatol* 1992;**26**:585–9.

6. Khumalo NP, Murrell DF, Wojnarowska F, Kirtschig G. A systematic review of treatments for bullous pemphigoid. *Arch Dermatol* 2002;**138**:385–9.

7. Bernard P. Bullous pemphigoid (BP): Topical or systemic treatment? (Abstract). *J Eur Acad Dermatol Venereol* 2000;**14**:8.

8. Zimmerman R, Faure M, Claudy A. Prospective study of treatment of bullous pemphigoid by a class I topical corticosteroid (see comments). *Ann Dermatol Venereol* 1999;**126**:13–16.

9. Westerhof W. Treatment of bullous pemphigoid with topical clobetasol propionate. *J Am Acad Dermatol* 1989;**20**:458–61.

10. Muramatsu T, Iida T, Shirai T. Pemphigoid and pemphigus foliaceous successfully treated with topical steroids. *J Dermatol* 1996;**23**:683–8.

11. Dreno B, Sassolas B, Lacour P *et al*. Methylprednisolone versus prednisolone methylsulphobenzoate in pemphigoid: a comparative multicenter study. *Ann Dermatol Venereol* 1993;**120**:518–21.

12. Morel P, Guillaime JC. Treatment of bullous pemphigoid with prednisolone only: 0·75mg/kg/day versus 1·25mg/kg/day. A multicenter randomised study. *Ann Dermatol Venereol* 1984;**111**:925–8.

13. Burton JL, Harman RR, Peachey RD, Warin RP. Azathioprine plus prednisolone in treatment of pemphigoid. *BMJ* 1978;**2**:1190–1.

14. Roujeau JC, Guillaume JC, Morel P *et al*. Plasma exchange in bullous pemphigoid. *Lancet* 1984;**2**:486–8.

15. Guillaume J-C, Vaillant L, Bernard P *et al*. Controlled trial of azathioprine and plasma exchange in addition to prednisolone in the treatment of bullous pemphigoid. *Arch Dermatol* 1993;**129**:49–53.

16. Fivenson D, Breneman D, Rosen G, *et al*. Nicotinamide and tetracycline therapy of bullous pemphigoid. *Arch Dermatol* 1994;**130**:753–8.

48
Pemphigus
Brain R Sperber and Victoria P Werth

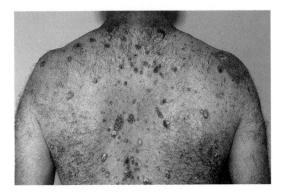

Figure 48.1   Patient with extensive erosions and flaccid bullae due to pemphigus vulgaris

Background
Definition

Pemphigus is an intra-epidermal autoimmune blistering disease involving the skin and mucous membranes. Pemphigus is conventionally divided into three distinct subtypes: pemphigus vulgaris, pemphigus foliaceus and paraneoplastic pemphigus. Pemphigus vulgaris is characterised by oral lesions and blistering skin lesions whereas patients with pemphigus foliaceus have only skin lesions with characteristic scaling. Patients with paraneoplastic pemphigus have painful oral lesions, conjunctival reactions and a widespread erythematous, sometimes blistering, skin eruption.

In this chapter we will exclusively address pemphigus vulgaris and foliaceus, except in the discussion of studies that included paraneoplastic pemphigus patients before it was recognised as a distinct clinicopathological entity, and was thus not distinguished from other forms of pemphigus.

Incidence/prevalence

The incidence of pemphigus ranges from approximately 1 per 1 000 000 to 1 per 100 000, depending on the population in question.[1] For instance, in regions with many Jewish residents or residents of Mediterranean origin, the incidence of pemphigus is estimated to be much higher than in regions with few people from these ethnic groups.[1]

Aetiology

As is the case with other autoimmune diseases, the exact pathophysiological mechanism that causes immune dysregulation in pemphigus is unknown. Pemphigus is a T-cell driven autoantibody-mediated disease, with T cells reacting to specific antigenic adhesion proteins in the skin. The production of autoantibodies to intercellular proteins in the epidermis, along with various inflammatory mediators, is believed to directly elicit acantholysis. The clinical phenotype of pemphigus is defined by the specific profile of intercellular autoantibodies. Patients with mucosal-dominant pemphigus vulgaris have only antidesmoglein 3 IgG autoantibodies. Patients with mucocutaneous pemphigus vulgaris have both antidesmoglein 3 and antidesmoglein 1 autoantibodies. Patients with pemphigus foliaceus, who have only skin lesions, have antidesmoglein 1 antibodies.[1]

Prognosis

The mortality of pemphigus decreased dramatically after corticosteroids were introduced as therapy in the 1950s. Before that time, mortality was approximately 70%[2] and usually resulted from sepsis. With corticosteroids and adjuvant therapy, mortality is now approximately 6%,[3] with most of the deaths related to side-effects of therapy.

Diagnosis

Diagnosis is based on three measures:

1. Clinical features – oral ulcers, flaccid blisters or erosions or scale
2. Histological features – acantholysis with loss of coherence between epidermal cells; upward growth of papillae lined by a single layer of epidermal cells
3. Direct and indirect immunofluorescence – detection of autoantibodies either in a biopsy specimen (direct) or in the patient's serum (indirect). The enzyme-linked immunosorbent assay (ELISA) is a new diagnostic modality that may prove to be effective for diagnosis as well as functioning as a prognostic indicator.

Aims of treatment

The main aims of treatment in pemphigus are to prevent or reduce new blister formation and promote the healing of old lesions whilst minimising the side-effects of treatment.

Relevant outcomes

Relevant outcome measures include the prevention of new blister formation, the healing of old lesions and a reduction in dose, or cessation, of treatment. Because there is no single definition of remission in the literature, for the purposes of this evaluation we will define a partial remission as a given period of time during which the patient is free of all lesions, and a complete remission as being free of all lesions and receiving no systemic therapy.

QUESTIONS

Is there an optimal initial dosing strategy for oral prednisolone that effectively controls disease progression in patients newly diagnosed with moderate-to-severe pemphigus?

Corticosteroids have been used extensively for the treatment of pemphigus, and are the mainstay of therapy. Many case series were published from the 1950s through the 1970s, and the results of a single randomised controlled trial (RCT) appeared in 1990. In the only RCT to address steroid dosing regimens, Ratnam *et al.* compared the efficacy of different prednisolone doses with respect to adequacy of disease control and side-effects.[4] Twenty-two previously untreated patients with severe disease (>50% of body surface area affected) were treated with either "high-dose" (120–150 mg/day) (n = 11) or "low-dose" (30–60 mg/day) (n = 11) prednisolone. Patients also received adjuvant therapy once formation of new blisters ceased. Patients were followed for 5 years. All patients were seronegative for pemphigus autoantibodies after 3 months of treatment (initial titres ranged from 1:40 to 1:160). The groups did not differ significantly in the duration of prednisolone therapy needed before "initial control of disease was achieved" (average 20 days). In addition, there was no significant correlation between duration of disease before treatment and duration of treatment necessary to achieve remission. Two patients in the low-dose regimen and four patients in the high-dose regimen required at least a 15 mg increase in prednisolone dose to control their disease. Although virtually all patients experienced complications, the incidence of complications was similar in the two groups. No deaths were reported in the study. Therefore, this trial suggested that with respect to initial disease control, relapse rate and length of time before relapse, a "high-dose" regimen offered no advantage over a "low-dose" regimen.

Because of the wide variation in disease course among patients, it is possible that the study of Ratnam et al.[4] simply had too few patients to demonstrate a statistically significant difference between the two dosing regimens. In addition, it is difficult to understand why, if the low-dose regimen can control severe disease as effectively as high-dose therapy, some of the patients on the high-dose regimen required an increase in the dose of steroid. If an initial daily dose of 30–60 mg prednisolone effectively controls the condition in one experimental group, why would 120 mg be insufficient? In support of this study, others have noted that most patients' disease could be controlled with moderate doses of prednisolone. Hirone[5] demonstrated that 56 of 64 patients (88%) with pemphigus, treated between 1970 and 1974, achieved control with initial daily doses of prednisone of 100 mg or less. Rates of remission in the series were not analysed, but overall mortality was only 8%. In a case series by Block et al.,[6] initial control of disease was achieved in 11 of 13 patients with 80–120 mg of prednisone per day. Mortality was 7·6%.

Previous studies also addressed the issue of the optimal initial dose of steroid. In response to the belief that mortality was often associated with undertreatment, Lever and White[7] suggested that "beginning with a too high daily dose [of prednisone] was preferable to beginning with too low a dose". In a case series of 32 patients with pemphigus vulgaris, treated between 1950 and 1959, each patient was given 180 mg prednisone daily for 6–8 weeks.[7] If a patient's condition did not improve rapidly, the dose was increased, often doubled. The mortality rate was 19%. Eight patients (25%) experienced a period of at least 2 months during which they were free of lesions and without therapy. It is not clear how long it took patients to achieve a disease-free state. Virtually all patients experienced serious side-effects from long-term use of corticosteroids.

In studies that attempted to follow the guidelines of Lever and White,[7] adverse effects of corticosteroids were often the major cause of death. Ryan[8] reported a mortality rate of 45% in 45 patients with pemphigus vulgaris treated between 1949 and 1969. In a large series of 107 consecutive cases of pemphigus seen between 1949 and 1970, Rosenberg et al.[9] found that deaths from corticosteroid complications were more frequent than deaths from uncontrolled pemphigus. Thus, Lever and Schaumburg-Lever[10] modified their earlier recommendation of rigid adherence to high-dose steroids for all patients, and suggested a two-tiered approach. Those patients "in the early, stable stage", presumably patients with mild disease, were treated with prednisone 40 mg daily in combination with an immunosuppressant. Patients with moderate or severe disease were still treated with high initial doses of prednisone (180 mg or higher). Using this approach in 63 patients with pemphigus vulgaris, treated between 1961 and 1975, mortality was 9%. Thirty-five per cent of patients experienced a complete remission during the study.[10] Therefore, compared with the previous study by Lever and White,[7] mortality and remission improved with the stratified approach.

While investigators were determining optimal steroid dosing regimens in the early 1970s, the first studies were being conducted on adjuvant therapy for the treatment of pemphigus. The rationale for adjuvant therapy was to employ a second therapeutic agent in an attempt to reduce the overall steroid dose. In some respects, this was unfortunate in that it confounded attempts to interpret the results of a new steroid regimen because it was not clear whether observed clinical benefits were the result of improved steroid dosing or the adjuvant therapy. In addition, it is not clear how the outcome was influenced by improvements in the management of the complications of steroid treatment that had occurred since earlier studies. Yet, it is evident that the stratification of patients according to disease severity and employing lower doses of steroids for patients with milder disease reduced complications and mortality associated with prolonged high-dose steroid treatment.

In summary, the evidence indicates that most patients achieve control with a daily dose of prednisolone below 100 mg/day. Apart from the study of Ratnam et al.,[4] there is no evidence that one dosing regimen is clearly indicated and effective in all patients. Moreover, there is a lack of studies attempting to identify factors that might aid in determining which patients will require higher doses. The treatment regimens used by many clinicians today originated, in large part, from observations made from the large case series, and from recommendations of the series' authors. The typical treatment regimen for a patient with moderate pemphigus consists of a dose of prednisolone of approximately 1 mg/kg/day. If there is no response in 5–7 days, the dose is increased in increments of 0·25–0·5 mg/kg/day until blistering ceases, complications arise or a dose of 2·0–2·5 mg/kg/day is reached.[3,11] Again, evidence for the efficacy of this specific dosing strategy comes from historical trends in observed rates of mortality and, in later studies, rates of remission, rather than from controlled clinical trials.

Reasons for the lack of controlled clinical trials are multiple. In part, the low incidence of pemphigus makes it difficult to recruit sufficient patients to generate substantial statistical power. A second issue that has hindered the progress of therapy for pemphigus is the lack of universally accepted criteria for assessing disease severity and for defining a remission. Without clear guidelines, therapeutic success will vary dramatically from patient to patient.

Do immunosuppressive drugs (azathioprine, cyclophosphamide, methotrexate, ciclosporin) in addition to corticosteroids reduce mortality and improve the rate of remission in patients with pemphigus vulgaris?

Two RCTs and a number of case series describe the use of immunosuppressive agents in the treatment of pemphigus. We have restricted our evaluation to controlled trials and selected case series (at least five patients) that represent the best available evidence for each treatment. In most studies, there is no direct comparison of corticosteroid treatment with and without immunosuppression, but it is the best evidence to support its use.

Azathioprine

There are no RCTs investigating the use of azathioprine in pemphigus, although it is probably the most commonly used adjuvant agent. The largest case series was reported by Aberer et al.[12] Twenty-nine patients with pemphigus vulgaris were treated with steroid plus azathioprine. Of eight additional patients excluded from the study because of insufficient follow up, two had been switched from azathioprine to cyclophosphamide as a result of inadequate disease control and later dropped out of the study. All patients were treated initially with corticosteroids (80–200 mg daily) plus azathioprine (2–3 mg/kg). Patients were followed for a minimum of 4 years, during which time there was only one (3%) disease- or therapy-related death. Partial remission was induced in all patients. Complete remission of at least 2 months (average 4 years) was achieved in 45% of patients. The duration of treatment needed to achieve either partial or complete remission was not reported. Sixty-six per cent of patients had a relapse, which the authors ascribed to too rapid a reduction in drug dose.

In another case series, Lever and Schaumburg-Lever[13] treated 21 patients with pemphigus vulgaris initially with one of two steroid regimens plus azathioprine. Thirteen patients with milder disease received prednisone 40 mg every other day plus azathioprine 100 mg daily. Eight patients with more severe disease initially received high-dose corticosteroid (200–400 mg/day) for 5–10 weeks, followed by tapering of the steroid and initiation of the combined regimen described above for patients with mild disease. Overall, no deaths occurred between 1976 and 1981, and complete remission was induced in 12 patients (57%). The duration of treatment required to achieve remission was not reported. Five patients had relapses, all of which were reportedly mild and were sensitive to either combined therapy or steroid alone.

Five earlier case series also reported no deaths using azathioprine, but reported lower rates of remission than the series summarised above.[12,13] The range in results may reflect the small number of patients in individual studies, and highlights the lack of reliability of the available data and the need for controlled studies. The higher rates of remission in more recent studies may reflect improved management of issues unrelated to azathioprine, such as improved management of steroid dosing regimens and complications resulting from therapy.

Cyclosphosphamide

Cyclophosphamide is another adjuvant drug often used in the treatment of pemphigus. A single small RCT and a few case series report on the use of cyclophosphamide in pemphigus vulgaris. Although there are a few reports of successful treatment with cyclophosphamide monotherapy, the most substantive evidence in support of its use comes from studies in which cyclophosphamide is used in combination with corticosteroids. Chrysomallis et al.[14] studied 28 patients with newly diagnosed pemphigus vulgaris restricted to the oral cavity. Patients were randomly allocated to treatment with prednisone equivalent 40 mg daily (n = 10) alone or in combination with either cyclophosphamide 100 mg/day (n = 10), or ciclosporin 5 mg/day (n = 8). All patients were followed for 5 years. There was no significant difference in the duration of treatment required to achieve partial remission or in the relapse rate in the three groups. All patients achieved partial remission within 40 days, and no patient died in the study. The incidence of complete remission in each group was not reported. The incidence of complications was higher with combination treatments.

In one of the largest case series, Piamphongsant[15] described 12 patients (six with pemphigus vulgaris and six with pemphigus foliaceus) treated with corticosteroid plus oral cyclophosphamide. Patients received an initial dose of prednisone of either 60 or 120 mg/day depending on disease severity. After 2 weeks, all patients were started on cyclophosphamide 100 mg daily. Each month both prednisone and cyclophosphamide were gradually tapered. Three patients (25%) achieved complete remission of at least a year after 2 years of therapy. All other patients achieved partial remission and at the time of publication were on a "maintenance dose" of prednisone <15 mg/day plus cyclophosphamide 50 mg on alternate days or once a week. There were no serious complications from cyclophosphamide therapy.

Block et al.[6] reported a series of 13 patients with "moderate-to-severe" pemphigus vulgaris treated with prednisone plus cyclophosphamide. Initially, patients were given prednisone alone until "control of acute generalised lesions was achieved". At that time, cyclophosphamide (dosage unspecified) was added. It is not clear how long patients were treated with prednisone before disease control was achieved, and rates of remission were not mentioned. There was one treatment-related death. Otherwise, side-effects were not addressed.

Pulse intravenous cyclophosphamide is a relatively recent use of cyclophosphamide in pemphigus. Because pulse cyclophosphamide has been shown in randomised trials to be more effective than oral cyclophosphamide in treating lupus nephritis[16,17] and autoimmune thrombocytopenic purpura,[18] it was anticipated that this mode of therapy might also be effective in treating pemphigus and may minimise the side-effects associated with prolonged daily oral therapy. However, to date no study has directly compared oral and intravenous cyclophosphamide. Three studies of five or more patients have investigated the use of pulse cyclophosphamide in pemphigus. Virtually all patients were simultaneously treated with either pulse or oral corticosteroids. Pasricha et al.[19] have summarised their experience with 300 patients over a 12-year period[20] using intravenous dexamethasone 100 mg on three consecutive days and intravenous cyclophosphamide 500 mg on one day, repeating these pulses every 2–4 weeks. Between pulses, patients received oral cyclophosphamide 50 mg every day and "generally no corticosteroids", although it is not known what percentage of patients received oral corticosteroids. They reported that 190 of the original 300 patients (63%) were in "remission", which was described as "disease-free" and on no medication. The remission lasted over 2 years in 123 patients. At the time of publication, 13 patients (4%) had continuing disease activity through the pulse treatments. It is not known how many pulses (i.e. months of treatment), on average, were required to achieve remission. Sixty-one patients (20%) were lost to follow up, and no other information about them was provided. Of the 12 patients who died during the study period, 11 (4%) died of possible treatment-related

causes. Forty patients relapsed during the study period; no average length of remission before relapse was given. Patients who relapsed were treated again with the pulse regimen. Infections, amenorrhoea, weight gain or loss and alopecia were common side-effects. There was one report of haemorrhagic cystitis.

Kaur and Kanwar[21] used an almost identical regimen of pulse dexamethasone plus cyclophosphamide to treat 50 patients with pemphigus over a course of 2 years. At the time of publication, almost half the patients had improved to some degree, but were still receiving monthly pulse treatments (range 2–15 months of treatment). Another five patients had responded well and were receiving only oral cyclophosphamide 50 mg/day. Six patients "did not respond" and 13 patients were lost to follow up, all of whom had reportedly improved on pulse treatment. Thus no patients achieved complete remission. Three patients (6%) died of septicaemia. Other side-effects reported included cardiac arrhythmias, "frequent" oral candidiasis and hair loss, and amenorrhoea in almost all women treated for at least 6 months. Haemorrhagic cystitis, sterility and avascular necrosis were not seen. It is difficult to know whether the beneficial results in this study and in that by Pasricha et al.[20] were due to cyclophosphamide or pulse steroids.

Fleischli et al.[22] studied the use of pulse cyclophosphamide without concomitant intravenous corticosteroids in nine patients. Monthly pulse treatments consisted of intravenous cyclophosphamide $0.5–1.0$ g/m^2. Between pulse treatments patients received oral cyclophosphamide 50 mg and all but one patient received prednisone (dose not specified). The number of pulses necessary to "control disease" ranged from three to 24. Six patients had an "excellent or good" response, but no objective criteria for this evaluation were described. One patient did not respond to therapy, even after

20 pulse treatments. One patient died of cardiac failure after three pulses, but her disease was reportedly under good control at the time of death.

Methotrexate

No controlled trials have tested the efficacy of methotrexate in pemphigus, but a few case series describe its use. Lever and Schaumburg-Lever[10] treated 20 patients with methotrexate alone or in combination with prednisone. Two of nine patients with mild disease who received methotrexate alone achieved complete remission. Another five patients with mild disease received prednisone plus methotrexate. One patient in this group achieved remission. Yet another treatment group consisted of patients with moderate-to-severe disease, all of whom received high-dose prednisone (>180 mg/day) followed by "maintenance" doses of prednisone plus methotrexate. Three of six patients were free of lesions at the time of publication and two of these three were also off medication. Overall, five of the 20 patients enrolled in the study achieved complete remission. One patient died of sepsis.

Reports of serious side-effects associated with methotrexate have largely precluded its use in pemphigus in recent years. These reports led many investigators to believe that methotrexate predisposed patients to sepsis. However, a recent report by Smith and Bystryn[23] suggested that the increased incidence of infection observed in previous studies may be attributed to higher than necessary doses of methotrexate (>20 mg/week). In a series of nine patients, all of whom had had been treated unsuccessfully with another adjuvant agent, Smith and Bystryn[23] reported that 17·5 mg/week or less was sufficient to induce a disease-free state in six patients, although there is no mention of the duration of methotrexate therapy required to achieve this. In all patients disease activity flared once methotrexate therapy was stopped. Corticosteroid therapy was discontinued once

disease control was achieved. No side-effects were mentioned.

Ciclosporin

Four studies of five or more patients have investigated the use of ciclosporin in the treatment of pemphigus. Ioannides et al.[24] recently published the results of a randomised controlled, but not blinded, trial of 33 patients with newly diagnosed pemphigus vulgaris (n = 29) or pemphigus foliaceus (n = 4). Patients were randomly assigned to treatment with prednisolone (n = 17) or prednisolone plus ciclosporin (n = 16). Both groups were treated with similar initial doses of prednisolone (prednisone equivalent 1 mg/kg), which were increased by 50% every 5–10 days depending on the persistence of disease activity. One group in addition received ciclosporin 5 mg/kg. The patients in each group were similar with respect to baseline clinical characteristics and disease severity. The groups did not differ significantly in any of the variables used to measure response to treatment or in total amount of corticosteroids administered. These variables included time to heal, time to achieve partial and complete remission, and total corticosteroid dose needed to control disease activity, to heal 80% of lesions or to induce partial or complete remission. Complications were more common among patients who received combination therapy. Thus this RCT demonstrated that ciclosporin is no more effective at inducing remission than corticosteroids alone, and is not effective as a corticosteroid-reducing agent.

Similar results were reported in another RCT of ciclosporin use in oral pemphigus.[14] The study consisted of 28 patients with newly diagnosed and confirmed pemphigus vulgaris restricted to the oral cavity. Patients were randomly allocated to treatment with prednisone equivalent 40 mg daily (n = 10) or to the same dose of corticosteroids in combination with either cyclophosphamide 100 mg/day (n = 10), or ciclosporin 5 mg/kg/day (n = 8). All patients were followed for 5 years. The duration of treatment required to achieve remission and the relapse rate did not differ significantly between the three groups. The incidence of complications was higher with combination treatment.

Lapidoth et al.[25] compared 16 patients treated with ciclosporin plus prednisone with a historical control group of 15 patients given prednisone alone. The study and control groups did not differ significantly in the time to healing of old lesions, but the authors claim that ciclosporin significantly shortened the time of new blister formation compared with the prednisone-only group. The mean total cumulative prednisone dose was significantly smaller in the ciclosporin group and the duration of hospitalisation was also shorter in that group than in the prednisone-only group. The two groups did not differ in the mean level of serum antibody titre before or after treatment. Overall more side-effects were reported in the ciclosporin treatment group and two patients treated with ciclosporin had to leave the study because of side-effects. The authors concluded that ciclosporin was more effective than prednisone alone in the treatment of pemphigus vulgaris.

Mobini et al.[26] described six patients with pemphigus vulgaris who were successfully treated with ciclosporin and prednisone. After at least 3 years of previous treatment failure, therapy with ciclosporin plus prednisone led to clearing of "most lesions" by 16–20 weeks. Over the next 1–2 years, ciclosporin was gradually reduced and eventually discontinued in all patients. The duration of follow up was 3.5–5 years and there had been no relapses during that time. The authors report "no serious side-effects", but give no details. They also say that corticosteroids were discontinued during the study, but they do not mention at what point this occurred.

Barthelemy et al.[27] published a small case series of nine patients treated with different regimens of ciclosporin with or without prednisone. None of the four patients treated with ciclosporin alone demonstrated clinical improvement. In four patients who showed no improvement after being treated for 2 months with prednisone, the addition of ciclosporin induced clearing of lesions within 3 weeks, but three of the four patients relapsed within an unspecified period. One patient was treated initially with ciclosporin plus prednisone. She demonstrated early improvement, but the disease worsened when the dose of prednisone was tapered. In all, three of nine patients achieved partial remission that lasted at least 18 months. In the four patients in whom ciclosporin was added after 2 months of prednisone, it is not clear whether the initial observed clinical improvement was the result of ciclosporin therapy or simply the time-dependent effects of continued prednisone treatment.

Overall, it is clear that further controlled studies are necessary to adequately evaluate the effectiveness of immunosuppressive therapy. However, most clinicians favour the early use of an immunosuppressive drug, at least in patients for whom steroid doses cannot be tapered without disease flare and in patients in whom steroids are contraindicated.

It is very difficult to evaluate the effectiveness of immunosuppressive drugs when there have been so few controlled studies. To differentiate the therapeutic benefits of immunosuppressive drugs from those of concurrently administered corticosteroids requires a comparison of clinical course, side-effects and cumulative corticosteroid dose administered to a large number of patients treated with and without immunosuppressive drugs. Unfortunately, no such studies have been performed. The few controlled trials that have been conducted are described above and demonstrate little or no benefit over steroid therapy alone. However, all of the trials are quite small and the patients are often heterogeneous with respect to age, disease severity, disease location and so on. In addition, the data regarding disease outcome and side-effects are often limited. Therefore, the results of the trials may need to be weighed more equally with some of the large case series in which beneficial effects were reported in a substantial percentage of patients.

In addition, it is important to move towards a standardised approach for each study. The methodology used to define previous studies was often incomplete, with omission of critical information such as time between onset of symptoms and treatment, length of previous treatments, or disease severity. Moreover, many investigators fail to stratify patients for other known risk factors that influence prognosis, such as age (older patients die more often and sooner) or type of pemphigus (the prognosis of pemphigus foliaceus is better than for pemphigus vulgaris).[8,28] Finally, a critical aspect of evaluating the effectiveness of immunosuppressive drugs is the comparison of side-effects in patients treated with combination therapy and those treated with corticosteroids alone. Unfortunately, apart from mortality data, this information is often unavailable.

> **Does intravenous pulse corticosteroid reduce morbidity and mortality in patients with severe widespread pemphigus vulgaris that is unresponsive to oral prednisone?**

Initially proposed for the treatment of acute rejection of kidney transplants, pulse corticosteroid therapy is now commonly used to treat a variety of inflammatory and immunological diseases. The treatment is based on the rationale that intravenous delivery of steroid may achieve more rapid control of disease and decrease cumulative steroid dose, thus reducing complications resulting from long-term usage.

One retrospective case-controlled trial and a few small case series are relevant. Werth[29] described 15 patients with pemphigus vulgaris who did not initially respond to prednisone and who were followed for at least 500 days after initiation of treatment. Nine patients received intravenous methylprednisolone 250–1000 mg every 24 hours for 1–5 days. The six patients assigned to the control group were selected on the basis of their similarity to patients in the experimental group except that they did not receive pulse steroid therapy. All patients in both groups received adjunctive therapy. Six (67%) of the nine patients who received pulse therapy improved during the pulse therapy. Four (44%) of the nine patients experienced complete remission lasting, on average, 2 years. None of the six control patients were in remission at the time of publication. In addition, the mean prednisone dose after 1 year of therapy was significantly lower in the pulse therapy group. One patient of the ten who underwent pulse steroid treatment died of candidal sepsis during therapy. Otherwise, patients tolerated pulse steroid therapy with minimal side-effects. Thus, the study suggests that pulse steroid therapy in combination with oral steroid and an immunosuppressive drug is more effective than a similar regimen without pulse steroids at inducing remission and lowering the requirements for oral steroids.

In a small case series of eight patients with severe or recalcitrant pemphigus vulgaris, Chryssomallis et al.[30] reported that all patients achieved partial remission following pulse steroid therapy. The treatment regimen consisted of 6–10 pulses of intravenous methylprednisolone 8–10 mg/kg plus oral prednisone and either azathioprine or cyclophosphamide. The follow up period ranged from 8 to 86 months. All patients achieved partial remission, but none could discontinue medication. Four patients relapsed within 16 months of pulse therapy. One patient died of cardiac arrest and one developed thrombophlebitis. Otherwise, side-effects were minimal.

Pulse steroid therapy has also been combined with pulse cyclophosphamide therapy (for example Pasricha et al.[19,20] – see section on cyclophosphamide). Because those studies lacked controls, and because pulse steroids were combined with potent immunosuppressive therapy, it is difficult to know what effects the pulse steroid therapy had on clinical outcome.

In summary, pulse steroid therapy may provide an effective means by which severe recalcitrant disease can be rapidly controlled, but data in support of its use are few. The results vary between studies conducted by Chryssomallis et al.[30] and Werth[29] with respect to remission, and may reflect the small number of patients in each study. Although remission may improve with pulse therapy, the average death rate reported from these studies (11%) does not differ significantly from the average rates reported in the most recent studies (all case series) in which only oral steroid was used (8.5%).[2] Therefore, pulse steroid treatment in combination with conventional therapy may increase the rate of remission, but it is important to pursue this question further in a larger prospective RCT.

> Does immunomodulatory therapy (i.e. plasmapheresis, or intravenous immunoglobulin (IVIG)) induce remission and reduce mortality more effectively than prednisone alone or in combination with immunosuppressive agents in patients with severe widespread pemphigus vulgaris that is unresponsive to oral prednisone?

The use of immunomodulatory agents is based on the hypothesis that effective therapy can be achieved through removal of autoantibodies (plasmapheresis) or by stimulation of autoantibody degradation (IVIG).

Plasmapheresis

Our search revealed an RCT of plasmapheresis, a case-controlled study and several case series. Guillaume et al.[31] enrolled 40 previously untreated patients in an RCT to determine the clinical efficacy of plasmapheresis in the treatment of pemphigus. Eighteen patients were treated with prednisolone alone (at least 0.5 mg/kg/day) and 22 with prednisolone plus 10 plasma exchanges over 4 weeks. There were no differences between the two groups with respect to clinical improvement or serum autoantibody titres. Eight patients, four in each group, did not achieve disease control with the highest steroid doses used in the study (2 mg/kg/day prednisolone). Four patients, all in the plasmapheresis group, died of sepsis or thromboembolism. The authors concluded that plasmapheresis, in association with "low" steroid doses, was not effective for treatment of pemphigus.

Although well designed, the study of Guillaume et al.[31] is difficult to interpret when one considers evidence that plasmapheresis without concurrent use of immunosuppressive agents results in antibody "rebound", or rapid synthesis of new autoantibody.[32-34] Therefore, it is possible that there was no evidence of clinical improvement due to "rebounding" antibody titres following plasmapheresis. In a case-controlled study, Tan-Lim and Bystryn[35] reported a more favourable conclusion regarding the effect of plasmapheresis on antibody titres when concurrently administered with corticosteroids and immunosuppressive agents. In 11 patients in the plasmapheresis group, three weeks of treatment resulted in a decrease in the average titres of autoantibodies of 83%. In contrast, titres decreased by only 18% among patients receiving the control regimen ($P = 0.037$). Although no clinical data were presented and long-term follow up was not reported, the drop in antibody titre is significant and represents a dramatic improvement over the results described by Guillaume et al.[31]

In a recent case series, Turner et al.[36] described their experience with plasmapheresis in seven patients with severe pemphigus vulgaris. All patients had been treated unsuccessfully with a variety of therapeutic agents for a period of 2 months to 10 years. Each patient underwent an average of nine plasma exchanges, during and immediately after which they received immunosuppressive therapy, pulse cyclophosphamide or pulse steroid, to prevent rebound autoantibody synthesis. Four patients achieved partial remission, two patients improved and were able to taper steroid dosage, and one patient showed initial improvement but relapsed within a month. Data concerning rates of remission and relapse are based on a follow up period of only 2 months. Because all patients received either pulse cyclophosphamide or pulse steroids, both believed to be effective for inducing remission in pemphigus, it is difficult to determine whether the observed benefits were the result of plasmapheresis or intensive immunosuppression.

In order to determine whether plasmapheresis is effective in controlling severe pemphigus, it is important to compare the clinical outcome in patients receiving immunosuppressive therapy with that in patients receiving immunosuppressive therapy plus plasmapheresis.

Intravenous immunoglobulin

Our search revealed no RCTs. We found a single case series of more than five patients that investigated the use of IVIG in the treatment of pemphigus. The study by Harman and Black[37] describes 14 patients with autoimmune blistering disorders who were treated with IVIG in conjunction with their previous therapy. Seven of these patients had pemphigus vulgaris.

Most patients had disease that was partially controlled with prednisolone with or without immunosuppressive agents. Patients received up to five IVIG treatments, 0.4 g/kg given on consecutive days. The addition of IVIG appeared to suppress blistering in two patients with pemphigus in whom the disease was severe and progressing rapidly. The other patients with pemphigus experienced some benefit initially, but the effect became less pronounced with subsequent treatments; all patients experienced a relapse within 6 weeks. All patients remained on medication. There was no mortality. Side-effects resulting from IVIG therapy were minimal.

Summary

Immunomodulatory therapy may be a very useful method of controlling severe or recalcitrant disease, but an RCT wherein patients receive either plasmapheresis (or IVIG) plus immunosuppressive agents, or immunosuppressive agents alone is needed. As it stands, plasmapheresis appears promising for its ability to eliminate what is assumed to be the source of disease – the autoantibodies. However, it is not clear whether plasmapheresis induces remission and prevents mortality more effectively than oral steroids alone. The literature on IVIG is even less conclusive. It may be an effective therapy in some patients, but further studies need to be conducted to establish its efficacy and to determine which patients may benefit from its use.

Does anti-inflammatory therapy (i.e. gold, dapsone, tetracycline) used as monotherapy or as a steroid-sparing agent effectively reduce symptoms and induce remission in patients with mild pemphigus vulgaris?

Anti-inflammatory agents are often prescribed for patients with relatively mild pemphigus, on the assumption that they are equally or more effective than other adjuvant agents, but pose less overall risk to the patient.

Gold

No controlled studies have tested the hypothesis that gold is an effective therapy for treatment of pemphigus. The largest and most recent case series, by Pandya and Dyke,[38] described 26 patients treated with gold, either alone or in combination with prednisone. Patients with severe disease requiring "aggressive" therapy and patients that had experienced "severe complications from steroid use" were excluded from the study. Eleven patients (42%) were able to discontinue steroids, seven of whom still required gold. The duration of gold therapy required before steroid dosages could be tapered was 3 months. There was no mortality, but toxic effects were noted in 11 patients, nine of whom discontinued therapy. Thus, a high percentage of patients improved during the study, but many were forced to discontinue the therapy because of toxic effects.

Similar results were reported by Poulin et al.[39] Thirteen patients, whose disease severity was not described, were treated with gold and prednisone. Three patients also received either dapsone or sulfapyridine. Seven patients (54%) experienced complete remission and one patient (8%) died. Gold therapy had to be discontinued in five patients (38%) because of toxic effects.

Because there are no controlled trials of gold therapy in pemphigus, it is difficult to determine whether the observed clinical improvement of patients receiving gold and steroids are, in fact, gold induced. Overall rates of remission and mortality reported for patients treated with gold and steroids are similar to rates that have been reported for patients treated with steroids alone or in combination with immunosuppressive agents.[3] Although side-effects related to gold therapy are often minor, a substantial proportion of patients are unable to tolerate treatment.

Dapsone

Dapsone is also reportedly effective in the treatment of mild pemphigus or as a steroid-sparing agent for maintenance therapy. The most substantial evidence in favour of dapsone therapy was reported by Basset et al.[40] Nine previously untreated patients received dapsone 200–300 mg/day and were followed up for an average of 22 months. Five patients, all with mild disease, responded with at least a 50% decrease in the extent of their disease within 15 days of starting therapy. One of these patients developed haemolytic anemia and discontinued dapsone. Although there are no controls, the finding that more than half of the patients responded to treatment with dapsone alone is noteworthy and indicates that dapsone provides significant clinical benefit. This issue is being followed up in a large international RCT sponsored by the Medical Dermatology Society and Jacobus Pharmaceuticals.

Tetracycline

As with other anti-inflammatory agents used to treat pemphigus, tetracycline is reportedly effective in patients with mild disease and offers a lower toxicity and broader safety profile than immunosuppressive agents. Calebotta et al.[41] conducted the only controlled study of tetracycline. Twenty patients were enrolled in the study. Thirteen prospective patients received tetracycline 2 g/day and prednisone 0·5–1·0mg/kg/day. The seven historical controls, all of whom had been treated with prednisone and azathioprine, were chosen at random. The duration of therapy before new blister formation ceased was significantly less in the treatment group (5·5 days versus 23 days). Interestingly, patients in the control group began the study with significantly higher dosages of prednisone and were unable to taper the dose as early as the patients in the treatment group. It is not clear whether this indicated a significant steroid-sparing effect, or whether patients in the treatment group had less severe disease. The range of disease severity was said to be similar in each group, but no objective criteria were reported. Regardless, the study suggested that the combination of tetracycline and steroid achieved more rapid control of disease than the combination of azathioprine and steroid. One patient in the experimental group discontinued the study because of sepsis and another because of gastrointestinal upset.

In another study by Alpsoy *et al.*,[42] 15 patients with pemphigus were treated with tetracycline and nicotinamide therapy. Almost half of the patients responded to the treatment. Thus, tetracycline (with or without nicotinamide), like dapsone, may be effective as monotherapy for a few select patients, thereby eliminating the need for steroids. Future studies may identify specific serological or molecular characteristics that distinguish responders.

Although the controlled study of tetracycline seems to suggest that more rapid control of disease can be achieved using tetracycline, when taken together, the evidence to support the efficacy of anti-inflammatory therapy is not substantial. The validity of historical controls is uncertain and the question remains whether the beneficial effects observed in patients treated with steroids and an adjuvant agent are the result of the adjuvant agent or are, in fact, due to the steroids. Anti-inflammatory agents such as dapsone and tetracycline may be of benefit in the treatment of mild cases of pemphigus or in the maintenance phase in steroid-dependent patients. However, large prospective controlled trials are necessary to recommend their use unequivocally.

Does mycophenolate mofetil, alone or in combination with corticosteroids, effectively reduce symptoms and induce remission in patients with pemphigus vulgaris?

Mycophenolate mofetil is an immunosuppressive drug recently introduced for use in preventing transplant rejection. Its potential usefulness in treating autoimmune or inflammatory skin conditions has generated much excitement, due in large part to its relatively minimal side-effects. A few small case series report on the treatment of pemphigus with mycophenolate. The largest series, reported by Enk and Knop,[43] described 12 patients with pemphigus vulgaris who received combination therapy with prednisone and mycophenolate. All patients had relapsed while being treated with prednisone and azathioprine. Disease severity was not reported. Patients initially received prednisone 2 mg/kg/day and mycophenolate 2 g/day. All but one patient improved, and in all responding patients the prednisone dose was reduced to at least 5 mg/day by the end of the study. However, all patients relapsed when steroid doses were tapered during the 12-month study. Thus, patients relapsed while taking mycophenolate, as they had done when they were taking azathioprine. Serum titres of pemphigus autoantibodies fell precipitously during the study to less than a half of their pretreatment level within a month, and all titres were undetectable by 2 months. Nearly all patients developed lymphopenia, but side-effects were not serious and there were no deaths.

There are two other case series of five patients each. Very little patient history, methods, and data are reported in either series. In the series by Enk and Knop,[44] patients enrolled in the study were described as having relapsed while taking azathioprine in the past. In the series by Nousari *et al.*[45] four of the five patients had experienced azathioprine-induced side-effects in the past. The patients in both series recieved prednisone, high dose in one study, in combination with mycophenolate. All patients responded to treatment, with partial remissions reported at the end of the follow up period (lasting 9 months[44] and >5 months,[45] respectively). Aside from lymphopenia and diarrhoea, no side-effects were reported.

The favourable results in each study are encouraging, and the prospect of a new and highly effective immunosuppressive agent is exciting, but so far no data indicate that mycophenolate plus prednisone is more effective than prednisone alone. Most patients in the studies either received very high-dose steroids, which may have been responsible for the observed improvement, or had mild disease that may have been responsive to lower doses of steroids. Thus, it is not surprising that most patients in the studies improved. In addition, the very rapid clinical and serological improvement, within a month, described by Enk and Knop[43] has been questioned. Other investigators found that at least 8 weeks' treatment was necessary to observe such serological improvement.[45] Regardless, further study of this interesting new drug is needed before it can be recommended as effective treatment for pemphigus.

Key points

- In most patients pemphigus can be controlled with a daily dose of prednisolone <100 mg/day. A typical dosage for a patient with moderate pemphigus is prednisolone 1 mg/kg/day. If there is no response in 5–7 days, the dosage is increased in increments of 0·25–0·5 mg/kg/day until blistering ceases, complications arise or a dosage of 2·0–2·5 mg/kg/day is reached. These dosages come from experience in large series; relevant RCTs have not been done.
- The addition of an immunosuppressant (azathioprine, cyclophosphamide, methotrexate, ciclosporin or mycophenolate mofetil) to prednisolone has not been shown to provide additional benefit, but does cause additional adverse effects. RCTs are needed to prove the benefit of adding immunosuppressant therapy.
- In patients with severe widespread pemphigus vulgaris not responding to oral prednisolone, intravenous pulse corticosteroid may help to bring the disease under control, but there is no reduction in mortality. Data on the value of intravenous pulse corticosteroid are scanty.
- Immunomodulatory therapy with plasmapheresis or IVIG may be useful for controlling severe or recalcitrant disease, but whether the results are better than with corticosteroid treatment alone remains unknown, and requires RCTs.
- A large RCT is testing whether dapsone can reduce symptoms and induce remission in mild and moderate pemphigus.

References

1. Stanley JR. Pemphigus. In: Freedberg IM, Eisen AM, Wolff A, eds. Fitzpatrick's *Dermatology in General Medicine, 5th ed.* New York: McGraw-Hill, 1999:654–66.
2. Bystryn JC. Adjuvant therapy of pemphigus. *Arch Dermatol* 1984;**120**:941–51.
3. Bystryn JC, Steinman NM. The adjuvant therapy of pemphigus. An update. *Arch Dermatol* 1996;**132**:203–12.
4. Ratnam KV, Phay KL, Tan CK. Pemphigus therapy with oral prednisolone regimens. A 5-year study. *Int J Dermatol* 1990;**29**:363–7.
5. Hirone T. Pemphigus: a survey of 85 patients between 1970 and 1974. *J Dermatol* 1978;**5**:43–7.
6. Block LJ, Caldarelli DD, Holinger PH, Pearson RW. Pemphigus of the air and food passages. *Ann Otol Rhinol Laryngol* 1977;**86**:584–7.
7. Lever WF, White H. Treatment of pemphigus with corticosteroids. *Arch Dermatol* 1963;**87**:52–66.
8. Ryan JG. Pemphigus. *Arch Dermatol* 1971;**104**:14–20.
9. Rosenberg FR, Sanders S, Nelson CT. Pemphigus: a 20-year review of 107 patients treated with corticosteroids. *Arch Dermatol* 1976;**112**:962–70.
10. Lever WF, Schaumburg-Lever G. Immunosuppressants and prednisone in pemphigus vulgaris: therapeutic results obtained in 63 patients between 1961 and 1975. *Arch Dermatol* 1977;**113**:1236–41.
11. Fine JD. Management of acquired bullous skin diseases. *New Engl J Med* 1995;**333**:1475–84.

12. Aberer W, Wolff-Schreiner EC, Stingl G, Wolff K. Azathioprine in the treatment of pemphigus vulgaris. A long-term follow-up. *J Am Acad Dermatol* 1987;**16**:527–33.

13. Lever WF, Schaumburg-Lever G. Treatment of pemphigus vulgaris. Results obtained in 84 patients between 1961 and 1982. *Arch Dermatol* 1984;**120**:44–7.

14. Chrysomallis F, Ioannides D, Teknetzis A *et al*. Treatment of oral pemphigus vulgaris. *Int J Dermatol* 1994;**33**:803–7.

15. Piamphongsant T. Treatment of pemphigus with corticosteroids and cyclophosphamide. *J Dermatol* 1979;**6**:359–63.

16. Austin HA, Klippel JH, Balow JE *et al*. Therapy of lupus nephritis. Controlled trial of prednisone and cytotoxic drugs. *Ncw Engl J Mcd* 1986;**314**:614–19.

17. Boumpas DT, Austin HA, Vaughn EM *et al*. Controlled trial of pulse methylprednisolone versus two regimens of pulse cyclophosphamide in severe lupus nephritis. *Lancet* 1992;**340**:741–5.

18. Reiner A, Gernsheimer T, Slichter SJ. Pulse cyclophosphamide therapy for refractory autoimmune thrombocytopenic purpura. *Blood* 1995;**85**:351–8.

19. Pasricha JS, Thanzama J, Khan UK. Intermittent high-dose dexamethasone-cyclophosphamide therapy for pemphigus. *Br J Dermatol* 1988;**119**:73–7.

20. Pasricha JS, Khaitan BK, Raman RS, Chandra M. Dexamethasone-cyclophosphamide pulse therapy for pemphigus. Int J Dermatol 1995;**34**:875–82.

21. Kaur S, Kanwar AJ. Dexamethasone-cyclophosphamide pulse therapy in pemphigus. *Int J Dermatol* 1990;**29**:371–4.

22. Fleischli ME, Valek RH, Pandya AG. Pulse intravenous cyclophosphamide therapy in pemphigus. *Arch Dermatol* 1999;**135**:57–61.

23. Smith TJ, Bystryn JC. Methotrexate as an adjuvant treatment for pemphigus vulgaris. *Arch Dermatol* 1999;**135**:1275–6.

24. Ioannides D, Chrysomallis F, Bystryn JC. Ineffectiveness of cyclosporin as an adjuvant to corticosteroids in the treatment of pemphigus. *Arch Dermatol* 2000;**136**:868–72.

25. Lapidoth M, David M, Ben-Amitai D *et al*. The efficacy of combined treatment with prednisone and cyclosporin in patients with pemphigus: preliminary study. *J Am Acad Dermatol* 1994;**30**:752–7.

26. Mobini N, Padilla TJ, Ahmed AR. Long-term remission in selected patients with pemphigus vulgaris treated with cyclosporin. *J Am Acad Dermatol* 1997;**36**:264–6.

27. Barthelemy H, Frappaz A, Cambazard F *et al*. Treatment of nine cases of pemphigus vulgaris with cyclosporin. *J Am Acad Dermatol* 1988;**18**:1262–6.

28. Krain LS. Pemphigus. Epidemiologic and survival characteristics fo 59 patients, 1955–1973. *Arch Dermatol* 1974;**110**:862–5.

29. Werth VP. Treatment of pemphigus vulgaris with brief, high-dose intravenous glucocorticoids. *Arch Dermatol* 1996;**132**:1435–9.

30. Chryssomallis F, Dimitriades A, Chaidemenos GC *et al*. Steroid-pulse therapy in pemphigus vulgaris long term follow-up. *Int J Dermatol* 1995;**34**.438–42.

31. Guillaume JC, Roujeau JC, Morel P *et al*. Controlled study of plasma exchange in pemphigus. *Arch Dermatol* 1988;**124**:1659–63.

32. Bystryn JC, Graf MW, Uhr JW. Regulation of antibody formation by serum antibody. II. Removal of specific antibody by means of exchange transfusion. *J Exp Med* 1970;**132**:1279–87.

33. Roujeau JC, Andre C, Joneau FM *et al*. Plasma exchange in pemphigus. Uncontrolled study of ten patients. *Arch Dermatol* 1983;**119**:215–21.

34. Derksen RHWM, Schurman HJ, Gmelig-Meyling FH *et al*. Rebound and overshoot after plasma exchange in humans. *J Lab Clin Med* 1984;**104**:35–43.

35. Tan-Lim R, Bystryn JC. Effect of plasmapheresis therapy on circulating levels of pemphigus antibodies. *J Am Acad Dermatol* 1990;**22**:35–40.

36. Turner MS, Sutton D, Sauder DN. The use of plasmapheresis and immunosuppression in the treatment of pemphigus vulgaris. *J Am Acad Dermatol* 2000;**43**:1058–64.

37. Harman KE, Black MM. High-dose intravenous immune globulin for the treatment of autoimmune blistering diseases: an evaluation of its use in 14 cases. *Br J Dermatol* 1999;**140**:865–74.

38. Pandya AG, Dyke C. Treatment of pemphigus with gold. *Arch Dermatol* 1998;**134**:1104–7.

39. Poulin Y, Perry HO, Muller SA. Pemphigus vulgaris: results of treatment with gold as a steroid-sparing agent in a series of thirteen patients. *J Am Acad Dermatol* 1984;**11**:851–7

40. Basset N, Guillot B, Michel B *et al.* Dapsone as initial treatment in superficial pemphigus. Report of nine cases. *Arch Dermatol* 1987;**123**:783–5.

41. Calebotta A, Saenz AM, Gonzalez F *et al.* Pemphigus vulgaris: benefits of tetracycline as adjuvant therapy in a series of thirteen patients. *Int J Dermatol* 1999;**38**: 217–21.

42. Alpsoy E, Yilmaz E, Basaran E *et al.* Is the combination of tetracycline and nicotinamide therapy alone effective in pemphigus? *Arch Dermatol* 1995;**131**: 1339–40.

43. Enk AH, Knop J. Mycophenolate is effective in the treatment of pemphigus vulgaris. *Arch Dermatol* 1999;**135**:54–6.

44. Enk AH, Knop J. Treatment of pemphigus vulgaris with mycophenolate mofetil. *Lancet* 1997;**350**:494.

45. Nousari HC, Anhalt GJ. The role of mycophenolate mofetil in the management of pemphigus. *Arch Dermatol* 1999;**135**:853–4.

49

Cutaneous manifestations of sarcoidosis

Anne Hawk and Joseph C English III

Background

Definition

Sarcoidosis is a systemic, idiopathic disease characterised by the formation of non-caseating epitheliod granulomas that disrupt underlying tissue function.[1] While sarcoidosis can affect virtually any organ system, pulmonary (>90%), hepatosplenic (50–80%), haematological (40%), musculoskeletal (39%), ocular (30–50%), cutaneous (25%), cardiac (5%) and neurological (5–10%) manifestations are most common.[1]

Cutaneous manifestations of sarcoidosis typically present at disease onset, and with the exception of erythema nodosum, do not correlate with the severity of disease. Erythema nodusum tends to be associated with acute, benign, spontaneously resolving sarcoidosis.[2] Skin lesions in sarcoidosis can be divided into specific lesions (i.e. skin biopsy demonstrates non-caseating granulomas) and non-specific lesions (i.e. reactive states). Specific lesions include papules, nodules, plaques, subcutaneous nodules, infiltrative scars and lupus pernio. Plaques and papules are the most common cutaneous lesions, while lupus pernio is most specific for sarcoidosis.[3] Lupus pernio tends to affect the face, manifesting as brownish-red, dusky, swollen and shiny infiltrated plaques.[1]

Incidence/prevalence

Sarcoidosis affects all ethnic groups, ages and both sexes, but incidence peaks in adults under 40 years of age.[4] Sarcoidosis is most common in African-American females, and they are typically afflicted with a more acute and severe form of the disease than others.[5,6] In the US, incidence is 10–14 per 100 000 for whites, and 35·5–64 per 100 000 for African-Americans.[7]

Aetiology

The aetiology of sarcoidosis remains elusive; with immune, genetic, infectious and environmental factors all postulated to contribute. The role of genetics is supported by the existence of positive family clusters of sarcoidosis, and serological studies demonstrating that patients with certain class I and II HLA types are more susceptible.[8–10] Mycobacteria have been investigated as a possible aetiological agent because of the granulomatous nature of the disease, but no definitive evidence has emerged thus far.[1]

Prognosis

Sarcoidosis has a variable course, with both limited/spontaneously resolving and chronic/progressive forms of the disease. Most patients with sarcoidosis do well. Up to 60% of cases spontaneously resolve, and only about 5% of patients with sarcoidosis will eventually die of their disease.[11,12] In the US, patients are most likely to die of pulmonary complications, such as pneumonia, pulmonary fibrosis progressing to cor pulmonale, and chronic obstructive pulmonary disease.[13]

Diagnostic tests

Because no specific diagnostic test exists, sarcoidosis is a diagnosis of exclusion. Evaluation of a patient for sarcoidosis may include[1,12]:

- **Detailed history and physical:** emphasis on lungs, skin, eyes, nervous system and heart
- **Chest radiograph:**

  - Stage 1: bilateral hilar with or without paratracheal adenopathy
  - Stage 2: adenopathy with pulmonary infiltrate
  - Stage 3: pulmonary infiltrates only
  - Stage 4: pulmonary fibrosis

- **Pulmonary function tests:** restrictive pattern with decreased diffusing capacity (DLCO)
- **Biopsy of affected tissue:** demonstrates non-caseating granulomas
- **Serum chemistry:** elevated alkaline phosphatase and/or hypercalcaemia may be found, but these are not specific for sarcoidosis
- **Angiotensin converting enzyme (ACE):** measurement is generally not a useful guide for diagnosis or therapeutic response

Aims of treatment

Treatment for cutaneous sarcoidosis is indicated if the skin findings are disfiguring. Available treatment modalities include topical and intralesional steroids, oral steroids, antimalarials and various immunosuppressive agents. Because cutaneous sarcoidosis may spontaneously regress and the available therapeutic modalities have the potential for substantial toxicity, it is important to carefully weigh the risks of treatment against the benefits. However, patients often seek treatment because of the poor cosmesis of cutaneous sarcoidosis, especially on the face, even if it is not disfiguring. The dermatologist therefore needs to be aware of the evidence-based treatment options available for cutaneous sarcoidosis.

Relevant outcomes

The outcome measures in cutaneous sarcoidosis are limited to evaluating if therapy decreased or resolved active skin lesions. No area and severity index scoring is available to date for this disease. The definition of disfiguring lesions is not well established among different investigators, and with polymorphic cutaneous manifestations, clinical endpoints are not uniform in measuring a response to therapies.

Methods of search

We searched the *Cochrane Library* for "sarcoidosis or sarcoid". We searched Medline from 1966 to 2001 using the terms "cutaneous sarcoidosis or sarcoidosis" and "therapeutics" or "treatment" or "prednisone" or "steroids" or "glucocorticoids" or "allopurinol" or "chloroquine" or "hydroxychloroquine" or "antimalarial" or "methotrexate" or "tretinoin" or "isotretinoin" or "tetracyclines" or "minocycline" or "phonophoresis" or "surgery" or "intralesional" or "pulse dye laser" as subject heading or title or key word.

QUESTIONS

Case scenario

The patient is a 44-year-old African–American woman with a 14-year history of sarcoidosis. The patient has pulmonary involvement that is asymptomatic and does not require treatment. However, she is requesting treatment for noticeable facial lesions (Figure 49.1).

> What are the effects of oral therapeutic interventions in patients with cutaneous sarcoidosis?

Oral steroids
Benefits

Oral glucocorticoids are postulated to work in systemic sarcoidosis by virtue of their

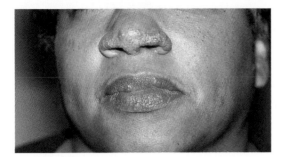

Figure 49.1 Cutaneous sarcoidosis

anti-inflammatory and immunosuppressant capabilities. For the same reasons, they are often offered as first-line treatment for lesions of cutaneous sarcoidosis.[14,15] However, there is very little evidence to support their use for this indication. Several studies have been conducted to evaluate the efficacy of steroids (particularly long-term steroids) for treatment of pulmonary sarcoidosis. Although some study participants were noted to have skin findings, none of these studies evaluated resolution or improvement of skin lesions as a clinical endpoint.[16–23] In 1967, James et al.[24] conducted a randomised prospective, placebo-controlled trial in which they compared the efficacy of prednisolone, 20 mg/day, with oxyphenbutazone, 400 mg/day, and placebo for the treatment of sarcoidosis with multisystem involvement. Seventy-five patients were included in the study (27 prednisolone, 24 oxyphenbutazone, 24 placebo), and therapy was administered to all patients for 6 months. Eleven patients in the prednisolone group, seven in the oxyphenbutazone group, and eight in the placebo group had skin manifestations of sarcoidosis at the start of the study. At the end of 6 months, two of 11 patients in the prednisolone group had improvement of their skin lesions compared with one of seven patients in the oxyphenbutazone group. In the placebo group, skin lesions improved in one patient, and deteriorated in two. Several open non-randomised non-controlled trials have been

published. Sharma et al.[25] published a summary of the management and clinical course of 41 patients with sarcoidosis treated at the University of Southern California's Sarcoidosis Clinic. Of the six patients with lupus pernio, five received oral corticosteroids, and only one had improvement of her lesions. Of the nine patients with skin plaques, seven received corticosteroids or chloroquine or both; however, only one patient had improvement of his skin lesions. Corticosteroids were either not administered or their effects were not included for the remaining patients. Johns et al.[26] reported the results of an unpublished retrospective review by Hackett and Hambrick describing treatment of cutaneous sarcoidosis at Johns Hopkins Sarcoid Clinic. Systemic prednisone was used in 32 patients with cutaneous manifestations, and improvement of lesions was noted in 12 patients. Verdegem et al.[27] reported on four patients with ulcerative sarcoidosis. Case one had partial improvement of her lesions with oral methylprednisone, 48 mg/day; case two had resolution of her lesions with a combination of prednisone, 10 mg/day, and hydroxychloroquine sulphate, 200 mg/day; case three had resolution of her lesions with a combination of prednisone, 30 mg/day, hydroxychloroquine sulphate, 200 mg/day and antibiotics; case 4 had resolution of her lesions with prednisone, 60 mg/day.

Harms

The list of complications of steroid therapy is long, and the likelihood and severity of complications increase with increasing length of administration. Complications may include glucose intolerance, increased susceptibility to infection, osteoporosis, avascular necrosis of bone, cataracts and neuropsychiatric changes.[28]

Comment/implications for clinical practice

Randomised controlled data exist to support the use of oral steroids for the pulmonary manifestations of sarcoidosis; however, very little objective data exist to support the use of steroids for the cutaneous manifestations of sarcoidosis. In the articles reviewed 56 patients were treated with oral steroids alone, of whom 17 had positive results. In patients with sarcoidosis for whom the main indication for treatment is cutaneous lesions, there is insufficient evidence to conclude that oral steroids are beneficial. Large randomised placebo-controlled therapeutic trials will be necessary for definitive proof.

Despite the lack of randomised-controlled data on oral steroids for cutaneous sarcoidosis, many dermatologists use it as first-line therapy. This is based on steroids reversing the manifestations of pulmonary and other extrapulmonary changes of sarcoidosis.[4,28–30]

Antimalarials
Benefits
Antimalarials such as chloroquine and hydroxychloroquine are 4-aminoquinolones and have been shown to be effective in treating connective tissue diseases. While no randomised placebo-controlled studies exist to evaluate their effectiveness in cutaneous sarcoidosis, a number of open non-randomised non-controlled prospective studies and one comprehensive literature review have been conducted. In 1991, Zic et al.[29] published a literature review of studies evaluating the use of antimalarials for treatment of sarcoidosis. They concluded that while corticosteroids should remain first-line treatment for patients with extracutaneous sarcoidosis, chloroquine should be strongly considered in patients for whom the main indication for treatment is disfiguring cutaneous lesions. Zic et al. recommended an initial 14-day course of chloroquine, 500 mg/day, followed by long-term therapy with 250 mg/day. These conclusions were based on the following studies.

Morse et al.[31] conducted the first open prospective trial of chloroquine for the treatment of cutaneous sarcoidosis in 1961. The trial included seven patients with chronic cutaneous sarcoidosis (i.e. 2 or more years duration) treated with chloroquine, 500 mg/day for 6 months. All had improvement of their skin lesions. Four out of seven relapsed after treatment was withdrawn, but responded again when therapy was reinstated.

Hirsch et al.[32] presented a case series of eight patients with chronic sarcoidosis (i.e. 5–15 years duration) treated with chloroquine, 500 mg/day, for 6 months. Seven of the eight patients had cutaneous lesions, which all improved with therapy. Six of the eight patients also had pulmonary disease – only two of the six pulmonary lesions improved.

Stilzbach et al.[33] conducted an open prospective study of 43 patients with pulmonary sarcoidosis treated with chloroquine, 500 mg/day. Fourteen of the 43 patients also had skin lesions, all of whom saw improvement of their skin lesions with therapy. In contrast, only 31 of the 43 patients had improvement of their pulmonary lesions.

Brodthagen et al.[34] published a study of 15 patients with cutaneous sarcoidosis treated with hydroxychloroquine, 500–1000 mg/day. Only two patients had improvement of their lesions after 6 months of therapy.

Johns et al.[35] report on an open prospective trial of 25 black patients on maintenance corticosteroid therapy who had regression of their skin lesions with the addition of chloroquine, 500 mg/day.

Finally, Jones et al.[36] report the results of a non-randomised open study of 17 patients with steroid-resistant cutaneous sarcoidosis treated with hydroxychloroquine, 2–3 mg/kg/day, for at least 3 months. Twelve patients improved and were able to discontinue other therapies. Five patients did not improve and three had worsening of their cutaneous disease. Of the twelve patients who were successfully treated, six discontinued the hydroxychloroquine and had re-emergence of their lesions, which again regressed when hydroxychloroquine was reinstated.

In addition to studies mentioned in the literature review by Zic *et al.*, Johns *et al.*[26] reported the results of an unpublished retrospective review by Hackett and Hambrick describing treatment of cutaneous sarcoidosis at the Johns Hopkins Sarcoid Clinic. In this study, 15 of 18 patients treated with chloroquine had improvement of their lesions. Chloroquine was typically administered for 6 months, followed by 6 months off treatment to avoid ocular toxicity. Multiple courses of therapy were often required.

Harms

Long-term administration of either chloroquine or hydroxychloroquine can lead to ocular complications ranging from corneal opacity, to transient visual changes, to irreversible retinopathy and blindness.[29] Hydroxychloroquine has a lower risk of ocular toxicity, but it may not be as effective in treating sarcoidosis.[12,29] When prolonged therapy with any antimalarial compound is contemplated, baseline and periodic ophthalmological examinations should be performed.[37,38] Other side-effects include nausea and vomiting, gastrointestinal upset, central nervous system toxicity (irritability, nervousness, depression), neuromuscular reactions (skeletal muscle palsies, myopathy or neuromyopathy) and cutaneous pigmentation. Millard *et al.*[39] report on a male patient treated with chloroquine for sarcoidosis who developed a widespread bullous eruption after 3 months of therapy consistent with drug-induced bullous pemphigoid.

Comment/implications for clinical practice

Articles written to date describe experience with a total of 103 patients treated with antimalarials,

82 of whom had positive results. While none of these articles represents a large randomised placebo-controlled trial, these studies as a whole suggest that chloroquine and hydroxychloroquine are reasonable for patients with cutaneous sarcoidosis without substantial systemic involvement.

Methotrexate

Methotrexate is a dihydrofolate reductase inhibitor used in the treatment of neoplastic diseases and as a non-steroidal immunosuppressant in chronic inflammatory conditions.

Benefits

There are no systematic reviews or RCTs of the role of methotrexate in the treatment of cutaneous sarcoidosis.[40,41] Baughman *et al.*[40] performed a double-blind placebo-controlled trial investigating whether methotrexate was steroid sparing in acute sarcoidosis. Although the study included three patients with skin manifestations of sarcoidosis, the results did not include information on whether the lesions had resolved, so no conclusions can be drawn from this study regarding the efficacy of methotrexate for this indication. Several open non-randomised non-controlled studies have been published. Veien *et al.*[41] conducted the first study of methotrexate for cutaneous sarcoidosis, and found that in 12 of 16 patients, skin lesions cleared with 25 mg/week. Two patients discontinued the medicine because of nausea. Lower *et al.*[42] reported on 55 patients with symptomatic sarcoidosis who were treated with methotrexate (average dose 28 mg/day) for over 2 years as a steroid-sparing agent. Clinical response was measured by improvement in affected organs and reduction in use of steroids. Sixteen of the 17 patients with cutaneous lesions had improvement of their lesions while taking methotrexate. Kaye *et al.*[43] report on five patients with severe steroid-resistant sarcoidosis treated with methotrexate, 10 mg/week, for 30 months. Of the four patients with skin lesions, three had at least 60% regression, and one had complete regression of lesions with methotrexate. Gedalia et al.[44] presented the results of methotrexate, 10–15 mg/week, in seven paediatric patients with sarcoidosis. Of the three patients with cutaneous lesions, two had resolution of their skin findings with methotrexate. Mean dose of prednisone for all study participants was tapered from an average of 49 mg/day to 7·3 mg/day at 6 months.[44] Lacher[45] published the first case report of methotrexate for cutaneous sarcoidosis, describing a patient in whom prednisone failed, but who responded to a combination of prednisone, 75 mg three times weekly, and methotrexate, 40 mg twice weekly. The dose of prednisone was eventually tapered and the patient maintained on methotrexate, 7·5 mg twice weekly. Webster et al.[46] presented case reports on three patients who had improvement of their severe steroid-resistant cutaneous sarcoidosis with methotrexate, 15–22·5 mg/week. Henderson et al.[47] presented a case report of a man with steroid-resistant laryngeal and cutaneous sarcoidosis who responded to methotrexate, 10 mg/week.

Harms
Complications of methotrexate therapy include bone marrow suppression, nausea and vomiting, hepatotoxicity, and hypersensitivity pneumonitis.[28] Albertini et al.[48] described a patient with severe systemic and ulcerative sarcoidosis who was started on methotrexate, 25 mg per week. Although her ulcerative lesions initially regressed, she soon developed anaemia, leucopenia and elevated aspartate transaminase level, necessitating the withdrawal of methotrexate. The patient subsequently died of her disease. Major toxic effects noted by Lower et al. were hepatotoxicity, leucopenia and cough.[42]

Comment/implications for clinical practice
Articles written to date describe experience with a total of 46 patients with cutaneous sarcoidosis

treated with methotrexate, of whom 39 had positive results. While none of these articles represents a large RCT, and there is very little consistency across trials in terms of patient population, dosage or clinical endpoints, these studies suggest that methotrexate might be useful as a steroid-sparing agent in people requiring or not responding to other therapies.

Thalidomide
Thalidomide is an inhibitor of tumour necrosis factor (TNF)-alpha. It was originally marketed as a sedative, but was withdrawn in 1962 because of its teratogenic effects.[49] It has recently been found to be effective at low doses in the treatment of inflammatory diseases such as lupus erythematous and erythema nodosum leprosum.[50]

Benefits
No systematic reviews or RCTs of the role of thalidomide in the treatment of cutaneous sarcoidosis were found. One retrospective study was identified by Estines et al.[51] on data collected on 10 patients with severe disfiguring lesions treated with thalidomide, 1·84 mg/kg, who were resistant to conventional therapy. Outcomes measured were: complete regression (total disappearance); incomplete regression (remaining signs) and treatment failure (no change, or worsening). Three of the study participants had complete regression, four had incomplete regression, and treatment failed in three. The thalidomide dose was gradually reduced for five of the seven patients for whom thalidomide was effective; three of the five patients relapsed, but the drug was efficacious at re-introduction at the same dose.

Three case reports of patients successfully treated with thalidomide for lesions resistant to other forms of therapy were found.[49,50,52] Carlisimo et al.[49] report on a 56-year-old woman with cutaneous sarcoid unresponsive to steroids who had clinical improvement after taking thalidomide, 200 mg/day for 2 weeks followed by 100 mg/day for 11 weeks. Rousseau et al.[50] report on a 30-year-old woman resistant to intralesional steroids, hydroxychloroquine, isotretinoin and isoniazid; she improved with thalidomide, 100 mg/day for 2 months, gradually tapered to a maintenance dose of 50 mg/day. Lee et al.[52] report on a 59-year-old patient who had clinical improvement of all lesions after taking thalidomide 200mg/day for 2 months and 300 mg/day for 4 months.

Harms
Thalidomide therapy can be complicated by neurosensory, gastrointestinal and teratogenic effects.[49,52] Neuropathy is a common and dangerous side-effect of thalidomide use, and was noted in two out of 10 patients in the study by Estines et al.[51] and in the patient discussed in the case report by Lee et al.[52]

Comment/implications for clinical practice
Articles written to date describe experience with a total of 13 patients treated with thalidomide, 10 of whom had positive results. This is insufficient evidence to conclude that thalidomide is beneficial for treatment of cutaneous sarcoidosis, particularly because sarcoidosis often resolves spontaneously. Large randomised placebo-controlled trials will therefore be necessary for definitive proof.

Tetracyclines
Tetracyclines are antibiotics that have been found to inhibit T-cell proliferation and granuloma formation in vitro, which is the rationale for their use in cutaneous sarcoidosis.[53]

Benefits
No systematic reviews or RCTs were found. One non-randomised non-controlled open prospective study of 12 patients treated with minocycline, 200 mg/day, for 12 months was found.[53] Notably, antimalarial therapy had failed in most patients prior to entering the study. Eight of the study participants had complete regression of their lesions, two had partial regression and treatment failed in two (one progressed and one remained stable). After withdrawal of therapy, three out of the 10 responders relapsed.

Harms
Side-effects of minocycline include nausea and vomiting, hypersensitivity reactions, blue skin pigmentation and vertigo.[53] Hypersensitivity was noted in one patient in this study.[53]

Comment/implications for clinical practice
Articles written to date describe experience with a total of 12 patients treated with tetracyclines, 10 of whom had positive results. This is insufficient evidence to conclude that tetracyclines are beneficial for treatment of cutaneous sarcoidosis, particularly because cutaneous sarcoidosis often resolves spontaneously. Therefore large randomised placebo-controlled trials will be necessary for definitive proof.

Allopurinol
Allopurinol is a xanthine oxidase inhibitor used in the treatment of gout and some inflammatory diseases. Its anti-inflammatory capabilities are the basis for its use in cutaneous sarcoidosis.

Benefits
No systematic reviews or RCTs describing the use of allopurinol for treatment of cutaneous sarcoidosis were found. One non-randomised non-controlled open prospective study of six patients with cutaneous sarcoidosis reported treatment with allopurinol, 100 mg/day,

increased by 100 mg every 2–4 weeks to 600 mg/day. Four of the six patients in the initial report had improvement of their lesions.[54]

Additional information was found in several case reports. Pfau et al.[55] treated two patients with scar sarcoidosis and two patients with nodular sarcoidosis with allopurinol 300 mg/day over a 3–7-month period. Lesions completely resolved in the patients with scar sarcoidosis and partially resolved in the patients with nodular sarcoidosis. Rosof et al.[56] observed remission of cutaneous sarcoidosis in two patients treated with allopurinol. Pollock[57] reported on two patients with cutaneous sarcoidosis; one treated with allopurinol, 100 mg/day, and the other with 300 mg/day; both patients experienced marked improvement in their lesions. Brechtel et al.[58] reported on a patient who had disseminated cutaneous sarcoidosis refractory to chloroquine treatment that responded to allopurinol, 300 mg/day. Voelter-Mahlknect et al.[59] observed a patient with subcutaneous sarcoidosis who was treated with allopurinol, 200 mg/day (later increased to 600 mg/day). Allopurinol failed, and the patient's lesions actually progressed. Antony et al.[60] reported on a case of cutaneous acral sarcoidosis unresponsive to other therapies that responded to allopurinol, 300 mg/day.

Harms
Allopurinol therapy can be associated with drug rash (severe as toxic epidermal necrosis) as well as nausea and vomiting, hepatotoxicity and bone marrow suppression.[57] No significant side-effects were noted in the patients reported.

Comment/implications for clinical practice
Articles written to date describe experience with a total of 18 patients treated with allopurinol, 15 of whom had positive results. This is insufficient evidence to conclude that allopurinol is beneficial for treatment of cutaneous

sarcoidosis, particularly because cutaneous sarcoidosis often resolves spontaneously. Large randomised placebo-controlled therapeutic trials will be necessary for definitive proof.

Isotretinoin
Isotretinoin, a retinoid that inhibits sebaceous gland function and keratinisation, is useful for treatment of many dermatological conditions, and is proposed as a treatment for cutaneous sarcoidosis because of its immunomodulatory effects.[61]

Benefits
No systematic reviews or RCTs describing use of isotretinoin for treatment of cutaneous sarcoidosis were found. However, four cases of isotretinoin use in cutaneous sarcoidosis were identified. Georgiou et al.[61] described a 31-year-old woman with a 3-year history of cutaneous sarcoid unresponsive to intralesional steroids, oral steroids and hydroxychloroquine. She experienced complete resolution of her skin lesions after 8 months' treatment with oral isotretinoin, 1 mg/kg/day. Waldinger et al.[62] described a woman with severe disfiguring lesions of 4 years duration in whom treatment with oral prednisone and allopurinol had failed. She was treated with isotretinoin for 30 weeks (initially 40 mg/day for 6 weeks, increased to 80 mg/day for 16 weeks, decreased back to 40 mg/day for the last 8 weeks because of side-effects), and had resolution or improvement of many of her lesions. Spiteri et al.[63] reported a case of a woman with chronic sarcoidosis treated with isotretinoin, 75 mg/day (decreased to 50 mg/day because of cheilitis) who had little resolution of her sarcoid nodules, and was withdrawn from the drug after 7 weeks because of the development of a severe exfoliative dermatitis. Vaillant et al.[64] report on a woman with cutaneous sarcoid unresponsive to steroids, allopurinol, and antimalarials. She had improvement of her lesions after 6 months'

treatment with oral isotretinoin, 0·4–1·0 mg/kg/day.

Harms

Isotretinoin is a teratogenic drug and must not be used by woman who are pregnant or who become pregnant while undergoing treatment. Other side-effects include depression, vision impairment, hepatic dysfunction and pancreatitis. Side-effects noted by study participants included myalgia, xerosis, dryness of nasal mucosa, cheilitis and exfoliative dermatitis.[61,62,64]

Comment/implications for clinical practice

Articles written to date describe experience with four patients treated with isotretinoin, three of whom had a positive result. This is insufficient evidence to conclude that isotretinoin is beneficial for treatment of cutaneous sarcoidosis, particularly because cutaneous sarcoidosis often spontaneously resolves and because isotretinoin is associated with severe side-effects. Large randomised placebo-controlled trials will be necessary for definitive proof.

Conclusions

After reviewing the available data on the oral therapy of cutaneous sarcoidosis, there is sparse evidence-based medicine. There is a desperate need for RCTs in this cutaneous disorder. Although oral steroids have been "grandfathered in" as the first-line treatment on the basis of many clinicians' personal experience on sarcoidosis, it has not been proven in clinical trials for cutaneous sarcoidosis.

The available reported evidence-based data suggest that chloroquine or hydroxychloroquine are the most effective agents available for the treatment of cutaneous sarcoidosis. Additional agents, in order of available evidence and side-effects, would include: methotrexate, allopurinol, minocycline, isotretinoin and thalidomide.

Several other drugs have been reported in isolated case reports (1–3 patients) as successful; these include tranilast,[65] melatonin,[66] clofazimine,[67] mepacrine[68] and infliximab.[69] Levamisole was studied in 16 patients with cutaneous sarcoid and was found to be effective in only two of the 13 patients completing the course of treatment. It was concluded not to be useful in the treatment of cutaneous sarcoidosis.[70]

> What are the effects of non-oral therapeutic interventions in patients with cutaneous sarcoidosis?

Flashlamp pulsed dye laser therapy

Flashlamp pulsed dye laser therapy has been successful in the treatment of portwine stains and telangiectasias, where it works by selective ablation of the affected dilated and inflamed vessels.[71] It is postulated to work by a similar mechanism in lupus pernio, a disfiguring cutaneous manifestation of sarcoidodis.

Benefits

There are no systematic reviews or RCTs of the role of flashlamp pulsed dye laser therapy in the treatment of cutaneous sarcoidosis. Four case reports were found. Goodman[71] reported a woman with a 5-year history of lupus pernio of the nose who responded to laser therapy at an energy level of 7–8 J/cm^2. The improvement induced by the laser was temporary: the erythema and papules returned 7 months after the first treatment, and 6–15 months after the second treatment, but both times responded again to laser therapy. She received three sessions altogether, and no side-effects of therapy (such as atrophy, scarring or hypopigmentation) were noted in any session.

Cliff et al.[72] described a patient with lupus pernio of the nose, who improved following six treatment sessions at 6-week intervals with flashlamp pulsed dye laser at a setting of 5·6–7·3 J/cm². A biopsy of her nose after treatment noted the continued presence of non-caseating sarcoid granulomas, leading the authors to conclude that laser therapy was effective in improving the appearance of the lesions, but not the underlying disease process. Dosik et al.[73] report on a woman with a 3-year history of topical and intralesional steroid-resistant lupus pernio who responded successfully to flashlamp pulsed dye laser at an energy of 7·25 J/cm². The therapy was given for nine sessions at 1–2-month intervals.

Harms

Goodman, Cliff et al. and Dosik et al. did not report any side-effects of laser therapy in their patients. In contrast, Green et al.[74] report on a 62-year-old black woman who was treated for lupus pernio with flashlamp-pumped pulsed dye laser (6·0–7·1 J/cm²) and developed worsening of her cutaneous sarcoidosis. Ulcerative lesions appeared in both the treated and untreated plaques within 3 weeks of receiving laser treatment.

Because of the inherent risk of eye damage from laser therapy, protective eyewear should be employed.

Comment/implications for clinical practice

Articles written to date describe experience with four patients with treatment-resistant chronic lupus pernio treated with flashlamp pulsed dye laser therapy, three of whom had a positive result). This is insufficient evidence to conclude that this therapy is beneficial for treatment of cutaneous sarcoidosis. Randomised placebo-controlled therapeutic trials will be necessary for definitive proof.

Plastic surgery
Benefits

There are no systematic reviews or RCTs of the role of plastic surgery in the treatment of cutaneous sarcoidosis; however, several case reports were found. In 1970, O'Brien described two patients successfully treated with plastic surgery for lupus pernio.[75] In 1984, Shaw et al.[76] described a man with a 6-year history of treatment-resistant lupus pernio successfully treated with surgical excision and split skin grafting; the result remained good 2·5 years after surgery. Collison et al.[77] described a man with extensive ulcerative nodules of the lower extremities, which were resistant to topical/intralesional steroids, oral steroids, hydroxychloroquine and methotrexate. He was treated with vigorous operative debridement and partial-thickness skin grafting. While the grafts were well accepted (80%), the patient developed new ulcerating nodules in previously uninvolved skin 2 months after surgery. Stack et al.[78] report on a black male with extensive facial lesions who was treated with CO_2 laser excision, followed by steroid injection. The wounds healed well, and the patient had no recurrence of lesions 2 years after surgery. Streit et al.[79] report the case of a woman with widespread ulcerative cutaneous sarcoidosis treated with Apligraf (graftskin), a bilayered human skin equivalent, with good results.

Harms

No complications were noted in the above studies. However, inherent risks of general anaesthesia and the operation (bleeding, scarring, postoperative infection) should be considered.

Comment/implications for clinical practice

Articles written to date describe experience with six patients with treatment-resistant chronic lupus pernio treated with plastic surgery, all of whom had a positive result. This is insufficient evidence to conclude that this therapy is beneficial for treatment of cutaneous sarcoidosis.

Topical corticosteroids and intralesional injections

While topical corticosteroids and intralesional injections are often recommended as first-line treatment for the cutaneous manifestations of sarcoidosis,[12,14,15,30] little evidence is presented regarding their efficacy for this indication. Khatri et al.[80] describe a case of lupus pernio which improved with topical 0.05% halobetasol propionate twice daily for 10 weeks. Volden et al.[81] describe three cases of cutaneous sarcoidosis that went into remission within 3–5 weeks of treatment with once-weekly clobetasol propionate covered with hydrocolloid dressing. The use of intralesional hydrocortisone and cortisone were reported in 1953 by Sullivan et al.[82] Eighteen skin lesions in five patients with cutaneous sarcoidosis were injected with 2.5 mg doses of hydrocortisone. All lesions developed evidence of regression by 14 days after the injection, with no evidence of recurrence 14 weeks later. Seven skin lesions in four patients were injected with 2.5 mg cortisone. All lesions improved but not to the same extent as was noted with intralesional hydrocortisone. Liedtka reported on a sarcoid patient who had cutaneous lesions affecting the face, back and upper extremities that responded to multiple injections of chloroquine hydrochloride, 50 mg/ml.[83]

Harms

No major side-effects were reported in any of the study participants. Post-inflammatory hypopigmentation and hyperpigmentation were noted after the intralesional hydrocortisone injections in the review of Sullivan et al.[82] Minimal bleeding from the needle puncture, and cutaneous atrophy from the steroids are inherent risks to intralesional steroid injections.[84]

Comment/implications for clinical practice

Articles written to date describe a limited number of patients (n = 15) with cutaneous sarcoidosis treated with intralesional injections or topical steroids. This is insufficient evidence to conclude that this therapy is beneficial for treatment of cutaneous sarcoidosis.

Conclusions

The evidence-based data on non-oral therapies for cutaneous sarcoidosis are extremely sparse. There are no RCTs published proving that intralesional or topical steroids are effective in the treatment of cutaneous sarcoidosis. Intralesional and topical steroids, as with oral steroids, have been accepted as first-line therapies on the basis of clinicians' experience, with no definitive dosage or duration of therapy identified. The physical modalities of laser and plastic surgery have been reported as successful in isolated treatment-resistant cases, but larger studies are lacking.

Phototherapy (PUVA and UVA1)[85,86] and phonophoresis[87] are other modalities reported in isolated case reports to be beneficial.

Key points

- There are no randomised, controlled trials of any therapy for the treatment of cutaneous sarcoidosis.
- Having reviewed the literature on oral therapies for cutaneous sarcoidosis, only antimalarials and methotrexate have been shown to be of benefit.
- Having reviewed the literature on non-oral therapies for cutaneous sarcoidosis, no therapy can be recommended at this time.

References

1. English JC, Patel PJ, Greer KE. Sarcoidosis. *J Am Acad Dermatol* 2001;**44**:725–43.

2. Mana J, Salazar A, Manresa F. Clinical factors predicting persistence of activity in sarcoidosis: a multivariate analysis of 193 cases. *Respiration* 1994;**61**:219–25.

3. Mana J, Marcoval J, Graells J, Salazaar A, Pyri J, Pujol R. Cutaneous involvement in sarcoidosis: relationship to systemic disease. *Arch Dermatol* 1997;**133**:882–8.

4. Newman LS, Rose CS, Maier LA. Sarcoidosis. *N Engl J Med* 1997;**336**:1224–34.

5. Edmonstone WM, Wilson AG. Sarcoidosis in Caucasians, blacks and Asians in London. *Br J Dis Chest* 1985;**79**:27–36.

6. Rybicki BA, Major M, Popovich J, Maliarik MJ, Iannuzzi MC. Racial differences in sarcoidosis incidence: a 5-year study in a health maintenance organization. *Am J Epidemiol* 1997;**145**:234–41.

7. Reich JM, Johnson R. Incidence of clinically identified sarcoidosis in a northwest United States population. *Sarcoid Vasc Diffuse Lung Dis* 1996;**13**:173–7.

8. Rybicki BA, Harrington D, Major M *et al*. Heterogeneity of familial risk in sarcoidosis. *Genet Epidemiol* 1996;**13**:23–33.

9. Rybicki BA, Maliarik MJ, Major M, Popovich J Jr, Iannuzzi MC. Epidemiology, demographics, and genetics of sarcoidosis. *Semin Respir Infect* 1998;**13**:166–73.

10. Ishihara M, Ohno S. Genetic influences on sarcoidosis. *Eye* 1997;**11**:155–61.

11. Peckham DG, Spiteri MA. Sarcoidosis. *Postgrad Med J* 1996;**72**:196–200.

12. American Thoracic Society. Statement on sarcoidosis. *Am J Respir Care Med* 1999;**160**:736–55.

13. Gideon NM, Mannino DM. Sarcoidosis mortality in the United States 1979–1991: an analysis of multiple cause mortality data. *Am J Med* 1996;**100**:423–7.

14. Russo G, Millikan LE. Cutaneous sarcoidosis: diagnosis and treatment. *Comp Therapy* 1994;**20**:418–21.

15. Wilson NJ, King CM. Cutaneous sarcoidosis. *Postgrad Med J* 1998;**74**:649–52.

16. Pietinalho A, Tukiainen P, Haahtela T, Persson T, Selroos O. Oral prednisolone followed by inhaled budesonide in newly diagnosed pulmonary sarcoidosis: a double-blind, placebo-controlled multicenter study. *Chest* 1999;**116**:424–31.

17. Rizzato G, Riboldi A, Imbimbo B, Torresin A, Milani S. The long-term efficacy and safety of two different corticosteroids in chronic sarcoidosis. *Respir Med* 1997;**91**:449–60.

18. Selroos O, Sellergren TL. Corticosteroid therapy of pulmonary sarcoidosis. A prospective evaluation of alternate day and daily dosage in stage II disease. *Scand J Respir Dis* 1979;**60**:215–21.

19. Eule H, Roth I, Ehrke I, Weinecke W. Cortocosteroid therapy of intrathoracic sarcoidosis stages I and II – results of a controlled clinical trial. *Zeitschrift fur Erkankungen der Atmunsorgane* 1977;**149**:142–7.

20. Johns CJ, Zachary JB, Ball WC. A ten year study of corticosteroid treatment of pulmonary sarcoidosis. *Johns Hopkins Med* 1974;**134**:271–83.

21. Israel HL, Fouts DW, Beggs RA: A controlled trial of prednisone treatment of sarcoidosis. *Am Rev Respir Dis* 1973;**107**:609–14.

22. Sharma OP, Colp C, Williams MH. Course of pulmonary sarcoidosis with and without corticosteroid therapy as determined by pulmonary function studies. *Am J Med* 1966;**41**:541–51.

23. Zaki MH, Lyons HA, Leilop L, Huang CT. Corticosteroid therapy in sarcoidosis: a five year controlled follow-up. *NY State J Med* 1987;**87**:496–9.

24. James DG, Carstairs LS, Trowell J, Sharma OP. Treatment of sarcoidosis: report of a controlled therapeutic trial. *Lancet* 1967;**2**:526–8.

25. Sharma OP. Cutaneous sarcoidosis: clinical features and management. *Chest* 1972;**61**:320–5.

26. Johns CJ, Michele TM. The clinical management of sarcoidosis: a 50-year experience at the Johns Hopkins Hospital. *Medicine* 1999;**78**:65–111.

27. Verdegem TD, Sharma OP. Cutaneous ulcers in sarcoidosis. *Arch Dermatol* 1987;**123**:1531–4.

28. Baughman RP, Sharma OP, Lynch III JP. Sarcoidosis: Is therapy effective. *Semin Respir Infect* 1998;**13**:255–73.

29. Zic JA, Horowitz DH, Arzubiaga C, King LE. Treatment of cutaneous sarcoidosis with chloroquine: review of the literature. *Arch Dermatol* 1991;**127**:1034–40.

30. Veien NK. Cutaneous sarcoidosis: prognosis and treatment. *Clin Dermatol* 1986;**4**:75–87.

31. Morse SI, Cohn ZA, Hirsch JG, Sheadler RW. The treatment of sarcoidosis with chloroquine. *Am J Med* 1961;**30**:779–84.

32. Hirsch JG. Experimental treatment with chloroquine. *Am Rev Respir Dis* 1961;**2**:947–8.

33. Siltzbach LE, Teirstein AS. Chloroquine therapy in 43 patients with intrathoracic and cutaneous sarcoidosis. *Acta Med Scand* 1964;**176**:302–8.

34. Brodthagen H. Hydroxychloroquine in the treatment of sarcoidosis. In: Turiaf J, Chabot J, eds. *La Sarcoidose: Rapports de la IV Conference International*. Paris: Mason & Co 1967:764–7.

35. Johns CJ, Schonfeld SA, Scott PP, Zachary JB, MacGregor MI. Longitudinal study of chronic sarcoidosis with low-dose maintenance corticosteroid therapy: outcome and complications. *Ann NY Acad Sci* 1986;**465**:702–12.

36. Jones E, Callen JP. Hydroxychloroquine is effective therapy for control of cutaneous sarcoidal granulomas. *J Am Acad Dermatol* 1990;**23**:487–9.

37. Baughman RP, Lower EE. Alternatives to corticosteroids in the treatment of sarcoidosis. *Sarcoid Vas Diffuse Lung Dis* 1997;**14**:121–30.

38. Baughman RP, Lower EE. Steroid sparing alternative treatments for sarcoidosis. *Clin Chest Med* 1997;**18**:853–64.

39. Millard TP, Smith HR, Black MM, Barker JN. Bullous pemphigoid developing during systemic therapy with chloroquine. *Clin Exp Dermatol* 1999;**24**:263–5.

40. Baughman RP, Winget DB, Lower EE. Methotrexate is steroid sparing in acute sarcoidosis. Results of a double blind, randomized trial. *Sarcoid Vas Diff Lung Dis* 2000;**17**:60–6.

41. Veien NK, Brodthagen H. Treatment of sarcoid with methotrexate. *Br J Dermatol* 1977;**97**:213–16.

42. Lower EE, Baughman RP. Prolonged use of methotrexate for sarcoidosis. *Arch Intern Med* 1995;**155**:846–51.

43. Kaye O, Palazzo E, Grossin M, Bourgeois P, Kahn MF, Malaise MG. Low-dose methotrexate: an effective corticosteroid-sparing agent in the musculoskeletal manifestations of sarcoidosis. *Br J Rheum* 1995;**34**:632–44.

44. Gedalia A, Molina JF, Ellis GS, Galen W, Moore C, Espinoza LR. Low-dose methotrexate therapy for childhood sarcoidosis. *J Pediatr* 1997;**130**:25–9.

45. Lacher MJ. Spontaneous remission or response to methotrexate in sarcoidosis. *Ann Intern Med* 1968;**69**:1247–8.

46. Webster GF, Razsi LK, Sanchez M, Shupack JL. Weekly low-dose methotrexate therapy for cutaneous sarcoidosis. *J Am Acad Dermatol* 1991;**24**:451–4.

47. Henderson CA, Ilchyshyn A, Curry AR. Laryngeal and cutaneous sarcoidosis treated with methotrexate. *J R Soc Med* 1994;**87**:632–3.

48. Albertini JG, Tyler W, Miller F. Ulcerative sarcoidosis: case report and review of the literature. *Arch Dermatol* 1997;**133**:215–19.

49. Carlesimo M, Giustini S, Rossi A, Bonaccorsi P, Calvieri S. Treatment of cutaneous and pulmonary sarcoidosis with thalidomide. *J Am Acad Dermatol* 1995;**32**:866–9.

50. Rousseau L, Beylot-Barry M, Doutre MS, Beylot C. Cutaneous sarcoidosis successfully treated with low doses of thalidomide. *Arch Dermatol* 1998;**134**:1045–6.

51. Estines O, Revuz J, Wolkenstein P, Bressieux JM, Roujeau JC, Cosnes A. Sarcoidosis: thalidomide treatment in ten patients. *Ann Dermatol Venereol* 2001;**128**:611–13.

52. Lee JB, Koblenzer PS. Disfiguring cutaneous manifestation of sarcoidosis treated with thalidomide: a case report. *J Am Acad Dermatol* 1998;**39**:835–8.

53. Bachelez H, Senet P, Cadranel J, Kaoukhov A, Dubertret L. The use of tetracyclines for the treatment of sarcoidosis. *Arch Dermatol* 2001;**137**:69–73.

54. Samuel M, Allen GE, McMillan SC, Burrows D, Corbett JR, Beare JM. Sarcoidosis: initial results on six patients treated with allopurinol. *Br J Dermatol* 1984;**111**(Suppl. 26):20.

55. Pfau A, Stolz W, Karrer S, Szeimies RM, Landthaler M. Allopurinol in treatment of cutaneous sarcoidosis. *Hautarzt* 1998;**49**:216–18.

56. Rosof BM. Allopurinol for sarcoid? *N Engl J Med* 1976;**294**:447.

57. Pollock JL. Sarcoidosis responding to allopurinol. *Arch Dermatol* 1980;**116**:273–4.

58. Brechtel B, Haas N, Henz BM, Kolde G. Allopurinol: a therapeutic alternative for disseminated cutaneous sarcoidosis. *Br J Dermatol* 1996;**135**:307–9.

59. Voelter-Mahlknecht S, Benez A, Metzger S, Fierlbeck G. Treatment of subcutaneous sarcoidosis with allopurinol. *Arch Dermatol* 1999;**135**:1560–1.

60. Antony F, Layton AM. A case of cutaneous acral sarcoidosis with response to allopurinol. *Br J Dermatol* 2000;**142**:1052–3.

61. Georgiou S, Monastirli A, Pasmatzi E, Tsamboas D. Cutaneous sarcoidosis: complete remission after oral isotretinoin therapy. *Acta Dermatol Venereol* 1998;**78**;457–8.

62. Waldinger TP, Ellis CN, Quint K, Voorhees JJ. Treatment of cutaneous sarcoidosis with isotretinoin. *Arch Dermatol* 1983;**119**:1003–5.

63. Spiteri MA, Taylor SJ. Retinoids in the treatment of cutaneous sarcoidosis (letter). *Arch Dermatol* 1985;**121**:1486.

64. Vaillant L, Le Marchand D, Bertrand S, Grangeponte MC, Lorette G. Sarcoidose cutanee annulaire du front: traitement par isotretinoine. *Ann Dermatol Venereol* 1986;**113**:1089–92.

65. Yamada H, Ide AA, Suigiura M. Treatment of cutaneous sarcoidosis with tranilast. *J Dermatol* 1995;**22**:149–52.

66. Cagnoni ML, Lombardi A, Cerinic MM *et al*. Melatonin for treatment of chronic refactory sarcoidosis. *Lancet* 1995;**346**:1229–30.

67. Schwarzenbach R, Djawari D. Disseminated small-node cutaneous sarcoidosis. *Dtsch Med Wochenschr* 2000;**125**:560–2.

68. Hughes JR, Pembroke AC. Cutaneous sarcoidosis treated with mepacrine. *Clin Exp Dermatol* 1994;**19**:448.

69. Baughman RP, Lower EE. Infliximib for refractory sarcoidosis. *Sarcoid Vas Diff Lung Dis* 2001;**18**:70–4.

70. Veien NK. Cutanoeus sarcoidosis treated with levamisole. *Dermatologica* 1977;**154**:185–9.

71. Goodman MM, Alpern K. Treatment of lupus pernio with the flashlamp pulsed dye laser. *Lasers Surg Med* 1992;**12**:549–51.

72. Cliff S, Felix RH, Singh L, Harland CC. The successful treatment of lupus pernio with the flashlamp pulsed dye laser. *J Cutan Laser Ther* 1999;**1**:49–52.

73. Dosik JS, Ashinoff R. Treating lupus pernio with the 585 nm pulsed dye laser. *Skin Aging* 1999;93–94.

74. Green JJ, Lawrence N, Heymann WR. Generalized ulcerative sarcoidosis induced by therapy with the flashlamp-pumped pulsed dye laser. *Arch Dermatol* 2001;**137**:507–8.

75. O'Brien P. Sarcoidosis of the nose. *Br J Plast Surg* 1970;**23**:242–7.

76. Shaw M, Black MM, Davis PKB. Disfiguring lupus pernio successfully treated with plastic surgery. *Clin Exp Dermatol* 1984;**9**:614–17.

77. Collison DW, Novice F, Banse L, Rodman OG, Kelly AP. Split thickness skin grafting in extensive ulcerative sarcoidosis. *J Dermatol Surg Oncol* 1989;**15**:679–83.

78. Stack BC, Hall PJ, Goodman AL, Perez IR. CO_2 laser excision of lupus pernio of the face. *Am J Otolaryngol* 1996;**17**:260–3.

79. Streit M, Bohlen LM, Braathen LR. Ulcerative sarcoidosis successfully treated with apligraf. *Dermatology* 2001;**202**:367–70.

80. Khatri KA, Chotzen VA, Burrall BA. Lupus pernio: successful treatment with a potent topical corticosteroid. *Arch Dermatol* 1995;**131**:617–18.

81. Volden G. Successful treatment of chronic skin diseases with clobetasol propionate and a hydrocolloid occlusive dressing. *Acta Derm Venereol* 1992;**72**:69–71.

82. Sullivan RD, Mayock RL, Jones Jr. *et al*. Local injection of hydrocortisone and cortisone into skin lesions of sarcoidosis. *JAMA* 1953;**152**:308–12.

83. Liedtka JE. Intralesional chloroquine for the treatment of cutaneous sarcoidosis. *Int J Dermatol* 1996;**35**:682–3.

84. Verbov J. The place of intralesional steroid therapy in dermatology. *Br J Dermatol* 1976;**94**(Suppl. 12):51–8.

85. Patterson JW, Fitzwater JE. Treatment of hypopigmented sarcoidosis with 8-methoxypsoralen and long wave ultraviolet light. *Int J Dermatol* 1982;**21**:476–80.

86. Graefe T, Konrad H, Barta U *et al*. Successful ultraviolet A1 treatment of cutaneous sarcoidosis. *Br J Dermatol* 2001;**145**:354–6.

87. Gogstetter DS, Goldsmith LA. Treatment of cutaneous sarcoidosis using phonophoresis. *J Am Acad Dermatol* 1999;**40**:797–9.

50
Erythema multiforme

Pierre Dominique Ghislain and J Claude Roujeau

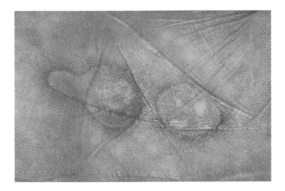

Figure 50.1 Acral lesions (palm)

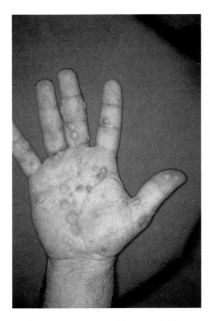

Figure 50.2 Typical targets with central blisters

Background
Definition

Erythema multiforme (EM) is an acute, self-limited, feverish eruption characterised by target cutaneous lesions, with a symmetric and mainly acral distribution. Lesions are rounded, with three zones: a central area of dusky erythema or purpura, sometimes bullous, a middle paler zone of oedema and an outer ring of erythema with a well-defined edge. Hands and feet are habitually the most affected areas and are sometimes selectively involved. Mucous membrane erosions are frequent and distinguish EM major from EM minor. Histopathological examination shows a predominantly inflammatory pattern characterised by a lichenoid infiltrate and limited epidermal necrosis that affects mainly the basal layer.

Incidence/prevalence

Unknown.

Aetiology/risk factors

The principal cause is infection with herpes simplex virus (HSV), which probably explains 40–70% of all cases. Many other infections can induce occasional cases. According to recent classification, EM-like drug eruptions are related to Stevens–Johnson syndrome (SJS), the clinical signs being quite similar.

Prognosis

EM has low morbidity and no mortality. A spontaneous resolution occurs in 1–6 weeks.

Ocular sequelae may also occur. Recurrences are frequent. Rarely recurrences overlap, leading to "continuous" or "persistent" EM. Mouth erosions may strongly impair the quality of life of patients.

Aims of treatment

- To reduce the duration of fever, eruption and hospitalisation
- To prevent or reduce recurrences

Outcomes

- Duration of fever, eruption and hospitalisation
- Frequency of recurrences
- Number of days with symptoms per year

Methods of search

Clinical Evidence search and appraisal, June 2001 (Cochrane databases of randomised controlled trials (RCTs) and controlled clinical trials; Medline 1966–June 2001).

QUESTIONS

What are the effects of treatment of an acute attack?

Short course of systemic corticosteroids

Based on retrospective series or small RCTs, corticosteroids seem to shorten the duration of fever and eruption but increase the duration of hospitalisation because of the risk of complications.

Benefits and harms

Sixteen children with EM major were included in a prospective RCT within 3 days of the onset of rash. Ten received bolus infusions of methylprednisolone, 4 mg/kg/day, while six had supportive treatment only. Corticosteroids reduced the period of fever (4·0 versus 9·5 days), reduced the period of acute eruption (7·0 versus 9·8 days) and signs of prostration were milder. Complications were minimal in both groups. The authors suggest that an early short course of corticosteroids favourably influences the course of EM major in children.[1]

In an RCT including nine adults with mild, uncomplicated EM major, four received prednisolone, 30 mg daily, reduced by 5 mg each day, and five received placebo. The mean length of stay in hospital was longer in the corticosteroid group (9·5 versus 8 days). Diagnoses were not clear: histology was consistent with EM; a drug-induced reaction was suspected in five cases; no information about HSV was given.[2]

In a retrospective study, Rasmussen compared 17 children with EM treated with systemic corticosteroids with 15 children who received supportive care only. Both groups were comparable in age, sex, length of prodrome, exposure to drugs, initial fever, extent of oral and cutaneous involvement and frequency of isolation of pathogens. The group treated with corticosteroids had a shorter fever period (1·8 versus 5·5 days) but a longer mean length of hospitalisation (21 versus 13 days) because of more frequent complications (53% versus 0%).[3]

In a series of 51 children, corticosteroids were claimed to worsen the prognosis: 74% of patients treated with corticosteroids had complications, versus 28% of the patients who did not receive corticosteroids.[4]

In a series of 25 patients with EM minor, corticosteroids allowed no clinical improvement except a shorter duration of fever (2·7 versus 5·6 days).[5]

Comment

Corticosteroids appear to be of little use, and side-effects are frequent. However, the methodology of most studies is poor: patient numbers are small and there is often a mix of idiopathic or viral-associated EM and drug-induced SJS.

Erythromycin

We found no evidence on the usefulness of erythromycin. Erythromycin is claimed to be useful only when *Mycoplasma pneumoniae* infection is suspected.

Aciclovir

There were no RCTs, but several series stated that initiating aciclovir for the *treatment* of full-blown post-herpetic EM was of no benefit.

> **What are the effects of treatment to prevent recurrence?**

Sun protection

We found no evidence on the effects of protection from sun.

Benefits

Ultraviolet light may induce recurrence of HSV infection. We found no good evidence on the effects of protection from sun on the recurrence of EM.

Harms

Interestingly, PUVA has been proposed as a treatment for persistent EM. We found no good evidence on its effectiveness.

Comment

The effects of ultraviolet light are not clear.

Aciclovir

We found one RCT showing effectiveness of continuous oral aciclovir in the prevention of EM

recurrences.[6] Another RCT showed that topical aciclovir is not effective.[7]

Benefits

We found one RCT. Nineteen patients with more than four attacks of EM per year were enrolled in a 6-month double-blind, placebo-controlled trial of aciclovir, 400 mg twice daily. There were no attacks in the aciclovir group (range 0–2), compared with a median of three (1–6) in the placebo group ($P<0.0005$). At the time of inclusion, five patients had no clinical evidence of disease precipitation by HSV; two of them were in the aciclovir group; one showed complete disease suppression.[6]

We found another RCT, which showed that topical aciclovir therapy used in a prophylactic manner is not successful in preventing recurrent herpes-associated EM.[7]

Harms

We found no evidence.

Comment

Continuous oral aciclovir is effective in prevention of recurrences of herpes-associated EM but it may also be useful for patients without clinical evidence that herpes is the precipitating factor.

Dapsone

We found no evidence on effects of dapsone.

Antimalarials

We found no evidence on the effects of antimalarials.

Azathioprine

We found no RCTs of azathioprine. We found one small series showing benefit of azathioprine. In a series of 65 patients with recurrent EM, 11 were treated with azathioprine when all other treatments had failed. Azathioprine was successful in all 11 patients.[8] Another series reported five cases in whom complete or almost complete remission was achieved.[9]

Comment
Further trials are needed.

Ciclosporin
We found no good evidence of the use of ciclosporin.

Thalidomide
We found one retrospective analysis of thalidomide prescription (1981–1993), which shows good efficacy for treatment of recurrent or subintrant EM.[10] However, the data were uncontrolled and the findings have not been confirmed. Side-effects were not described.

Potassium iodide
We found insufficient evidence on potassium iodide.

Benefits
In a retrospective study, potassium iodide 300 mg three times daily was used for 16 patients with EM. Complete remission was noted in 14 patients, including those with concomitant HSV.[11]

Harms
We found no evidence.

Comment
No conclusion is possible to date.

Levamisole
Levamisole appeared useful in one RCT.

Benefits
We found a double-blind placebo-controlled crossover trial, which included 14 patients with chronic or recurrent EM resistant to corticosteroid therapy. Levamisole was used at a dose of 150 mg/day for three consecutive days each week, for at least 4 weeks after first appearance of a lesion. Levamisole allowed decrease of severity, duration and frequency of EM attacks.[12]

An open comparative trial showed similar efficacy of levamisole used alone (17 patients; 76% complete response) versus a combination of prednisone and levamisole (22 patients; 82% complete response).[13]

Harms
Because agranulocytosis is a severe and not exceptional adverse effect, levamisole is not admitted by all national drug agencies.

Comment
The benefit/risk ratio is probably too low to support the use of levamisole in EM.

Cimetidine
We found insufficient evidence.

Immunoglobulin
We found no evidence.

Key points
- We found one RCT which shows usefulness of aciclovir in preventing the recurrence of EM.
- We found little or controversial evidence on the effects on corticosteroids in the treatment of an acute attack of EM. Early administration reduces the duration of fever but may cause many side-effects.
- While levamisole showed some benefit, the benefit/risk ratio was considered too low.
- We found no good evidence on all other therapeutic choices (erythromycin, dapsone, antimalarials, azathioprine, ciclosporin, thalidomide, potassium iodide, cimetidine, immunoglobulins).

References

1. Kakourou T, Klontza D, Soteropoulou F, Kattamis C. Corticosteroid treatment of erythema multiforme major (Stevens–Johnson syndrome) in children. *Eur J Pediatr* 1997;**156**:90–3.

2. Wright S. The treatment of erythema multiforme major with systemic corticosteroids. *Br J Dermatol* 1991;**124**:612–13.

3. Rasmussen JE. Erythema multiforme in children. Response to treatment with systemic corticosteroids. *Br J Dermatol* 1976;**95**:181–6.

4. Ginsburg CM. Stevens–Johnson syndrome in children. *Pediatr Infect Dis* 1982;**1**:155–8.

5. Ting HC, Adam BA. Erythema multiforme – response to corticosteroid. *Dermatologica* 1984;**169**:175–8.

6. Tatnall FM, Schofield JK, Leigh IM. A double-blind, placebo-controlled trial of continuous acyclovir therapy in recurrent erythema multiforme. *Br J Dermatol* 1995;**132**:267–70.

7. Fawcett HA, Wansbrough-Jones MH, Clark AE, Leigh IM. Prophylactic topical acyclovir for frequent recurrent herpes simplex infection with and without erythema multiforme. *BMJ* (Clin Res Ed) 1983;**287**:798–9.

8. Schofield JK, Tatnall FM, Leigh IM. Recurrent erythema multiforme: clinical features and treatment in a large series of patients. *Br J Dermatol* 1993;**128**:542–5.

9. Farthing PM, Maragou P, Coates M, Tatnall F, Leigh IM, Williams DM. Characteristics of the oral lesions in patients with cutaneous recurrent erythema multiforme. *J Oral Pathol Med* 1995;**24**:9–13.

10. Cherouati K, Claudy A, Souteyrand P *et al.* Traitement par thalidomide de l'érythéme polymorphe chronique (formes récidivantes et subintrantes). Etude rétrospective de 26 malades. *Ann Dermatol Venereol* 1996;**123**:375–7.

11. Horio T, Danno K, Okamoto H, Miyachi Y, Imamura S. Potassium iodide in erythema nodosum and other erythematous dermatoses. *J Am Acad Dermatol* 1983;**9**:77–81.

12. Lozada F. Levamisole in the treatment of erythema multiforme: a double-blind trial in fourteen patients. *Oral Surg Oral Med Oral Pathol* 1982;**53**:28–31.

13. Lozada-Nur F, Cram D, Gorsky M. Clinical response to levamisole in thirty-nine patients with erythema multiforme. An open prospective study. *Oral Surg Oral Med Oral Pathol* 1992;**74**:294–8.

51

Stevens–Johnson syndrome and toxic epidermal necrolysis

Pierre Dominique Ghislain and J Claude Roujeau

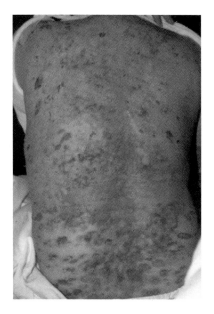

Figure 51.1   Patient with Stevens–Johnson syndrome

Background
Definition

Stevens–Johnson syndrome (SJS) and toxic epidermal necrolysis (TEN) are variants of the same process, presenting as severe mucosal erosions with widespread purpuric cutaneous macules (atypical targets), often confluent with positive Nikolsky's sign and epidermal detachment. In SJS, epidermal detachment involves less than 10% of total body skin area; transitional SJS–TEN is defined by an epidermal detachment between 10% and 30%, and TEN by

a detachment greater than 30%. A full-thickness epidermal necrosis is observed on pathological examination.

Incidence/prevalence

On the basis of case registries and observational studies, the incidence of TEN is estimated at 1–1·4 cases per million inhabitants per year. The incidence of SJS is probably of the same order (1–3 cases per million inhabitants per year).[1–3]

Aetiology/risk factors

SJS–TEN is essentially drug induced (70–90% of cases). Graft versus host disease is another well-established aetiology, independent of drugs. A few cases are related to infection (*Mycoplasma pneumoniae*); other cases remain unexplained ("idiopathic" forms). The most extensive study of medication use and SJS–TEN pointed mainly to sulfonamides, anticonvulsant agents, non-steroidal anti-inflammatory drugs, allopurinol and chlormezanone.[4] HIV infection dramatically increases the risk. A predisposing effect of autoimmune disorders, such as lupus, and an HLA-linked genetic susceptibility have been also suggested.

Prognosis

SJS–TEN is an acute self-limiting disease, with high morbidity and is potentially life-threatening. Mortality rates are 5% with SJS, 30–35% with

TEN and 10–15% with transitional forms. Epidermal detachment may be extensive, possibly the entire skin surface. As in severe burns, fluid losses are massive, with electrolyte imbalance. Superinfection, impairment of thermoregulation, energy expenditure, alteration of immunological function and haematological abnormalities are usual systemic complications. Mucous membrane involvement (oropharynx, eyes, genitalia and anus) require attentive nursing. The gastrointestinal and tracheobronchial epithelia can be involved and cause high morbidity.

Age, percentage of denuded skin, neutropenia, serum urea nitrogen level and visceral involvement are prognostic factors. There are different scoring systems for vital prognosis estimation, such as simplified acute physiology score (SAPS) and SAPS II, which are not specific. A new score – SCORTEN – has been proposed as a TEN-specific severity-of-illness score and validated in a single centre.[5]

After healing, scars, pigmentation disorders, conjunctival lesions and Sjögren-like syndrome are the main long-term complications.

Aims of treatment

- to reduce mortality
- to block the extent of the disease
- to reduce associated morbidity
- to prevent sequelae

Outcomes

- mortality rate
- percentage of epidermal detachment at the acme of the disease
- infectious complications
- length of healing
- length of stay in hospital
- ocular sequelae

Methods of search

Clinical Evidence search and appraisal – June 2001. We used the Cochrane databases of RCTs and controlled clinical trials and Medline 1966–June 2001. We found no systematic review and only one placebo-controlled trial. Therefore, we have also included observational studies and open trials.

QUESTIONS

What are the effects of specific treatments?

Prompt withdrawal of potential culprit drugs

We found limited evidence that early withdrawal of the drug(s) that cause(s) TEN/SJS alters the clinical course of the disease.

Benefits

We found one observational study, which showed that death rates were lower when causative drugs with short elimination half-lives were withdrawn no later than the day when blisters or erosions first occurred: 2/44 (5%) compared with 11/42 (26%) when withdrawn later. No difference was seen for drugs with long half-lives.[6]

Harms

We found no controlled data.

Comment

Since it would be unethical to perform an RCT of the effect of prolonging drug administration, observational studies will probably remain the only available clinical evidence for this question.

Corticosteroids

We found no good evidence about the use of corticosteroids in TEN/SJS. Beneficial effects are doubtful and are accompanied by many side-effects.

Benefits

We found only uncontrolled series in which fourteen patients with 45–100% skin detachment were treated with high doses of corticosteroids (400 mg prednisone/day (six patients) and 200 mg/day (eight patients), gradually decreased over a 4–6-week period). Only one death occurred, which was considered much fewer than expected, considering the extent of the disease.[7]

A series of 67 patients with SJS/TEN treated with corticosteroids (from prednisolone, 40 mg, to methylprednisolone, 750 mg) claimed an excellent survival rate and minor side-effects. But diagnoses were not clear: only some patients had mucous involvement.[8–12] In a small retrospective study of 14 patients, no difference in mortality rates or infectious complications was noted in patients who received steroids before referral.[13] In a retrospective analysis of 39 patients with TEN, steroid treatment was not significantly related to the mortality rate.[14]

Harms

We found poor evidence that corticosteroid use is detrimental. It is suggested that corticosteroids provoke prolonged wound healing, increased risk of infection, masking of early signs of sepsis, severe gastrointestinal bleeding and increased mortality. Thirty patients with SJS or TEN were included in an uncontrolled prospective study. The first 15 patients received corticosteroids, and the mortality rate was 66%. Therefore, the next 15 patients were treated without corticosteroids, and the mortality rate was 33%. Both groups were similar in other aspects. However, 11 of the 15 patients treated without corticosteroids had taken corticosteroids before referral. Thus no conclusion can be drawn about exclusive early administration of corticosteroids.[15]

In a retrospective study, a multivariate analysis of prognosis factors showed that corticosteroid therapy is an independent factor for increased mortality.[16] Other series seem to come to the same conclusion.[17] Moreover, many cases of TEN occur during treatment with high doses of corticosteroids for pre-existing disease. Data from 216 patients with TEN were investigated in a retrospective study; 11 of them had been treated with corticosteroids for at least a week before the first sign of TEN (from 1 week to several months, at doses of 7·5–325 mg prednisolone/day).[18] In another series of 179 patients, 13 were undergoing long-term glucocorticosteroid therapy before TEN developed. Compared with 166 other cases, these patients had a longer delay between the introduction of the suspect drug and the onset of TEN, and a longer time elapsed between the first symptom of TEN and hospital admission. No other differences were observed.[19]

Comment

These data, although uncontrolled, suggest that corticosteroids are more detrimental than useful in most severe cases of TEN and should be avoided in these cases and after the first days of clinical course. We found no evidence about their effects early in the disease.

The results of many studies are difficult to analyse because cases of drug-induced SJS and erythema multiforme are often mixed in the same series.

Intravenous immunoglobulins (IVIG)

We found no good evidence on the effects on IVIG in TEN.

Benefits

We found one uncontrolled clinical trial. It was based on in vitro demonstration that IVIG can inhibit Fas–Fas ligand mediated apoptosis. Ten consecutive patients with TEN of moderate severity were treated with different doses of IVIG (0·2–0·75 g/kg/day for four consecutive days); all survived.[20] But this study was uncontrolled, and other authors did not obtain same results.

Harms
We found no clinical TEN-specific evidence.

Comment
Enthusiasm for IVIG is premature.

Plasmapheresis
We found no good evidence about plasmapheresis/plasma exchanges in TEN/SJS.

Benefits
We found a few retrospective or uncontrolled trials about plasmapheresis, but no good evidence of positive effect.

Harms
We found one open trial with historical controls: eight consecutive patients with TEN received plasma exchange. This series showed no significant difference in mortality, duration of hospital stay and time to re-epithelialisation.[21]

Comment
The usefulness of plasmapheresis is unknown and doubtful.

Ciclosporin
We found no sufficient evidence on the effects of ciclosporin.

Benefits
We found a case series of TEN treated with ciclosporin. The treatment was safe and was associated with a more rapid re-epithelialisation

rate and a lower mortality rate (0/11 versus 3/6) in comparison with a historical series of patients treated with cyclophosphamide and corticosteroids.[22]

Harms
We found no evidence.

Comment
A controlled trial is needed to evaluate the real value of ciclosporin.

Cyclophosphamide
We found insufficient evidence of the therapeutic benefits of cyclophosphamide.

Benefits
We found some trials using historical controls. Eight patients with TEN were treated with cyclophosphamide alone (initial dose 300 mg/day); all survived.[23] We found some series of combined therapy with cyclophosphamide and corticosteroids but they were not interpretable.

Harms
Some cases of cyclophosphamide-induced TEN were reported, of which one was with positive rechallenge test.

Comment
No conclusion is possible.

N-acetylcysteine (NAC)
NAC increases the clearance of several drugs and their metabolites and *in vitro* inhibits production of tumour necrosis factor (TNF)-α and interleukin-1β. We found no evidence of clinical effectiveness in TEN.

Benefits

We found no evidence concerning SJS or TEN.

Harms

High doses of NAC may inactivate not only the culprit drug but also other drugs, which is potentially useful for the patient.

A randomised trial has shown that NAC is ineffective in preventing hypersensitivity reactions to trimethoprim-sulfamethoxazole in patients with HIV infection.[24]

Comment

The usefulness of NAC is unknown and doubtful.

Other medications

We found no evidence on granulocyte colony stimulating factor, heparin, monoclonal antibodies against cytokines, or pentoxifylline.

Benefits

We found only case reports.

Harms

We found no evidence.

Thalidomide

We found one RCT comparing thalidomide with placebo, which showed an excess of mortality with thalidomide.

Benefits

Thalidomide has been proposed as treatment for TEN because it is a potent inhibitor of TNF-α action. We found no clinical evidence about the benefits of thalidomide in TEN/SJS.

Harms

We found a double-blind randomised placebo-controlled study of thalidomide, 400 mg daily for 5 days, in patients with TEN. Twenty-two patients were included, but the study was stopped because there was an unexplained excess

mortality in the thalidomide group (10 of 12 patients died, compared with 3 of 10 in the placebo group). There was no significant difference in origin of death between both groups.[25]

Comment

Based on a unique RCT, thalidomide seems to be detrimental in TEN.

What are the effects of symptomatic treatments?

Early referral to specialised medical units

We found several retrospective studies, which show a lower risk of infection and a lower mortality if patients are referred early to a specialised unit.

Benefits

Three retrospective studies pointed out the interest of prompt referral. In the first study, the patients transferred to a specialised centre more than 7 days after the onset of epidermal slough had a period of hospitalisation that was more than twice as long as for patients transferred before 7 days, despite other comparable risk factors.[16] In another study of 44 patients, delayed transfer was associated with high morbidity and mortality rates.[26] Finally, a third retrospective analysis summarised the data of 36 patients with TEN; it showed that patients who survived had been referred earlier than non-survivors (4·0 versus 11·5 days). Patients referred before 7 days had a mortality rate of 4%, compared with 83% for those referred after 7 days. Increased risk of infection in outside facilities was claimed to be the critical factor,[27] but in a previously mentioned small retrospective study, there was no difference in the infection or mortality rate in patients who were transferred late.[13]

Harms

We found no evidence.

Comment

Early referral is a priority during treatment, even if good evidence is still lacking.

Supportive care

Most symptomatic treatments are similar (but not identical) to those used for severe burns. We found no controlled study of specific care for TEN/SJS.

Benefits

Main aspects of symptomatic treatment are: careful handling, intravenous fluid replacement (quantity adjusted daily) by peripheral access distant from the affected areas (no central venous line), oral rehydration started as soon as possible (by nasogastric support) and nutrition, aseptic care, warming of environment, pain and anxiety control, prevention of sequelae and so on. It is claimed that the fluid requirements of patients with TEN is two-thirds to three-quarters of that of patients with burns covering the same area. We found no RCT or controlled clinical trial on this.

We found many trials on techniques to help skin healing – epidermal stripping, biological skin covering (porcine xenografts or cadaveric allografts), synthetic dressings, and so on – but none was comparative. In comparison with burns, skin necrosis is more superficial.

It is suggested that wearing gas-permeable scleral contact lenses reduces photophobia and discomfort; these lenses improved visual acuity and healed corneal epithelial defects in half of patients.[28]

Harms

The nature of intravenous fluid replacement is not specific (macromolecules and saline solutions). A systematic review of human albumin in critically ill patients proposed to substitute albumin and colloids with crystalloids, because an excess of mortality was observed with albumin.[29]

Comment

By contrast to TEN, many RCTs on burn care have been published. Several recent trials are potentially useful for TEN/SJS.

Enteral feeding

Twenty-two patients were randomly assigned into two groups (early enteral feeding versus delayed enteral feeding). Early enteral feeding had a beneficial effect on the reduction of enterogenic infection, by decreasing intestinal permeability.[30]

Supplementation

Oxandrolone is an anabolic agent. Compared with placebo, it is effective for decreasing weight loss and net nitrogenous loss and increasing donor site wound healing.[31] Compared with human growth hormone, oxandrolone was equally effective but induced fewer complications (hyperglycaemia and hypermetabolism).[32] The effectiveness of ornithine alpha-ketoglutarate supplementation of enteral feeding was assessed against an isonitrogenous control. Wound healing time was reduced by 33% with ornithine supplementation.[33] High-dose ascorbic acid (66 mg/kg/hour) for the first 24 hours for >30% burns reduces volume of rehydration fluid required.[34]

Topical treatment

A controlled right–left comparative and randomised study showed that frozen cultured human allogeneic epidermal sheets reduced healing time of partial-thickness burns by 44%.[35] A living skin equivalent, Apligraf, was applied over meshed split-thickness autografts in 38 patients while a control site in each patient was treated with split-thickness autograft alone.

There was no difference in the per cent and delay of graft take, but Apligraf-treated sites were rated superior to control sites in 58% and worse in 16%. Pigmentation and vascularity were significantly better.[36] In 89 children with <25% burns, Biobrane decreased healing time without increasing the risk of infection.[37] In a trial of 20 children, Biobrane was superior to topical 1% silver sulfadiazine in pain, requirements for analgesics, wound healing time and length of hospital stay.[38] TransCyte is composed of human newborn fibroblasts cultured on the nylon mesh of Biobrane. Sites treated with TransCyte healed more rapidly (11 versus 18 days) and with less hypertrophic scarring than sites treated with silver sulfadiazine in 14 patients.[39] In an RCT of 600 patients with second-degree burns, topical recombinant bovine basic fibroblast growth factor allowed faster granulation tissue formation and epidermal regeneration than with placebo.[40] The effect of systemic growth hormone is still debated.

Prophylactic antibiotics

We found no evidence on the effects of prophylactic antibiotics.

Most authors do not use prophylactic antibiotics. Preventive isolation, aseptic handling and use of sterile fields are suggested to be better. We found no clinical evidence on the benefits or harms of early antibiotic therapy.

Is there any test to prove drug culpability?

We found no evidence for a reliable test to prove the link between a single case and a specific drug.

Benefits

A study of patch tests and drug reactions showed only two patients among 22 SJS/TEN cases with a relevant positive test: one with sulphonamide and one with phenobarbital. Healthy volunteers were used as controls.[41] In a series of 14 patients, seven patch tests were performed, three of which were positive (ethylbutylmalonylureum, phenazone, phenylbutazone). Among the four negative tests, three intracutaneous tests were performed, two of which were positive (phenacetine, chloramphenicol).[7]

We found only case reports and no clinical trial about *in vitro* tests (essentially lymphocyte transformation tests).

Harms

Even though theoretically possible, no reactivation of SJS/TEN was reported from patch tests. We found only a few case reports of generalised erythema or irritation.

Comment

The usefulness and specificity of patch tests – and thus their clinical usefulness – remain to be determined. *In vitro* tests are not performed routinely.

What happens in case of rechallenge with the causative drug or a related drug?

We found no good evidence on the risk of re-use of a culprit drug or on the possibility of desensitisation in patients with TEN. Some data are available for prevention and desensitisation in benign cutaneous adverse drug reactions.

Benefits

Primary prevention is the avoidance of the culprit drug and of closely related drugs. We found two RCTs about prevention of drug reactions (not specifically for TEN). In the first trial, the incidence of rash complicating the first few weeks of treatment with nevirapine was significantly diminished by adding corticosteroids

(50 mg every other day) for 2 weeks, or by using a slowly escalating dose.[42] The second RCT demonstrated a lower incidence of adverse reactions to sulfamethoxazole in the prevention of pneumocystosis in HIV-infected individuals by using a slowly escalating dose.[43] These two RCTs were concerned only with primary prevention and did not include patients with previous drug reactions.

By contrast, desensitisation with low doses of culprit drug and progressive increases concern patients with a history of benign drug eruption. We found one RCT: HIV patients with history of reaction to trimethoprim-sulfamethoxazole were rechallenged with oral trimethoprim. If no reaction was seen (59 cases of 73), patients were randomised to sulfamethoxazole with either a treatment scheme of desensitisation, or immediately at the dosage commonly used in prophylaxis. Adverse effects occurred in 28% of patients in the desensitisation group compared with 20·5% in the other group. This difference was not statistically significant.[44]

Harms

We found one publication with a series of provocation tests in patients with TEN (10 cases) or SJS (8 cases). The dose was progressively increased to a commonly used daily dose and then continued at this level for 2–9 days. Only one test was positive in the TEN patients (maculopapular eruption) and four in the SJS patients (with two recurrences of SJS). Hypotheses to explain this low rate of recurrence are misdiagnosis, desensitising effect by use of progressive dose or real lack of systematic recurrence.[45]

Comment

Even if the rate of recurrence was only 10%, risk for life was so high that rechallenge with a highly suspect drug is not ethically acceptable.

Summary of interventions

- **Likely to be beneficial:** prompt withdrawal of potentially causative drugs
- **Trade-off between benefits and harms:** systemic corticosteroids
- **Unknown effectiveness:** intravenous immunoglobulins, plasmapheresis, ciclosporin, cyclophosphamide, N-acetylcysteine, granulocyte colony stimulating factor, heparin, monoclonal antibodies against cytokines, pentoxifylline
- **Harmful:** thalidomide

Key points

- Erythema multiforme, SJS and TEN are still used with different definitions. This does not allow correct literature analysis.
- We found insufficient evidence about effective treatments.
- We found only one placebo-controlled RCT, which showed a higher mortality with thalidomide.
- We found no good evidence on the effects of corticosteroids.
- We found no evidence of the value of tests.
- We found insufficient evidence of the effect of drug reintroduction.

References

1. Rzany B, Mockenhaupt M, Baur S et al. Epidemiology of erythema exsudativum multiforme majus, Stevens–Johnson syndrome, and toxic epidermal necrolysis in Germany (1990–1992): structure and results of a population-based registry. J Clin Epidemiol 1996;**49**:769–73.

2. Roujeau JC, Guillaume JC, Fabre JP, Penso D, Flechet ML, Girre JP. Toxic epidermal necrolysis (Lyell syndrome). Incidence and drug etiology in France, 1981–1985. Arch Dermatol 1990;**126**:37–42.

3. Chan HL, Stern RS, Arndt KA et al. The incidence of erythema multiforme, Stevens–Johnson syndrome, and toxic epidermal necrolysis. A population-based study with particular reference to reactions caused by drugs among outpatients. Arch Dermatol 1990;**126**:43–7.

4. Roujeau JC, Kelly JP, Naldi L *et al.* Medication use and the risk of Stevens–Johnson syndrome or toxic epidermal necrolysis. *N Engl J Med* 1995;**333**:1600–7.

5. Bastuji-Garin S, Fouchard N, Bertocchi M, Roujeau JC, Revuz J, Wolkenstein P. SCORTEN: a severity-of-illness score for toxic epidermal necrolysis. *J Invest Dermatol* 2000;**115**:149–53.

6. Garcia-Doval I, LeCleach L, Bocquet H, Otero XL, Roujeau JC. Toxic epidermal necrolysis and Stevens–Johnson syndrome: does early withdrawal of causative drugs decrease the risk of death? *Arch Dermatol* 2000;**136**:323–7.

7. Tegelberg-Stassen MJ, van Vloten WA, Baart de la Faille. Management of nonstaphylococcal toxic epidermal necrolysis: follow-up study of 16 case histories. *Dermatologica* 1990;**180**:124–9.

8. Patterson R, Dykewicz MS, Gonzales A *et al.* Erythema multiforme and Stevens–Johnson syndrome. Descriptive and therapeutic controversy. *Chest* 1990;**98**:331–6.

9. Patterson R, Grammer LC, Greenberger PA *et al.* Stevens–Johnson syndrome (SJS): effectiveness of corticosteroids in management and recurrent SJS. *Allergy Proc* 1992;**13**:89–95.

10. Patterson R, Miller M, Kaplan M *et al.* Effectiveness of early therapy with corticosteroids in Stevens–Johnson syndrome: experience with 41 cases and a hypothesis regarding pathogenesis. *Ann Allergy* 1994;**73**:27–34.

11. Cheriyan S, Patterson R, Greenberger PA, Grammer LC, Latall J. The outcome of Stevens–Johnson syndrome treated with corticosteroids. *Allergy Proc* 1995;**16**:151–5.

12. Tripathi A, Ditto AM, Grammer LC *et al.* Corticosteroid therapy in an additional 13 cases of Stevens–Johnson syndrome: a total series of 67 cases. *Allergy Asthma Proc* 2000;**21**:101–5.

13. Engelhardt SL, Schurr MJ, Helgerson RB. Toxic epidermal necrolysis: an analysis of referral patterns and steroid usage. *J Burn Care Rehabil* 1997;**18**:520–4.

14. Schulz JT, Sheridan RL, Ryan CM, MacKool B, Tompkins RG. A 10-year experience with toxic epidermal necrolysis. *J Burn Care Rehabil* 2000;**21**:199–204.

15. Halebian PH, Corder VJ, Madden MR, Finklestein JL, Shires GT. Improved burn cenrer survival of patients with toxic epidermal necrolysis managed without corticosteroids. *Ann Surg* 1986;**204**:503–12.

16. Kelemen JJ, Cioffi WG, McManus WF, Mason ADJ, Pruitt BAJ. Burn center care for patients with toxic epidermal necrolysis. *J Am Coll Surg* 1995;**180**:273–8.

17. Kim PS, Goldfarb IW, Gaisford JC, Slater H. Stevens–Johnson syndrome and toxic epidermal necrolysis: a pathophysiologic review with recommendations for a treatment protocol. *J Burn Care Rehabil* 1983;**4**: 91–100.

18. Rzany B, Schmitt H, Schopf E. Toxic epidermal necrolysis in patients receiving glucocorticosteroids. *Acta Derm Venereol* 1991;**71**:171–2.

19. Guibal F, Bastuji-Garin S, Chosidow O, Saiag P, Revuz J, Roujeau JC. Characteristics of toxic epidermal necrolysis in patients undergoing long-term glucocorticoid therapy. *Arch Dermatol* 1995;**131**:669–72.

20. Viard I, Wehrli P, Bullani R *et al.* Inhibition of toxic epidermal necrolysis by blockade of CD95 with human intravenous immunoglobulin. *Science* 1998;**282**:490–3.

21. Furubacke A, Berlin G, Anderson C, Sjoberg F. Lack of significant treatment effect of plasma exchange in the treatment of drug-induced toxic epidermal necrolysis? *Intensive Care Med* 1999;**25**:1307–10.

22. Arevalo JM, Lorente JA, Gonzalez-Herrada C, Jimenez-Reyes J. Treatment of toxic epidermal necrolysis with cyclosporin A. *J Trauma* 2000;**48**:473–8.

23. Trautmann A, Klein CE, Kampgen E, Brocker EB. Severe bullous drug reactions treated successfully with cyclophosphamide. *Br J Dermatol* 1998;**139**:1127–8.

24. Walmsley SL, Khorasheh S, Singer J, Djurdjev O. A randomized trial of N-acetylcysteine for prevention of trimethoprim-sulfamethoxazole hypersensitivity reactions in Pneumocystis carinii pneumonia prophylaxis (CTN 057). Canadian HIV Trials Network 057 Study Group. *J Acquir Immune Defic Syndr Hum Retrovirol* 1998;**19**:498–505.

25. Wolkenstein P, Latarjet J, Roujeau JC *et al.* Randomised comparison of thalidomide versus placebo in toxic epidermal necrolysis. *Lancet* 1998;**352**:1586–9.

26. Murphy JT, Purdue GF, Hunt JL. Toxic epidermal necrolysis. *J Burn Care Rehabil* 1997;**18**:417–20.

27. McGee T, Munster A. Toxic epidermal necrolysis syndrome: mortality rate reduced with early referral to regional burn center. *Plast Reconstr Surg* 1998;**102**:1018–22.

28. Romero-Rangel T, Stavrou P, Cotter J, Rosenthal P, Baltatzis S, Foster CS. Gas-permeable scleral contact lens therapy in ocular surface disease. *Am J Ophthalmol* 2000;**130**:25–32.

29. Cochrane Injuries Group. Human albumin administration in critically ill patients: systematic review of randomised controlled trials. *BMJ* 1998;**317**:235–40.

30. Peng YZ, Yuan ZQ, Xiao GX. Effects of early enteral feeding on the prevention of enterogenic infection in severely burned patients. *Burns* 2001;**27**:145–9.

31. Demling RH, Orgill DP. The anticatabolic and wound healing effects of the testosterone analog oxandrolone after severe burn injury. *J Crit Care* 2000;**15**:12–17.

32. Demling RH. Comparison of the anabolic effects and complications of human growth hormone and the testosterone analog, oxandrolone, after severe burn injury. *Burns* 1999;**25**:215–21.

33. Coudray-Lucas C, Le Bever H, Cynober L, De Bandt JP, Carsin H. Ornithine alpha-ketoglutarate improves wound healing in severe burn patients: a prospective randomized double-blind trial versus isonitrogenous controls. *Crit Care Med* 2000;**28**:1772–6.

34. Tanaka H, Matsuda T, Miyagantani Y, Yukioka T, Matsuda H, Shimazaki S. Reduction of resuscitation fluid volumes in severely burned patients using ascorbic acid administration: a randomized, prospective study. *Arch Surg* 2000;**135**:326–31.

35. Alvarez-Diaz C, Cuenca-Pardo J, Sosa-Serrano A, Juarez-Aguilar E, Marsch-Moreno M, Kuri-Harcuch W. Controlled clinical study of deep partial-thickness burns treated with frozen cultured human allogeneic epidermal sheets. *J Burn Care Rehabil* 2000;**21**:291–9.

36. Waymack P, Duff RG, Sabolinski M. The effect of a tissue engineered bilayered living skin analog, over meshed split-thickness autografts on the healing of excised burn wounds. The Apligraf Burn Study Group. *Burns* 2000;**26**:609–19.

37. Lal S, Barrow RE, Wolf SE *et al.* Biobrane improves wound healing in burned children without increased risk of infection. *Shock* 2000;**14**:314–18.

38. Barret JP, Dziewulski P, Ramzy PI, Wolf SE, Desai MH, Herndon DN. Biobrane versus 1% silver sulfadiazine in second-degree pediatric burns. *Plast Reconstr Surg* 2000;**105**:62–5.

39. Noordenbos J, Dore C, Hansbrough JF. Safety and efficacy of TransCyte for the treatment of partial-thickness burns. *J Burn Care Rehabil* 1999;**20**:275–81.

40. Fu X, Shen Z, Chen Y *et al.* Randomised placebo-controlled trial of use of topical recombinant bovine basic fibroblast growth factor for second-degree burns. *Lancet* 1998;**352**:1661–4.

41. Wolkenstein P, Chosidow O, Flechet ML *et al.* Patch testing in severe cutaneous adverse drug reactions, including Stevens–Johnson syndrome and toxic epidermal necrolysis. *Contact Dermatitis* 1996;**35**:234–6.

42. Barreiro P, Soriano V, Casas E *et al.* Prevention of nevirapine-associated exanthema using slow dose escalation and/or corticosteroids. *AIDS* 2000;**14**:2153–7.

43. Para MF, Finkelstein D, Becker S, Dohn M, Walawander A, Black JR. Reduced toxicity with gradual initiation of trimethoprim-sulfamethoxazole as primary prophylaxis for *Pneumocystis carinii* pneumonia: AIDS Clinical Trials Group 268. *J Acquir Immune Defic Syndr* 2000;**24**:337–43.

44. Bonfanti P, Pusterla L, Parazzini F *et al.* The effectiveness of desensitization versus rechallenge treatment in HIV-positive patients with previous hypersensitivity to TMP-SMX: a randomized multicentric study. C.I.S.A.I. Group. *Biomed Pharmacother* 2000;**54**:45–9.

45. Kauppinen K. Cutaneous reactions to drugs with special reference to severe bullous mucocutaneous eruptions and sulphonamides. *Acta Derm Venereol* 1972;**68**:1–89.

52
Focal hyperhidrosis

Berthold Rzany and Daniel M Spinner

Background

Sweating helps control body temperature.[1] However, excessive sweating (hyperhidrosis) can cause physical and social problems. People with excessively sweaty palms may not be able to handle paper without soaking it. They may also experience social stigmatism and discrimination, especially when shaking hands, since their hands may be wet and clammy. People who suffer from excessive underarm sweating have to change clothes frequently. Their clothes may show stains and may not last long (Figure 52.1). Since sweating is commonly associated with insecurity, people with excessive localised sweating may be stereotyped as lacking in confidence.

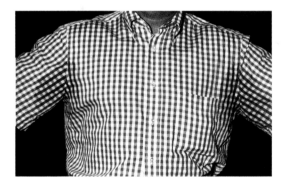

Figure 52.1   A 24-year-old man with excessive axillary hyperhidrosis. Note the significant sweat stains around the axillae.

Definition

There are no precise criteria for the definition of hyperhidrosis. Hyperhidrosis is defined on the basis of clinical findings and gravimetry as excessive sweating at rest and during normal temperature. On the basis of the size of the area affected, excessive sweating can be divided into generalised and focal.

In addition, there is no accepted severity grading system for hyperhidrosis. Reinauer et al.[2] suggested a four-grade score palmar hyperhidrosis on the basis of gravimetry and clinical appearance. No such grading system exists for axillary hyperhidrosis.

Incidence/prevalence

Good epidemiological studies are lacking. Localised excessive sweating occurs in adolescence and may persist in some people throughout their life. No sex or ethnic differences have been documented.

Aetiology

Generalised excessive sweating can occur over most of the body and may be caused by underlying infections, malignancies or hormonal imbalances. In contrast, apart from some known trigger factors such as emotional challenges,[3] the reasons for localised (focal) sweating are not readily apparent. It is therefore described as idiopathic. Idiopathic sweating seams to have a genetic background as patients with focal hyperhidrosis often report a family history of hyperhidrosis. In a study on the effects of sympathectomy, 54% of 91 patients were found to have a positive family history.[4]

Prognosis

No good data are available on the prognosis of focal hyperhidrosis. Incidence and prevalence are presumed to decrease with age. In an experimental setting, Kenney et al.[5] found a decrease in methylcholine-activated eccrine sweating in men of 58–67 years compared with men of 22–24 years.

Diagnostic tests

Focal hyperhidrosis is a clinical diagnosis, diagnosable by a hand shake or stained clothes. In severe localised excessive sweating, pearls of sweat form even when the person is resting. In addition, the amount of sweat and the area affected can be measured. The amount of sweat can be measured by gravimetry (milligrams of sweat produced over a period of time). However there is no standardisation on the time period for which sweat should be collected. In the two randomised clinical trials (RCTs) on botulinum toxin A, Heckmann et al.[6] report the sweat rate in mg/minute whereas Naumann et al.[7] used units of mg/5 minutes. In other trials a volume per 10 minutes has been used.[8,9] The area that is affected by increased sweating can be defined by the ninhydrin test or the iodine starch test. Both tests use a change in colour to indicate the hyperhidrotic area. Studies on validity or reproducibility are not available for either test.

In most studies – especially the studies evaluating surgical interventions – patient satisfaction is used as a marker of therapeutic success.[3,10]

Aims of treatment

The aim of treatment is to reduce the amount of sweating and to produce patient satisfaction.

Relevant outcomes

Relevant outcomes for success of treatment are the reduction of sweating as measured by gravimetry, or the iodine starch or ninhydrin tests.

Methods of search

The following key words were used for a systematic search of the literature: "hyperhidrosis", "focal", "localised", "palmar", "hands", "plantar", "feet", "therapy", "treatment", "topical", "surgery", "surgical", "aluminium-chloride", "anticholinergic drugs", "methenamine", "bornaprine", "methanthelinum bromide", "botulinum toxin", "triethanolamine", "iontophoresis", "sympathectomy" and "sweat".

QUESTIONS

Which interventions reduce sweating efficiently in patients with *axillary* hyperhidrosis?

Case scenario 1

A 24-year-old patient enters the outpatient department complaining about excessive axillary sweating. Significant sweat stains can be found around the axillae (Figure 52.1).

Aluminium chloride
Benefits

There are no systematic reviews or good RCTs on aluminium chloride treatments (25–30% aluminium chloride hexahydrate, 10% aluminium chloride in combination with 5% propantheline bromide) in focal hyperhidrosis. The following treatments have been reported to be beneficial in axillary hyperhidrosis in case series. Graber[9] reported the successful treatment of axillary hyperhidrosis using a 30% aluminium chloride solution in 10 patients. Sweat production was reduced from 201 mg/10 minutes to 44 mg/10 minutes (22% of baseline value). Brandrup et al.[8] reported on 23 women with axillary hyperhidrosis treated with 25% aluminium chloride hexahydrate, with (n = 11) and without occlusion (n = 12). The treatment was considered to be effective, the amount of sweat produced in 10 minutes (measured by gravimetry) decreasing by 60–80% even during exercise for both groups. Ewert et al.[11] reported a good or very good effect in 34 of 49 (70%) soldiers with clinical hyperhidrosis of the axillae, palms and plantar surfaces by combining 10% aluminium chloride and 5% propantheline bromide in a solution. The effect was less obvious, however, in additional 27 soldiers who lived in the tropics.

Harms

No serious side-effects were reported for aluminium chloride. However, reversible skin irritations can occur, and some patients have to discontinue the treatment. Graber[9] reported that one of 10 treated patients had to discontinue treatment. In the study of Brandrup et al.[8] itching was reported in all 23 patients, leading to discontinuation of therapy in two. Irritation and itching were worsened by occlusive dressing. Occlusive dressing had to be discontinued in all 11 patients.

Comment/implications for clinical practice

Although there is no good RCT, 10–30% aluminium-chloride hexahydrate seems likely to be effective. There is a trade-off between efficacy and side-effects (i.e. local irritation of the skin). Occlusive dressings seem to increase irritation.

Botulinum toxin A

Botulinum toxin A is a bacterial toxin that paralyses muscles and decreases sweating by blocking the release of the acetylcholine from presynaptic vesicles. It is given by injection into the deeper part of the skin where the sweat glands are located.

Benefits

There is no systematic review. Besides a small RCT that demonstrated the efficacy of 200 units of botulinum toxin A (Dysport),[12] two large RCTs have demonstrated the efficacy of this treatment in axillary hyperhidrosis. Heckmann et al.[6] investigated the efficacy of botulinum toxin A 200 units (two-fifths of a vial Dysport) in 145 participants with axillary hyperhidrosis. After 2 weeks the rate of sweating was reduced below 25 mg/minute in 64·8% of the axillae treated with botulinum toxin compared with 1·4% of the axillae treated with placebo. At least 50% reduction in sweating (compared with baseline) could be achieved in 134/145 of the axillae treated with botulinum toxin and 22/145 of the axillae treated with placebo. Based on this data, the numbers needed to treat (NNT) can be calculated as 1·3 to 1 (i.e. from four patients treated with 200 units Dysport, three patients will obtain at least a 50% reduction in sweating). In another RCT, 320 patients with axillary hyperhidrosis were treated with 50 units of a different strain of botulinum toxin A (half a vial of Botox). After 3 weeks, 95% (95% confidence intervals 91·5 to 97·4) in the active-treatment group and 32·1% (21·9, 43·6) in the placebo group reported at least a 50% reduction in sweating.[7] Based on this data the NNT for 50 units Botox can be calculated as 1·7 to 1 (of four patients treated, two would obtain at least a 50% reduction in sweating).

Harms

There is no evidence for systemic side-effects. In the study of Naumann et al.,[7] 11 (4.5%) patients reported an increased non-axillary (compensatory) sweating after treatment. Heckmann et al.[6] reported one (<1%) patient with increased sweating.

Comment/implications for clinical practice

Botulinum toxin A is the only drug with proven efficacy for hyperhidrosis of the axilla. There are two products on the market: Botox and Dysport, Botox in vials of 100 units and Dysport in vials of 500 units. These units are not comparable. Based on the available studies, 50 units of Botox, or 100 or 200 units of Dysport seem to be effective in the treatment of axillary hyperhidrosis.

Oral anticholinergics

There are no systematic reviews or RCTs on the efficacy of oral anticholinergics (bornaprin, methantelinum bromide) in axillary hyperhidrosis. There are a few case series of patients with palmar and plantar hyperhidrosis (see below).

Iontophoresis
Benefits

In contrast to palmar and plantar hyperhidrosis (see below), there is little evidence on the efficacy of iontophoresis in axillary hyperhidrosis. Akins et al.[13] reported eight of 27 sites in 22 patients with focal hyperhidrosis treated with iontophoresis. Iontophoresis was not effective in two of the eight axillae. Three of eight axillae (37·5%) showed a 50% decrease in sweating after 2 weeks, as measured by the starch iodine test. In another case series, Hölzle et al.[14] reported an excellent or moderate reduction in one of five patients with axillary sweating.

Harms

In the study of Akins et al.[13] two of eight treated sites developed vesicles, four developed erythematous papules and three developed scaling. For three sites the discomfort was defined as moderate or severe.

Comment/implications for clinical practice

There is little evidence that iontophoresis works in axillary hyperhidrosis. Local side-effects such as discomfort and skin inflammation limit the use of iontophoresis in some patients.

Surgical interventions – curettage of the axilla

Several local surgical interventions can be used for hyperhidrosis of the axilla. The idea is to reduce the number of active sweat glands by removing them or by disturbing the anatomical integrity of the skin. This procedure is only used for axillary hyperhidrosis and cannot be used for palmar or plantar hyperhidrosis.

Benefits

We found no RCT. The largest case series so far compared subcutaneous curettage (n = 90) with injection of botulinum toxin A (n = 20), and reported equally good results for both interventions.[10] Sixty-seven per cent of patients reported a good or very good outcome after subcutaneous curettage in this study. Hasche et al.[15] reported a reduction of the area of sweating as shown by the starch iodine test. However, no quantitative efficacy data were reported. Subjectively, 18 of 20 patients considered that the intervention had led to good results.

Harms

As with any surgery, curettage of the axillary sweat glands might be accompanied by local infections, haematoma and scarring. However, the prevalence of these adverse effects seems to be low.[10,15]

Comment/implications for clinical practice

There is no good evidence on the efficacy of axillary surgery on hyperhidrosis. Subjective data from various studies suggest that it is beneficial. Clinical trials using objective outcome measures such as gravimetry are needed.

Surgical interventions – sympathectomy

Sympathectomy is the dissection or coagulation of sympathetic nerve nodes and may be done to reduce excessive sweating of the axillae. This procedure is now done by endoscopy (introducing instruments through the skin via a narrow tube) rather than by opening the chest surgically, but a general anaesthetic is still required. The lungs are collapsed by pumping in carbon dioxide, and the sympathetic nerve nodes that transmit the nervous signals to the sweat glands in the upper limb and the face (T1–T4) are destroyed.

Benefits

In a retrospective study of the long-term efficacy and side-effects in 270 patients with a total of 480 T1–T4 sympathectomies, Herbst *et al.*[3] reported results in 39 patients with axillary hyperhidrosis. After surgery 30 (77%) reported immediate success. However, after a mean follow up of 14·6 years, only 13 patients (33%) with axillary hyperhidrosis remained completely satisfied, in contrast to 167 (73·2 %) with palmar hyperhidrosis (see comment below under Harms).

Harms

Acute side-effects include bleeding (1 of 48 sites) and transient or persistent Horner's syndrome (3 of 48 sites).[16] Long-term side-effects include compensatory sweating and gustatory sweating, which is reflected in a decrease in long-term satisfaction. The results of Herbst *et al.*[3] (i.e. a decreased proportion of completely satisfied patients) are a reflection of increases in compensatory and gustatory sweating, not loss of efficacy.

Comment/implications for clinical practice

There is insufficient evidence for sympathectomy for axillary hyperhidrosis. The long-term side-effects are compensatory or gustatory sweating.

Other interventions – salvia

Salvia is a herb given in the form of tea or tablets. There are no systematic reviews or RCTs of its use, and no evidence for harm. There is insufficient evidence that salvia works in patients with hyperhidrosis.

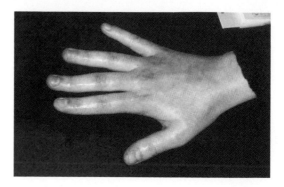

Figure 52.2 Dropping sweat pearls in a 22-year-old woman with grade III hyperhidrosis

Which interventions reduce sweating efficiently in patients with *palmar* hyperhidrosis?

Case scenario 2

A 22-year-old woman complains of severe sweating of the palms. Both palmar areas are covered with sweat drops. Paper is stained as soon as the patient touches it (Figure 52.2).

Topical agents
Benefits

There are no studies treating patients with palmar hyperhidrosis with exclusively topical agents (10% aluminium chloride, 5% methenamine, 5% glutaraldehyde, 5% propantheline bromide). There was one placebo-controlled RCT of 5% methenamine based on 109 patients with palmar and plantar hyperhidrosis.[17] In this study the mean ± SEM hyperhidrosis score was 1·39 ± 0·11 for patients treated for 28 days with 5% methenamine, compared with 2·52 ± 0·9 in the placebo group (P ≤ 0·001). Of the treated patients, 71/109 (65·1%) rated the result as good or excellent, compared with 19/109 (17%) of the placebo group. In another study by Phadke *et al.*,[18] 60 patients were randomised to treatment with topical 10% methenamine aqueous solution, 5% glutaraldehyde, or tap water iontophoresis with direct current. After 4 weeks, 19 of 20 patients treated with methenamine, 13 of 20 patients treated with glutaraldehyde and 11 of 20 treated with iontophoresis described good or excellent results.

The case series of Ewert et al.[11] on the efficacy of 10% aluminium chloride plus 5% propantheline bromide in a solution included patients with axillar hyperhidrosis as well as palmar and plantar hyperhidrosis. In this European study the efficacy was reported to be good or very good.

Harms

As in the treatment of axillary hyperhidrosis, reversible skin irritations can occur, causing some patients to discontinue the treatment. In the study of Phadke et al.,[18] hyperpigmentation occurred in 8 or 20 patients treated with methenamine and in 12 of 20 patients treated with glutaraldehyde. Scaling was provoked in five of 20 patients treated with methenamine.

Comment/implications for clinical practice

There is insufficient data that 10–30% aluminium chloride (hexahydrate) is beneficial. Local irritation of the skin may occur.

Botulinum toxin A
Benefits

There are no good RCTs demonstrating the efficacy of botulinum toxin A for palmar hyperhidrosis. Two RCTs, one of Dysport 120 units and of Botox, comparing 50 units versus 100 units, had significant flaws in the design or analysis of the study.[19,20] Therefore evidence is based on case series. The largest case series comprise 23 patients treated with Botox 50 units (half a vial)[21] and 21 patients treated with Dysport 240 units (approximately half a vial) per hand.[22] Vadoud-Seyedi et al.[21] reported "significant improvement". Schnider et al.[22] reported a median reduction of sweat production, as

measured by the ninhydrin test, of 42% compared with the baseline values. The median overall satisfaction was "very good".

Harms

A decrease in finger pinch strength, resulting from diffusion of the toxin to the palmar muscles, has been documented. Schnider et al.[22] reported a transient measurable reduction in finger power in five of 21 patients after the first treatment. Finger pinch strength seems to decrease with increasing dosage (50 units versus 100 units Botox.[20]

Comment/implications for clinical practice

Although the available data is limited to case series, botulinum toxin A seems to be beneficial in patients with palmar hyperhidrosis. The injections are very painful, regional anaesthesia with medial, ulnar and radial nerve blocks should be performed before the injection of the toxin. However, topical local anaesthesia with Emla cream does not seem to be sufficient to reduce the pain of the injection.

Oral anticholinergics
Benefits

Evidence on anticholinergics (bornaprin, methanthelinum bromide) is based on case series. In the study of Castells Rodellas et al.,[23] six of 12 patients (50%) with palmar or plantar hyperhidrosis reported that the response to bornaprin was excellent after the first week. In a small pilot study, methanthelinum bromide was found to reduce sweating in four patients by 24–80% from baseline values.[24]

Harms

Oral anticholinergics have well-known systemic side-effects (for example, dry mouth and eyes). Only one patient of 10 in the case series of Castells Rodellas et al. had to discontinue bornaprin because of dizziness, and dryness of the mucosa.

Comment/implications for clinical practice

So far there is no good evidence on the efficacy of oral anticholinergics. There certainly is a trade-off between efficacy and anticholinergic side-effects. One RCT focusing on the efficacy on methanthelinum bromide is under way.

Iontophoresis
Benefits

In contrast to axillary hyperhidrosis, there are more studies on the efficacy of iontophoresis in palmar and plantar hyperhidrosis. There are two RCTs, one double-blind, comprising a total of 31 patients. Dahl et al.[25] demonstrated in 11 patients that iontophoresis with direct current reduced sweat production by 38% (median quartiles: 7%, 53%) compared with placebo. Phadke et al.[18] reported a good or excellent response in 11 of 20 patients after 4 weeks of iontophoresis with direct current. Iontophoresis was compared with glutaraldehyde and topical methenamine in this study (see above).

Akins et al.,[13] using the Drionic unit, reported a 50% decrease in sweating compared with the control site in eight of ten hands. In a non-randomised study, Hölzle et al[14] reported that sweating was reduced to normal or to a moderate extent using the Drionic unit in 7 of 12 patients. The average reduction of spontaneous palmar sweating was $19 \pm 17\%$ compared with the untreated site after 3 weeks' treatment. In another study by Reinauer et al.,[2] different types of current (4·3 kHz and 10 kHz pulsed direct current versus direct current) were investigated in a total of 30 patients. All patients were reported to return to normal sweat rate after an average of 10–12 sessions. Treatment failed in two patients in the 4·3 kHz pulse group. However, the generalisability of this study is

limited as only patients with moderate palmar hyperhidrosis were included.

Harms

Dahl et al.[25] reported that one of 11 patients had multiple bullae after direct contact with electrodes. Phadke et al.[18] report scaling in two of 20 patients, but no irritant dermatitis. Akins et al.[13] reported moderate-to-severe discomfort in six of 10 hands. Reinauer[2] reported that the pulsed current was well tolerated.

Comment/implications for clinical practice

There is some evidence, based mostly on smaller studies, that iontophoresis reduces hyperhidrosis of the palms. Treatment has to be performed once or twice daily. The treatment is usually safe. However, burns and blisters might occur.

Iontophoresis with 2% aluminium chloride and 0·01% glycopyrrolate
Benefits

A small trial based on 10 patients reported a greater decrease in severity of sweating (scored on a five-point scale from −3 to +1): −3·1 for the combination therapy versus −1·5 for iontophoresis alone.[26]

Harms

One patient reported transient mouth dryness. Some patients noted peeling or vesiculation after 3–4 days of treatment.

Comment

Combination therapy may increase the efficacy of iontophoresis. However, there are a lack of good data to prove it.

Surgical interventions – sympathectomy
Benefits

Sympathectomy is mostly used for palmar hyperhidrosis. When performed correctly, it is effective in almost all patients, resulting in dry hands.[16] In a retrospective study on 270 patients with a total of 480 T1–T4 sympathectomies, sweating was relieved in the majority of patients (98·1%),and 95·5% were satisfied initially.[3]

Harms

In a large study,[3] T1–T4 endoscopic thoracic sympathectomies in 270 patients were found to be associated with rare acute severe side-effects such as pneumothorax (n = 11; 2%) Horner syndrome (n = 12; 2%), and ptosis (n = 7; 1%). These data are supported by other smaller studies. Chiou et al.[4] reported a haemothorax in one of 91 patients with transaxillar T2 sympathectomy.

There is a systematic review looking at the current indications for this intervention and the incidence of late complications, collectively and per indication. A total of 135 articles (no RCT) up to April 1998 reporting 22 458 patients were identified. The main indication found was hyperhidrosis, accounting for 84·3% of procedures. Compensatory hyperhidrosis occurred in 52·3% of patients, gustatory sweating in 32·3%, phantom sweating in 38·6% and Horner's syndrome in 2·4%. Compensatory sweating occurred three times more often after sympathectomy for hyperhidrosis.[27]

In the recent study of Herbst et al.,[3] 182 (67·4%) patients reported compensatory sweating, mostly on the feet and face. In the study of Chiou et al.,[4] 97% of 91 patients reported compensatory sweating in the first year, mostly on the upper back. Some patients might regret this procedure (13% of 91) because of this side-effect.[4] In addition to compensatory sweating, Herbst et al.[3] reported gustatory sweating in 50·7% of patients. In the same study 10% of patients reported an increased susceptibility to influenza and rhinitis.

Comment/implications for clinical practice

So far there is no good evidence on the efficacy of sympathectomy. Although it is quite likely that, when performed correctly, sympathectomy is effective in palmar hyperhidrosis, there is increasing evidence on harms, especially long-term harms. Therefore, sympathectomy should never be considered as first-line therapy.

Other interventions – salvia

No additional comments can be made for salvia in palmar hyperhidrosis. It is unlikely to be an effective drug.

Key points

- Limited data suggest that 10–30% aluminium chloridehexahydrate is effective but there is a trade-off between efficacy and side-effects (local irritation of the skin).
- Evidence from RCTs suggests the efficacy of botulinum toxin A in focal hyperhidrosis. Botulinum toxin A is a highly effective treatment for axillar hyperhidrosis.
- There is limited evidence on the efficacy of oral anticholinergics, bornaprin and methanthelinum bromide. These are associated with anticholinergic side-effects.
- Iontophoresis of the palm may be moderately effective. The efficacy of iontophoresis of the axillae is questionable. Local irritation is common.
- There is little evidence in support of the surgical removal of axillar sweat glands. No hard outcome criteria had been used in any of the published studies. Therefore the real efficacy is not clear.
- There is some evidence for the efficacy of sympathectomy, although there is a lack of objective criteria to measure efficacy. Sympathectomy for axillar and palmar sweating is associated with long-term side-effects such as compensatory and gustatory sweating. Because of the unknown long-term side-effects, sympathectomy should be only considered in very severe cases.

References

1. Lopez M, Sessler DI, Walter K, Emerick T, Ozaki M. Rate and gender dependence of the sweating, vasoconstriction, and shivering thresholds in humans. *Anesthesiology* 1994;**80**:780–8.

2. Reinauer S, Neußer A, Schauf G, Hälzle E. Die gepulste Gleichstrom-Iontophorese als neue Behandlungsmöglichkeit der Hyperhidrosis. *Hautarzt* 1995;**46**:538–75.

3. Herbst F, Plas EG, Fägger R, Fritsch A. Endoscopic thoracic sympathectomy for primary hyperhidrosis of the upper limbs. A critical analysis and long-term results of 480 patients. *Ann Surg* 1994;**220**:86–90.

4. Chiou TSM, Chen SC. Intermediate-term results of endoscopic transaxillary T2 sympathectomy for primary palmar hyperhidrosis. *Br J Surg* 1999;**86**:45–7.

5. Kenney LW, Fowler SR. Methylcholine-activated eccrine sweat gland density and output as a function of age. *J Appl Physiol* 1988;**65**:1082–6.

6. Heckmann M, Ceballos-Baumann AO, Plewig G. Botulinum toxin A for axillary hyperhidrosis (excessive sweating). *N Engl J Med* 2001;**344**:488–93.

7. Naumann M, Lowe NJ. Efficacy and safety of botulinum toxin A in the treatment of bilateral primary axillary hyperhidrosis: a randomised, placebo controlled study. *BMJ* 2001;**323**:596–9.

8. Brandrup F, Larsen PO. Axillary hyperhidrosis: local treatment with aluminium chloride hexahydrate 25% in absolute ethanol. *Acta Derm Venerol* 1978;**58**:461–5.

9. Graber W. Ein einfache, wirksame Behandlung der axillären Hyperhidrose. *Schweiz Rundschau Med (Praxis)* 1977;**66**:1080–4.

10. Rompel R, Scholz S. Subcutaneous curretage *v.* injection of botulinum toxin A for treatment of axillary hyperhidrosis. *Eur J Dermatol* 12001;**15**:207–11.

11. Ewert L, Link A. Neuartiges Antihidrotikum in der Erprobung bei Soldaten der Bundeswehr. *Derm u Kosmet* 1976;**17**:10–14.

12. Schnider P, Binder M, Kittler H, Birner P, Starkel D, Wolff K, Auff E. A randomized, double-blind placebo controlled trial of botulinum toxin A for severe axillary hyperhidrosis. *Br J Dermatol* 1999;**140**:677–80.

13. Akins DL, Meisenheimer JL, Dobson RL. Efficacy of the Drionic unit in the treatment of hyperhidrosis. *J Am Acad Dermatol* 1987;**16**:828–32.

14. Hölzle E, Alberti N. Long-term efficacy and side effects of tap water iontophoresis of palmoplantar hyperhidrosis – the usefulness of home therapy. *Dermatologica* 1987;**175**:126–35.

15. Hasche E, Hagedorn M, Sattler G. Die subkutane Schweißdräsensaugkärettage in Tumeszenzlokalanästhesie bei Hyperhidrosis axillaris. *Hautarzt* 1997;**48**:817–19.

16. Hashmonai M, Kopelman D, Schein M. Thoracoscopic versus open supraclavicular upper dorsal sympathectomy: a prospective randomised trial. *Eur J Surg Suppl* 1994;**572**:13–16.

17. Bergstresser P, Quero R. Treatment of hyperhidrosis with topical methenamine. *Intern J Dermatol* 1976;**15**;452–5.

18. Phadke VA, Joshi RS, Khopar US, Wadhwa SL. Comparision of topical methenamine, glutaraldehyde and tap water iontophoresis for palmoplantar hyperhidrosis. *Ind J Dermatol Venerol Leprol* 1995;**61**:346–8.

19. Schnider P, Binder M, Auff E, Kittler H, Berger T, Wolff K. Double-blind trial of botulinum A toxin for the treatment of focal hyperhidrosis of the palms. *Br J Dermatol* 1997;**136**:548–52.

20. Saadia D, Voustianiouk A, Wang AK, Kaufmann H. Botulinum toxin type A in primary palmar hyperhidrosis: randomized, single blind, two dose study. *Neurology* 2001;**57**:2095–9.

21. Vadoud-Seyedi J, Heenen M, Simonart T. Treatment of idiopathic palmar hyperhidrosis with botulinum toxin. Report of 23 cases and review of the literature. *Dermatology* 2001;**203**:318–21.

22. Schnider P, Moreau E, Kittler H, Binder M, Kranz M, Voller B, Auff E. Treatment of focal hyperhidrosis with botulinum toxin type A: longterm follow-up in 61 patients. *Br J Dermatol* 2001;**145**:289–93.

23. Castells Rodellas A, Moragon Gordon M, Ramiresz Bosca A. Efecto de la Bornaprina en las Hiperhidrosis localizadas. *Med Cut ILA* 1987;**15**:303–5.

24. Fuchslocher M, Rzany B. Orale anticholinerge Terapie der fokalen Hyperhidrose mit Methanthelinumbromid

(Vagantin). Erste Daten zur Wirksamkeit. *Hautarzt* 2002;**53**:151–2.

25. Dahl CJ, Glent-Madsen L. Treatment of hyperhidrosis manuum by tap water iontophoresis. *Acta Derm Venerol* 1989;**69**:343–8.

26. Shen JL, Lin GS, Li WM. A new strategy of iontophoresis for hyperhidrosis. *J Am Acad Dermatol* 1990;**22**:239–41.

27. Furlan AD, Mailis A, Papagapiou M. Critical review: Are we paying a high price for surgical sympthectomy? A systematic review of late complications. *J Pain* 2000;**1**:287–9.

53
The idiopathic photodermatoses

Robert S Dawe and James Ferguson

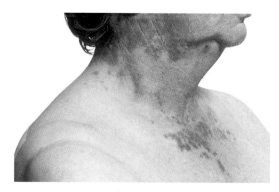

Figure 53.1   Typical papular polymorphic light eruption

This group of photosensitivity disorders includes polymorphic light eruption (PLE), hydroa vacciniforme, chronic actinic dermatitis (also called photosensitivity dermatitis and actinic reticuloid syndrome), solar urticaria, actinic prurigo and juvenile springtime eruption. The causes of each of these conditions remain unknown, although there are suggestions that the mechanism for some, especially PLE, might be autoimmune. For the purposes of this book, we discuss PLE, the commonest of these conditions on which there is the largest volume of published literature. Where appropriate, for example when discussing differential diagnosis, we mention other photodermatoses. Other photodermatoses such as cutaneous porphyrias, DNA-repair disorders (such as xeroderma pigmentosa) and drug induced photosensitivity will be dealt with in future editions of the book and accompanying website.

Background
Definition
PLE is a recurrent abnormal reaction to sunlight (or artificial UV radiation) that occurs after a delay following exposure and heals without scarring.[1-3]

Prevalence
Questionnaire surveys have found 10–21% of selected North European and North American populations to be affected.[4-6] PLE is less frequent closer to the equator.[7-9]

Aetiology
A commonly postulated mechanism is that PLE could be an autoimmune disorder in which there is an abnormal delayed hypersensitivity to an endogenous molecule rendered antigenic by UV exposure.[10]

Prognosis
Spontaneous resolution can occur, but is probably infrequent amongst those affected severely enough to be assessed in hospital.[11]

Diagnostic tests
The diagnosis is usually made on the basis of the clinical history. The following investigations are sometimes indicated:

- **Lupus serology** when cutaneous lupus erythematosus is considered in the differential diagnosis, particularly if treatment with prophylactic phototherapy is considered, antinuclear antibody and anti-Ro and La antibodies should be requested.[12]
- **Histopathology** when a superficial and deep, perivascular, dermal inflammatory

infiltrate is seen. Histopathology and direct immunofluorescence can help differentiate PLE and lupus erythematosus.[13,14]

- **Phototesting** Monochromator phototesting is usually normal in PLE, but can be useful in excluding solar urticaria or chronic actinic dermatitis if these are considered possible alternative, or concomitant, diagnoses. Repeated irradiation provocation testing to 4 × 4 cm or larger areas is positive in a proportion (<50% in some series) of patients, but can be helpful in cases of diagnostic uncertainty.

- **Patch testing and photopatch testing to sunscreens**. These are useful when sunscreen photoallergy or contact allergy is suspected as a co-existent diagnosis.[15–18]

- **Porphyrin plasma spectrofluorimetry** Cutaneous porphyrias occasionally feature as differential diagnoses, and can be excluded if this simple test is negative.

- **HLA class II typing** This can help to distinguish actinic prurigo (see below).[19,20]

Aims of treatment

Treatments can be divided into prophylactic and suppressive. Prophylactic measures include sunlight avoidance and "desensitisation" prophylactic phototherapy. Sunlight avoidance measures include advice on behaviour (for example, avoiding outdoor exposure between 10 am and 3 pm), clothing (long sleeves and hat), topical broad-spectrum sunscreens, and environmental measures (such as applying UV-absorbing "museum film" to house and car windows for those severely sensitive to UV wavelengths). The aim of these measures is to reduce the frequency of and severity of the eruption.

The aim of prophylactic phototherapy is to increase the duration of sunlight exposure required to elicit PLE, and so improve quality of life for those severely affected patients who cannot carry out normal activities (for example putting out washing during day time) because very limited sunlight exposure triggers the eruption. Suppressive treatment should alleviate symptoms (particularly itch), and speed resolution of PLE when it occurs.

Relevant outcomes

For prophylactic treatments important outcomes are number of episodes of PLE (and their severity), and quality of life. For symptomatic suppressive therapies, the main outcomes are symptom (primarily itch) severity, and speed of resolution of the eruption.

Methods of search

Studies were identified using Medline (1966 to January 2001) and Embase (1988 to January 2001) databases, with search terms including "polymorphic/polymorphous light eruption AND treatment OR prognosis". Abstracts were read to determine which were likely to be relevant.

QUESTIONS

What is the prognosis for resolution of PLE for a severely affected patient living in a temperate country?

Follow up of 94 Finnish patients (by questionnaire, supplemented by repeat clinical assessments of a subgroup) up to a mean of 32 years after onset found 24% (95% confidence interval (CI) 16–34%) to have experienced resolution of their PLE, and 51% (CI 41–62%) to have milder PLE.[11] A recent report suggested that those with negative provocation tests may be more likely to proceed to remission than those with positive provocation tests.[21]

Comment

We have very limited information on PLE prognosis, and this one well-conducted follow up study[11] involved a selected group of patients – those assessed in a hospital department, and willing to attend for review. Our experience in Dundee (based on another severely affected patient group) is that a substantial proportion of those with PLE severe enough to require repeated yearly prophylactic phototherapy do, after several years, experience resolution, or marked improvement, so that they can then stop attending for treatment.[22] We do not know whether this is spontaneous resolution, or whether it is a result of repeated phototherapy courses.

Implications for practice

We can advise patients that spontaneous resolution is possible, but cannot reliably indicate how likely it is to occur. We still do not know whether repeated yearly courses of prophylactic phototherapy influence long-term prognosis.

Which form of prophylactic phototherapy – psoralen-UVA photochemotherapy or UVB monotherapy – should be prescribed for severely affected patients?

Efficacy

A randomised, patient-masked, controlled trial[23] involving 25 adults found narrow-band (TL-01) UVB to be as effective as PUVA in preventing episodes of PLE following a treatment course, and to possibly be more effective in reducing post-treatment subjective PLE severity scores. PUVA is more effective than broad-band UVB.[24]

Drawbacks

Both TL-01 UVB and PUVA produced PLE during the treatment course in about half of those treated.[23] High cumulative PUVA exposures administered to psoriasis patients increases the risk of later development of skin cancers, particularly squamous cell carcinomas.[25]

Although the risks with UVB have not been well defined, it is probable that high cumulative UVB exposure will also result in a higher skin cancer risk.

Comment

The analysis of each of these studies comparing PUVA with UVB (narrow band and broad band) as prophylactic therapies for PLE took into account polysulphone-badge-determined natural UV exposure after the treatment courses. Even with randomisation (methods for which were not defined in either paper), differences in subsequent sunlight seeking or avoidance behaviour in the groups compared could have influenced findings. Insufficient raw data are presented to allow retrospective calculations of the power of either study. Nevertheless, it can be safely concluded that PUVA is not much more effective than TL-01 UVB, and may even be less effective.

Implications for practice

TL-01 UVB is the prophylactic phototherapy of choice for patients severely affected by PLE. When this fails to provide useful benefit, or when repeated episodes of PLE are provoked during therapy, PUVA can be considered.

Should corticosteroids be prescribed for a mildly affected patient to use if PLE develops while he or she is on holiday?

Efficacy

A randomised controlled trial of prednisolone, 25 mg daily in a presumably mildly affected group (only 10 of 21 patients needed to take the study drug while on vacation) showed that it had an effect. PLE resolved more quickly (by a mean of 3·6 days (95% CI 0·6 to 6·1 days)) with prednisolone than with placebo, despite the fact that for this study patients were encouraged to continue sun exposure after they developed PLE.[26]

It is unclear whether moderately potent or potent topical steroids help to suppress established PLE, but potent topical steroids may be of value prophylactically if applied immediately after exposure.[27]

Drawbacks
One of 10 patients who took a short course of oral prednisolone for PLE experienced "mild gastrointestinal disturbance and slight depression of mood".[26]

Comment
For most patients with mild PLE, it is doubtful whether the small improvement produced by systemic prednisolone is sufficient to outweigh concerns about side-effects. We do not know whether a potent topical steroid is of benefit for established PLE, but as systemic steroids have an effect it is possible that, at least for some patients, this may be beneficial.

Implications for practice
Corticosteroids can have a small-to-modest effect on established PLE. While lacking evidence that topical steroids have a similar effect, it may be appropriate to prescribe a potent topical steroid to use if PLE develops for patients whose problem is mild and confined to episodes induced by holiday sunlight.

Can HLA class II typing distinguish PLE from actinic prurigo?

Actinic prurigo is strongly associated with HLA-DR4, and particularly HLA-DRB1*0407 in the UK[19,20] and Mexico.[28]

Comment
Polymorphic light eruption is distinguished from actinic prurigo on the basis of history and clinical features. The finding of a strong HLA association with actinic prurigo but not PLE strengthened the evidence that these are distinct diseases. A study to determine the value of HLA class II typing as a diagnostic test in cases of clinical uncertainty about diagnosis has not been performed, but such testing could be helpful.

Implications for practice
In cases where the diagnosis is in doubt, a negative HLA-DR4 test makes actinic prurigo less likely than PLE, while a positive HLA-DR4 is of limited value as this antigen is common (about 25%) in most populations. A positive HLA-DRB1*0407 test (rare in most populations) may help to rule in a diagnosis of actinic prurigo (and exclude PLE), whereas a negative test result (found in almost 40% of UK cases of actinic prurigo) is of limited value.

Key points

- PLE can improve over the years. This improvement may be spontaneous, or partly due to repeated prophylactic phototherapy.
- Narrow-band UVB and PUVA are similarly effective in preventing episodes of PLE.
- Oral prednisolone has a small or modest beneficial effect in PLE.
- Is not clear whether topical corticosteroids are of help.
- HLA typing may occasionally be helpful in classifying a photodermatosis with features of both PLE and actinic prurigo.

References

1. Elpern DJ, Morison WL, Hood AF. Papulovesicular light eruption. A defined subset of polymorphous light eruption. *Arch Dermatol* 1985;**121**:1286–8.
2. Holzle E, Plewig G, von Kries R, Lehmann P. Polymorphous light eruption. *J Invest Dermatol* 1987;**88**(Suppl. 3):32s–8s.
3. Dover JS, Hawk JLM. Polymorphic light eruption sine eruptione. *Br J Dermatol* 1988;**118**:73–6.

4. Morison WL, Stern RS. Polymorphous light eruption: a common reaction uncommonly recognized. *Acta Derm Venereol* 1982;**62**:237–40.

5. Millard TP, Bataille V, Snieder H, Spector TD, McGregor JM. The heritability of polymorphic light eruption. *J Invest Dermatol* 2000;**115**:467–70.

6. Ros AM, Wennersten G. Current aspects of polymorphous light eruptions in Sweden. *Photodermatology* 1986;**3**:298–302.

7. Pao C, Norris PG, Corbett M, Hawk JLM. Polymorphic light eruption: Prevalence in Australia and England. *Br J Dermatol* 1994;**130**:62–4.

8. Olumide YM. Photodermatoses in Lagos. *Int J Dermatol* 1987;**26**:295–9.

9. Khoo SW, Tay YK, Tham SN. Photodermatoses in a Singapore skin referral centre. *Clin Exp Dermatol* 1996;**21**:263–8.

10. Norris PG, Morris J, McGibbon DM, Chu AC, Hawk JL. Polymorphic light eruption: an immunopathological study of evolving lesions. *Br J Dermatol* 1989;**120**:173–83.

11. Hasan T, Ranki A, Jansen CT, Karvonen J. Disease associations in polymorphous light eruption. A long-term follow-up study of 94 patients. *Arch Dermatol* 1998;**134**:1081–5.

12. Murphy GM, Hawk JL. The prevalence of antinuclear antibodies in patients with apparent polymorphic light eruption. *Br J Dermatol* 1991;**125**:448–51.

13. Panet-Raymond G, Johnson WC. Lupus erythematosus and polymorphous light eruption – differentiation by histochemical procedures. *Arch Dermatol* 1973;**108**:785–7.

14. Weedon D. Polymorphous light eruption. In: *Skin Pathology*. Melbourne: Churchill Livingstone, 1997: 509–10.

15. Green C, Norris PG, Hawk JL. Photoallergic contact dermatitis from oxybenzone aggravating polymorphic light eruption. *Contact Dermatitis* 1991;**24**:62–3.

16. Bilsland D, Ferguson J. Contact allergy to sunscreen chemicals in photosensitivity dermatitis/actinic reticuloid syndrome (PD/AR) and polymorphic light eruption (PLE). *Contact Dermatitis* 1993;**29**:70–3.

17. Thune P. Contact and photocontact allergy to sunscreens. *Photodermatology* 1984;**1**:5–9.

18. Allan SJR, Ray RE, Savin JA. The optimal management of polymorphic light eruption in a non-photobiological unit. *J Dermatol Treat* 1999;**10**:3–6.

19. Grabczynska SA, McGregor JM, Kondeatis E, Vaughan RW, Hawk JLM. Actinic prurigo and polymorphic light eruption: Common pathogenesis and the importance of HLA-DR4/DRB1*0407. *Br J Dermatol* 1999;**140**: 232–6.

20. Dawe RS, Collins P, O'Sullivan A, Ferguson J. Actinic prurigo and HLA-DR4 1. *J Invest Dermatol* 1997;**108**: 233–4.

21. Leroy D, Dompmartin A, Faguer K, Michel M, Verneuil L. Polychromatic phototest as a prognostic tool for polymorphic light eruption. *Photodermatol Photoimmunol Photomed* 2000;**16**:161–6.

22. Man I, Dawe RS, Ferguson J. Artificial hardening for polymorphic light eruption: Practical points from ten years' experience. *Photodermatol Photoimmunol Photomed* 1999;**15**:96–9.

23. Bilsland D, George SA, Gibbs NK, Aitchison T, Johnson BE, Ferguson J. A comparison of narrow band phototherapy (TL-01) and photochemotherapy (PUVA) in the management of polymorphic light eruption. *Br J Dermatol* 1993;**129**:708–12.

24. Murphy GM, Logan RA, Lovell CR, Morris RW, Hawk JL, Magnus IA. Prophylactic PUVA and UVB therapy in polymorphic light eruption – a controlled trial. *Br J Dermatol* 1987;**116**:531–8.

25. Stern RS, Lunder EJ. Risk of squamous cell carcinoma and methoxsalen (psoralen) and UV-A radiation (PUVA). A meta-analysis. *Arch Dermatol* 1998;**134**: 1582–5.

26. Patel DC, Bellaney GJ, Seed PT, McGregor JM, Hawk JLM. Efficacy of short-course oral prednisolone in polymorphic light eruption: a randomized controlled trial. *Br J Dermatol* 2000;**143**:828–31.

27. Man I, Dawe RS, Ibbotson SH, Ferguson J. Is topical steroid effective in polymorphic light eruption? *Br J Dermatol* 2000;**143**(Suppl. 57):113.

28. Hojyo-Tomoka T, Granados J, Vargas-Alarcon G *et al.* Further evidence of the role of HLA-DR4 in the genetic susceptibility to actinic prurigo. *J Am Acad Dermatol* 1997;**36**:935–7.

Part 4: The future of evidence-based dermatology

Editor: Luigi Naldi

54

Where do we go from here?

Hywel Williams

What is the point of discussing evidence-based dermatology?

The idea that doctors should base their treatment decisions on good evidence seems such an obvious and common sense notion that it might be taken for granted. If the practice of evidence-based medicine (EBM) goes without saying, what is point of discussing and promoting EBM? Medicine is advancing very rapidly, creating major changes in the way we treat our patients. We must keep up with such changes. Although we need to keep up to date with such new external evidence, we frequently fail to do this when we rely on passive sources such as a visit from a pharmaceutical representative or an occasional flick through the main journals. This leads to a deterioration of our knowledge with time. Systematic reviews which have searched for all relevant data are needed nowadays to update dermatologists on current best treatment. Attempts to overcome this deficiency by attending clinical education programmes fail to improve our performance, whereas the practice of EBM has been shown to keep its practitioners up to date.[1] This does not mean that information technology skills replace those attributes of being a good doctor, such as history and examination skills. As the original definition in Chapter 2 implies, the practice of EBM is a synthesis of knowledge management skills with clinical skills. The aim is to create an emergent skilful, caring and efficient doctor.

What exactly are the advantages of evidence-based dermatology?
Being explicit and systematic

At the top of the evidence hierarchy tree discussed in Chapter 7 lies the systematic review. Systematic reviews of randomised clinical trials (RCTs) developed after it was realised that traditional reviews were done in quite arbitrary ways. They are to some extent synonymous with evidence-based dermatology (EBD) in that they inform practitioners on treatment efficacy and harms. Systematic reviews, such as those produced by the Cochrane Collaboration, summarise accurate, up-to-date, high-quality external evidence of the effectiveness of interventions for treating and preventing human disease.[2] Put more simply, systematic reviews can be thought of as the science of summarising other studies. The key difference from other more traditional reviews is in the word *systematic*. Just as those conducting clinical trials follow an explicit and exhaustive protocol of clearly laid-out steps to conduct their trial, systematic reviewers describe precisely how they will search, appraise and synthesise data concerning a specific clinical question. This explicit structure and methodology means that another researcher could replicate the review if necessary. As Chapter 8 emphasises, systematic reviews are done systematically along a series of well-defined steps that are outlined in a protocol. Another important advantage is that some reviews, such as those

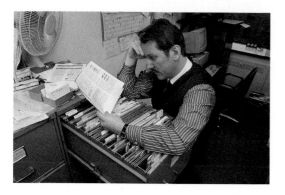

Figure 54.1 The good old "file drawer" method for locating studies is still the method used and preferred by some authors of traditional "expert" reviews

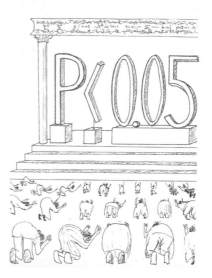

Figure 54.2 As dermatologists, we must overcome our slavish obsession for dividing the results of all clinical trials into those that are statistically significant at the 5% level and those that are not, and instead use confidence intervals to estimate a range of likely effects

conducted within the Cochrane Collaboration, are updated as new evidence and criticisms become available.

Traditional expert reviews are fine for raising issues for discussion, but they are less suitable for summarising treatment efficacy. The unsystematic approach used in such traditional reviews often means that they are more prone to bias and hidden agendas.[3] We have all done this in our "traditional" review articles in the past, and I admit having used the "file drawer" method to search for articles for my review of atopic eczema in 1995 (Figure 54.1).[4]

Keeping up to date and increasing precision

Evidence from cardiovascular medicine has shown that doctors failed to use effective treatments, such as intravenous streptokinase, for acute myocardial infarction even when there is overwhelming evidence for their effectiveness.[5] Conversely, they continued to recommend medicines such as intravenous lidocaine for post-infarction arrhythmias long after the evidence suggested that they were ineffective or even harmful.[6] With over 200 specialist dermatology journals, it has become increasingly difficult for the dermatologist to

keep up with the literature.[7] Systematic reviews such as those supported by the Cochrane Skin Group that track down all possible published and unpublished studies are needed to keep us up to date.

Such systematic reviews can reduce uncertainty produced by the conflicting results of several small inconclusive studies by combining their results – provided they are sufficiently similar. This may overcome our current obsession with dividing all clinical trials into those that are significant at the arbitrary 5% level and those that are not (Figure 54.2), instead of estimating a range of plausible treatment effects by means of confidence intervals and pooling studies that are sufficiently alike in terms of patients, interventions and outcomes. Studies that reach the "magic" $P<0.05$ significance are commonly claimed as being "positive" and those that fail to reach that level are often considered "negative",

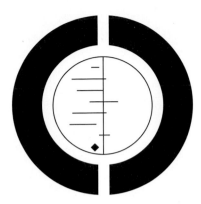

Figure 54.3 The Cochrane Collaboration logo depicts a systematic review of seven placebo-controlled trials evaluating the efficacy of a short course of oral corticosteroids for women in premature labour to prevent fetal death. Each horizontal line represents a single RCT – the shorter the line the more certain are the results. If an RCTs touches the vertical line, it means that particular trial found no clear evidence of treatment benefit. The diamond at the bottom represents the combined results, and its position to the left of the vertical line of no treatment difference indicates that the treatment was clearly beneficial in reducing premature infant mortality by 30–50%.

The first of these RCTs was done in 1972. The figure depicts what would have been revealed had a systematic review of the available evidence been done a decade later. By 1991, another seven RCTs had been done. Because no systematic review of these studies had been produced until 1989, most obstetricians had not realised that the treatment was so effective, but instead, interpreted each individual study as "conflicting". As a result, tens of thousands of premature babies around the world have probably died or suffered unnecessarily. This is an example of the human costs of failing to perform an up-to-date systematic review of apparently "conflicting" studies

Source: The cochrane collaboration

whereas in reality many of the latter trials are far too small to detect even quite large changes.[8] Instead of concluding that such studies are "conflicting", a meta-analysis performed within the context of a carefully conducted systematic review may show that they are all compatible with a clear overall treatment benefit. The Cochrane Collaboration logo shows a good example of this (Figure 54.3).

Minimising bias and identifying research gaps

Systematic reviews are powerful tools to minimise bias because they use explicit methods. In assessing an intervention for skin disease, the pre-published protocols provide an opportunity to state which participants should ideally be studied, which comparators are appropriate, and which outcomes would make a difference clinically. This "bottom up" and non-reductionist approach also provides the opportunity of consulting consumers (people with a condition or their carers) to ensure that the outcome measures capture something that is important to them. The beneficial role of such consumer involvement was extolled in Chapter 3. Such a pre-planned protocol helps to avoid the problem of being driven by the data already out there and thereby amplifying outcomes that may interest the pharmaceutical industry more than patients and doctors. Even for rare skin diseases, producing a systematic review which finds no reliable evidence to inform practice may still be useful in that one is not missing some important new development, and also highlights the area as a possible research gap for future study.[9–11]

The basic unit of analysis in most systematic reviews is the RCT. As pointed out in Chapter 9, like any study design, this can be done badly and used in the wrong situations.[12] Nevertheless, the RCT remains one of the strongest designs in modern medicine for assessing treatment efficacy because of its potential to minimise bias. As Bigby points out in his essay on "snake oil for the 21st century", studies of inferior design, such as case series, have many times led to overly optimistic claims of treatment efficacy in dermatology which were not borne out by subsequent RCTs.[13]

Influencing the agenda of future dermatology trials

Perhaps the most important and subtle advantage of EBD is its propensity to help change the RCT agenda. It is quite clear from the systematic review of 300 or so RCTs in atopic eczema that most trials have reflected the agenda of the drug industry in order to license a particular "me-too" product, and that many questions that are important to clinicians and patients remain unanswered.[10] Many of the outcome measures used in these trials are clinical scoring systems that may show up treatment effects, yet their clinical significance in practice is often obscure.

What are the potential limitations of evidence-based dermatology?

Poor coverage

Given that groups such as the Cochrane Skin Group are less than 5 years old, it is not surprising that many of the questions that interest dermatologists have not yet been the subject of a systematic review. Such lack of comprehensiveness is a phenomenon of time rather than intent, and one hopes that an evidence base as comprehensive as that for perinatal medicine will be achieved within 5 years if the current trends continue. This book is itself an attempt at filling in some of the evidence gaps from existing systematic reviews. Even so, there is still a large number of rarer skin diseases that are not covered in this book. This issue will be partly addressed by including them on the website accompanying this book and future editions of the hard-copy version.

A threat of reductionism

Meta-analysis, which refers to the statistical pooling of results drawn from several studies, is prone to dangerous reductionism in terms of adding together studies that it does not make sense to combine.[14,15] Thus, before contemplating playing with any statistics, it may seem sensible *not* to combine studies of childhood atopic dermatitis with those dealing exclusively with adult atopic dermatitis, as they

may belong to a different disease group in terms of the aetiology of treatment responsiveness. It may also be sensible *not* to combine studies of atopic eczema that evaluate one sort of dietary exclusion with another. It may not make any sense to pool a clinically obscure outcome measure such as a "doctor-assessed itch" simply because it was the only outcome that was common to all trials.[10] Meta-analyses are only as good as the data from the individual studies that make up such analyses, and great care needs to be taken to avoid adding together things that should not be combined, especially when the statistical output may give rise to a spurious air of precision to those less experienced in assessing the quality of such analyses. It is for this reason that we recommend that meta-analyses are always performed within the context of a systematic review.[16] The involvement of "consumers" with the condition being reviewed is also another important aspect that groups such as the Cochrane Skin Group use to protect against reductionism in choice of outcomes.

Cheating

Like any research methodology, it is possible for those with a vested interest to twist the conclusions of a systematic review to their own advantage. Thus, one could conveniently fail to include one crucial study that went against the results you wanted to show, or if it is declared within the review, find a weak excuse to exclude it *post hoc*. Because many trials never see the light of day in terms of publication and are held as "data on file" by many pharmaceutical companies, it is possible for a review done by a company to include additional unpublished studies that favour their product (whereas similar studies from competitors remain buried). As with any written document assessing drug treatments, there is plenty of scope for undue emphasis on positive effects and lack of discussion of relevant adverse events. As with any other study, readers need to develop a "good nose" for what constitutes a good systematic review and clinical trial; some pointers are given in Chapters 8 and 9. This includes a peep at the acknowledgements to see who sponsored the review/study, if, in fact, sponsorship has been declared.[17]

Overreliance on RCTs

Whilst RCTs may be the most robust study design for minimising bias for conventional evaluation of the effectiveness of interventions for skin diseases, they have their limitations.[18] In some circumstances, it may be impossible or unethical to perform an RCT. For example, it is unlikely that mothers will agree to be randomised to breastfeeding or bottle-feeding to see whether either prevents atopic eczema. Similarly, it would be impractical to randomise medical students to one form of education and others to another within the same class, because they would not be blinded to the interventions, and there may be considerable "contamination" of the intervention from one group as students talk together. Just because it is an RCT does not mean that it is a good RCT, and attention to quality is important here rather than just blindly following the concept of the hierarchy of evidence.[12] Rare but serious events, which are extremely important when evaluating the pros and cons of a new treatment, are not well characterised in RCTs, but instead require other approaches such as case reports, case-control studies and widescale pharmaceutical surveillance methods, as Naldi points out in Chapter 10. Frequently, there is asymmetry in the way that systematic reviews devote a lot of space to treatment efficacy and less or none to issues such as potentially serious side-effects.[19]

Also, the concept of only using RCTs as evidence for systematic reviews has been criticised because it implies that all other evidence that contributes to our understanding of treatment efficacy, such as case series, case reports and "clinical experience", are not valid.[20] This is clearly inappropriate. Ideally, the totality of evidence should be considered when conducting a systematic review so that evidence from observational studies can contribute to the conclusions from RCTs. Approaches such as hierarchical modelling, likelihood estimations and bayesian statistics have been used in attempts to address these gaps. It is likely that the concept of good informative study design is more of a continuum representing risk of bias, rather than a dichotomy of "good" (i.e. RCTs) and "bad" (for example, a large case series). This continuum needs to be tempered by the added but crucial dimension of study quality.

It is true that there are challenges for future systematic reviewers to find ways of incorporating informative data from non-randomised studies, and a methodology group has been set up within the Cochrane Collaboration specifically to address this (http://www.cochrane.dk/nrsmg). In the meantime, it is best that we learn to walk before we run by adhering to the RCT as the basic building block for assessing treatment efficacy in dermatology, at least until better methodological approaches have evolved that enable us to integrate evidence from a wider range of designs.

It should be remembered that EBD is not just based on judging the effectiveness of treatments, even though this is the emphasis in this book. Often, dermatologists want to know "What is the best diagnostic test?", or "What is the prognosis?" or "What is the most cost-effective treatment?". These questions are best addressed using other study designs such as comparison of tests with reference standards in appropriate populations, cohort studies for disease prognosis, and economic studies.[1] Some of these are discussed in more detail in Chapters 10 and 11, and more will be added to future editions of the book.

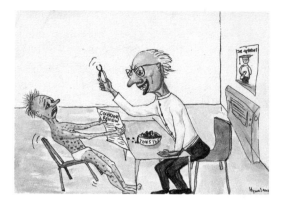

Figure 54.4 A recent Cochrane systematic review found no good evidence to support the use of antistreptococcal interventions (prolonged antibiotics or tonsillectomy) for treating guttate psoriasis. Sometimes such a "negative" systematic review can be useful by empowering patients to question doctors on the evidential basis for their treatment decisions

Reviews always end with the phrase "insufficient evidence"

A common criticism of Cochrane skin reviews by dermatology trainees, is that they always end up with the same conclusion of "insufficient evidence" to inform current practice. Whilst this may be true for some reviews, a glance at those reviews on the *Cochrane Database of Systematic Reviews* shows that at least 50% of those relevant to a practising dermatologist make specific and clear recommendations for therapy.[21] Even "null reviews" that do not find any good evidence to make specific treatment recommendations have their uses. Thus, a recent systematic review evaluating the evidence for antistreptococcal treatments for guttate psoriasis found no reliable evidence despite confident textbook recommendations in favour of such a treatment approach.[11] Not only does this identify a major gap needing research, it also reassures doctors and their patients that they are not missing some important study. It empowers doctors to feel more confident in relying on other levels of evidence such as case series and empirical reasoning based on mechanism until better studies are done. It also empowers patients with guttate psoriasis by allowing them to challenge doctors who insist that they must take prolonged courses of antibiotics or who threaten to take out their tonsils (Figure 54.4).

Evidence-based paralysis

The other important corollary of the evidence hierarchy is that absence of RCT evidence does not mean we become paralysed into doing nothing.[22] Failure to find any RCTs for the treatment of necrobiosis lipoidica does not mean that we tell our patients to go away because there is no treatment. We may come across a well-conducted case series, a convincing case report, or trust the anecdotal evidence of a senior colleague – all of forms of evidence that are entirely appropriate to *use in the absence of better sources*. It is just that for many years, the evidence hierarchy has been used the other way around in practice – starting with asking a colleague and usually ending up by referring to an out-of-date textbook.

Conclusion

The potential limitations of EBD are diverse and only partly justified.[20] Some such as inadequate coverage are a function of time, and some such as reductionism, a refusal to consider non-RCT evidence and cheating belong to those conducting systematic reviews. Other aspects such as evidence-based paralysis are a misunderstanding that belongs to those using the evidence. Many of the commonly cited criticisms such as "all skin reviews are negative" fall down when challenged by objective data and when the original tenets of evidence-based practice are revisited.

So is it all just another fashion that will come and go?

For some, the whole concept of EBD might seem like just another new management-driven fad that will come and go like others.[14] Perhaps it is the shame in admitting that some of our previous treatments might be wrong that prevents progress – the "elephant in the front room" that doctors keep bumping into without seeing.[23] Yet what is the alternative to EBD? Is it anecdote-based medicine ("I once treated a patient with such and such with remarkable effect…"), entropy-based medicine, or propaganda-based dermatology driven by powerful cartels with vested interests? I cannot believe that any caring dermatologist would not wish to base his or her treatments on the best external evidence. Two studies have already shown that dermatologists use as much high-quality external evidence to inform their treatment decisions as other specialists.[24,25]

It is reasonable at this point to ask "What is the evidence for EBD?". This is a tautological question as it implies that there is a group of doctors who are evidence based and another group who are not, whereas the reality is that we conform to a dynamic and complex continuum. Some are *more* EBM-orientated than others, but we *all* practise EBM to some degree, this rendering traditional comparisons through designs such as RCTs difficult to interpret, quite apart from ethical issues.[15]

Perhaps it is the name "evidence-based medicine" that is at fault here since it implies that anyone who does not call himself or herself an EBM physician is not one. This binary thought disorder is clearly an inaccurate reflection of real life. Like Moliáre's bourgeois gentilhomme, who, after 40 years, discovered that he had been speaking prose without realising it, many dermatologists have been practising, and will continue to practice, high-quality EBD. Yet we all need to learn new skills in searching, appraising and translating the evidence. Now it's up to you.

References

1. Sackett DL, Richardson WS, Rosenberg Q, Haynes RB. *Evidence-based Medicine. How to practise and teach EBM*. London: Churchill Livingstone, 1997.

2. Greenhalgh T. *How to read a paper*. London: BMJ Publishing Group, 1997.

3. Ladhani S, Williams HC. The management of established postherpetic neuralgia: a comparison of the quality and content of traditional *v.* systematic reviews. *Br J Dermatol* 1998;**139**:66–72.

4. Williams HC. Atopic eczema – we should look to the environment. *BMJ* 1995;**311**:1241–2.

5. Lau J, Antman EM, Jimenez-Silva J, Kupelnick B, Mosteller F, Chalmers TC. Cumulative meta-analysis of therapeutic trials for myocardial infarction. *N Engl J Med* 1992;**327**:248–54.

6. Echt DS, Liebson PR, Mitchell LB *et al.* Mortality and morbidity in patients receiving encainide, flecainide, or placebo. The Cardiac Arrhythmia Suppression Trial. *N Engl J Med* 1991;**324**:781–8.

7. Delamere FM, Williams HC. How can hand searching the dermatological literature benefit people with skin problems? *Arch Dermatol* 2001;**137**:332–5.

8. Williams HC, Seed P. Inadequate size of "negative" clinical trials in dermatology. *Br J Dermatol* 1993;**128**:317–26.

9. Griffiths CEM, Clark CM, Chalmers RJG, Li Wan Po A, Williams HC. A systematic review of treatments for severe psoriasis. *Health Technol Assess* 2000;**4**(40).

10. Hoare C, Li Wan Po A, Williams H. Systematic review of treatments for atopic eczema. *Health Technol Assess* 2000;**4**(37).

11. Owen CM, Chalmers RJG, O'Sullivan T, Griffiths CEM. Antistreptococcal interventions for guttate and chronic plaque psoriasis (Cochrane Review). In: Cochrane Collaboration. *Cochrane Library*. Issue 3. Oxford: Update Software, 2001.

12. Barton S. Which clinical studies provide the best evidence? The best RCT still trumps the best observational study. *BMJ* 2000;**321**:255–6.

13. Bigby M. Snake oil for the 21st century. *Arch Dermatol* 1998;**134**:1512–14.

14. Rees J. Evidence-based medicine: the epistemology that isn't. *J Am Acad Dermatol* 2000;**43**:727–9.

15. Goodman NW. Who will challenge evidence-based medicine? *J R Coll Phys Lond* 1999;**33**:249–51.

16. Egger M, Smith GD, Sterne JA. Uses and abuses of meta-analysis. *Clin Med* 2001;**1**:478–84.

17. Bero LA. Accepting commercial sponsorship. Disclosure helps – but is not a panacea. *BMJ* 1999;**319**:653–4.

18. Hampton JR. Evidence-based medicine, practice variations and clinical freedom. *J Eval Clin Pract* 1997;**3**:123–31.

19. Ernst E, Pittler MH. Assessment of therapeutic safety in systematic reviews: literature review. *BMJ* 2001;**323**:546.

20. Straus SE, McAlister FA. Evidence-based medicine: a commentary on common criticisms. *Can Med Assoc J* 2000;**163**:837–41.

21. Parker ER, Schilling LM, Diba V, Williams HC, Dellavalle RP. What's the point of databases of reviews in dermatology if all they find is "insufficient evidence". *J Am Acad Dermatol* 2003 (in press).

22. Hill D. Efficacy of sunscreens in protection against skin cancer. *Lancet* 1999;**354**:699–700.

23. Davidoff F. Shame: the elephant in the room. *BMJ* 2002;**324**:623–4.

24. Jemec GB, Thorsteinsdottir H, Wulf HC. Evidence-based dermatologic out-patient treatment. *Int J Dermatol* 1998; **37**:850–4.

25. Abeni D, Girardelli CR, Masini C *et al.* What proportion of dermatological patients receive evidence-based treatment? *Arch Dermatol* 2001;**137**:771–6.

Index

Note: Subentries called "background" refer to definition, epidemiology, aetiology and risk factors, prognosis, treatment aims and study methods/outcomes. *v* denotes differential diagnosis or comparisons.

RCT – randomised controlled trial